Prostate Brachytherapy
MADE COMPLICATED

THIRD EDITION

Prostate Brachytherapy
MADE COMPLICATED

THIRD EDITION

Kent Wallner
Gregory Merrick
John C. Blasko
Michael Dattoli

SmartMedicine Press
Seattle, Washington

Third Edition

ISBN 10: 0-9648991-6-7
ISBN 13: 978-0-9648991-6-2

Published by SmartMedicine Press, Seattle, Washington
Cover design by Deborah Rust, New York, New York
Distributed by Pathway Books, Gilsum, NH 800-345-6665

Printed in Canada

Dedicated to our patients—
pioneers in prostate brachytherapy

Acknowledgments

The following people helped in various aspects with this book. Their insightful comments and suggestions were invaluable:

Jesse Aronowitz, MD
Carl Bergsagel, MS
Jason, Dominitz, MD
Kathryn Elliott, MD
Paul Herstein, MD
Felix Mick, PhD
T. Tydings Robin, Jr. PhD, LLB
Steven Sutlief, PhD
Lawrence True, MD
Joseph Walker

Kent Wallner, M.D.
Chief, Radiation Oncology
Puget Sound Health Care System, Veterans Administration
Staff physician, Group Health Cooperative
Associate Professor
University of Washington Medical Center
Seattle, Washington

Gregory Merrick, M.D.
Chief, Radiation Oncology
Wheeling Hospital Schiffler Cancer Center
Wheeling Jesuit University
Wheeling, West Virginia

John Blasko, M.D.
Seattle Prostate Institute
Clinical Professor
Department of Radiation Oncology
University of Washington Medical Center
Seattle, Washington

Michael J. Dattoli, M.D.
Physician in Chief
Dattoli Cancer Center and Brachytherapy Research Institute
Sarasota, Florida

Contents

1

Why a 3rd edition

When we wrote the first edition of this book in 1996, prostate brachytherapy was in the midst of a rebirth, fueled by improvements in transrectal ultrasound, computer-planning, and the pioneering efforts of physicians and patients willing to question and defy traditional wisdom. By 2000, prostate brachytherapy had been reborn into *conventional* therapy. Even the most diehard former critics have implemented prostate brachytherapy programs within their practices.

We wrote the first and second editions primarily because no other comprehensive textbook of prostate brachytherapy was available at the time.

There is now a rapidly growing body of journal articles regarding prostate brachytherapy. But there are still few comprehensive information sources to help sort out the hype from the legitimate, or the sensible from the ridiculous. Having spent so much time wrestling with these issues, we believe that a 3rd edition will be valuable to the growing number of physicians, patients, and attorneys with an interest in brachytherapy.

TOUGH POLITICS

Prostate brachytherapy has always been controversial. There remains an almost visceral dislike of it among many mainstream, otherwise rational radiation oncologists and urologists. The reasons are varied and include residual skepticism borne from inferior results with older retropubic techniques, as well as a natural disdain toward a newer modality viewed as competition for more established procedures. In this book, we have the luxury of freely sharing our experiences, impressions, musings, and gripes without concern for "getting past the reviewer."

IMPLANTS AREN'T FOR EVERY PATIENT

While prostate cancer control rates generally look good and morbidity rates are generally low, it has become clear that brachytherapy is not for every patient, something that we've sometimes learned the hard way. In the pages ahead, we provide detailed information about potential complications and what we have learned about who is more likely to experience them. But one of the most frustrating aspects of our experience with brachytherapy has been the difficulty in identifying ahead of time the occasional patient who will develop more serious implant-related problems—and there's no end in sight to this dilemma.

IMPLANTS AREN'T FOR EVERY PHYSICIAN

Performing good prostate brachytherapy requires skill, attention to detail, and tolerance for tedium. Given the current technological limits, there is still a substantial dependence on manual dexterity and familiarity with the physics of brachytherapy—the title of this book was chosen to emphasize this fact. Even as more and more technical information is available to guide newcomers to the field, we still believe that physicians who are too busy with other responsibilities to put a substantial effort into a brachytherapy practice should leave it to someone else.

PERMANENT VERSUS TEMPORARY IMPLANTS

Permanent implants with either of two radioactive isotopes, I-125 or Pd-103, are the predominant form of prostate brachytherapy in the United

States. They're favored over temporary Ir-192 brachytherapy due to more encouraging tumor control rates and greater convenience (both for patients *and* physicians). Because of the continued overwhelming preference for permanent implants, we again declined to add in-depth discussions of temporary implants.

THIS BOOK SHOULD HELP

We witnessed a remarkable re-emergence of brachytherapy in the 1990s, and it likely will assume an even bigger role in the future. But we believe that a lot of fine-tuning is still to be done. This text gives us a platform to continue to share our experiences and advice. The descriptions, data, opinions, and ruminations ahead should be helpful to brachytherapists who are just getting started, and to those with established practices who are looking for ways to improve their techniques. We hope that this 3rd edition helps you to improve your brachytherapy skills and the results that you can achieve for your patients.

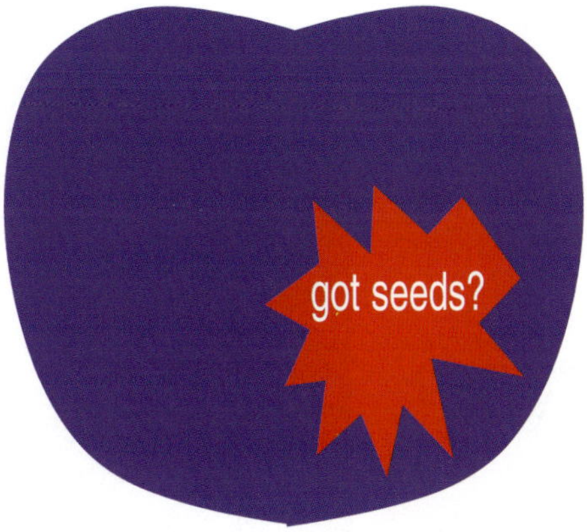

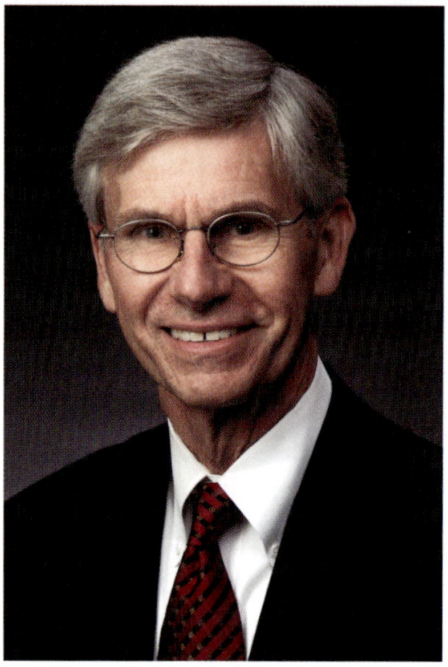

John Blasko

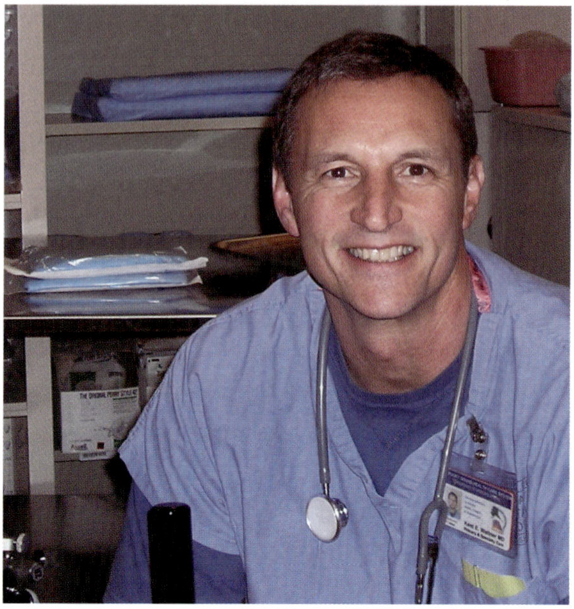

Kent Wallner

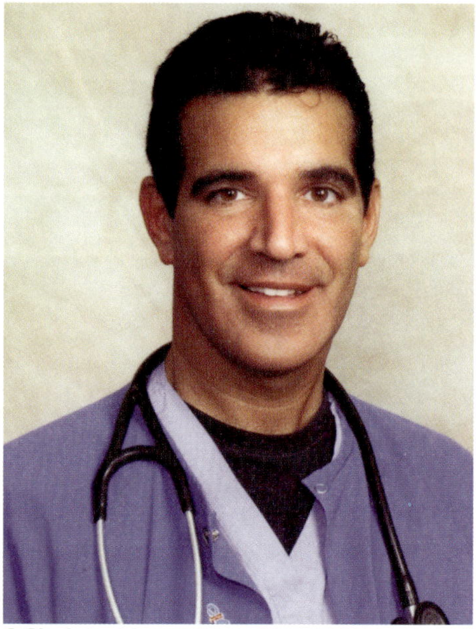

Michael
Dattoli

Gregory Merrick

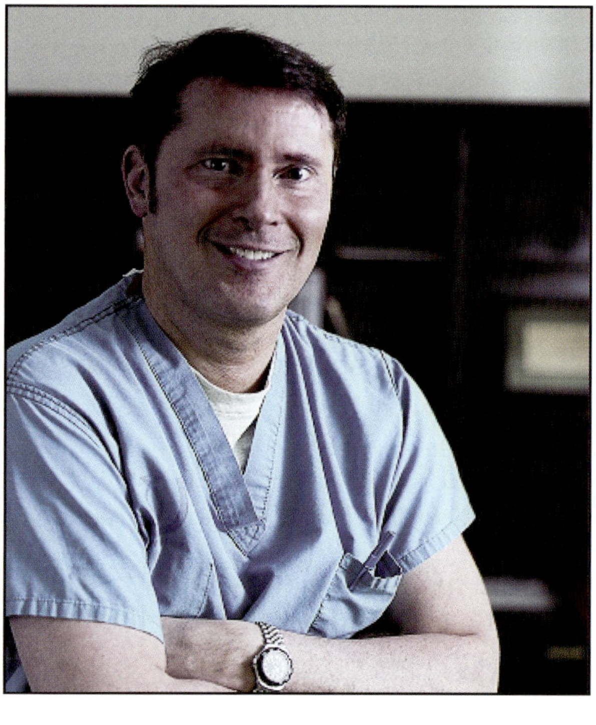

2

1895–2006

In the ten years since we wrote the first edition of this text, we have seen a remarkable shift toward brachytherapy as the treatment of choice for early-stage prostate cancer.(COOPERBERG) While many expected brachytherapy to grow, few expected it to happen so rapidly. Widespread resistance largely melted away as favorable 5-year and 10-year reports appeared in the late 1990s.(DATTOLI 07, CRITZ, BLASKO 00, ZELEFSKY)

THE EARLY DAYS

Prostate brachytherapy, in various forms, has fluctuated in popularity for more than 100 years (**Figure 2-1**). During most of that time, it was more a

Century time line

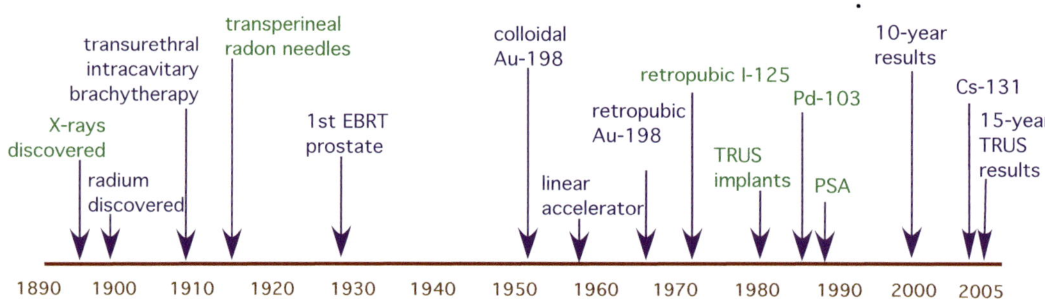

Figure 2-1. Major developments in prostate brachytherapy and external beam radiation (EBRT) from 1890 through 2006.

curiosity than a generally accepted method of treatment. Until the late 1990s, it had never been widely accepted by the medical community, for a variety of reasons.

Barringer, chief of Urology at what is now Memorial Sloan-Kettering Cancer Center in New York (MSKCC), was among the first to espouse use of transperineal prostate brachytherapy.(BARRINGER) He was impressed with his results with radon needles, concluding his 1917 JAMA report with:

> "*[B]ecause of the initial success of radium treatment, I now take the stand that no patient with prostate cancer should be operated on*"

Since Barringer's time, the evolution of prostate brachytherapy has been punctuated by a few basic ideas, re-implemented in various ways as technology has evolved.

RETROPUBIC IMPLANTS

The first widespread adoption of prostate brachytherapy occurred in the 1970s, when the open, retropubic method using I-125 was popularized by Hilaris and Whitmore at MSKCC.(WHITMORE) Early reports appeared favorable, but subsequent reports with longer follow-up were not.(FUKS, SCHELL-

1978 1999

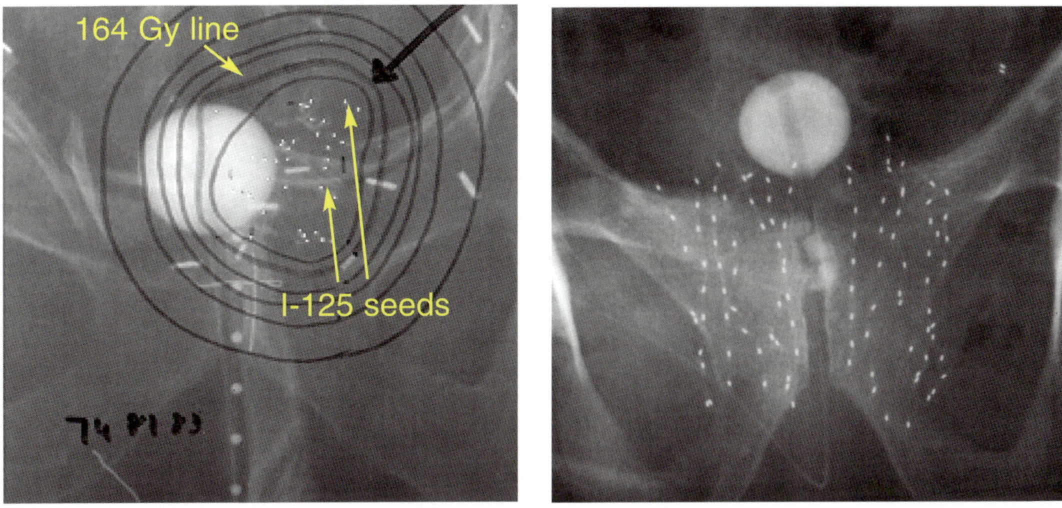

Figure 2-2. On the left is an anterior radiograph of a retropubic implant performed at MSKCC in 1978. You don't need a Ph.D. in physics to recognize that the I-125 seeds could not possibly be distributed throughout the prostate. This obviously inadequate implant (along with many others like it) was included in long-term retropubic implant reports from MSKCC.(FUKS) Unfavorable tumor control rates with poor quality retropubic implants initiallly dimmed enthusiasm for modern implant techniques. The implant on the right was performed in 1999 with modern transperineal techniques at the Puget Sound Health Care System VA Hospital.

HAMMER) In retrospect, the introduction of the retropubic method was probably a step backward from Barringer's transperineal needle placement. The quality of retropubic implants was terrible (**Figure 2-2**), due to technical limitations and lack of dosimetric quality assessment.

Although it seemed simple enough to do an implant under direct visualization of the exposed prostate, it was not. The prostate was not well exposed, the operative field was bloody, and without transrectal ultrasound (TRUS) it was impossible to visualize the seed location within the prostate—brachytherapists would have had little idea whether placement was properly performed. To compound the technical difficulties, quality assurance was almost non-existent. Post-implant radiation doses were

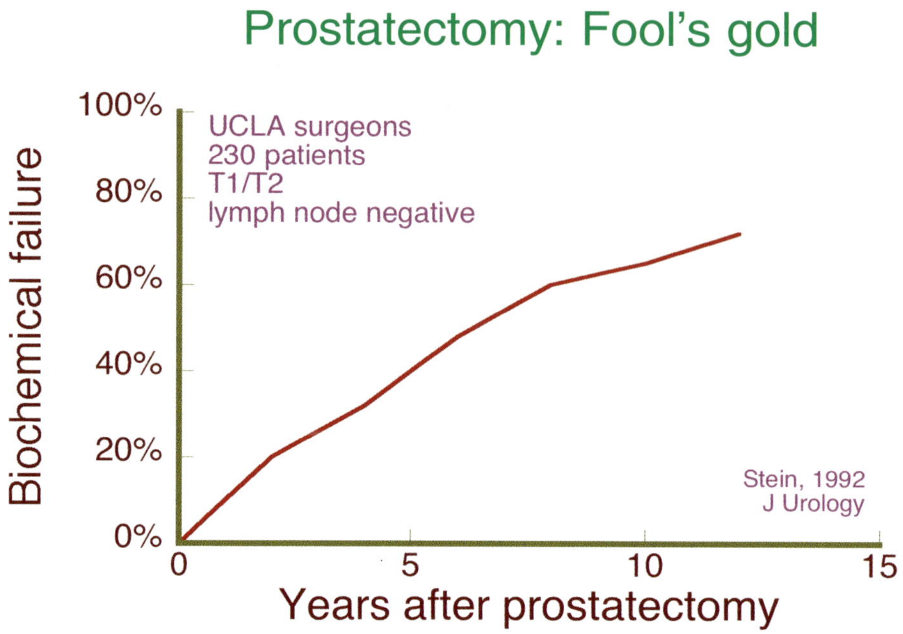

Figure 2-3. First PSA-based tumor control rates with prostatectomy, reported in 1992. The results were dismal, with no plateau on the cancer-free curves. Oncologists began to question whether any patient could be cured surgically.(STEIN)

calculated from plain X-rays, without knowledge of their relationship to the prostatic margins (see Chapter 11). Without a system of quality assurance, brachytherapists did not know how badly they were doing with the retropubic method (although they should have had some idea!).

THE BABY AND THE BATH WATER

Understandably, when unfavorable long-term results for retropubic implants were published, the urologic oncology community went from being enthusiastic to becoming highly suspicious of brachytherapy. With introduction of nerve-sparing surgery and widespread availability of linear accelerators, interest in brachytherapy plummeted in the 1980s. Less understandable is the use of unfavorable reports of retropubic implants to vigorously oppose modern transperineal brachytherapy. We were often reminded (sometimes with a certain glee) that the results of I-125 prostate brachytherapy, even at its birthplace (MSKCC), were suboptimal. But wait.

1980–2006

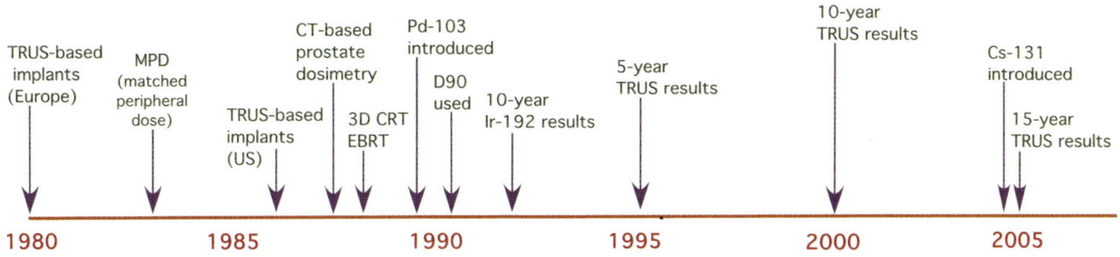

Figure 2-4. Time line showing some of the major developments in prostate brachytherapy from 1980 through 2006.

The retropubic implants of the 1970s were so bad technically, it was obvious to some of us early on that the clinical results would be much better with modern transrectal ultrasound, computer technology, and transperineal approach.

(FOOL'S) GOLD STANDARD

Widespread adoption of improved surgical techniques in the 1990s generated renewed enthusiasm for prostatectomy. However, the introduction of PSA-based follow-up showed how ineffective surgery can be in eradicating even early stage cancers, forcing a reassessment of the alternatives (**Figure 2-3**).(STEIN, ZIETMAN)

NEW TECHNOLOGIES ARRIVE

The last 15 years have witnessed a tremendous surge in prostate brachytherapy. CT scanners were introduced in the mid-1970s and TRUS in the early 1980s. Computer-based treatment planning became widely available in the late 1970s. By the mid-1980s, these technologies had been combined with the old idea of transperineal implantation, to allow high-quality outpatient prostate brachytherapy.(CHARYULU, HOLM, BLASKO 87, OSIAN)(**Figures 2-4 & 2-5**)

IR-192 BRACHYTHERAPY

While the rise and fall of retropubic implants was playing out, some brachytherapists took up temporary implants, the most influential and innovative being Nisar Syed, Ajmel Puthawala, Alvaro Martinez and Tim Mate. They treated patients with 30 to 40 Gy external beam radiation plus a tem-

The stats

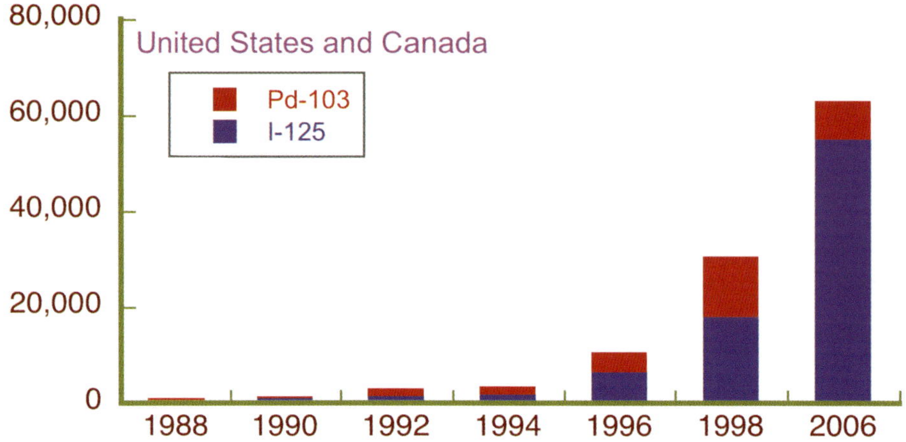

Figure 2-5. Approximate number of implants performed annually in the United States and Canada (courtesy of Theragenics Corporation and Oncura).

porary Ir-192 boost for an additional 30 to 35 Gy. Source loading was based on CT scan reconstruction of the prostate after the source guides were in place, allowing the radiation dose to be conformed to the geometry of the prostate. Accordingly, it should be as accurate a system for dose delivery as current TRUS-guided transperineal methods.(SYED)

Despite the pioneering work of Syed and colleagues, the popularity of temporary Ir-192 implants declined substantially in the 1980s. Like permanent retropubic implants, it was eclipsed by "nerve-sparing" prostatectomy, by conformal radiation, and by permanent transperineal implants. Modern high dose rate (HDR) methodology and encouraging five-year results, however, have fueled renewed interest in Ir-192 (**Figure 2-6**).(MARTINEZ, MATE, YOSHIOKA)

WHERE THE CONTROVERSIES WILL GROW

Several groups are reaching the 15-year follow-up mark for transperineal methods, with biochemical-based cancer-free rates that compare favorably with surgery.(DATTOLI 07, GRIMM) But brachytherapy has now entered mid-

HDR versus permanent implants

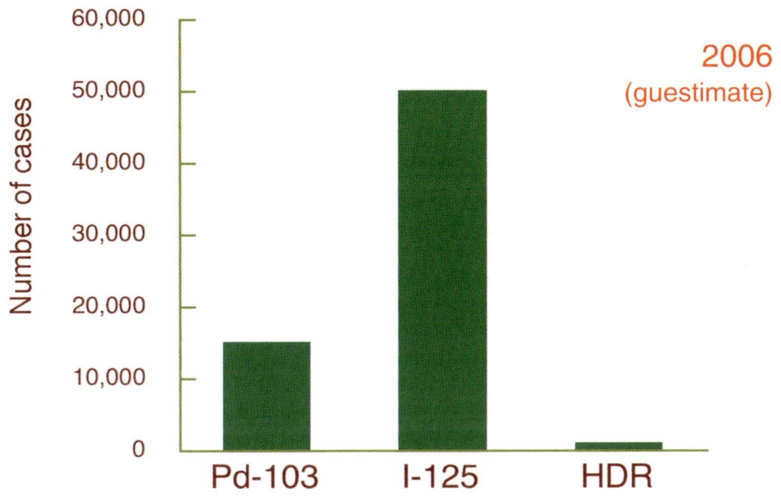

Figure 2-6. Approximate number of permanent implants versus HDR implants in 2005 (HDR estmiates courtesy of Dr. Philip Devlin). Precise numbers are not available due to fragmentation of the seed maufacturing market.

dle age, and it is being widely scrutinized by more conventional investigators from varied disciplines.

Brachytherapy has some obvious advantages over prostatectomy or external beam radiation, including patient convenience and the potential for far lower cost. Where controversy will continue over the next few years is how much of an impact brachytherapy has on patients' quality of life (QOL), compared to surgery or external radiation. Mounting evidence shows that brachytherapy, especially if not optimally performed, can have more adverse effects than first appreciated. Potency preservation, in particular, has been less favorable than believed in the early 1990s.(MERRICK) And it is increasingly apparent that good outcomes are dependent on good technique. Quality of life and dosimetric quality assurance are likely to dominate investigators' interest for the next few years.

BOLD PHYSICIANS AND PATIENT AND INDUSTRY ACTIVISM

The wide acceptance of modern prostate brachytherapy was largely due to a handful of physicians determined to proceed despite the admonitions of much of the medical establishment. Drs. Blasko, Ragde, Grimm, and Sylvester were the first prominent advocates in the United States. They were considered for almost 10 years to be out of the mainstream. Now they find themselves center stage before the oncology community.

Resurgent interest in prostate brachytherapy is also largely due to direct patient involvement. In the 1990s patients increasingly began to investigate their treatment options and pass information to other prospective patients through formal (support groups, news articles) and informal (Internet, personal contact) channels. These patient-directed efforts had a substantial impact on the public's awareness of brachytherapy.

Taking the brachytherapy message to the public was boosted by industry—companies that needed to *get the message out* in order to sell their products. Industry advertising incorporated traditional methods of printed materials, and higher-tech vehicles like video, CDs and websites (**Figures 2.7 to 2.9**).

Many physicians have grumbled about patients and industry taking the lead in promoting brachytherapy. But for better or worse, patients are taking a larger role in their medical decision-making. We think it is mostly for the better.

EVOLVING FROM AN "ART" TO A "SCIENCE"

One common criticism of brachytherapy has been that it is too much of an *art*, without hard data to support precise seed placement strategies. We couldn't agree more. We, the authors of this textbook, have dedicated much of our last 15 years to gathering and disseminating outcomes data and technical dosimetric analyses to better define the effect of dose distribution throughout the prostate and adjacent organs.(MERRICK) Progress is being made. Prostate brachytherapy is gradually transforming from an *art* to a *science*.

VERY GOOD, BUT NOT PERFECT

As a result of technological developments and clinical testing over the last 15 years, brachytherapy is gaining an increasingly prominent role in the fight against prostate cancer. Much of the prior skepticism has melted

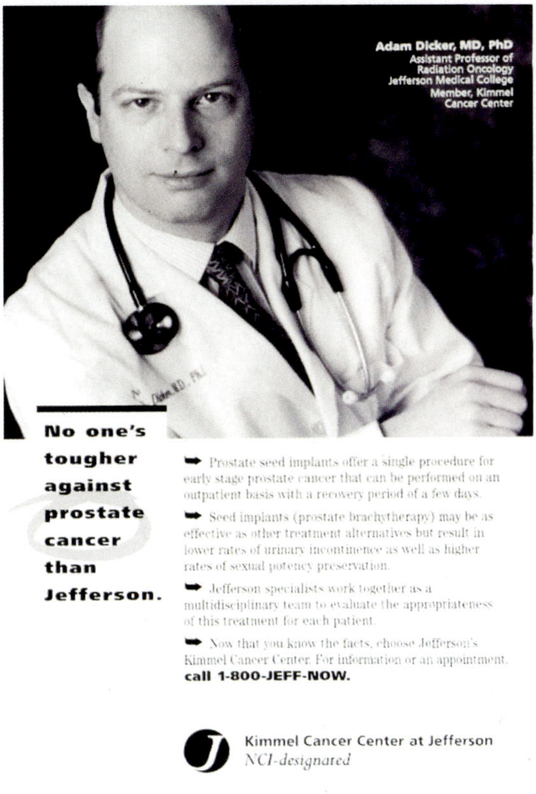
Adam Dicker, MD, PhD
Assistant Professor of Radiation Oncology
Jefferson Medical College
Member, Kimmel Cancer Center
No one's tougher against prostate cancer than Jefferson.
➡ Prostate seed implants offer a single procedure for early stage prostate cancer that can be performed on an outpatient basis with a recovery period of a few days.
➡ Seed implants (prostate brachytherapy) may be as effective as other treatment alternatives but result in lower rates of urinary incontinence as well as higher rates of sexual potency preservation.
➡ Jefferson specialists work together as a multidisciplinary team to evaluate the appropriateness of this treatment for each patient.
➡ Now that you know the facts, choose Jefferson's Kimmel Cancer Center. For information or an appointment, call 1-800-JEFF-NOW.
Kimmel Cancer Center at Jefferson
NCI-designated
Thomas Jefferson University Hospital • 11th and Walnut Streets, Philadelphia, PA 19107 • Jefferson Health System

Figure 2-7. Newsprint adverstisement (left) and pamphlet (below) used to promote prostate brachytherapy in the 1990s.

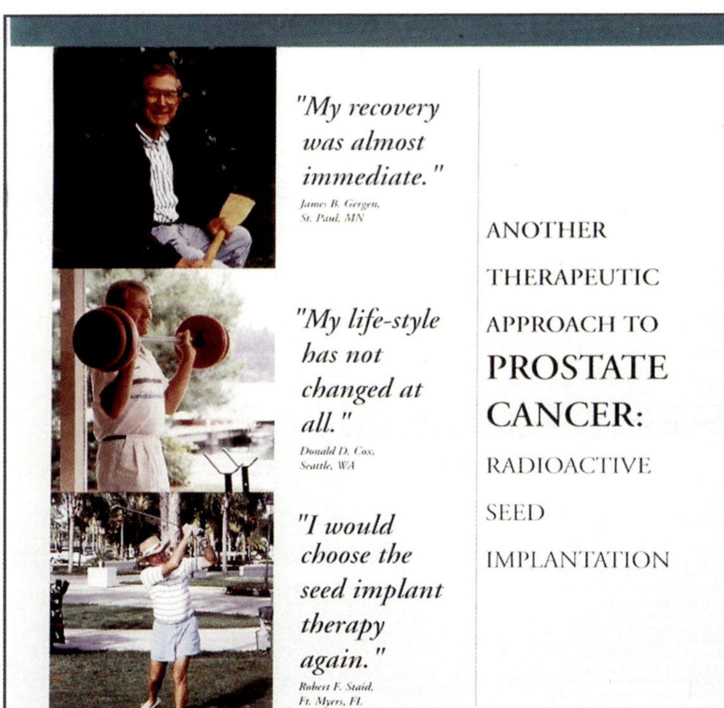
"My recovery was almost immediate."
James B. Gergen, St. Paul, MN
"My life-style has not changed at all."
Donald D. Cox, Seattle, WA
"I would choose the seed implant therapy again."
Robert F. Staid, Ft. Myers, FL
ANOTHER THERAPEUTIC APPROACH TO PROSTATE CANCER: RADIOACTIVE SEED IMPLANTATION

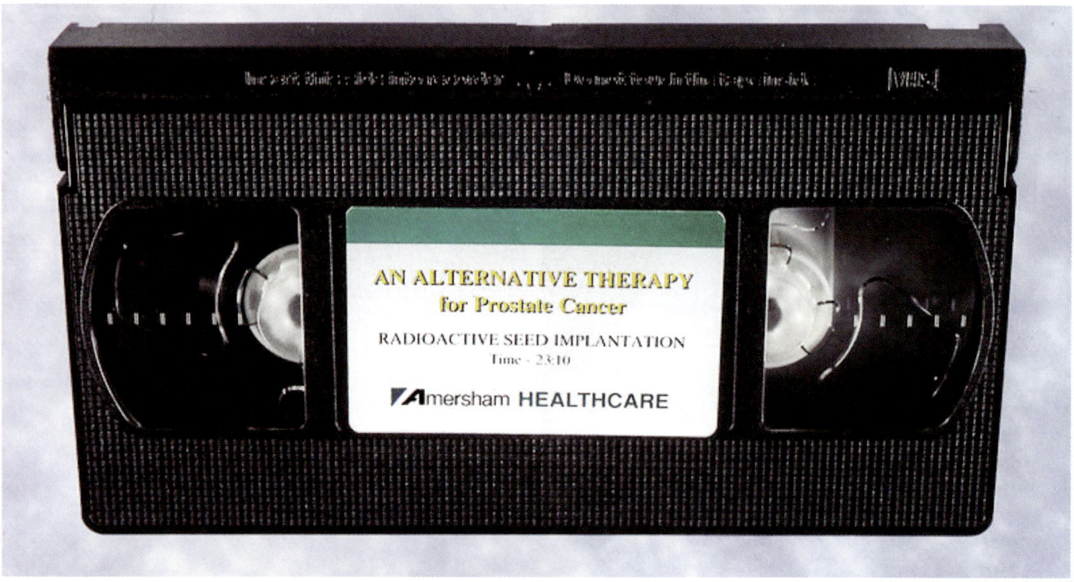

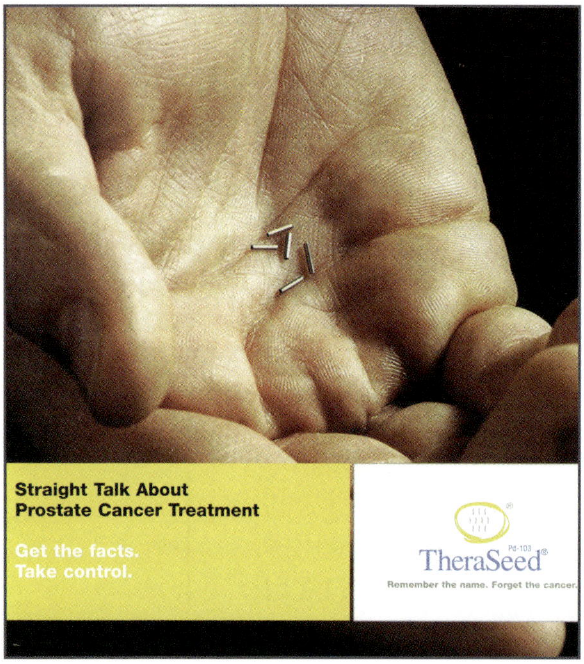

Figure 2-8. Video (1990s) and CD (2006) used to promote prostate brachytherapy directly to patients.

away. But with increasing experience, it's clear that brachytherapy is not the runaway best treatment that a few zealots believed it to be. There *are* some brachytherapy patients who develop treatment-related problems that severely impact on their lifestyle. Most of the problems resolve with time, but doctors and patients should understand that there are pitfalls to this

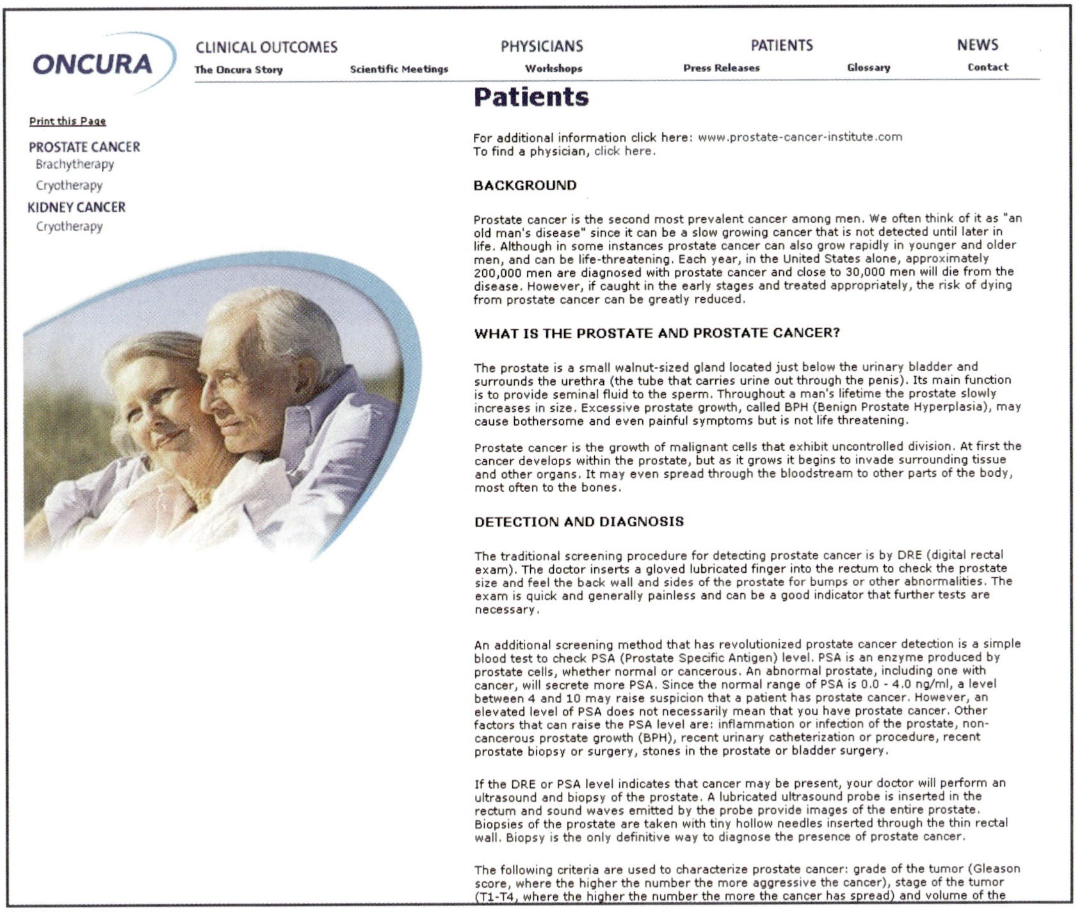

ONCURA

CLINICAL OUTCOMES PHYSICIANS PATIENTS NEWS

The Oncura Story Scientific Meetings Workshops Press Releases Glossary Contact

Print this Page

PROSTATE CANCER
Brachytherapy
Cryotherapy
KIDNEY CANCER
Cryotherapy

Patients

For additional information click here: www.prostate-cancer-institute.com
To find a physician, click here.

BACKGROUND

Prostate cancer is the second most prevalent cancer among men. We often think of it as "an old man's disease" since it can be a slow growing cancer that is not detected until later in life. Although in some instances prostate cancer can also grow rapidly in younger and older men, and can be life-threatening. Each year, in the United States alone, approximately 200,000 men are diagnosed with prostate cancer and close to 30,000 men will die from the disease. However, if caught in the early stages and treated appropriately, the risk of dying from prostate cancer can be greatly reduced.

WHAT IS THE PROSTATE AND PROSTATE CANCER?

The prostate is a small walnut-sized gland located just below the urinary bladder and surrounds the urethra (the tube that carries urine out through the penis). Its main function is to provide seminal fluid to the sperm. Throughout a man's lifetime the prostate slowly increases in size. Excessive prostate growth, called BPH (Benign Prostate Hyperplasia), may cause bothersome and even painful symptoms but is not life threatening.

Prostate cancer is the growth of malignant cells that exhibit uncontrolled division. At first the cancer develops within the prostate, but as it grows it begins to invade surrounding tissue and other organs. It may even spread through the bloodstream to other parts of the body, most often to the bones.

DETECTION AND DIAGNOSIS

The traditional screening procedure for detecting prostate cancer is by DRE (digital rectal exam). The doctor inserts a gloved lubricated finger into the rectum to check the prostate size and feel the back wall and sides of the prostate for bumps or other abnormalities. The exam is quick and generally painless and can be a good indicator that further tests are necessary.

An additional screening method that has revolutionized prostate cancer detection is a simple blood test to check PSA (Prostate Specific Antigen) level. PSA is an enzyme produced by prostate cells, whether normal or cancerous. An abnormal prostate, including one with cancer, will secrete more PSA. Since the normal range of PSA is 0.0 - 4.0 ng/ml, a level between 4 and 10 may raise suspicion that a patient has prostate cancer. However, an elevated level of PSA does not necessarily mean that you have prostate cancer. Other factors that can raise the PSA level are: inflammation or infection of the prostate, non-cancerous prostate growth (BPH), recent urinary catheterization or procedure, recent prostate biopsy or surgery, stones in the prostate or bladder surgery.

If the DRE or PSA level indicates that cancer may be present, your doctor will perform an ultrasound and biopsy of the prostate. A lubricated ultrasound probe is inserted in the rectum and sound waves emitted by the probe provide images of the entire prostate. Biopsies of the prostate are taken with tiny hollow needles inserted through the thin rectal wall. Biopsy is the only definitive way to diagnose the presence of prostate cancer.

The following criteria are used to characterize prostate cancer: grade of the tumor (Gleason score, where the higher the number the more aggressive the cancer), stage of the tumor (T1-T4, where the higher the number the more the cancer has spread) and volume of the

Figure 2-9. Website used to promote prostate brachytherapy directly to patients.

exciting modality. We, the authors of this text, are not blind to the limitations of brachytherapy. We'll spend the next 600+ pages describing the negatives as well as the positives of prostate brachytherapy.

REFERENCES

1. Barringer BS. Radium in the treatment of carcinoma of the bladder and prostate. JAMA 1917; 68:1227-1230.

2. Blasko JC, Ragde H, Schumacher D. Transperineal percutaneous iodine-125 implantation for prostatic carcinoma using transrectal ultrasound and template guidance. Endo/Hypertherm 1987; 3:131-139.

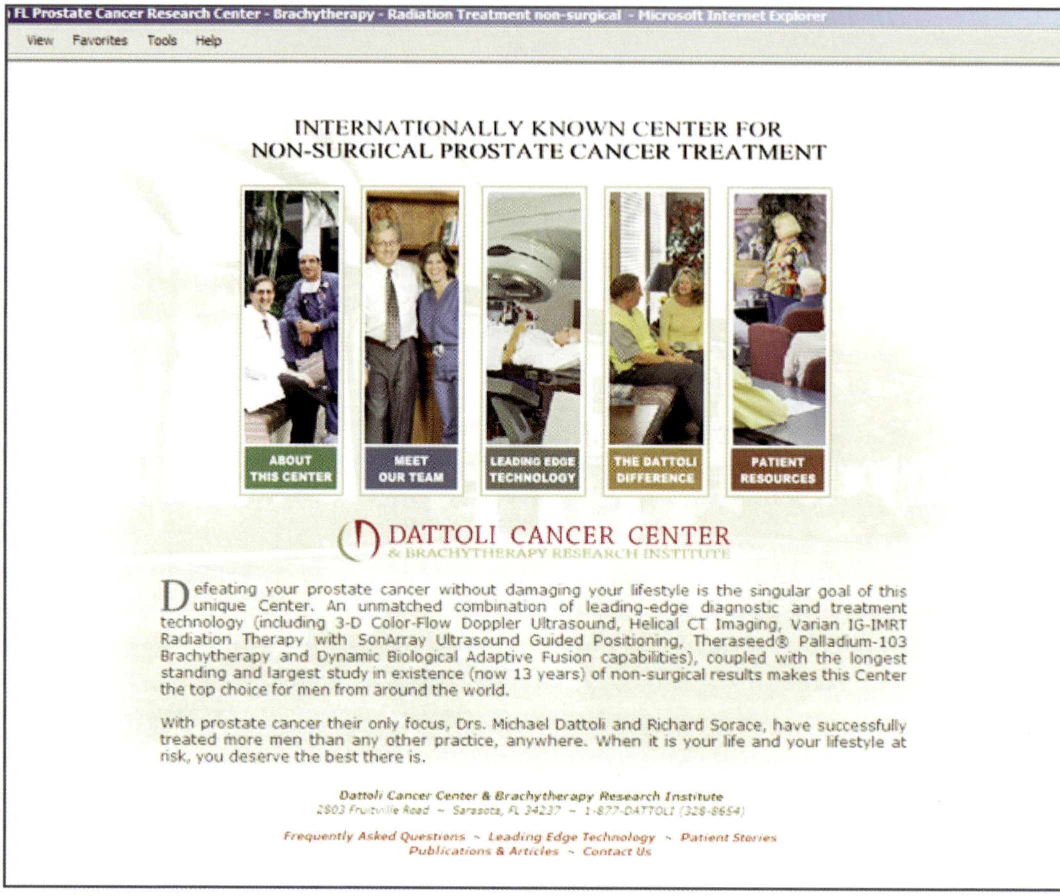

Figure 2-10. Informational Website for patients.

3. Blasko JC, Wallner KE, Grimm PD, Ragde H. PSA-based disease control following ultrasound-guided I-125 implantation for stage T1/T2 prostatic carcinoma. J Urol 1995; 154:1096-1099.

4. Charyulu KKN. Transperineal interstitial implantation of prostate cancer: A new method. Int J Rad Oncol Biol Phys 1980; 6:1261-1266.

5. Cooperberg M, Lubeck D, Meng M, Mehta S, Carroll P. The changing face of low-risk prostate cancer: Trends in clinical prsentation and primary management. J Clin Oncol 2004; 22:2141-2149.

6. Critz FA, Williams H, Holladay CT, Levinson AK, al e. Post-treatment PSA 0.2 ng/ml defines disease freedom after radiotherapy for prostate cancer using modern techniques. Urol 1999; 54:968-971.

7. Dattoli M, Wallner K, True L, Cash J, Sorace R. Long-term prostate cancer control using Palladium-103 brachytherapy and external beam radiotherapy in patients with a high likelihood of extracapsular cancer extension. Urology 2007.

8. Dattoli M, Wallner K, True L, Sorace R, Koval J, al e. Prognostic role of serum prostatic acid phosphatase for 103-Pd-based radiation for prostatic carcinoma. Int J Rad Oncol Biol Phys 1999; 45:853-856.

9. Fuks Z, Leibel SA, Wallner KE, et al. The effect of local control on metastatic dissemination in carcinoma of the prostate: Long term results in patients treated with 125-I implantation. Int J Radiat Oncol Biol Phys 1991; 21:337-347.

10. Holm HH, Juul N, Pederson JF, Hansen H, Stroyer I. Transperineal 125-Iodine seed implantation in prostatic cancer guided by transrectal ultrasonography. J Urol 1983; 130:283-286.

11. Martinez A, Gustafson G, Gonzales J, et al. Dose escalation using conformal high-dose-rate brachytherapy improves outcome in unfavorable prostate cancer. Int J Rad Oncol Biol Phys 2002; 53:316-327.

12. Mate TP, Gottesman JE, Hatton J, al e. High dosed-rate after-loading iridium-192 prostate brachytherapy: feasibility report. Int J Rad Oncol Biol Phys 1998; 41:525-533.

13. Merrick G, Butler WM, Wallner K, et al. Erectile function after prostate brachytherapy. Int J Rad Oncol Biol Phys 2005; 62:437-447.

14. Merrick G, Wallner K, Butler W. Minimizing prostate brachytherapy-related morbidity. Urol 2003; 62:786-792.

15. Osian AD, Anderson LL, Linares LA, Nori D, Hilaris BS. Treatment planning for permanent and temporary percutaneous implants with custom made templates. Int J Rad Oncol Biol Phys 1989; 16:219-223.

16. Schellhammer PF, El-Mahdi AM, Wright GL, Kolm P, Ragle R. Prostate-specific antigen to determine progression-free survival after radiation therapy for localized carcinoma of prostate. Urology 1993; 42:13-20.

17. Stein A, deKernion JB, Smith RB, Dorey F, Patel H. Prostate specific antigen levels after radical prostatectomy in patients with organ confined and locally extensive prostate cancer. J Urol 1992; 147:942-946.

18. Syed AM, Puthawala A, Austin P, Cherlow J. Temporary iridium-192 implant in the management of carcinoma of the prostate. Cancer 1992; 69:2515-2524.

19. Sylvester J, Grimm P, Blasko J, et al. 15-year biochemical relapse free survival in clinical stage T1-T3 prostate cancer following combined external beam radiotherapy and brachytherapy: Seattle experience. Int J Rad Oncol Biol Phys 2007; 67:57-64.

20. Whitmore WF, Hilaris B, Grabstald H. Retropubic implantation of Iodine 125 in the treatment of prostatic cancer. J Urol 1972; 108:918-920.
21. Yoshioka Y, Nose T, Yoshida K, al e. High-dose-rate interstitial brachytherapy as a monotherapy for localized prostate cancer: treatment description and preliminary results of a Phase I/II clinical trial. Int J Rad Oncol Biol Phys 2000; 48:675-681.
22. Zelefsky MJ, Wallner KE, Ling CC, Raben A, al e. Comparison of the 5-year outcome and morbidity of three-dimensional conformal radiotherapy versus transperineal permanent iodine-125 implantation for earl-stage prostatic cancer. J Clin Oncol 1999; 17:517-522.
23. Zietman AL, Coen JJ, Shipley WU, Willett CG, Efird JT. Radical radiation therapy in the management of prostatic adenocarcinoma: The initial prostate specific antigen value as a predictor of treatment outcome. J Urol 1994; 151:640-645.

3

Radiobiology

FEW FACTS, STRETCHED THIN

Radiobiology is a fascinating area of study. Unfortunately, its applicability to clinical decision-making is tenuous. Most radiobiologic concepts are theoretical or based on *in vitro* experiments. *In vivo* work has nearly all been derived from transplantable mouse (murine) tumors, which typically behave far differently than spontaneously occurring human tumors (**Table 3-1**).

Nearly all radiobiological data regarding prostate brachytherapy is purely theoretical.(LING 92) While such work is important to guide clinical investi-

Table 3-1. Radiobiologic factors that likely affect the degree of cell killing, and how much is known about each for human prostate cancers.

Factor	Quantifiable in vivo?
Dose	no*
Dose rate	no*
Damage repair	no
Oxygen enhancement ratio	no
RBE	no
Apoptosis	no
Repopulation	no
Reassortment	no

*even the dose and dose rate can't be quantified precisely, due to rapid fall-off near the sources

gators, its practical relevance to clinical practice is highly questionable. The point here is not to belittle such theoretical efforts, but to keep them in proper perspective.

BRACHYTHERAPY VERSUS EXTERNAL BEAM RADIATION

Brachytherapy and external beam irradiation differ in three principal respects:

- dose localization
- total dose
- dose rate

All three factors *may* be advantages for brachytherapy over external beam radiation, but data regarding their clinical relevance are scarce.

Dose localization

The rectum is relatively sensitive to radiation, the anterior rectal wall being the principal dose-limiting structure for prostate radiation in any form. A small rectal area can tolerate a large dose, but as the area irradiated increases so does the risk of complications.(MUELLER,LEE,JACKSON) Even with conformal external radiation, the potential for prostate motion (typically 0.5 cm in the anterior-posterior direction) requires that a relatively large

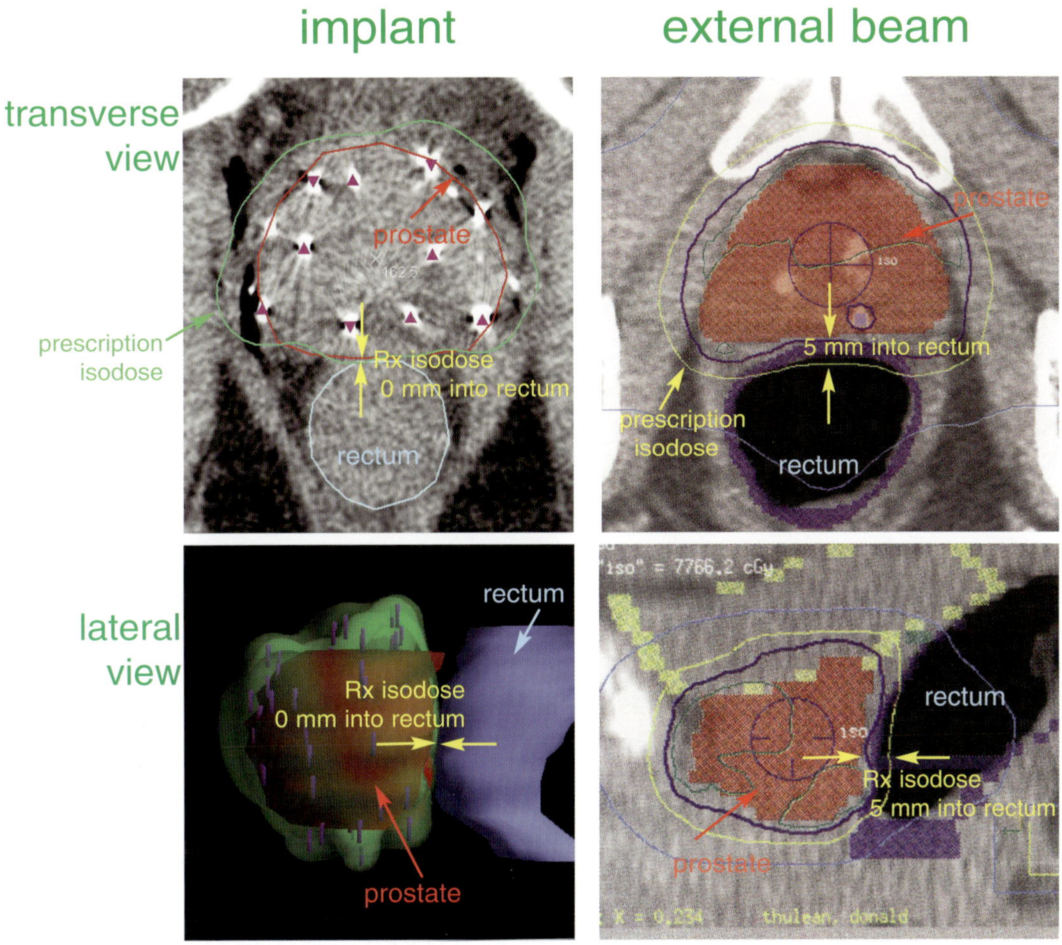

Figure 3-1. Prescription dose in relation to the prostate and rectum for brachytherapy versus beam radiation. Much more rectal surface is included in the high dose region with beam compared to brachytherapy. With brachytherapy, a smaller portion of the rectum receives the prescription dose because of rapid dose fall-off and because no allowance needs to be made for prostate motion.(HAN)

IMPORTANT POINT

The fact that brachytherapy does not require a posterior margin to account for prostate motion is the primary reason the biologic dose can be substantially higher than with beam radiation.

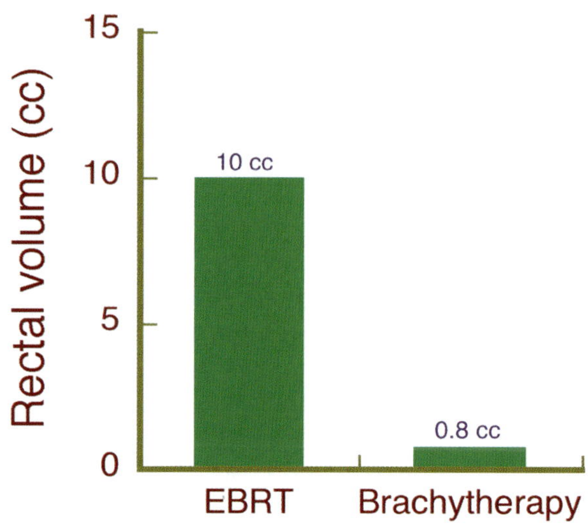

Figure 3-2. Typical rectal volume treated to prescription dose or higher with conformal external beam radiation versus brachytherapy. With beam, approximately 20 times as much volume receives the prescription dose or higher. (KUPELIAN 02, MUELLER)

portion of the anterior rectal wall is included in the target volume to avoid underdosing the posterior prostate.

Using brachytherapy, a higher radiation dose can be given to the prostate, mostly due to the rapid dose fall-off at the prostatic margins, limiting the rectal surface area that receives the prescription dose or higher (**Figure 3-1**). With a well-executed implant, less than 1.0 cm^3 of rectal volume receives the prescription dose or higher (R100). With a typical conformal external beam plan, approximately 10 cm^3 of anterior rectal wall receives the prescription dose or higher (**Figure 3-2**).

Bladder tolerance is *not* a dose-limiting concern with prostate brachytherapy or conformal external beam radiation. Because of rapid dose fall-off, no more than 1.0 cm of bladder wall receives the brachytherapy prescription dose. Even with combined brachytherapy plus supplemental beam radiation, bladder irradiation (40 to 50 Gy) is probably of little consequence. Brachytherapy-related urinary morbidity is predominantly due to *urethritis* and *prostatitis*, not *cystitis*.

Total dose

Nominal brachytherapy doses are approximately twice those given with external beam radiation (**Figure 3-3**). Total doses of 76 Gy for beam, 144 Gy with I-125, and 124 Gy with Pd-103 all produce high rates of biochem-

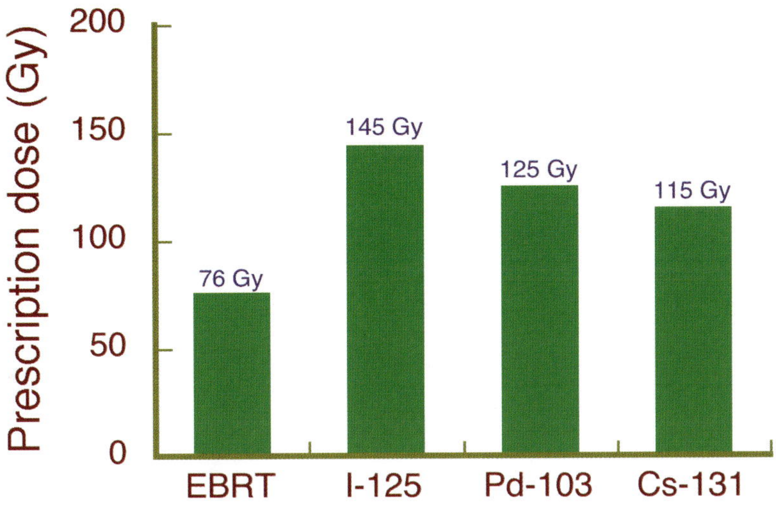

Figure 3-3. Typical external beam prescription dose versus those for I-125, Pd-103 and Cs-131. Brachytherapy doses are approximately 50% higher than that deliverable with beam radiation.

ical control for patients with pre-treatment PSA below 10 ng/ml.(ZELEFSKY 99)

A modification of the TDF tables (time, dose, fractionation) has been made to allow interconvertability between beam radiation and low dose rate brachytherapy.(ORTON) While it reflects current prescription doses, its clinical applicability for designing alternate dose schedules is unclear.

Dose rate

The most dramatic difference between beam radiation and brachytherapy is in dose rates. The typical initial dose rate of an I-125 or Pd-103 implant is less than 1 percent of the typical 2 to 4 Gy per minute of a linear accelerator (**Figure 3-4**). This marked difference dwarfs the moderate differences in total dose, and may entail substantial differences in radiation damage repair, reassortment, reoxygenation, and redistribution in the cell cycle.

With few exceptions, lower dose rates yield lower cell killing, given the same total dose. As the dose rate gets low enough, its effect diminishes,

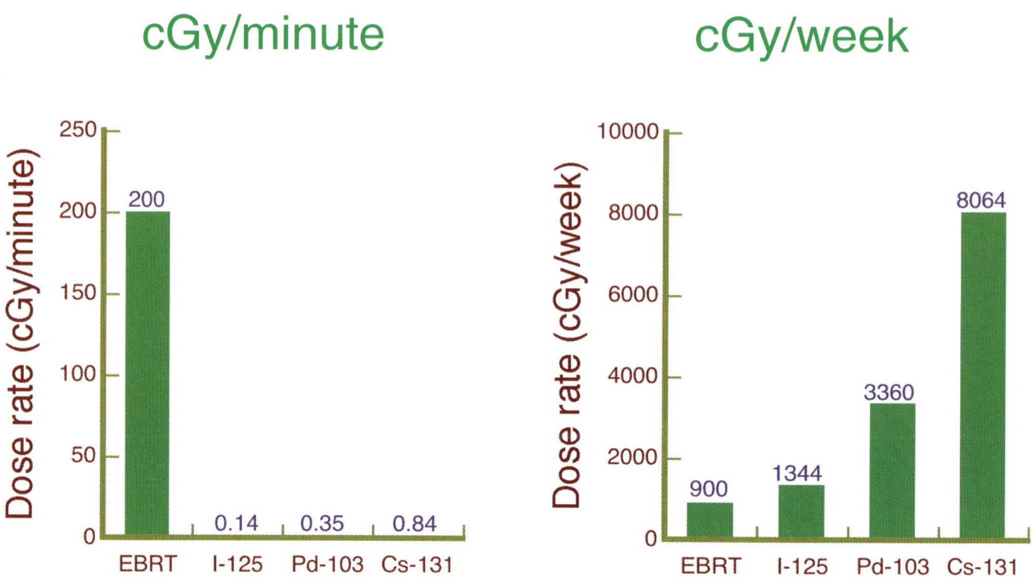

Figure 3-4. The instantaneous dose rate of a linear accelerator is far higher than the dose rate at the periphery of a I-125, Pd-103 or Cs-131 implant (left). However, when compared over a longer time interval, brachytherapy dose rates are similar or greater than that of beam radiation (right). The clinical relevance of how dose rates are expressed is not understood.

presumably due to dominance of single hit cell killing. In fact, very little work has been done with dose rates as low as those of I-125/Pd-103 brachytherapy.(LING 95) The comparability of high and low dose rate radiation effects on human tumors specifically is unknown.

Comparing brachytherapy versus beam dose rates is even more confused due to the fact that the rates can be calculated for different time intervals. Nominal dose rates are markedly different depending on the time interval chosen for the denominator. For example, the beam dose rate is typically 10 Gy per week, versus 13 Gy per week for an I-125 implant (**Figure 3-4**). For slow-growing tumors like those of the prostate, dose rates expressed in terms of the longer denominators may be more clinically relevant than those expressed in minutes.

OXYGEN ENHANCEMENT RATIO (OER)

Sterilizing poorly oxygenated (hypoxic) tumors requires 2.5 to 4.0 times as much radiation as is needed for fully oxygenated tumors. The low dose rate radiation of I-125 or Pd-103 brachytherapy may decrease hypoxia-related radiation resistance.(HALL 74) However, the relationship between the OER and dose rate is complicated, depending on both cell type and the dose rate tested.(LING 85)

While brachytherapy might offer an advantage in eradication of hypoxic tumors, little is known about OER with low dose rate brachytherapy. A wide range of oxygen tensions has been reported in human prostate tumors.(RASEY, MOVSAS 00 & 99) However, judging from the almost uniformly viable appearance of prostate tumors on microscopy, it's unlikely that substantial areas of severe hypoxia exist in most patients' tumors, in contrast to the classic portrayals of histologically evident hypoxic cancer tissue.(HALL 94)

α/β RATIO

Much has been written about the α/β ratio for prostate cancer. The ratio is considered as the dose at which the degree of single hit (alpha) killing equals multi-hit (beta) cell kill. The ratio for slow-turnover normal tissues is considered to be in the range of 1-5, while that for tumor tissues is believed to be higher. The flip-flop in expert opinions regarding the ratio for prostate cancer is almost comical. The α/β ratio du jour is in the 1.5-3.0 range.(WANG, FOWLER, BRENNER)

A lower α/β ratio argues for higher dose per treatment fraction—presumably HDR over LDR, or Pd-103 over I-125. The clinical relevance of numerical α/β ratio values is unclear and will not be considered further here.

APOPTOSIS

Apoptosis is "signal-induced, programmed" cell death, seemingly distinct from mitotic death due to indiscriminate DNA damage. It occurs as a natural involution process in lymphocytes, and to some extent in other tissues. It is probably the mechanism of prostate cell death following androgen deprivation.(MCDONNELL)

The role of apoptosis in radiation-related death of prostate cancer is unclear. It accounts for only a small percent of radiation cell killing in most human cell types, and there is scant evidence that it is important for radiation against prostate cancer.(ALGAN, POLLACK)

HYPERTHERMIA

Hyperthermia is the use of elevated temperature to enhance the cytotoxic effect of radiation. Hyperthermia may act primarily by suppressing sublethal damage repair.(BENHUR, PAULUS) The thermal enhancement ratio varies from 1.0 to 5.0, depending on the temperature and time the hyperthermia is given. Temperatures of 41° to 42°C for 30 to 90 minutes are most practical with the technology currently available.

Hyperthermia generated substantial enthusiasm in the 1980s, when a variety of external and interstitial heating devices were designed for clinical use. Prostate cancer was studied widely, due to its accessibility by interstitial heating with radiofrequency antennae. Unfortunately, only locally advanced or recurrent tumors were studied.(PRIONAS) Patients with locally advanced tumors were generally not curable with any local modality available at the time, and the chance of showing a benefit from hyperthermia would have been miniscule.

While there were anecdotal reports of good local response, patients did poorly overall, as would be expected. It is still unclear whether hyperthermia would add to local control.(ALGAN) In the meantime, it has generally fallen out of favor due to technical difficulties in achieving a homogeneous heat dose with available technology.

I-125 VERSUS PD-103

The half lives and dose rates of the commonly used isotopes are vastly different (see Figure 3-4). It has been argued that inferior results with the implants done with I-125 in the 1970s were due to suboptimal radiobiologic properties. Probably not. Retropubic implants were technically poor (see Chapter 2). Their high failure rates likely had little to do with the isotope choice. Despite the potential clinical implications, there is only a smattering of data available regarding the effect of different dose rates on cancer killing or normal tissue complications.

In vitro

Low energy photons have a higher linear energy transfer (LET), leading to higher radiobiologic effect (RBE). The higher RBE presumably results from more energy deposition per cell as photons traverse the tissue. With an

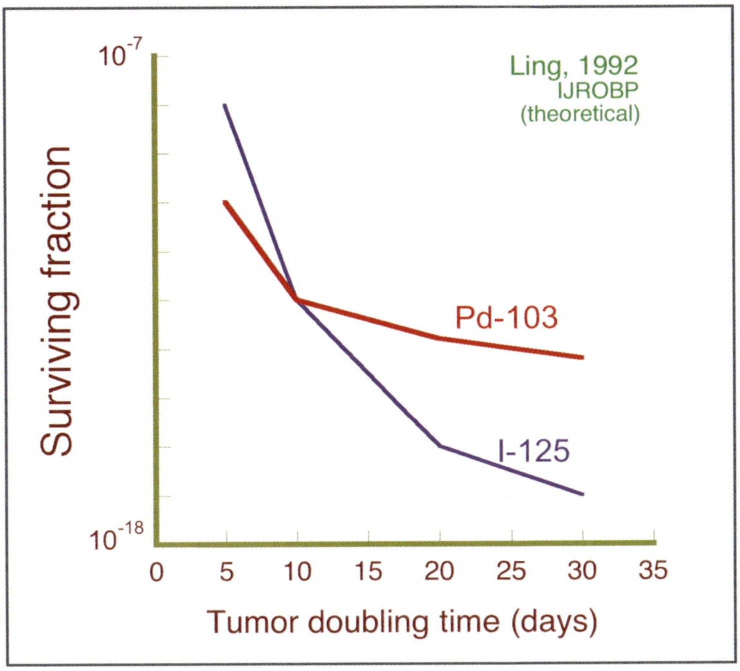

Figure 3-5. Surviving cell fractions following I-125 or Pd-103 versus tumor doubling times. Numbers are theoretical, based on biological equivalent dose calculations.(LING 92) *Below is the equation used to determine cell survival levels. The equation contains five variables, the values for which are unknown.*

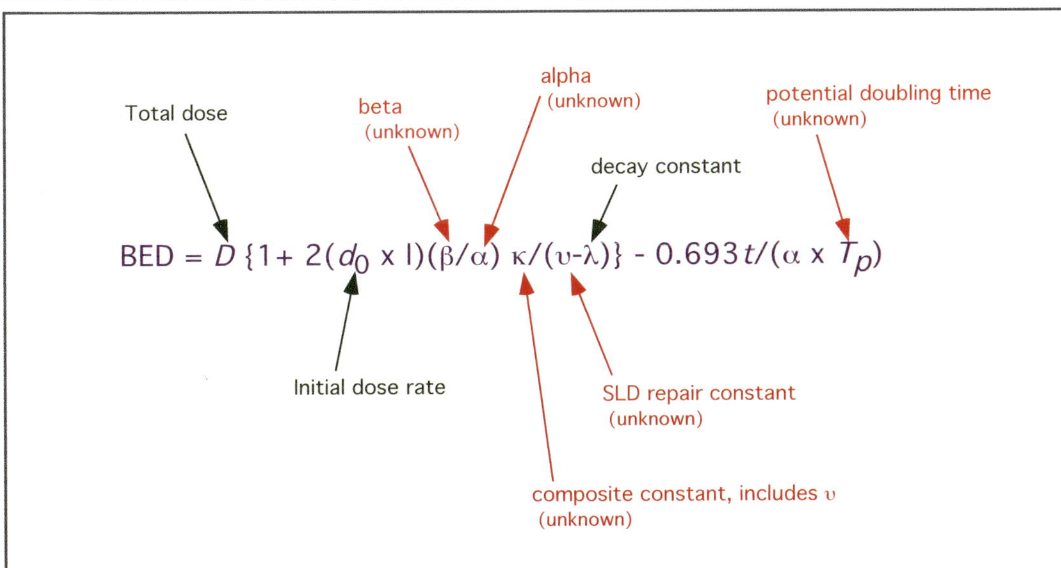

average 21 keV Pd-103 photon energy versus 30 keV for I-125, Pd-103 would be expected to have a slightly higher LET and RBE.

The RBE of I-125 versus Pd-103 has been compared in only one system—rat embryo cells transfected with Ha-ras oncogene.(LING 95) Using this system, Ling and colleagues reported an I-125 RBE of 1.4, compared to 1.9 for Pd-103. A difference of this magnitude is numerically substantial, and may justify a reduction in total dose by approximately 30 percent. Unfortunately, it has been studied in only one (in vitro) system, and likely has little relevance to human prostate tumors.

There are no in vitro studies comparing I-125 to Pd-103 against prostate cancer specifically, due in part to the limited number of cell lines available. There are several rodent models, and only a handful of human models. And the clincial relevance of laboratory-grown immortal murine cancer cell lines is highly questionable.

In vivo

Nag and colleagues studied the effect of I-125 versus Pd-103 in transplantable Nb AI-1 prostate tumors in Noble rats.(NAG) At similar doses, tumor growth delay and tumor eradication rates were increased by a factor of 2 or more with Pd-103 versus I-125. The increased tumorcidal effect of Pd-103 was higher than what would be expected by its higher RBE alone, suggesting an enhanced therapeutic ratio.

The results of Nag and colleagues, while intriguing, were based on a limited number of animals (five per group). Large inter-animal differences in tumor response to identical treatment require that experiments be repeated multiple times, to give more confidence in the findings. Their findings should also be viewed skeptically because of imprecise dosimetry and inconsistencies within the data, especially in that tumor control rates did not increase with increasing dose. To determine the generalizability of such findings, more in vivo work is needed, using larger numbers of animals and a variety of prostate tumor types.

Theoretical arguments

Based on the biologic effective dose (BED) formula, Ling calculated that Pd-103 would be more effective against faster-growing tumors—those with a shorter doubling time (**Figure 3-5**).(LING 92) While interesting and potentially valuable work, its applicability to the clinical setting is questionable due to its purelly theoretical nature. For instance, Ling calculated that a tumor doubling time of less than 10 days is a criterion for better tumor control with Pd-103. In fact, probably all prostate cancers have doubling times far in excess of 10 days.

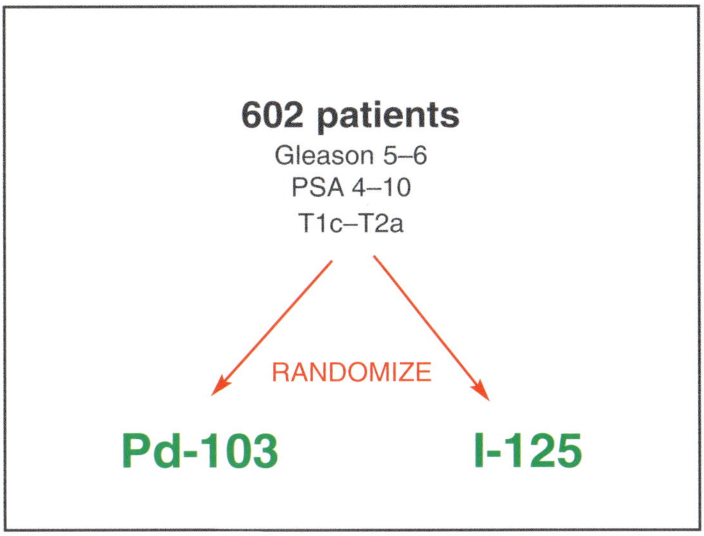

Figure 3-6. Design of randomized trial between I-125 and Pd-103 for early stage, low-risk cancers. The study has finished accrual of all 602 patients as of July 2005. (WALLNER)

Even more disturbing than the disconnect with actual tumor doubling times, the core equation used by Ling to calculate the surviving fraction with various isotopes includes five variables of which virtually nothing is known for prostate cancer in humans (**Figure 3-5**). Although the variables would presumably be equivalent for different patients and should essentially "cancel out" in the comparisons between isotopes, use of equations with so little basis in reality should raise skepticism about their clinical relevance. This work is of theoretical importance and a good starting point for planning in vitro and in vivo experiments. Basing clinical decisions on it, however, pushes against the limits of logical thinking.

I-125 versus Pd-103: Tpot

Potential tumor doubling time (Tpot) is a balance between cell proliferation rate and cell-loss rates. If the proliferation rate increases, or the loss rate decreases, Tpot decreases and tumors grow faster. Tpot can be estimated by the ratio of DNA synthetic phase (S-phase) and the labeling index.(BEGG)

Tpot variability could substantially affect time-related radiation effects. It has been argued that tumors with a more rapid proliferation rate, or shorter Tpot, should be treated with a shorter acting isotope to allow less time for cell repopulation during the radiation interval.(LING 92)

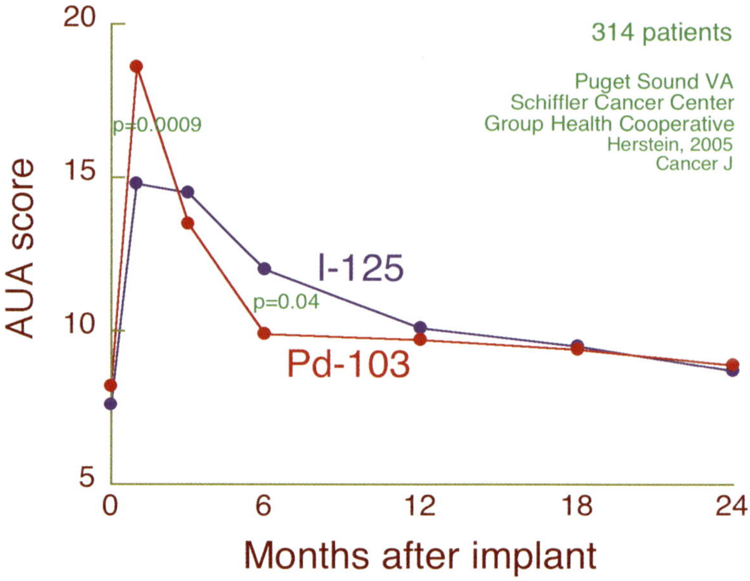

Figure 3-7. Mean AUA scores are higher in the first few weeks after Pd-103, but return toward baseline sooner with Pd-103 compared to than after I-125.

Unfortunately, determination of tumor doubling times is still in its infancy. Results with human tumors in general have been mixed.(BOURHIS) Using an antibromodeoxyuridine monoclonal antibody, the percentage of S-phase cells has been correlated with Gleason score.(NEMOTO) Using bromodeoxuridine administered prior to needle biopsy, Scrivner and colleagues showed that the labeling index correlated with Gleason score.(SCRIVNER) In contrast, Haustermans and colleagues found no correlation between Tpot and Gleason score.(HAUSTERMANS)

It is possible that such indexes of tumor growth rates could be used to guide isotope choice. Use of such tests, however, is clouded by tumor heterogeneity, by which different parts of a tumor have different S-phase fractions, just as there is heterogeneity of the Gleason score within a tumor. No clinical reports regarding Tpot and radiation response in human prostate cancer are available.

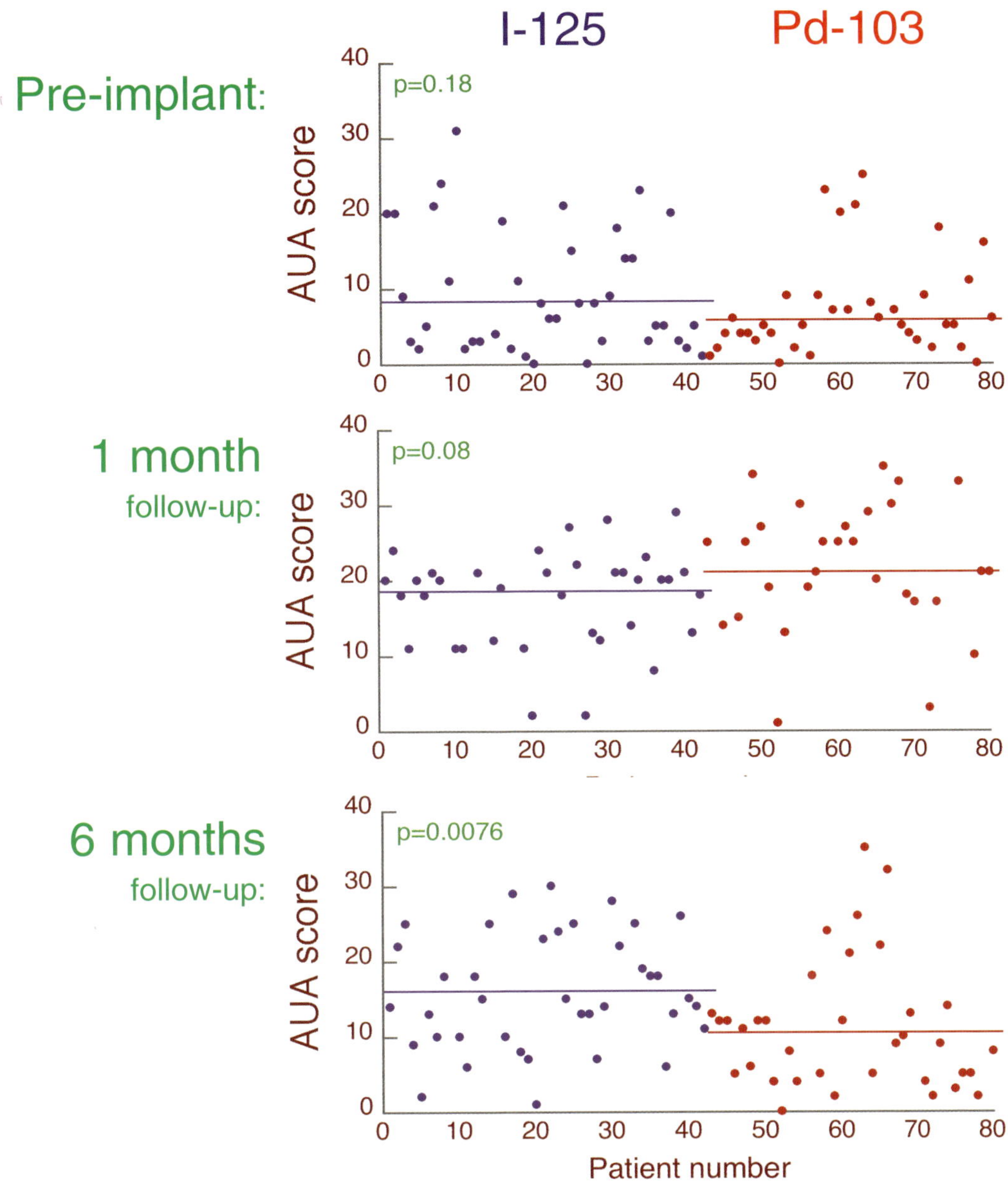

Figure 3-8. Data points for individual patients at the pre-implant, one and six month time points. Although the differences between isotopes are statistically different, note the large amount of scatter in the data.

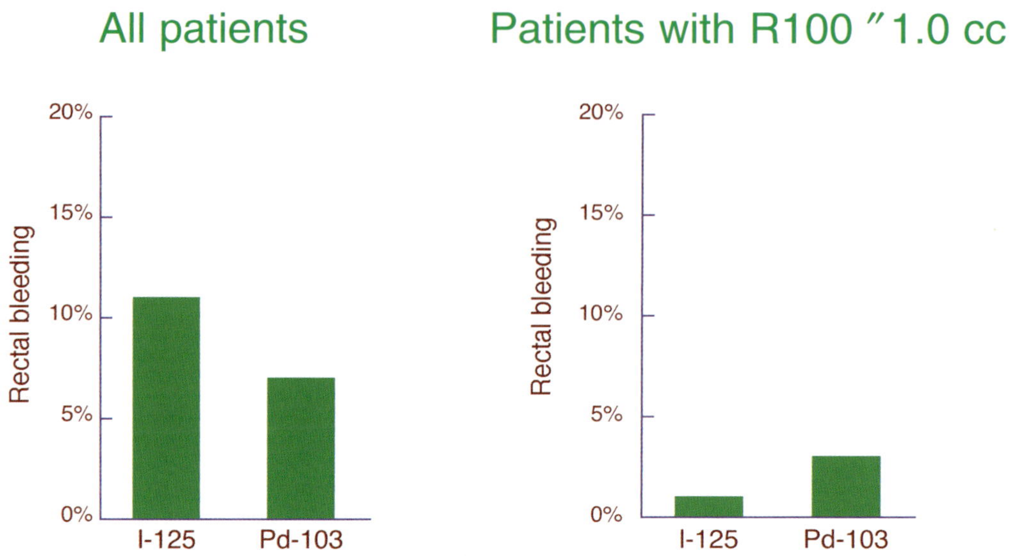

Figure 3-9. When all patients were considered, rectal bleeding was more common with I-125 (left panel). However, when analysis was limited to the 163 patients with R100 <1.0 cc, there was no statistically significant relationship between isotope and proctitis (right panel). This argues in favor of dose volume outweighing dose rate as the factor repsonible for differences in proctitis between I-125 and Pd-103.

I-125 versus Pd-103: Clinical
To date, retrospective studies have failed to show a clear difference in morbidity or tumor-control rates for low-risk patients.(CHA, GELBLUM, PESCHEL) In one retrospective study, Yale investigators showed a lower complication rate with Pd-103, but the Pd-103 patients were treated in the later time periods, such that any decrease in complications may have been due simply to better implantation technique, rather than a true difference in biology.(PESCHEL, REF) No rectal dosimetry was reported.

Because of patient-selection criteria related to preconceived notions regarding isotope choice, retrospective studies are unlikely to definitively answer questions regarding the effect of isotope choice on cure rates and morbidity. In a prospective randomized study led by Wallner and Merrick, 602 low-risk patients were randomized to I-125 versus Pd-103 (**Figure 3-**

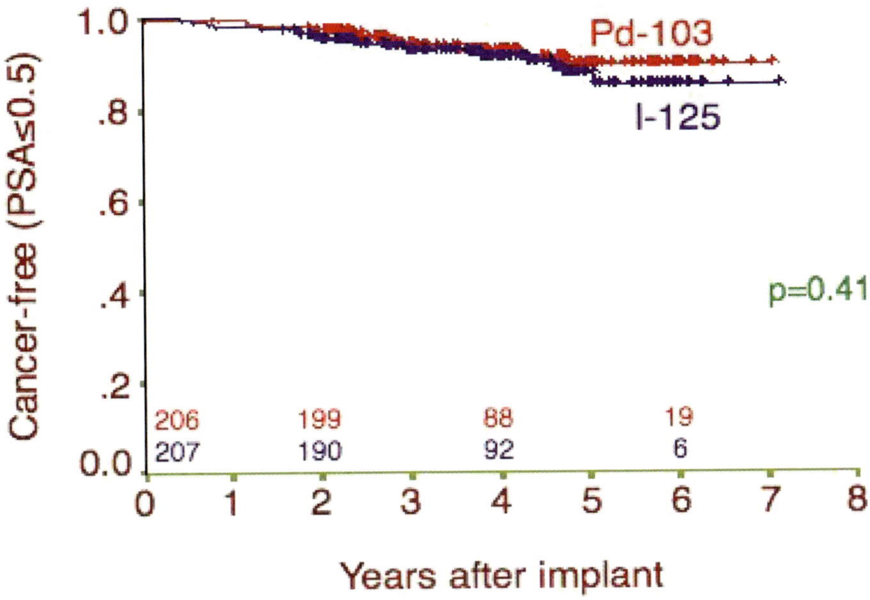

Figure 3-10. Preliminary analysis of biochemical control for I-125 versus Pd-103 in all eligible patients with minimum two years follow-up.

6). Quicker resolution of radiation-related symptoms was seen in the Pd-103 patient, but with substantial scatter in the data (**Figures 3-7 and 3-8**).

Late rectal complications were more common in I-125 patients overall, but Herstein and colleagues showed that the likelihood of grade 2 proctitis (persistent bleeding) was dependent on the rectal volume receiving 100% of the prescription dose, and independent of isotope when controlled for R100 (**Figure 3-9**)(HERSTEIN) With regard to minimizing rectal morbidity, it appears that proper source placement is more important than a difference in dose rate. Preliminary tumor control rates show similar overall biochemical control between isotopes (**Figure 3-10 through 3-12**).(WALLNER)

In addition to the 602 low risk patients randomized to I-125 versus Pd-103, Wallner, Merrrick and colleagues have randomized 600 higher risk patients to full dose I-125 versus Pd-103 monotherapy (**Figure 3-13**). Clinical outcomes should be available by 2009.

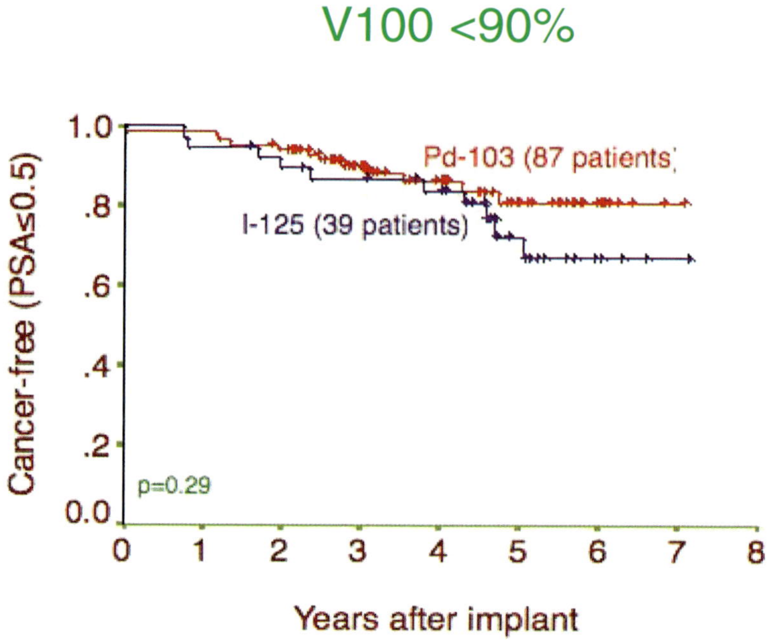

Figure 3-11. Preliminary analysis of biochemical control for I-125 versus Pd-103 in patients with a V100 less than 90%.

DO WE NEED A RADIATION SENSITIZER?
Much effort has been expended to develop chemical radiation sensitizers (enhancers), but without success. In fact, radiation sensitizers may be of limited value for prostate cancer, given the high negative biopsy rates after brachytherapy.(PRESTIDGE) It appears that local control can be achieved in most cases. The remaining impediment to increased cure rates will be the presence of micrometastases at the time of diagnosis. Better systemic cytotoxic agents would likely be more helpful than a radiation sensitizer.

HUMAN TUMORS—THE GREAT UNKNOWN
Almost nothing is known about radiobiology of brachytherapy against prostate human tumors specifically. Existing in vivo and in vitro work has been done primarily with rodent-derived cell lines, with questionable applicability to human prostate cancers. Work with more closely related tumor models might offer some insight as to how best to use the isotopes available, and perhaps how best to combine them with beam radiation. It is an opportunity for the radiation oncology community to revive classic radiobi-

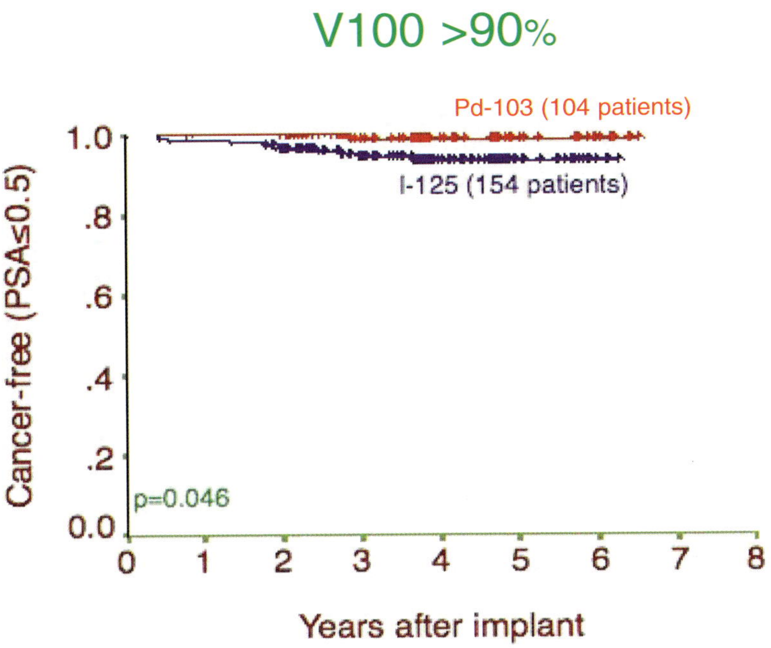

Figure 3-12. Preliminary analysis of biochemical control for I-125 versus Pd-103 in patients with a V100 greater than 90%. The trend toward better Pd-103 outcomes could represent a statistical artifact, since it is a subgroup analysis of a prospective randomized trial.

ology, an area that has been hard hit by cynicism and budgetary constraints.

REFERENCES

1. Algan O, Fosmire H, Hynynen K, et al. External beam radiotherapy and hyperthermia in the treatment of patients with locally advanced prostate carcinoma: Results of long term follow-up. Cancer 2000; 89:399-403.

2. Algan O, Stobbe CC, Helt AM, Hanks GE. Radiation inactivation of human prostate cancer cells: the role of apoptosis. Radiat Res 1996; 146:267-275.

3. Begg AC, McNally NJ. A method to measure the duration of DNA synthesis and the potential doubling time from a single sample. Cytometry 1997; 6:620-623.

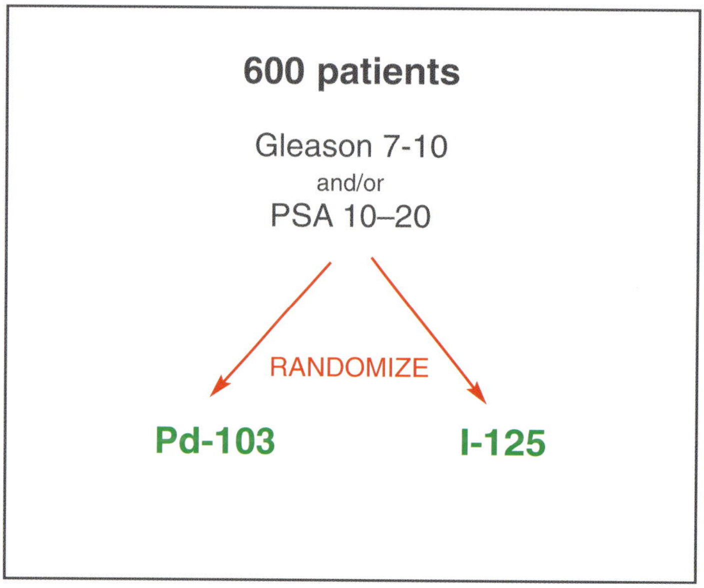

Figure 3-13. Design of a randomized trial comparing I-125 and Pd-103 for early stage, intermediate-risk cancers. The study was opened in 2003 and will have accrued all 600 patients by 2007.

4. BenHur E, Elkind MM, Bronk BV. Thermally enhanced radioresponse of cultured Chinese hamster cells: inhibition of repair of sublethal damage and enhancement of lethal damage. Radiat Res 1974; 58:38-51.
5. Bourhis J, Dendale R, Hill C, Bosq J. Potential doubling time and clinical outcome in head and neck squamous cell carcinoma treated with 70 Gy in 7 weeks. Int J Radiat Oncol Biol Phys 1996; 35:471-476.
6. Brenner D. Hypofractionation for prostate cancer radiotherapy—What are the issues? Int J Rad Oncol Biol Phys 2003; 57:912-914.
7. Cha CM, Potters L, Ashley R, al e. Isotope selection for patients undergoing prostate brachytherapy. Int J Rad Oncol Biol Phys 1999; 45:391-395.
8. Fowler J, Tome W, Fenwick J, Mehta M. A challenge to tradional radiation oncology. Int J Rad Oncol Biol Phys 2004; 60:1241-1256.
9. Gelblum DY, Potters L, Ashley R, Waldbaum R, Wang X, Leibel S. Urinary morbidity following ultrasound-guided transperineal prostate seed implantation. Int J Rad Oncol Biol Phys 1999; 45:59-67.
10. Hall EJ. Radiobiology for the radiologist. Philadelphia: J. B. Lippincott, 1994.
11. Hall EJ, Roizin-Towle LA, Colvett RD. RBE and OER determinations for Radium and Californium-252. Radiol 1974; 112:425-430.
12. Han B, Wallner K, Aggarwal S, Armstrong J, Sutlief S. Treatment margins for prostate brachytherapy. Seminars in Urol Oncol 2000; 18:137-141.

13. Haustermans KMG, Hofland I, Van Poppel H, al e. Cell kinetic measurements in prostate cancer. Int J Rad Oncol Biol Phys 1997; 37:1067-1070.
14. Herstein A, Wallner K, Merrick G, et al. I-125 versus Pd-103 for low-risk prostate cancer: Long-term morbidity outcomes from a prospective randomized multicenter controlled trial. Cancer J 2005; 11:385-389.
15. Jackson A, Skwarchuk MW, Zelefsky MJ, Cowen DM, al e. Late rectal bleeding after conformal radiotherapy of prostate cancer (II): Volume effects and dose-volume histograms. Int J Rad Oncol Biol Phys 2001; 49:685-698.
16. Kupelian P, Potters L, Khuntia D, et al. Radical prostatectomy, external beam radiotherapy <72 Gy, external beam radiotherapy ≥72 Gy, permenent seed implantation, or combined seeds/external beam radiotherapy for stage T1-T2 prostate cancer. Int J Rad Oncol Biol Phys 2004; 58:25-33.
17. Kupelian P, Reddy C, Carlson T, Willoughby T. Dose/volume relationship of late rectal bleeding after external beam radiotherapy for localized prostate cancer: absolute or relative rectal volume? Cancer J 2002; 8:62-66.
18. Lee WR, Hanks GE, Hanlon AL, Schultheiss TE, Hunt MA. Lateral rectal shielding reduces late rectal morbidity following high dose three-dimensional conformal radiation therapy for clinically localized prostate cancer: further evidence for a significant dose effect. Int J Rad Oncol Biol Phys 1996; 35:251-257.
19. Ling CC. Permanent implants using Au-198, Pd-103 and I-125: radiobiological considerations based on the linear quadratic model. Int J Radiat Oncol Biol Phys 1992; 23:81-87.
20. Ling CC, Li WX, Anderson LL. The relative biological effectiveness of I-125 and Pd-103. Int J Radiat Oncol Biol Phys 1995; 32:373-378.
21. Ling CC, Spiro IJ, Mitchell J, Stickler R. The variation of OER with dose rate. Int J Radiat Oncol Biol Phys 1985; 11:1367-1373.
22. McDonnell TJ, Troncoso P, Brisbay SM, Logothetis C. Expression of the protooncogene bel-2 in the prostate and its association with emergence of androgen-independent prostate cancer. Ca Res 1992; 52:6940-6944.
23. Movsas B, Chapman JD, Greenberg RE, Hanlon AL, al e. Increasing levels of hypoxia in prostate carcinoma correlate significantly with increasing clinical stage and patient age: an Eppendorf pO2 study. Cancer 2000; 89:2018-2024.

24. Movsas B, Chapman JD, Horwitz EM, al e. Hypoxic regions exist in human prostate carcinoma. Urol 1999; 53:11-18.
25. Mueller A, Wallner K, Merrick G, Cavanagh W, Butler W. Peri-rectal seeds as a risk factor for prostate brachytherapy-related rectal bleeding. Int J Rad Oncol Biol Phys 2004; 59:1047-1052.
26. Nag S, Sweeney PJ, Wienthjes MG. Dose-response study of Iodine-125 and Palladium-103 brachytherapy in a rat prostate tumor (Nb-Al-1). Endocur/Hypertherm 1997; 9:97-104.
27. Nemoto R, Uchida K, Shiimazui T, Hattori K. Immunocytochemical demonstration of S phase cells by anti-bromodeoyuridine monoclonal antibody in humna prostate adenocarcinoma. J Urol 1989; 141:337-340.
28. Orton CG, Webber BM. Time-dose factor (TDF) analysis of dose rate effects in permanent implant dosimetry. Int J Radiat Oncol Biol Phys 1977; 2:55-60.
29. Paulus JA, Tucker RD, Loening SA, Flanagan SW. Thermal ablation of canine prostate using interstitial temperature self-regulating seeds: New treatment for prostate cancer. J Endourol 1997; 11:295-300.
30. Peschel RE, Colberg JW, Chen Z, Nath R, Wilson LD. Iodine 125 versus palladium 103 implants for prostate cancer: Clinical outcomes and complications. Cancer J 2004; 10:170-174.
31. Pollack A, Ashoori F, Sikes C, al e. The early supra-additive apoptotic response of R3327-G prostate tumors to androgen ablation and radiation is not sustained with multiple fractions. Int J Rad Oncol Biol Phys 2000; 46:153-158.
32. Prestidge BR, Hoak DC, Grimm PD, Ragde H, Cavanagh W, Blasko JC. Posttreatment biopsy results following interstitial brachytherapy in early-stage prostate cancer. Int J Radiat Oncol Biol Phys 1997; 37:31-39.
33. Prionas SD, Kapp DS, Goffinet DR, Ben-Yosef R. Thermometry of interstitial hyperthermia given as an adjuvant to brachytherapy for the treatment of carcinoma of the prostate. Int J Radiat Oncol Biol Phys 1993; 28:151-162.
34. Rasey JS, Koh W-J, Evans ML, al e. Quantifying regional hypoxia in human tumors with positron emission tomography of fluoromisonidazole. Int J Rad Oncol Biol Phys 1996; 36:417-428.
35. Scrivner DL, Meyer JS, Rujanavech N, Fathman A. Cell kinetics by bromodeoxyuridine labeling and deoxyribonucleic acid ploidy in prostatic carcinoma needle biopsies. J Urol 1991; 146:1034-1039.
36. Wallner K, Merrick G, True L, Cavanagh W, Simpson C, Butler W. I-125 versus Pd-103 for low risk prostate cancer: Morbidity outcomes from a prospective randomized multicenter trial. Ca J Sci American 2002; 8:67-73.

37. Wallner K, Merrick G, True L, Sutlief S, Cavanagh W, Butler W. I-125 versus Pd-103 for low risk prostate cancer: Preliminary biochemical outcomes from a prospective randomized mulitcenter trial. Int J Rad Oncol Biol Phys 2003; 57:1297-1303.
38. Wang JZ, Guerrero M, Li A. How low is the alpha/beta ratio for prostate cancer? Int J Rad Oncol Biol Phys 2003; 55:194-203.

4

Prostate anatomy

The prostate is a glandular structure situated between the bladder base and the pelvic floor (**Figure 4-1**). It is roughly the shape of an inverted cone, or upright strawberry.

The prostate is considered to have five zones: peri-urethral, peripheral, transitional, central and anterior fibromuscular stroma (**Figure 4-2**). These zones have little significance in planning or executing brachytherapy, because cancer can arise and spread throughout the glandular portions of prostate.

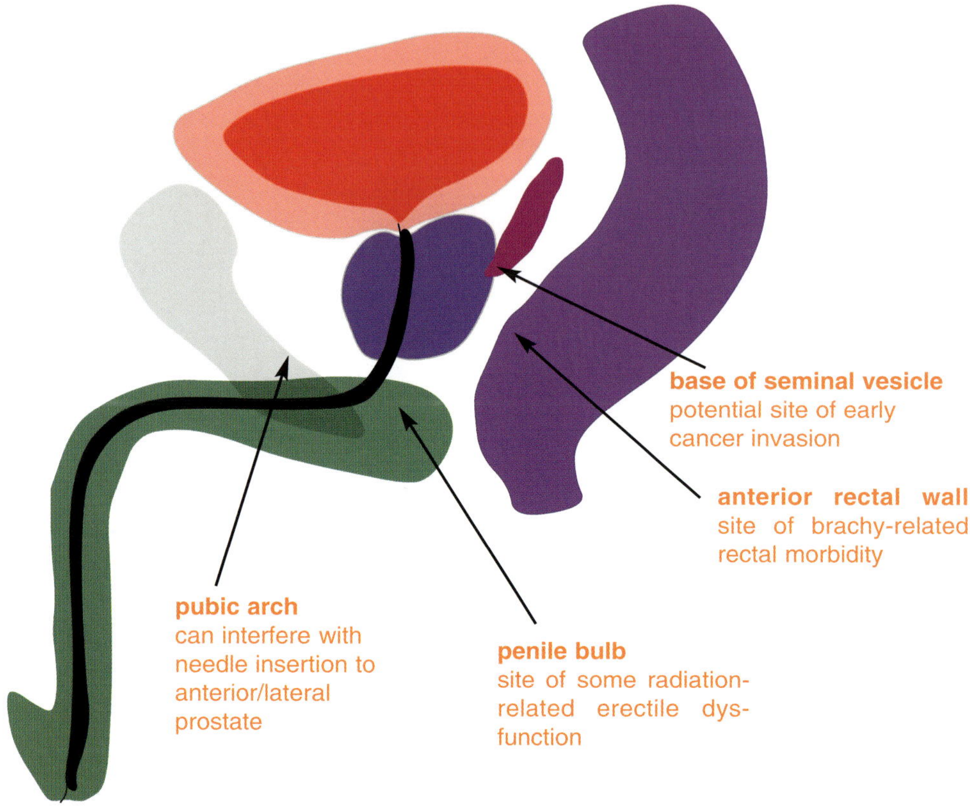

Figure 4-1. Lateral view of key structures to be considered in brachytherapy treatment planning.

In a normal, unenlarged prostate, the peripheral, transition and central zones make up approximately 70%, 5% and 25% of the prostate, respectively. However, the transition zone, as the principle site of benign prostatic enlargement, often composes a much higher percentage of the prostate volume in older men (**Figure 4-3**). The various glandular zonal tissues appear to have a similar predisposition to cancer formation, so that the percent of cancers arising in each zone mirrors the tissue mass of each (**Figure 4.4**).

Demarcation of the prostate zones is typically obscured on TRUS imaging (**Figure 4.5**). Typically, the best demarcation is the interface between the peripheral zone and enlarged transition zone often visible in patients with

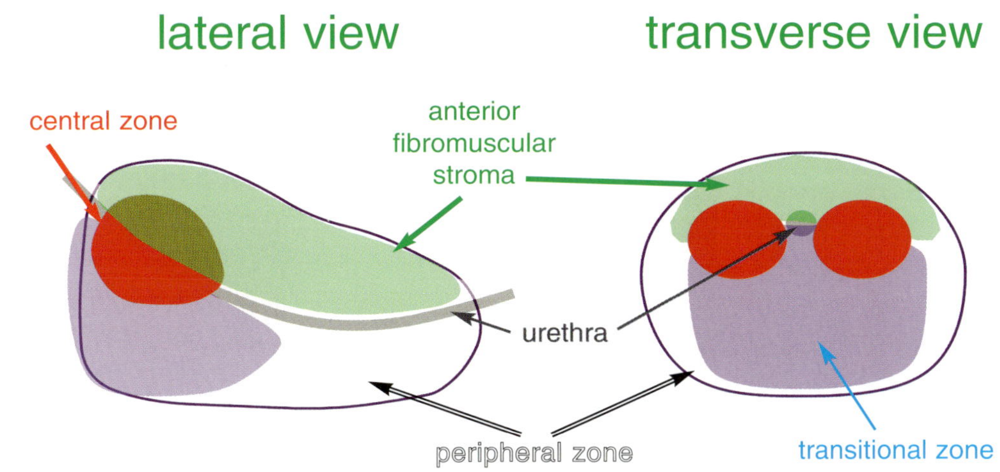

Figure 4-2. Diagrammatic lateral and cross-sectional views of normal prostate.

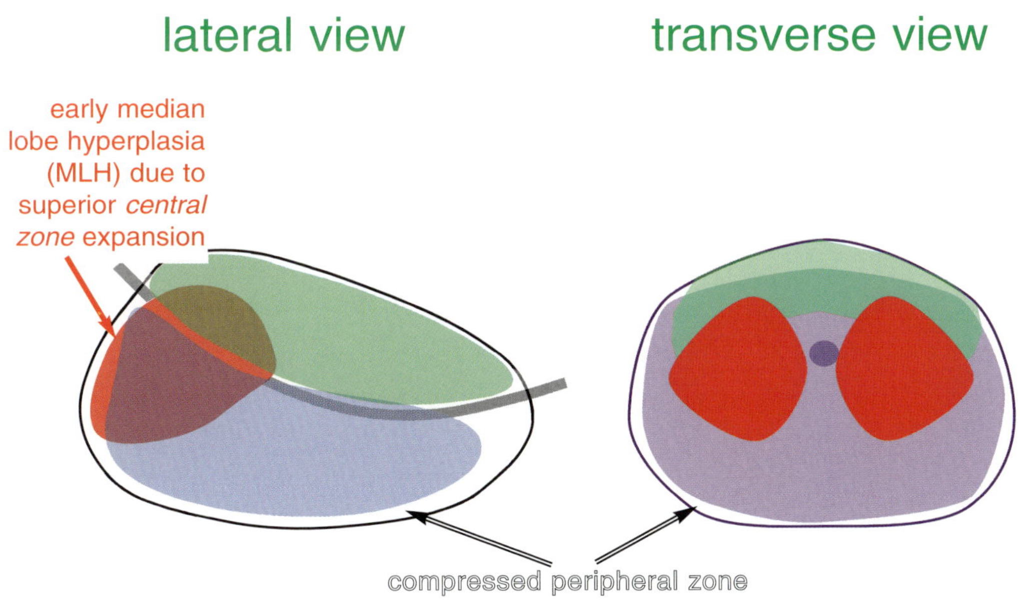

Figure 4-3. Diagrammatic lateral and cross-sectional views of prostate with substantial BPH.

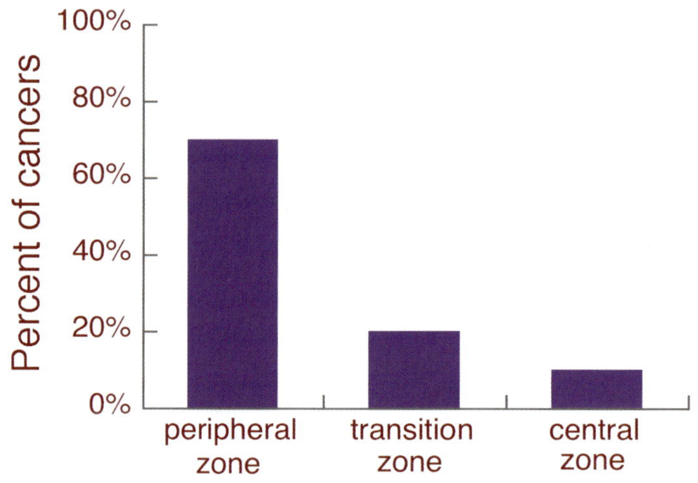

Figure 4-4. Glandular zones as sites of cancer origin.

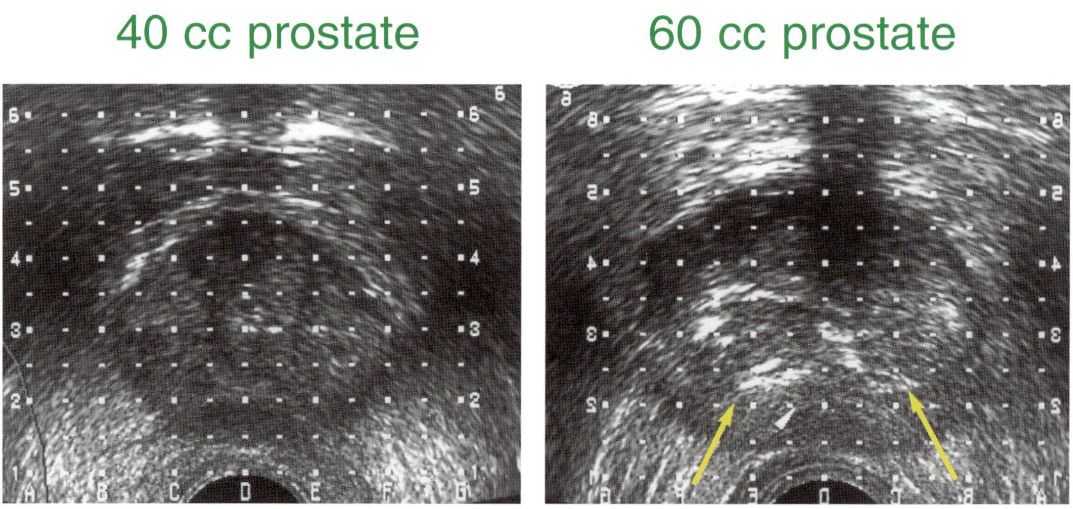

Figure 4-5. TRUS cross-sectional views of normal prostate versus one with substantial BPH. In smaller glands, the peripheral zone is not typically well visualized. With substantial BPH, the peripheral zone is more easily distinguishable from the the expanded transitional zone (yellow arrows).

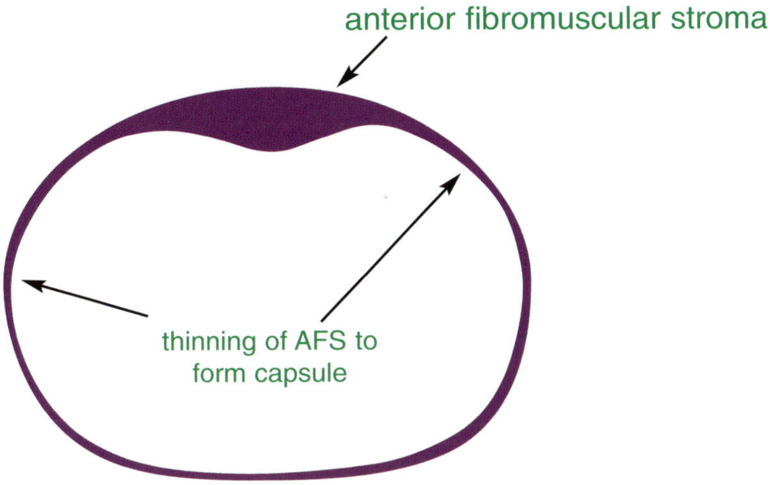

Figure 4-6. Schematic transverse view of prostatic capsule.

BPH (**Figure 4-5**). The transition zone is usually easier to delineate with realtime imaging than on the static images seen in Figure 4-5.

The anterior fibromuscular stroma, approximately 5-10 mm thick anteriorly, extends laterally and posteriorly to form a paper thin capsule around the prostate (**Figure 4-6**). It seems to act as a partial barrier to cancer spread.

TRUS ANATOMY
Ultrasound images do not reliably detect cancerous regions within the prostate, but they are remarkably effective at showing the sites of interest for brachytherapy treatment planning. The seminal vesicles, peripheral prostatic margins, and prostatic apex are easily visible (**Figures 4-7 and 4-8**). The anterior fibromuscular stroma is usually not well demarcated from the glandular tissue, and typically is included in the planning volume.

CANCER LOCATION WITHIN THE PROSTATE
Before the PSA era, most clinically detected prostate cancer occurred posteriorly, where they could be palpated. Their posterior location, however, reflected their accessibility to palpation, not that cancers preferentially arose posteriorly. McNeal showed that non-palpable, incidental cancers

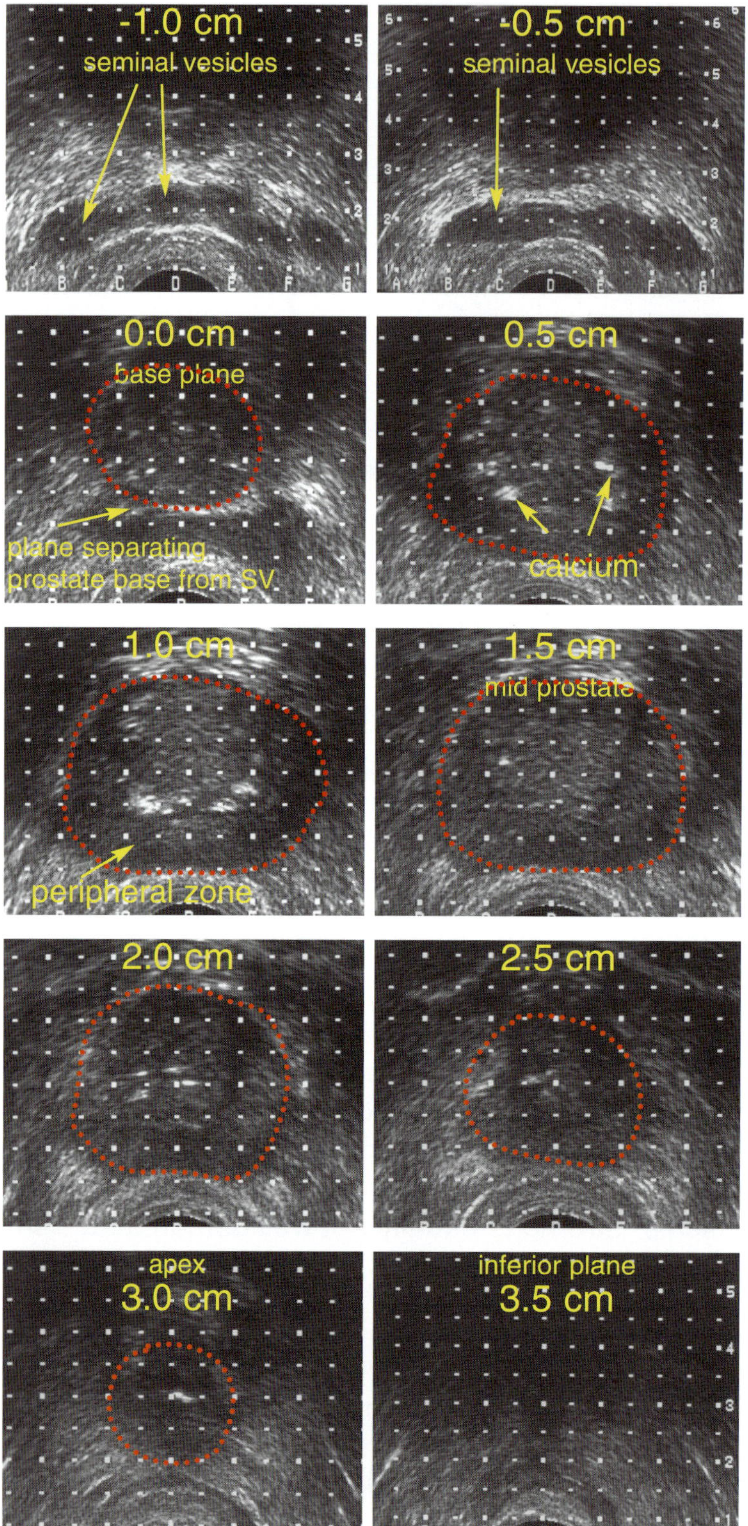

Figure 4-7. TRUS cross-sectional views of a typical 40 cc prostate. The centimeter values represent the distance from the base of the prostate.

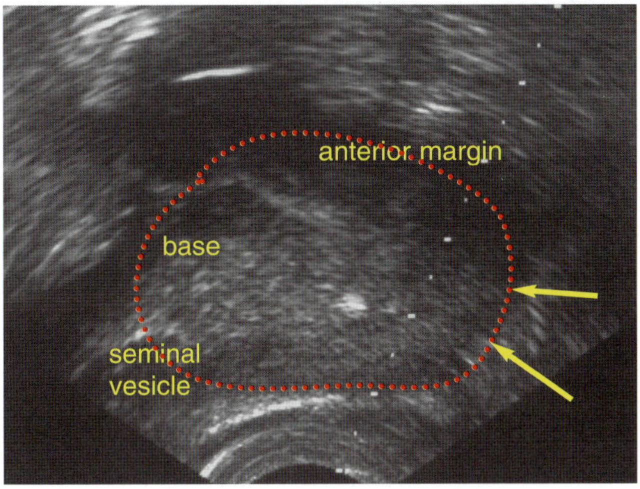

Figure 4-8. Sagittal TRUS view, with better visualization of prostatic apex (yellow arrows) than can be obtained with transverse images alone.

occur evenly throughout the prostate, irrespective of zonal glandular anatomy (**Figure 4-9**). There have been isolated reports advocating preferential treatment of one portion over another. While these concepts may have a place in treatment planning in the future, saturation biopsy studies universally show more diffuse cancer involvement than previously recog-

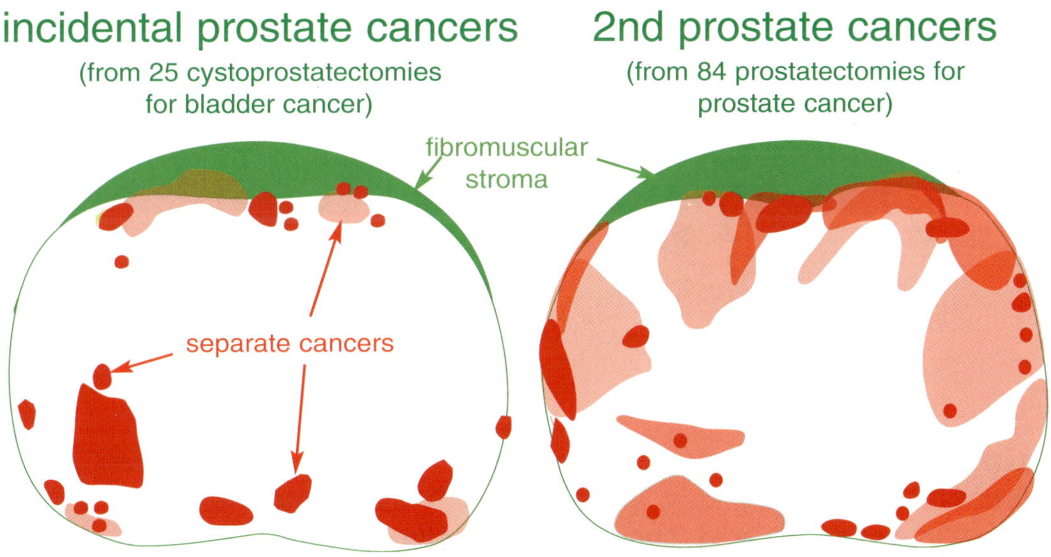

Figure 4-9. 25 incidental and 38 second adenocarcinomas seen in cystoprostatectomy or prostatectomy specimens, respectively. The different cancers are shown in various shades of red for clarity.(MCNEAL)

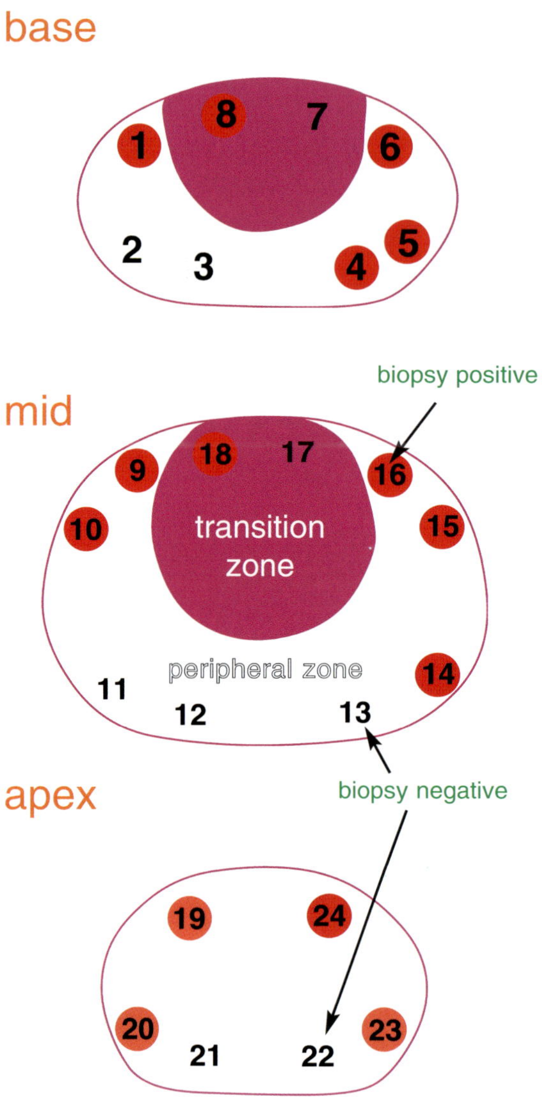

Figure 4-10. Example of anterior cancer detection in a 55 year-old patient with saturation biopsies by G. Merrick after three negative conventional biopsy sets. The saturation biopsies included two cores at each numbered site, yielding a total of 48 cores. This patient's PSA was 13.7 ng/ml at the time of saturation biopsy. Of the 48 total cores, 21 showed cancer(Gleason 7 and 8), primarily from the anterior portion of the gland.

nized (**Figure 4-10**).(MERRICK 07, STEWART) Considering the limitations of current imaging technology, all regions of the prostate are at risk of cancerous involvement and should be included in the treatment volume. (DEMURA)

Some investigators have advocated dropping the anterior base from the intended treatment region or targeting preferentially areas of involvement detected by radioimmunoguidance.(D'AMICO, ELLIS) These concepts are not in keeping with the classical works of McNeal and colleagues. Until there is a completely reliable method to image microscopic disease within the prostate, the margin of the *entire* prostate should dictate the region which should receive a cancercidal radiation dose.

REFERENCES

1. D'Amico AV, Davis A, Vargas SO, Renshaw AA, Jiroutek M, Richie JP. Defining the implant treatment volume for patients with low risk prostate cancer: does the anterior base need to be treated? Int J Rad Oncol Biol Phys 1999; 43:587-590.
2. Demura T, Hioka T, Furuno T, et al. Differences in tumor core distribution between palpable and nonpalpable prostate tumors in patients diagnosed using extensive transperineal ultrasound-guided template prostate biopsy. Cancer 2005; 103:1826-1832.
3. Ellis RJ, Zhou H, Kim E, et al. Biochemical disease-free survival rates following definitive low-dose-rate prostate brachytherapy with dose escalation to biologic target volume identified with SPECT/CT capromab pendetide. Brachytherapy 2007; 6:16-25.
4. McNeal JE, Price HM, Redwine EA, Freiha FS, Stamey TA. Stage A Versus Stage B Adenocarcinoma of the Prostate: Morphological Comparison and Biological Significance. J Urol 1988; 139:61-65.
5. Merrick G, Gutman s, Andreini H, et al. Prostate cancer distribution in patients diagnosed by transperineal template-guided saturation biopsy. submitted 2007.
6. Rifkin MD, Zerhouni EA, Gatsonis CA, Quint LE. Comparison of magnetic resonance imaging and ultrasonography in staging early prostate cancer. NEJM 1990; 323:621-626.
7. Stewart C, Leibovich B, Weaver A, Lieber M. Prostate cnacer diagnosis using a saturation needle biopsy technique after previous negative sextant biopsies. J Urol 2001; 166:86-92.
8. Villeirs G, Verstraete K, De Neve W, Meerleer G. Magnetic resonance imaging anatomy of the prostate and periprostatic area: a guide for radiotherapists. Radiother and Oncol 2005; 76:99-106.

5

TRUS, CT, or MR?

The introduction of transrectal ultrasound (TRUS) was the primary technological breakthrough behind the resurgence of prostate brachytherapy. TRUS made it possible to image the prostate for treatment planning and to monitor needle position during the implant procedure. Computerized tomography (CT) played a supporting role in the resurgence of prostate brachytherapy, being the basis for post-implant dosimetry (quality assurance).

Pre-implant or post-implant prostate contours, used to determine the number and arrangement of seeds, can be derived from TRUS, CT, or MR

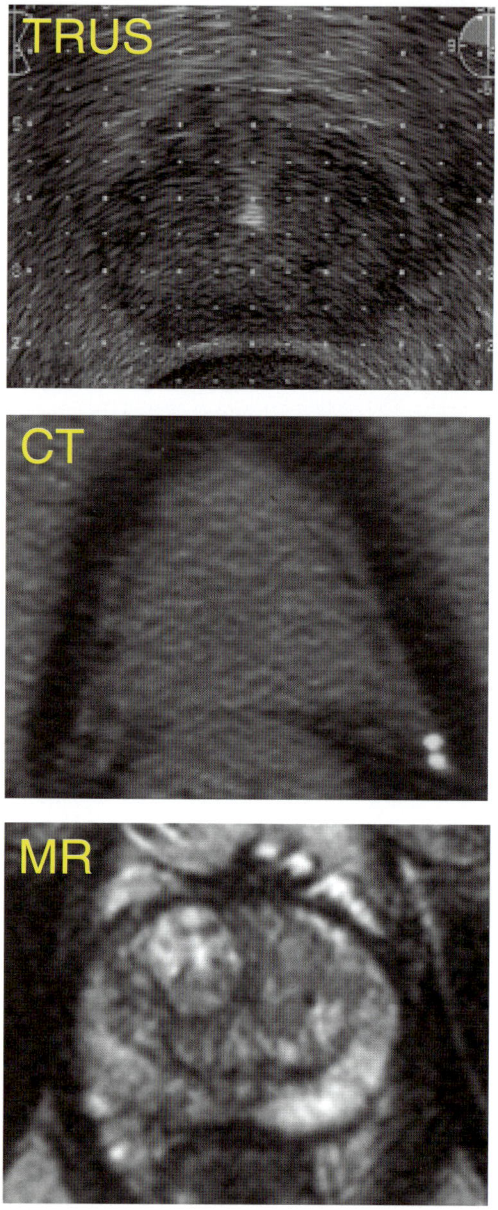

Figure 5-1. Cross section at mid prostate, viewed by TRUS, CT, and MR. TRUS usually gives the sharpest image of the prostate contour, while MR gives a better image of internal architecture. CT typically gives the least sharp image of internal architecture and outer contour but shows the spatial relationship between the prostate gland, pubic bones, and rectum.

images. Each modality has its advantages and disadvantages. Currently, nearly all brachytherapists use TRUS for planning and intra-operative visualization. However, there is some interest in substituting MR or CT for TRUS.(HURWITZ, ZAIDER, PICKETT)

The appearance of the prostate and the peri-prostatic region varies markedly between imaging techniques (**Figure 5-1**). But despite their qualitative differences, the prostate shape and size are fairly consistent between modalities, if interpreted correctly. Until we have a reliable way to image microscopic disease within the prostate, it is the prostatic *margins* that determine how many and in what arrangement the seeds should be placed.

Past reports of inconsistent prostate volume determinations with different imaging techniques were more likely due to image misinterpretation than to problems with the modalities per se. Unfortunately, interpretation pitfalls have led to a contradictory body of literature and a persistent, smoldering controversy regarding the best imaging modality. A chapter dedicated to this controversy seems warranted.

TRUS

Quick and easy real-time imaging is the most compelling aspect of TRUS, allowing visualization of needles within the prostate during the procedure. Whether you're doing pre- or intra-operative planning (see chapter 6), the volume defined by the prostate contour is the primary determinant of the radioactivity needed and how it is placed. The sharp contour of TRUS images minimizes inter-observer inconsistencies. In particular, the posterior prostate contour is sharply delineated, helping to optimize rectal doses.

Although real-time TRUS images show a fairly sharp prostatic margin, the images may underestimate the true prostatic size. Several conflicting reports describe the relation between TRUS-based volumes and those determined from prostatectomy specimens. Rahmouni and colleagues, from Johns Hopkins University (JHU), compared pre-operative TRUS and MR prostate volumes with the volumes of the resected glands.(RAHMOUNI) In their hands, the TRUS volume was only 70 percent of that measured at the time of prostatectomy (**Figure 5-2**).

The JHU investigators' finding that TRUS grossly underestimates the prostate volume might be criticized on the grounds that the prostatic volumes were calculated by the elliptical volume formula (.525 x D1 x D2 x D3 [where D1–D3 are the prostatic orthogonal dimensions]) rather than step-section planimetry. Stone and colleagues reported that prostate volumes are generally smaller with step-section planimetry than with an elliptical volume approximation. However, other investigators have reported that prostate volumes are similar, on average, when determined by step-section planimetry or elliptical volume estimation.(TERRIS)

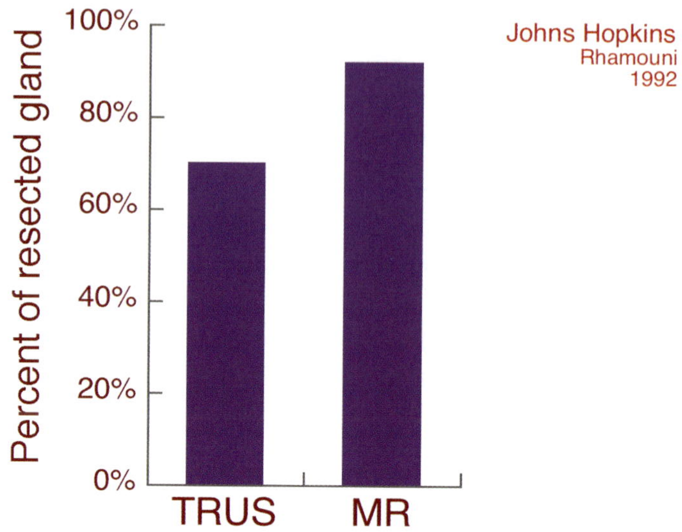

Figure 5-2. Prostate volume measured from prostatectomy specimens versus pre-op TRUS or MR.(RAHMOUNI)

Other investigators have found less discrepancy between TRUS volume and the volume of the resected prostate.(BARTSCH) Differences among investigators might be explained by disparity in how TRUS images are interpreted, formulas used to approximate the volume, equipment differences, or how the surgical specimens are processed.

The biggest disadvantage of TRUS is the potential for inter- and intra-observer variability. Average differences of 5% to 25% have been reported when patients are re-scanned by the same ultrasonographer on the same day.(BATES, BAZINET) For scans performed in succession by two different observers, a variability of about 10% has been reported.(BATES) The lack of reproducibility is not explained by image interpretation alone, because computer-assisted interpretation does not diminish the inter- or intra-observer variability.(NATHAN) Variability in prostate volume determinations is partially explained by differences in ultrasound probe angulation, which leads to 2 to 4% changes in the volume.(NATHAN) Another potential confounding issue is that prostate volume and shape may change in fully awake versus anesthetized patients. The degree of variability may be less if planimetry, rather than dimension-estimated volumes, is used.(AARNINK)

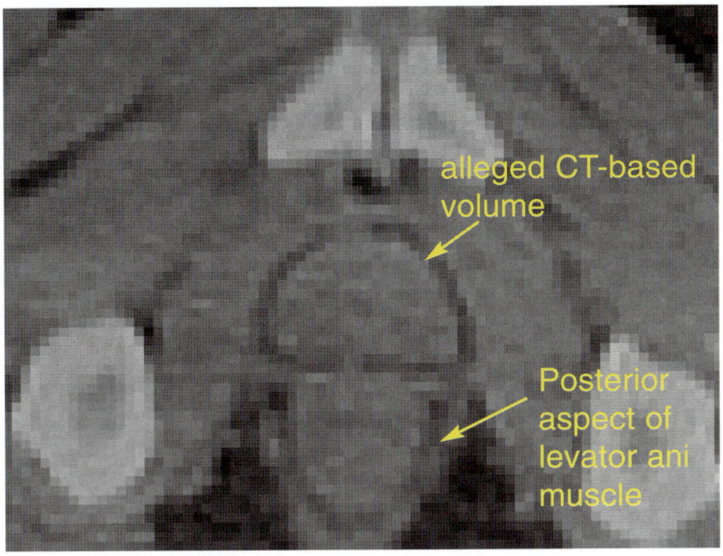

Figure 5-3. Magnification of previously published CT-based prostate margin drawn by Roach and colleagues at UCSF, comparing prostate volumes by CT versus MR.(ROACH) In this example from their publication, the levator muscles are included in the target volume, giving an artificially large CT prostate volume. Excluding non-prostatic tissue, like the levator ani, would yield a more accurate prostate volume determination. Dr. Roach agrees (personal communication).

Reproducibility problems may be partly explained by real, physiologic variations. Prostate volume, measured by TRUS or MR, has been reported to change by approximately 10% from day to day, a variation that is consistent between TRUS and MR; these are likely *real* changes in volume rather than an inconsistent TRUS technique.(AL-RIMAWI)

We have seen some surprising TRUS volume studies from various institutions, probably due to excessive probe pressure against the prostate (see chapter 6). The effect that reproducibility problems have on clinical outcomes is unknown, but it could be substantial. Falsely low prostate volumes could lead to inadequate dose coverage, and falsely high volumes could lead to complications from over-radiation of normal tissues.(NARAYANA)

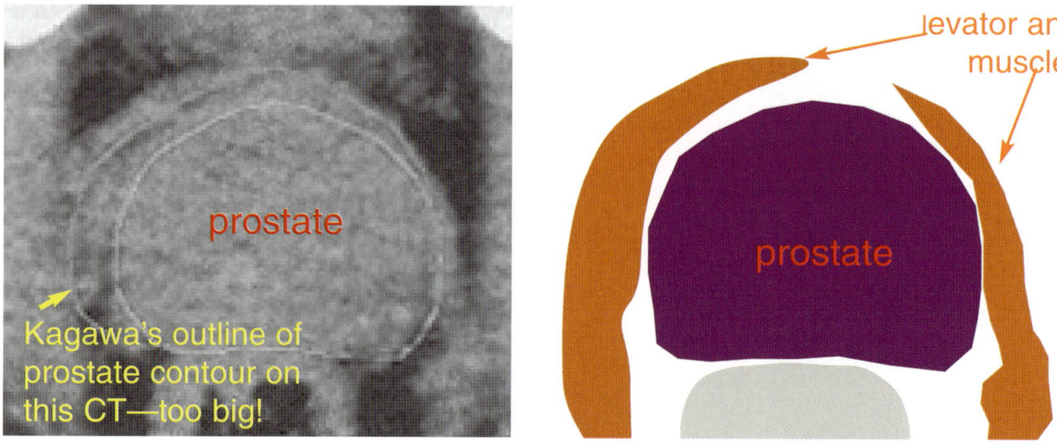

Figure 5-4. In this example of CT interpretation at Fox Chase Cancer Center, the levator ani muscle has been included with the authors' determination of the CT-based lateral prostatic margin, giving a falsely large prostate volume.(KAGAWA) The outer light line is their tracing of the prostate on the left, based on CT. The inner light line is their tracing of the prostate from MR, overlaid on the CT image. On the right is a line drawing of their published image, with K. Wallner's tracing of levator ani muscles and prostate as they appear on the Fox Chase CT image, nearly identical to the Fox Chase MR tracing!

Despite some early claims to the contrary, TRUS cannot reliably image the presence or extent of intra-prostatic cancers.(RIFKIN). Color doppler may offer a better appreciation for tumor vascular location. Its role in prostate brachytherapy has yet to be defined.

CT

The primary advantages of CT over other techniques are that CT can image seeds more clearly and delineate the pubic bones more precisely. Also, CT is far less operator-dependent than TRUS and requires minimal patient preparation.

Like TRUS, there are conflicting reports regarding the accuracy of CT prostate volume determination, with most investigators reporting that CT volumes are too large. Nonsense. Investigators who claim that CT grossly over-estimates the prostate volume are over-interpreting their CT scans.

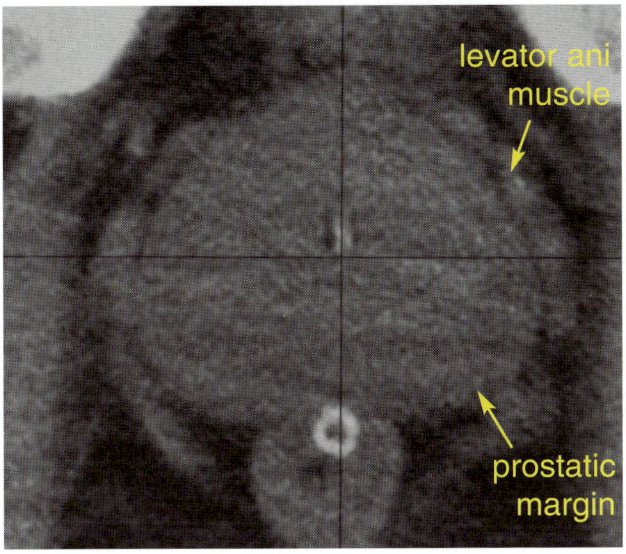

Figure 5-5. Unusually clear example of the separation between prostatic margin and levator ani musculature. This degree of clarity is not typical, but it serves to illustrate the potential to overdraw the prostatic volume if the levator ani muscles are included.

Roach and colleagues, for example, reported that CT volumes were approximately 30% larger than MR-based volumes.(ROACH) The CT volumes determined by the UCSF investigators, however, were probably excessive. Judging from the representative case shown in the Roach paper, the levator ani musculature was included within the target volume (**Figure 5-3**). Doing so would erroneously increase the prostatic volume. Similar over-estimation of the prostate contour was evident in a publication

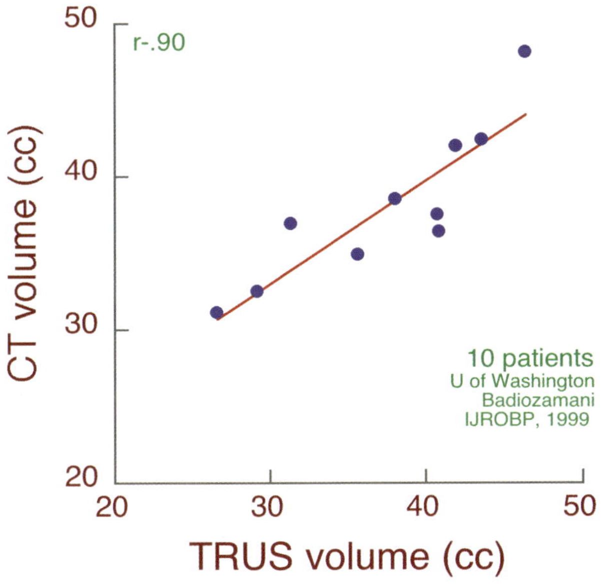

Figure 5-6. Prostate volume measured by TRUS versus CT. If the levator ani muscles are not included in the prostate volume, the volumes are almost identical. (BADIOZAMANI)

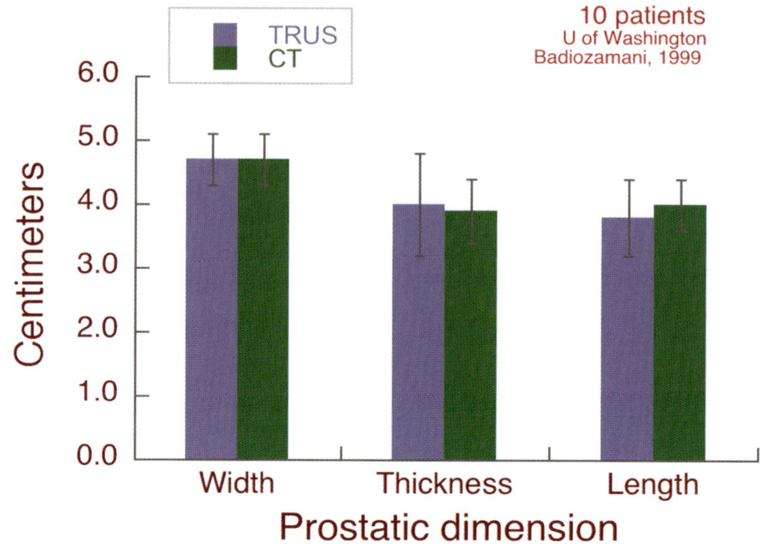

Figure 5-7. Anterior-posterior (thickness), lateral, and cranio-caudal dimensions determined by CT versus TRUS.

from Fox Chase Cancer Center (**Figure 5-4**). **Figure 5-5** shows an unusually striking example of the separation between the prostate and the levator ani musculature. More commonly, there is little or no separation, hence the risk of including the levators inappropriately in the prostate volume.

To clarify the use of CT versus TRUS for pre-planning, CT and TRUS images from ten consecutive, unselected patients from the University of Washington were analyzed by Badiozamani and colleagues.(BADIOZAMANI) Each patient underwent a pre-implant TRUS volume study and pelvic CT scan on the same day. To test for consistency between observers, the CT volumes were drawn independently by Badiozamani, Wallner, and Blasko. The CT-based volumes ranged from 31 cc to 48 cc and the TRUS-based volumes ranged from 27 cc to 46 cc. There was close agreement in the determinations between imaging modalities (**Figure 5-6**), including the anterior-posterior, lateral, and cranio-caudal prostatic dimensions (**Figure 5-7**). The measurements were consistent between observers (**Figure 5-8**). The practical significance of the University of Washington study is that CT and TRUS images can be substituted for each other in pre-implant prostate volume determinations, if the CT images are not over-interpreted.

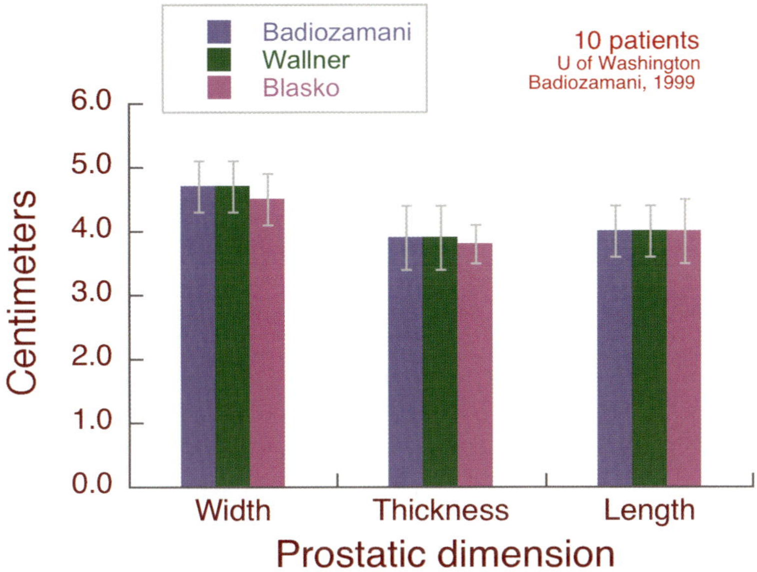

Figure 5-8. In the UW study of CT versus TRUS imaging, interpretation of prostate CT images in each dimension was consistent between the three physician authors.

The primary limitation of CT-based implants is the lack of real-time imaging. While intra-op CT scanning would offer some advantages over current TRUS-based methods, intra-op CT scanning is currently not practical due to technical costs and lack of working space in most CT facilities. Portable scanners are commercially available, but to date they have not generated much interest within the prostate brachytherapy community. With wider availability of faster scan reconstruction capability and smaller, portable scanners or CT simulators, real-time intra-operative CT scanning could catch on.

MR

MR images show a dramatically sharper prostatic margin than CT, potentially decreasing the subjectivity in image interpretation and making the planning and evaluation processes more reproducible. MR also shows the most detailed image of the internal architecture of the prostate. But while striking in its degree of detail, the clinical utility of parenchymal imaging is questionable, because nearly all of the prostate should still be treated to

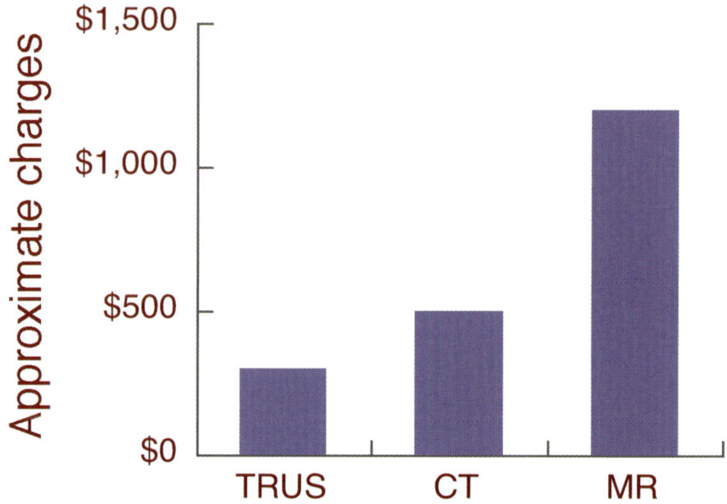

Figure 5-9. Approximate charges for diagnostic TRUS , CT, or MR.

prescription dose to sterilize areas of potential microscopic disease.(MCNEAL)

The primary disadvantage of MR, like that of CT, is that real-time MR is not readily available. However, there is some interest in developing easier access to real-time imaging, and more widespread adoption of MR techniques may occur.(HURWITZ, DUBOIS, AMDUR, MOERLAND, ZAIDER) Another disadvantage of MR, in the current clinical setting, is its price. Patient charges for a diagnostic pelvic MR are two to three times those for a TRUS or CT, extra charges that are difficult to justify in the absence of good quality data substantiating higher cure rates with MR versus TRUS-based implants (**Figure 5-9**).

NORMAL TISSUE DELINEATION

All three modalities have some advantages in normal tissue delineation. For brachytherapy, the most important structures are the prostate, rectum and penile bulb. There is strong data establishing relationships between dose to each of these structures and relevant clnical outcomes.(MERRICK 03) CT is probably best for rectal wall delineation. TRUS is not so useful for rectal dose determination, since the presence of the probe distorts the rectum into an unnatural shape (**Figure 5-10**).

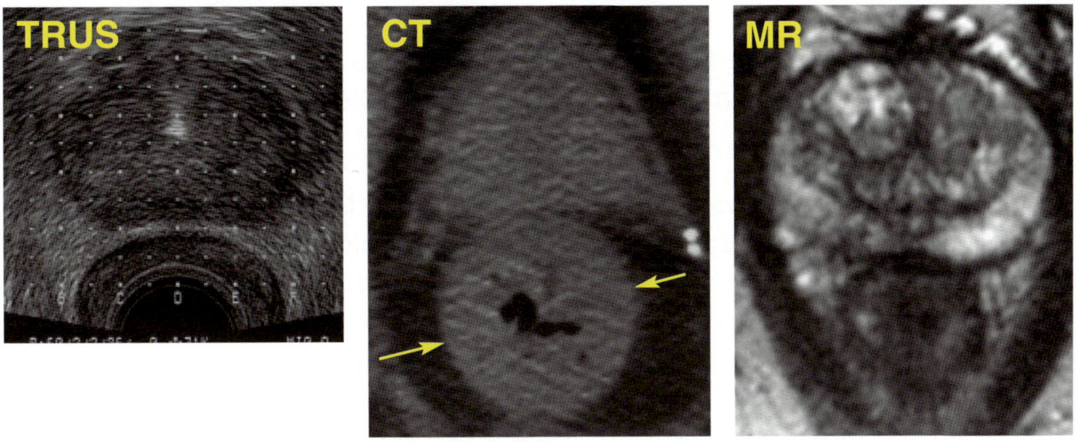

Figure 5-10. Rectal imaging is generally best on CT, because the peri-rectal fat sharpens its delineation (arrows). TRUS is not typically used for rectal imaging, because the probe distorts the rectal anatomy.

Imaging of the penile bulb has also become a subject of interest; doses to the bulb have been correlated with a higher likelihood of impotence. (MERRICK 05) There is little question that MR is optimal for imaging the penile bulb, but CT is adequate.(see Chapter 22).

TUMOR IMAGING

Tumor imaging remains the holy grail of prostate brachytherapy. MR has shown the most promise for macroscopic imaging, and MR spectroscopy has shown promise in microscopic tumor imaging.(ROACH) However, imaging of microscopic tumor extension remains inadequate for guiding dose placement. Until such imaging is substantially more reliable, it will not provide enough confidence in treatment planning.

PRACTICAL CONSIDERATIONS

One practical reason for clarifying the relative accuracy of the various imaging modalities is the ability to interchange prostate volume information between modalities. If CT, TRUS, and MR images give similar prostate volumes, one set of images can be substituted for the other, making the choice of modality more one of convenience. For instance, CT images are routinely used at the Veterans Administration Puget Sound Health Care System to plan TRUS-based implants. Doing so avoids more labor-intensive TRUS imaging for planning. Additionally, it allows for pre-planning of out-of-state patients without having them make a preliminary trip just to have a planning TRUS done to our specifications. Similarly, some might prefer MR-based planning, with TRUS-based implementation.

DOES IT MATTER?

Controversy continues as to the relative accuracy, reproducibility, and practical merits of the different prostate imaging modalities. Substantial differences in imaging technology or image interpretation could have serious consequences—underestimation of prostate volume could lead to substantial underdose of the prostatic periphery, and overestimation could increase the likelihood of complications.(NARAYANA) Prostate brachytherapy is not alone in suffering from inter-observer variability in image interpretation. The radiation oncology literature is filled with studies showing the lack of agreement in tumor and normal tissue identification, especially as it relates to potential outcomes with more precise radiation delivery techniques.(GEETS, CATTANEO) However, the fact that clinical results with modern transperineal brachytherapy are so favorable, even with widely varying techniques, probably means that the differences described above can be compensated for by good treatment planning. Operator skill is likely far more important than the particular imaging equipment used.

REFERENCES

1. Aarnink RG, De La Rosetter JJ, Debruyne FMJ, Wijkstra H. Reproducibility of prostate volume measurements from transrectal ultrasonography by an automated and a manual technique. Br J Urol 1996; 78:219-223.

2. Al-rimawi M, Griffiths DJ, Boake RC, Mador DR. Transrectal ultrasound versus magnetic resonance imaging in the estimation of prostatic volume. Br J Urol 1994; 74:596-600.

3. Amdur RJ, Gladstone D, Leopold KA, Harris RD. Prostate seed implant quality assessment using MR and CT image fusion. Int J Radiat Oncol Biolo Phys 1999; 43:67-72.

4. Badiozamani KR, Wallner KE, Cavanagh W, Blasko J. Comparability of CT-based and TRUS-based prostate volumes. Int J Rad Oncol Biol Phys 1999; 43:375-378.

5. Bartsch G, Egender G, Hubscher H, Rohr H. Sonometrics of the prostate. J Urol 1982; 127:1119-1121.

6. Bates TS, Reynard JM, Peters TJ, Gingell JC. Determination of prostatic volume with transrectal ultrasound: A study of intra-observer and interobserver variation. J Urol 1996; 155:1299-1300.

7. Bazinet M, Karakiewicz PI, Aprikian A, Trudel C. Reassessment of nonplanimetric transrectal ultrasound prostate volume estimates. Urol 1996; 47:857-862.

8. Cattaneo G, Reni M, Rizzo G, et al. Target delinieation in post-operative radiotherapy of brain gliomas: interobserver variability and impact of image registration of MR)pre-operative images on treatment planning CT scans. Radiother and Oncol 2005; 75:217-223.

9. Dubois FD, Prestidge BR, Hotchkiss LA, Bice WS, Prete JJ. Source localization following permanent transperineal prostate intersititial brachytherapy using magnetic resonance imaging. Int J Radiat Oncol Biol Phys 1997; 39:1037-1041.

10. Geets X, Daisne J, Arcangeli S, et al. Inter-observer variability in the delineation of pharyngo-laryngeal tumor, parotied glands and cervical spinal cord: Comparison between CT-scan and MRI. Radiother and Oncol 2005; 77:25-31.

11. Hurwitz MD, Cormack R, Tempany CM, al e. Three-dimensional real-time magnetic resonance-guided interstitial prostate brachytherapy optimizes radiation dose distribution resulting in a favorable acute side effect profile in patients with clinically localized prostate cancer. Techniques in Urology 2000; 6:89-94.

12. Kagawa K, Lee WR, Schultheiss TE, Hunt MA, Shaer AH, Hanks GE. Initial clinical assessment of CT-MRI image fusion software in localization of the prostate for 3D conformal radiation therapy. Int J Radiat Oncol Biol Phys 1997; 38:319-325.

13. McNeal JE, Price HM, Redwine EA, Freiha FS, Stamey TA. Stage A Versus Stage B Adenocarcinoma of the Prostate: Morphological Comparison and Biological Significance. J Urol 1988; 139:61-65.

14. Merrick G, Butler WM, Wallner K, et al. Erectile function after prostate brachytherapy. Int J Rad Oncol Biol Phys 2005; 62:437-447.

15. Merrick G, Wallner K, Butler W. Minimizing prostate brachytherapy-related morbidity. Urol 2003; 62:786-792.

16. Moerland MA, Wijrdeman HK, Beersma R, Bakker CJG. Evaluation of permanent I-125 prostate implants using radiography and magnetic resonance imaging. Int J Radiat Oncol Biol Phys 1997; 37:927-933.

17. Narayana V, Roberson PL, Winfield RJ, McLaughlin PW. Impact of ultrasound and computed tomography prostate volume registration on evaluation of permanent prostate implants. Int J Radiat Oncol Biolo Phys 1997; 39:341-346.

18. Nathan MS, Seenivasagam K, Mei Q, Wickham JEA. Transrectal ultrasonography: why are estimates of prostate volume and dimension so inaccurate? Br J Urol 1996; 77:401-407.

19. Pickett B, Vigneault E, Kurhanewicz J, Verhey L, Roach M. Static field intensity modulation to treat a dominant intra-prostatic lesion to 90 Gy compared to seven field 3-dimensional radiotherapy. Int J Rad Oncol Biol Phys 1999; 43:921-929.

20. Rahmouni A, Yang A, Tempany C, Frenkel T. Accuracy of in-vivo assessment of prostatic volume by MRI and transrectal ultrasonography. J Comp Assist Tomo 1992; 16:935-940.

21. Rifkin MD, Zerhouni EA, Gatsonis CA, Quint LE. Comparison of magnetic resonance imaging and ultrasonography in staging early prostate cancer. NEJM 1990; 323:621-626.

22. Roach M, Faillace-akazawa P, Malfatti C, Holland J. Prostate volumes defined by magnetic resonance imaging and computerized tomographic scans for three-dimensional conformal radiotherapy. Int J Rad Oncol Biol Phys 1996; 35:1011-1018.

23. Stone NN, Stock RG, DeWyngaert JK, Tabert A. Prostate brachytherapy: Improvements in prostate volume measurements and dose distribution using interactive ultrasound guided implantation and three-dimensional dosimetry. Radiat Oncol Invest 1995; 3:185-195.

24. Terris MK, Stamey TA. Determination of prostate volume by transrectal ultrasound. J Urol 1991; 145:984-987.

25. Zaider M, Zelefsky MJ, Lee EK, al e. Treatment planning for prostate implants using magnetic-resonance sprectroscopy imaging. Int J Rad Oncol Biol Phys 2000; 47:1085-1096.

6

Seeds

I-125, Pd-103, and Cs-131 are the radioisotopes currently used for low dose rate prostate brachytherapy. Radioactive gold (Au-198) has some theoretical appeal, but it is not widely available because of its short half-life and onerous radiation protection requirements due to its high energy.(BUTLER, LOENING)

TEMPORARY VERSUS PERMANENT IMPLANTS

Prostate brachytherapy can be done with permanent or temporary source placement. Ir-192 brachytherapy, with ribbons of sources placed inside plastic hollow catheters, is termed *temporary,* because the sources are

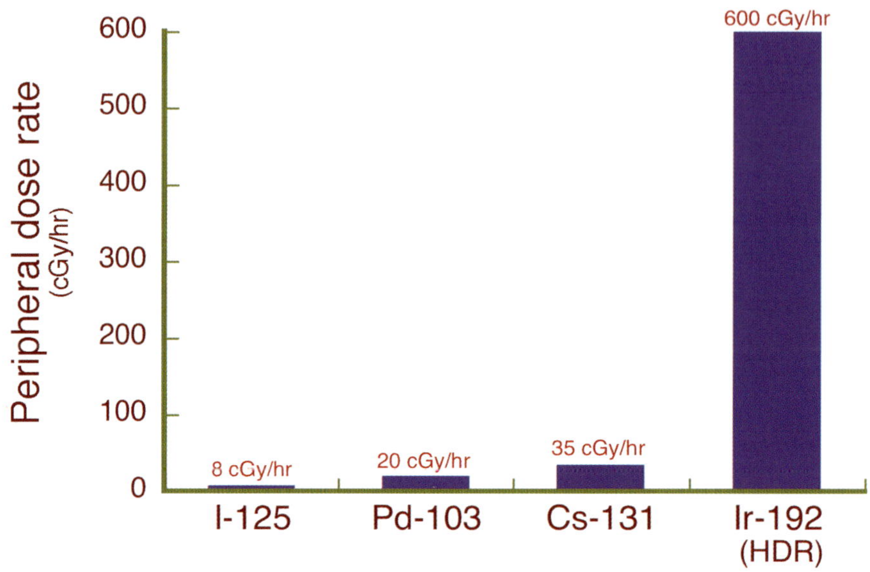

Figure 6-1. Initial dose rate to the prostate periphery with I-125, Pd-103, Cs-131 or HDR Ir-192 implants.

removed after the dose is delivered. Traditionally, Ir-192 seeds were left in place for two to four days, delivering a 20–30 Gy boost to an abbreviated course of external beam radiation (~40 Gy). The boost was delivered at about 50 cGy/hour, an *intermediate* dose rate. Intermediate dose rate temporary implants have been largely replaced by *high dose rate* (HDR) Ir-192 implants, delivering 10–20 Gy in a few minutes. While the dose rates for Ir-192 implants are far higher than those for permanent implants (**Figure 6-1**), the clinical implications are unclear (see Chapter 3). Results comparable to permanent implants have been reported.(MATE, MARTINEZ)

Temporary HDR brachytherapy has its practical advantages and disadvantages. The principal advantage is that seed insertion time can be modified to adjust for less-than-ideal needle placement, as determined from real-time CT or TRUS.(EDMUNDSON) The option to adjust the loading time is appealing because it allows modification of the implant dosimetry *after* needle placement. With permanent implants, the only way to modify dosimetry after the seeds are placed is to take the patient back to the operating room to place more seeds. And if too many permanent seeds are

Table 6.1. Pros and cons of permanent versus temporary implants.

	Pros	Cons
I/Pd/Cs	• Convenient • Substantial PSA-based data	• Can't alter source loading
Ir-192	• Can alter source loading • Re-use sources • No esposure to medical personnel	• Need for supplemental beam(?) • Less convenient

inadvertently placed, they cannot be removed, short of doing a prostatectomy.

A second advantage of temporary or *remote afterloading* techniques (HDR) is that after the seed is removed, no radioactivity remains and no radioprotection precautions are needed. A third advantage of HDR is the ability to reuse sources. Each Ir-192 source typically lasts for three to four months. At $10,000 per source change, reusing them offers a significant savings over I-125 or Pd-103 seeds, which can cost several thousand dollars per patient. (But a significant cost savings is seen only in a large patient volume practice, due to the purchase price and maintenance cost of the HDR machine.)

The biggest disadvantage of temporary implants is the routine use of supplemental external beam radiation. To date, long-term reports of Ir-192 brachytherapy have used it as a boost to 40–45 Gy external beam radiation. In contrast, permanent implants are typically used as sole therapy, avoiding the inconvenience and cost of supplemental beam radiation. There is interest in devising proper dose schemes to use temporary implants as stand-alone therapy, but meaningful tumor cure rate data for HDR alone are still a few years off.

A second disadvantage of HDR is the need for overnight hospitalization and or repeated needle placement on different days, as opposed to the one-time, outpatient I-125 or Pd-103 procedure. Another concern is that giving high implant doses (≥6 Gy) in a single day may create a higher risk

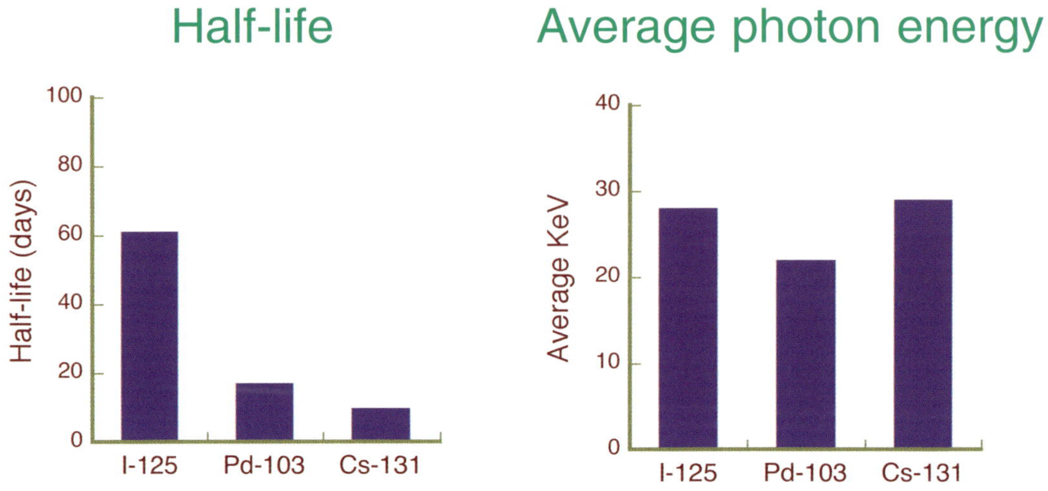

Figure 6-2. Physical characteristics of radionuclides used for prostate brachytherapy.

of complications. A third disadvantage of HDR is the need for radiation shielding of the treatment area, an expensive endeavor for some out-of-hospital patient-care centers. The use of temporary Ir-192 implants has fallen in popularity, relative to permanent implants (see Figure 2-6). While Ir-192-based implants have some appealing aspects, a significant shift back to their use in the near future seems unlikely.

PERMANENT IMPLANTS

I-125, Pd-103 and Cs-131 are all in general use for permanent prostate brachytherapy. They differ substantially in their half-life and photon energy, factors that may influence their biologic effects (**Figure 6-2**). The time to deliver a cancercidal dose is makedly shorter for Pd-103 and Cs-131, compared to I-125 (**Figure 6-3**).

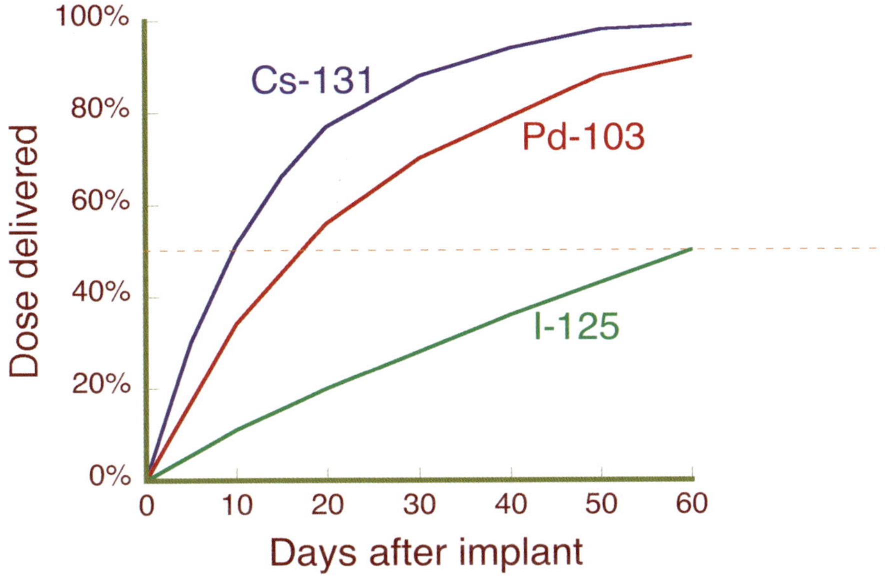

Figure 6-3. Dose delivered versus days after implant.

Iodine-125

I-125 is produced in a nuclear reactor, from Xe-124. I-125 decays, by electron capture and internal conversion, to Te-125. In the process, it emits photons of 27, 31, and 36 keV, for an average energy of 29 keV. I-125's low average energy of 29 keV minimizes shielding requirements. The half-value layer thickness of lead is only 0.02 mm.

The I-125 is adsorbed on a silver rod, which is encased in a titanium capsule (**Figure 6-4**). The inner wire or markers, not the outer titanium capsule, is radiographically visible (**Figure 6-5**). The outside dimensions of the seeds are 4.5 x 0.8 mm. I-125 is typically used at a seed strength of 0.4-1.2 U (0.4 to 0.9 mCi) (**Figure 6-6**).

I-125 has been the most widely used radionuclide. Its relatively long half-life of sixty days is a practical advantage in that it can be stored for several weeks prior to use. Additionally, due to less rapid dose fall-off, the aver-

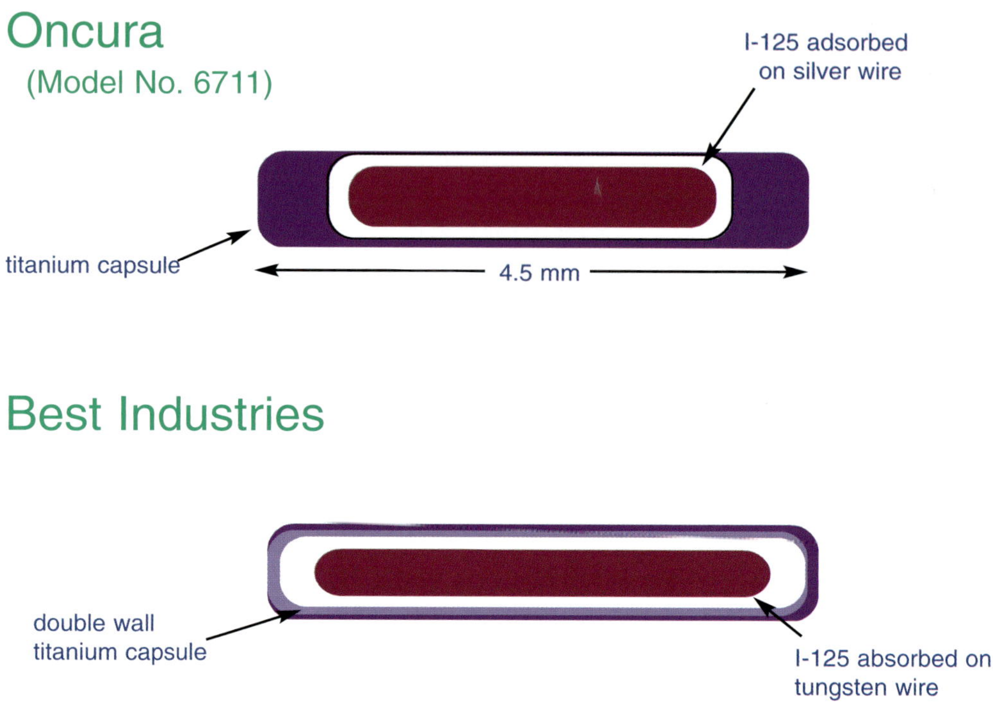

Figure 6-4. Construction of Oncura and Best Industries I-125 seeds.

age treatment margins achieved tend to be about 1 mm larger than those achieved with Pd-103 (see Chapter 7).

Some authors have attributed the inferior results with retropubic implants performed in the 1970s to the choice of I-125 as the isotope. No. Poor results in retropubic series were almost certainly due to poor seed placement, not the properties of the isotope (see chapter 2).

Until the 1990s, Oncura was the only company to manufacture I-125 seeds. Several companies have since introduced alternatives.(NATH 93, HEDTJARN)

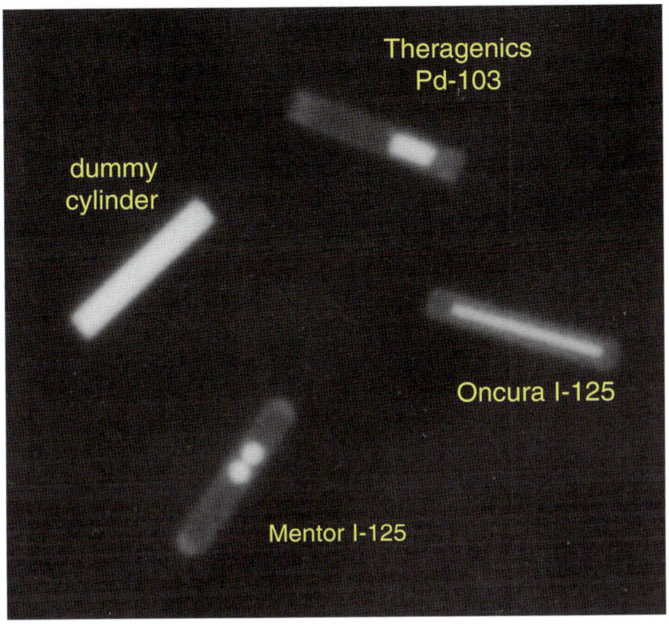

Figure 6-5. Distinct appearance of seeds on plain radiographs, due to use of different radio-dense markers.

Pd-103

Palladium-103 is the second most commonly used isotope for permanent implants. It was initially produced in a nuclear reactor, during a process in which Pd-102 absorbs a neutron, but it is currently produced in a cyclotron by bombarding rhodinium with protons. It decays by electron capture and internal conversion to Rhodium-103. Photons of 20, 23, 40 and 357 keV are emitted, with an average energy of 21 keV. Pd-103 seeds are the same size as I-125 seeds (4.5 x 0.8 mm), but they appear differently on radiographs, depending on the manufacturer.(LI, MEIGOONI) For TheraSeed®, the original and still dominant seed, Pd-103 is plated on radiolucent graphite rods at each end of the seed (**Figures 6-5 and 6-7**). A lead wire is added to the center of the seed to make it easily visible on X-ray films.

Pd-103 seeds are typically used at 1.5 to 4.5 U (NIST-99), with the lower activity seeds generally used for boost implants combined with supplemental external beam radiation (**Figure 6-6**).

Pd-103's shorter half-life of 17 days may be a radiobiologic advantage (**Table 6-2**). On average, it does shorten the duration of radiation prostatitis compared to I-125.(HERSTEIN) The difference in average energy between I-125 and Pd-103 has minor effects on most treatment planning parameters.(DICKER)

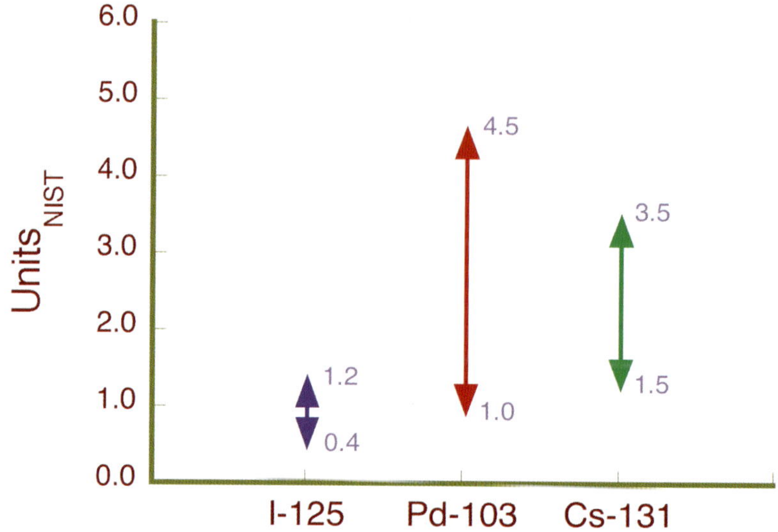

Figure 6-6. Activity ranges commonly used for I-125, Pd-103 and Cs-131. Some brachytherapists advocate use of the lower activity seeds for boost implants, combined with supplemental external beam radiation.

The biggest disadvantage of Pd-103 compared to I-125 is its short shelf life. Depending on the initial activity, Pd-103 can be held only for about 10 days before the activity is too low to be practical (too many seeds would be required). In general, achieving sufficient prostate coverage is a little more technically demanding, because the relatively rapid dose fall-off means that cold areas appear more readily if a few seeds are not properly placed (see Chapter 7).

CS-131

The newest seed to be marketed is Cesium-131, with a half-life of 9.7 days and an average energy of 29 keV (**Figure 6-8**). As such, it combines a relatively short half life with more gradual dose fall-off. Theoretically, it combines the advantages of higher RBE with better peripheral coverage of the prostate. A negative, however, could be higher rectal doses with more risk of rectal complications. Another negative, from a practical perspective, is its short shelf-life. It would be impractical to use the seeds more than one week after the date of delivery. Widspread adoption of Cs-131 will meet some resistance due to the fact that it is expensive to manufacture, and

Theragenics

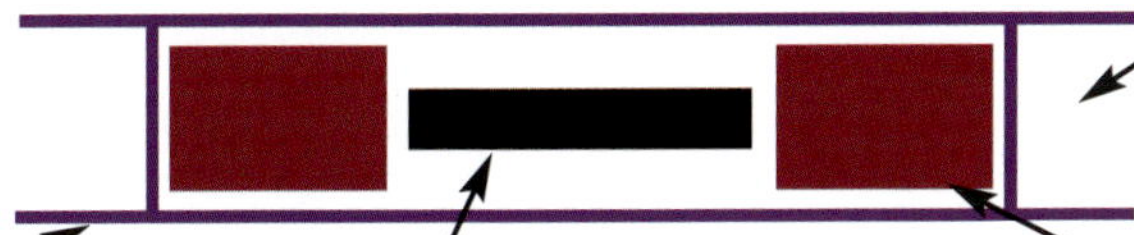

Figure 6-7. Construction of Theragenics Pd-103 seed.

was introduced long after I-125 and Pd-103 have been shown to be highly efficacious, with well-defined rectal toxicity.

UNITS OF MEASURE

Several changes in seed calibration that were made in the late 1990s affected I-125 and Pd-103 in different ways. For Pd-103, there were several alterations in the apparent activity, due to changing the international Cd-109 standardization seeds every three years, implementation of an air-kerma strength standard (S_k) and a change in the dose rate constant.(NATH, WILLIAMSON) The cumulative effect of these changes has been summarized in an American Brachytherapy Society article, recommending that the stated prescription dose for a Pd-103 implant be changed from 115 Gy to 125 Gy, with the simultaneous adoption of the NIST-99 air-kerma strength standard for Pd-103 using the new dose rate constants, which are unique for each seed manufacturer.(BEYER)

For I-125, the American Association of Physicists in Medicine (AAPM) Radiation Therapy Committee Task Group No. 43 (TG-43) recommended a switch to air-kerma parameters developed by the Interstitial Collaborative Working Group (ICWG).(NATH 95, YU) The clinical ramifications, apart from the fact that differences among manufacturers could be better accounted for, was a change from a stated prescription dose of 160 Gy to 144 Gy, assuming the TG-43 formalism was simultaneously implemented.(LUSE, BICE)

Isoray

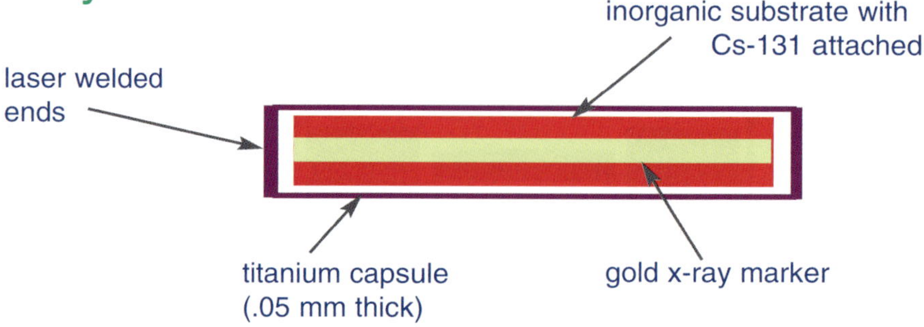

Figure 6-8. Construction of Isoray Cs-131 seed.

The changes in *nominal* doses for Pd-103 and I-125 amount to approximately an 8% increase for Pd-103 and a 10% decrease for I-125. Compared to the substantial variability in treatment margins used by brachytherapists around the world (see Chapter 7), these dose specification changes are probably not of major significance (see Chapter 7). This book includes some inconsistencies between quoted studies, because published data spans the time intervals in which the dosimetry changes have been made. Rather than go back and alter the stated doses, we have tried to specify, when necessary, the period from which the dose calculations were made. When implemented as recommended by the AAPM and ABS, these changes in stated doses, along with the appropriate dose formalisms, should result in the same long-term success already reported. And, yes, additional small adjustments in the NIST-99 calibration standard and associated dose rate constant are being considered but should have minimal clinical significance.(WILLIAMSON)

COST

The cost of seeds dropped dramatically in the late 1990s, as more manufacturers entered the market. As of 2007, the price of I-125 has fallen the most (Figure 6-9) The total seed cost for a given patient is largely dictated by the prostate size and the seed strength chosen.(MAGUIRE) Suture-mounted I-125 seeds (RAPID Strand™) cost about $4 more per seed than loose I-125 seeds (**Figure 6-9**).

ANISOTROPY

Both I-125 and Pd-103 seeds have more dose attenuation at the ends of the seeds than at the central plane due to absorption at the thick ends of

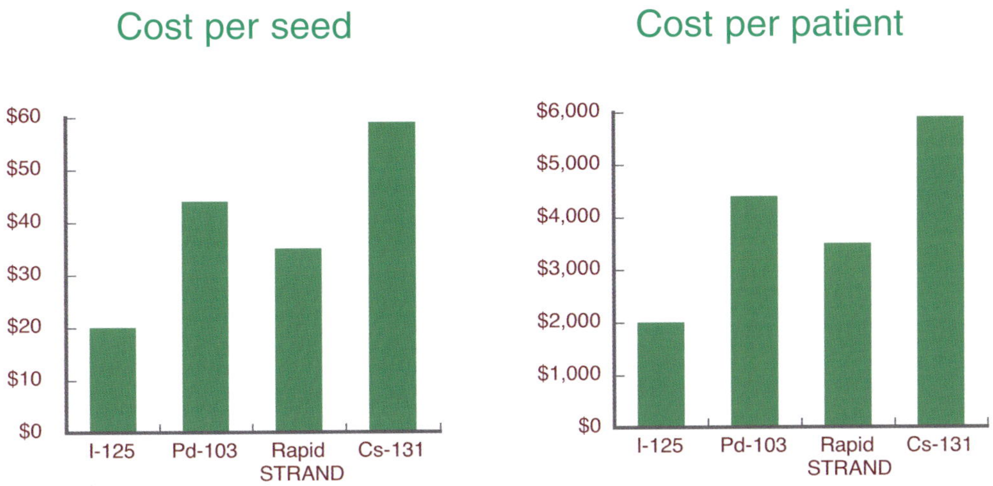

Figure 6-9. Cost of seeds, assuming 100 seeds to implant a 40 cc prostate gland (2007). These numbers may have changed subtantially by the time you read this textbook.

the metal capsule, and due to some absorption by the silver or aluminum carrier itself (**Figure 6-10**). Decreased dose at the ends of the seed could significantly affect the dose distribution of the implant itself, particularly if the seeds are uniformly aligned. In practice, seeds typically are more randomly oriented. Currently, the actual orientation is not taken into account for implant evaluation, because it would be technically difficult to enter precise orientation data. Instead, commercial planning programs employ a uniform correction factor, assuming random seed rotation from the longitudinal prostatic axis. Calculating the actual anisotropic effect would add a substantial degree of complexity to planning and evaluation of the dose

Table 6-2. Practical issues regarding I-125 versus Pd-103.

	Pros	Cons
I-125	Longer shelf life Less expensive	Low dose rate Longer duration side effects
Pd-103	Radiobiologic advantage(?) Shorter duration of side effects	Short shelf life (7 days)

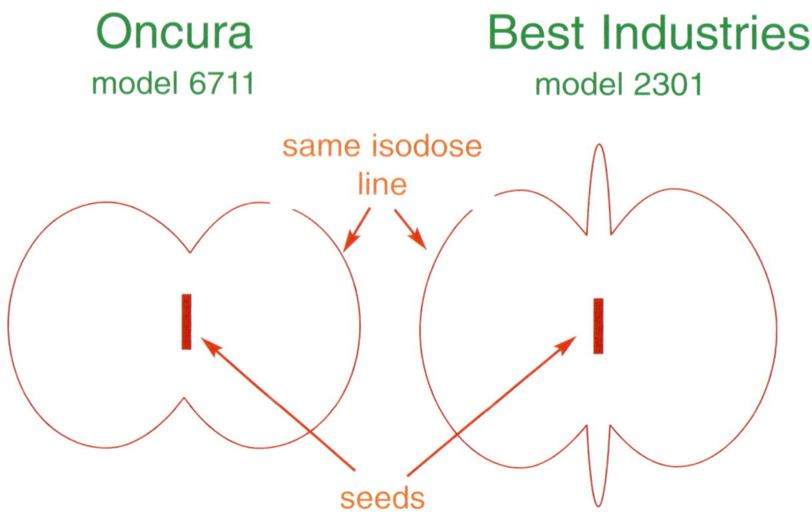

Figure 6-10. Effect of seed orientation on dose distribution. The isodose lines are constricted at the seed ends (anisotropy). Anisotropy could cause substantial underdosage in the longitudinal axis of an implant, when all seeds are closely aligned in the longitudinal direction.(MEIGOONI)

distribution, but it could be automated with the proper software. The clinical relevance of this, however, is likely minimal.

SEED INSERTION

There are two principle ways to insert seeds—with pre-loaded needles or by use of the Mick Applicator®. Each has its pros and cons. Most brachytherapists choose one or the other method, and use it exclusively.(PRESTIDGE)

Mick Applicator®

The Mick Applicator®, manufactured in various models since 1972, has a needle retraction mechanism through which seeds are fed from a magazine cartridge (**Figures 6-11 through 6-13**). The primary advantages of the applicator are: decreased radiation exposure to personnel, flexibility in changing seed spacing at the time of the implant, ease in adding extra seeds ad hoc, simplified sterilization procedures, and simpler seed loading into the device. Accordingly, the Mick is preferred for intra-operative treatment planning. Limitations of the Mick® Applicator are that it occasionally jams (easy to correct), and it requires some getting used to. About half of brachytherapists use a Mick® Applicator, and half use pre-loaded needles.(PRESTIDGE)

Pre-loaded needles
Pre-loaded 18-gauge needles are loaded with seeds before starting the case or intra-operatively. To provide gaps where needed, absorbable spacers (No. 3 chromic gut suture material) of appropriate multiples of 5.5 mm are placed between the seeds (**Figure 6-14 through 6-16**). With experience, manual needle loading can be done in a matter of minutes (**Figures 6-17 and 6-18**). Devices are also available to help with the tedious task of pre-loading seeds into the needles.

One advantage of pre-loaded needles is that they are easier to learn to use, with less operator-dependent seed spacing error. Disadvantages are that they are time-consuming and tedious to set up, offer less intra-operative seed placement flexibility, and increase radiation exposure to the staff.

Choosing a method
The choice between pre-loaded needles and the Mick® Applicator has substantial practical implications—give it serious thought before you buy (**Table 6-3**). In addition to the points mentioned above, there can be significant cost differences between the two methods, depending on the number of cases you do. The Mick has higher start-up costs, but avoids personnel time needed to load needles.

SUTURE-MOUNTED SEEDS
There are a variety of commercially available ways to link seeds into strands. The most widely used has been suture-mounting. Suture-mounted I-125 seeds (RAPID Strand™, Oncura) are mounted in #1 Vicryl™ (polyglactin 910). The suture is stiffened and sterilized with ethylene oxide gas prior to being shipped inside a plastic spacing jig, packed inside a stainless steel shielding tube (**Figure 6-19**). Suture-mounted seeds are more likely to maintain their position, and should not migrate if one or two seeds of the suture are protruding partly out of the prostate. Theoretically, they could allow for wider periprostatic coverage, but their true clinical benefit is unclear. While proper placement at one centimeter intervals is assured with RAPID Strand™, one centimeter spacing may not be the best

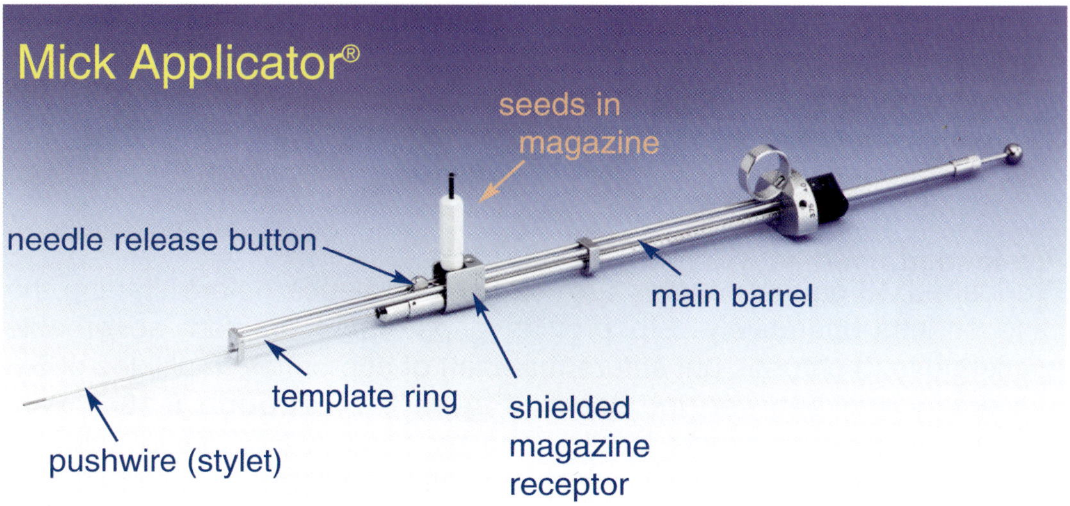

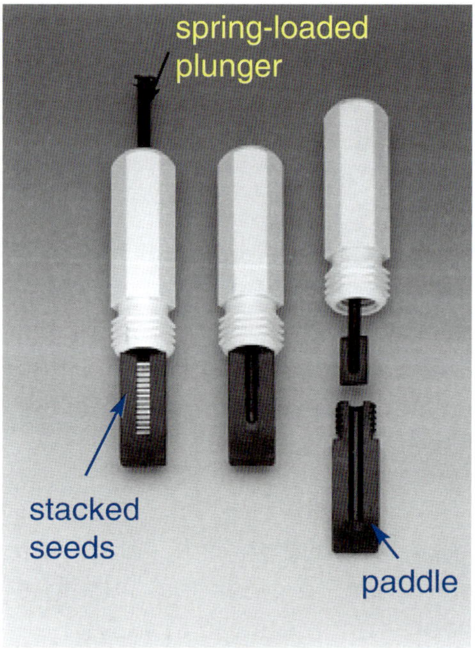

Figure 6-11. Mick Applicator® (top). Seeds are fed into the hollow needle by magazines that can hold 10 to 20 seeds (left).

Mick Applicator® needles

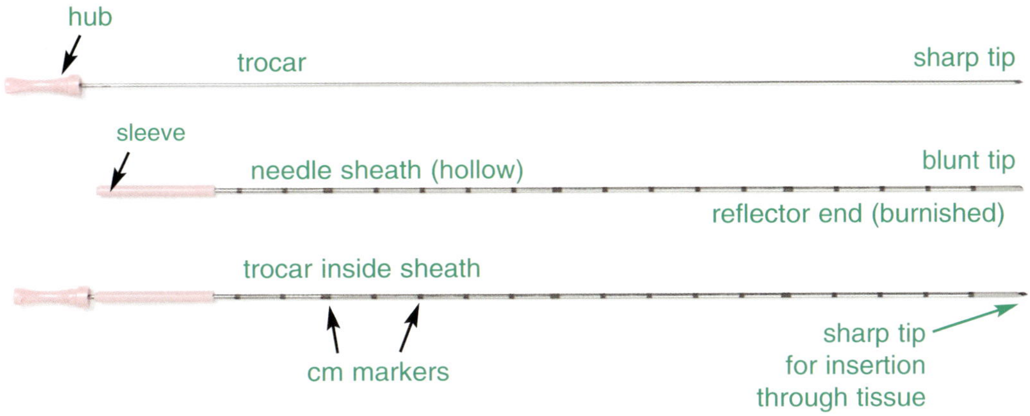

Figure 6-12. Mick Applicator® needles have a trocar that is placed inside the sheath to provide a sharp tip for insertion, and then removed prior to attaching the applicator to insert seeds through the hollow sheath.

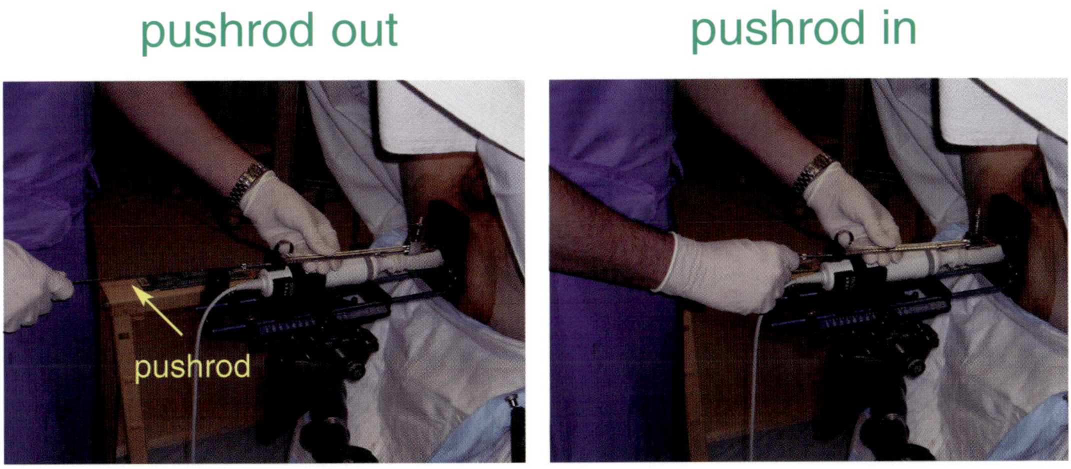

Figure 6-13. Mick Applicator® in action, with pushrod out (left) or in (right). Moving the pushrod in drives a seed from the magazine, out the tip of the hollow sheath.

Pre-loaded needles

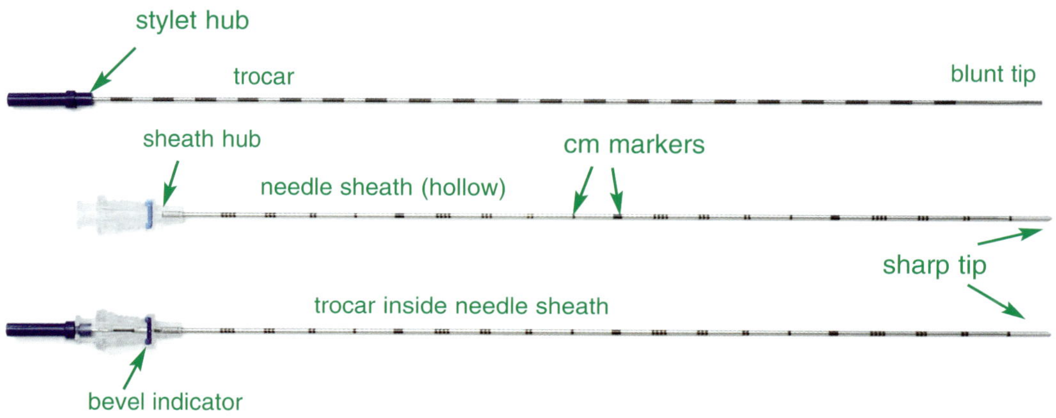

Figure 6-14. Pre-loaded needles have an inner stylet and hollow sheath. The seeds and spacers are loaded prior to starting the procedure (below). After insertion, the needle is withdrawn over the stylet, leaving the seeds in place. Centimeter markers on the stylet indicate how many seeds are in the needle, depending on how many cm of stylet protrude out the sheath. The bevel indicator shows which way the bevel tip points, which is the direction the needles tend to deviate as they pass through tissue. The sheath hub is funnel shaped to facilitate source pre-loading.

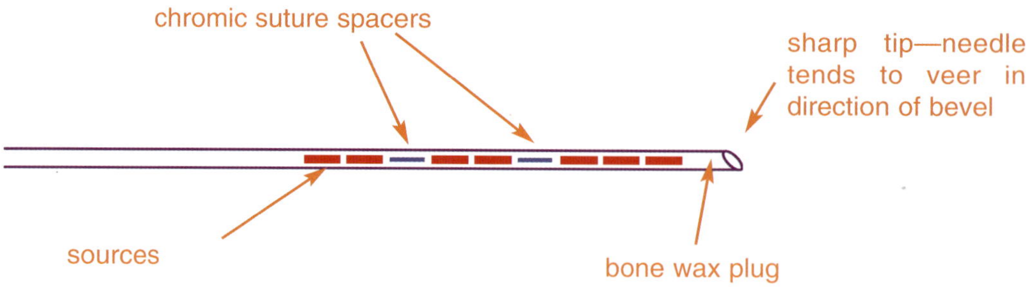

Pre-loaded needles: the sequence of events

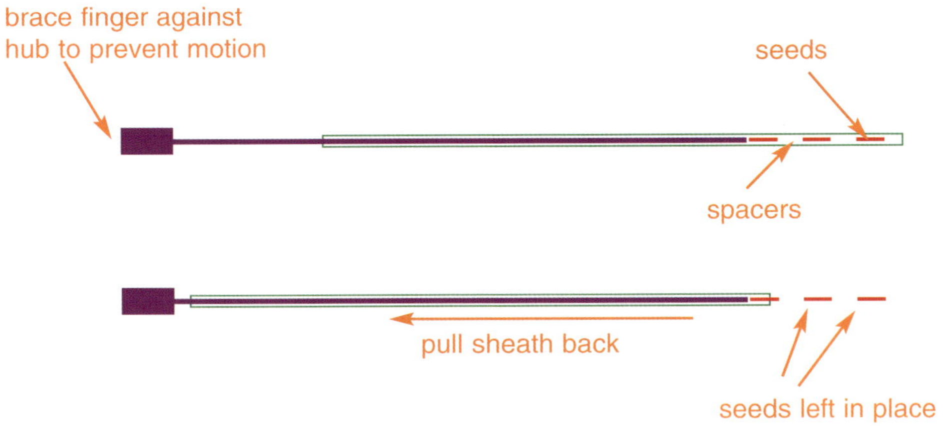

Figure 6-15. Schematic of pre-loaded needles. After insertion, the sheath is withdrawn over the stylet, leaving the seeds in place.

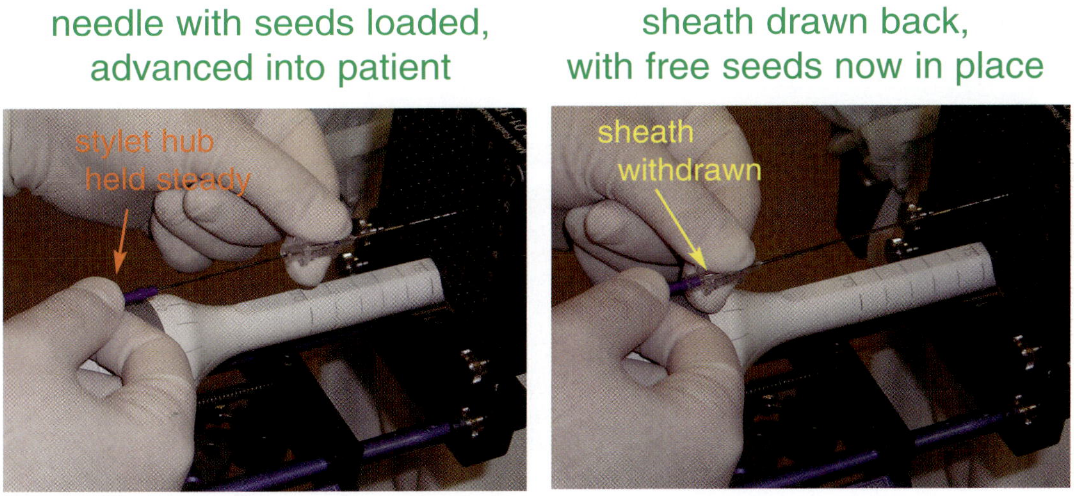

Figure 6-16. Pre-loaded needles, with stylet out (left) or in (right). Pulling the sheath back leaves the free seeds in place in the patient.

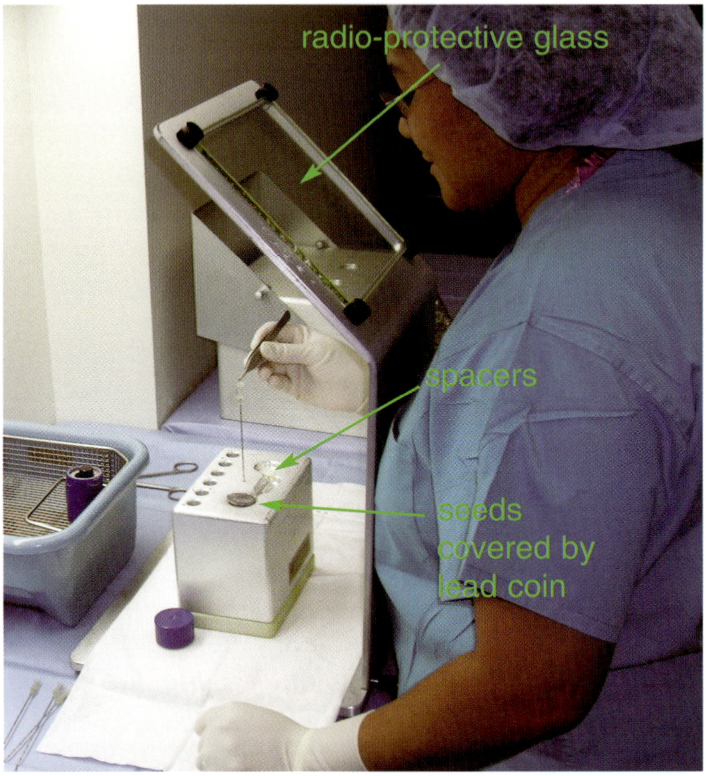

Figure 6-17. Manual seed loading.

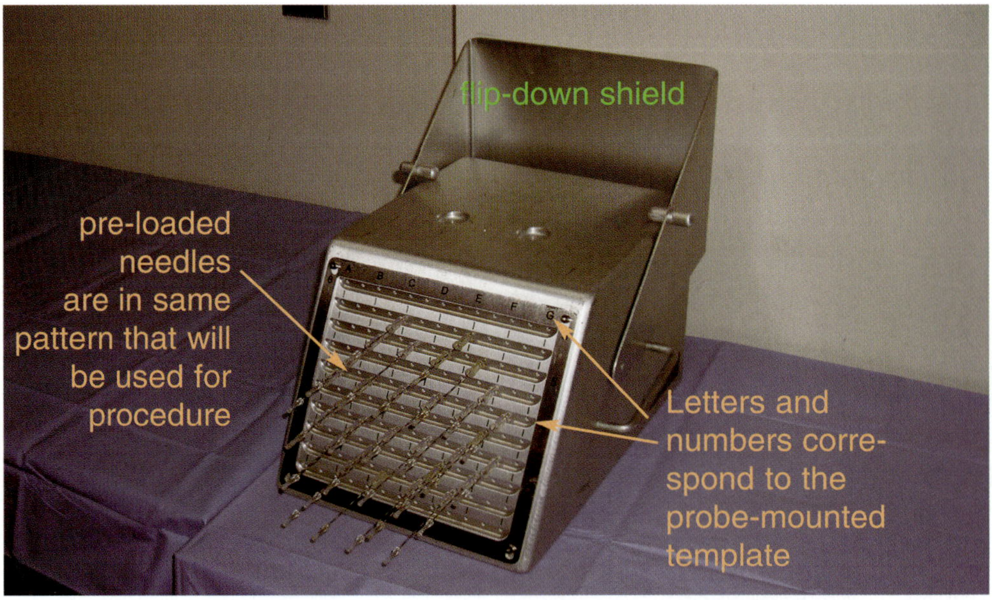

Figure 6-18. Hot box used to hold needles from time of loading until use. Numbers and letters on the margins of the box correspond to those on the TRUS template.

Table 6-3. Mick Applicator® versus pre-loaded needles.

Mick Applicator®	Pre-loaded needles
• Less preparation required - preloaded cartridges • More flexible -ad hoc source placement • Less radiation exposure	• Easier to learn(?) • suture-mounted I-125 (RAPID Strand™)

way to achieve coverage in certain parts of the prostate. If you need intraoperative flexibility in seed placement, you'll probably supplement RAPID Strand™ by placing some seeds with a Mick® Applicator.

The primary disadvantage of suture-mounted seeds has been their tendency to stick inside the needles. Plugging the needle tips with heated Anusol™ provides lubrication and helps prevent needle jamming problems. There is clearly an *art* to proper use of RAPID Strand™.(BUTLER) If you're thinking about using them, it would be wise to first spend some time observing a skilled brachytherapist with substantial experience. When properly performed, there is little question that stranded implants look better, because linear seed alignment is maintained (**Figure 6-20**). Whether the cleaner look of a stranded implant results in better outcomes, however, is still a subject of some dispute.

There have been several retrospective studies comparing loose versus stranded seeds. The effect on dosimetry has been mixed, with some investigators reporting an improvement.(TAPEN, AL-QAISIEH) However, the retrospective studies are probably unreliable because the implants were performed at different points on the practitioners' learning curves.

In a more rigorous comparison, Reed and colleagues randomized 61 patients to implantation with loose seeds versus RAPID Strand.(REED) Patients had plain x-rays for seed counting immediately following their implant, and 30 days later. CT and MR were obtained at each time, to compare dosimetry using image registration. Reed reported a small decrease in seed loss favoring patients implanted with Rapidstrand (**Figure 6-21**). In the investigators' hands, there was no difference in dosimetric parameters at day 0 or day 30. However, less seed loss with

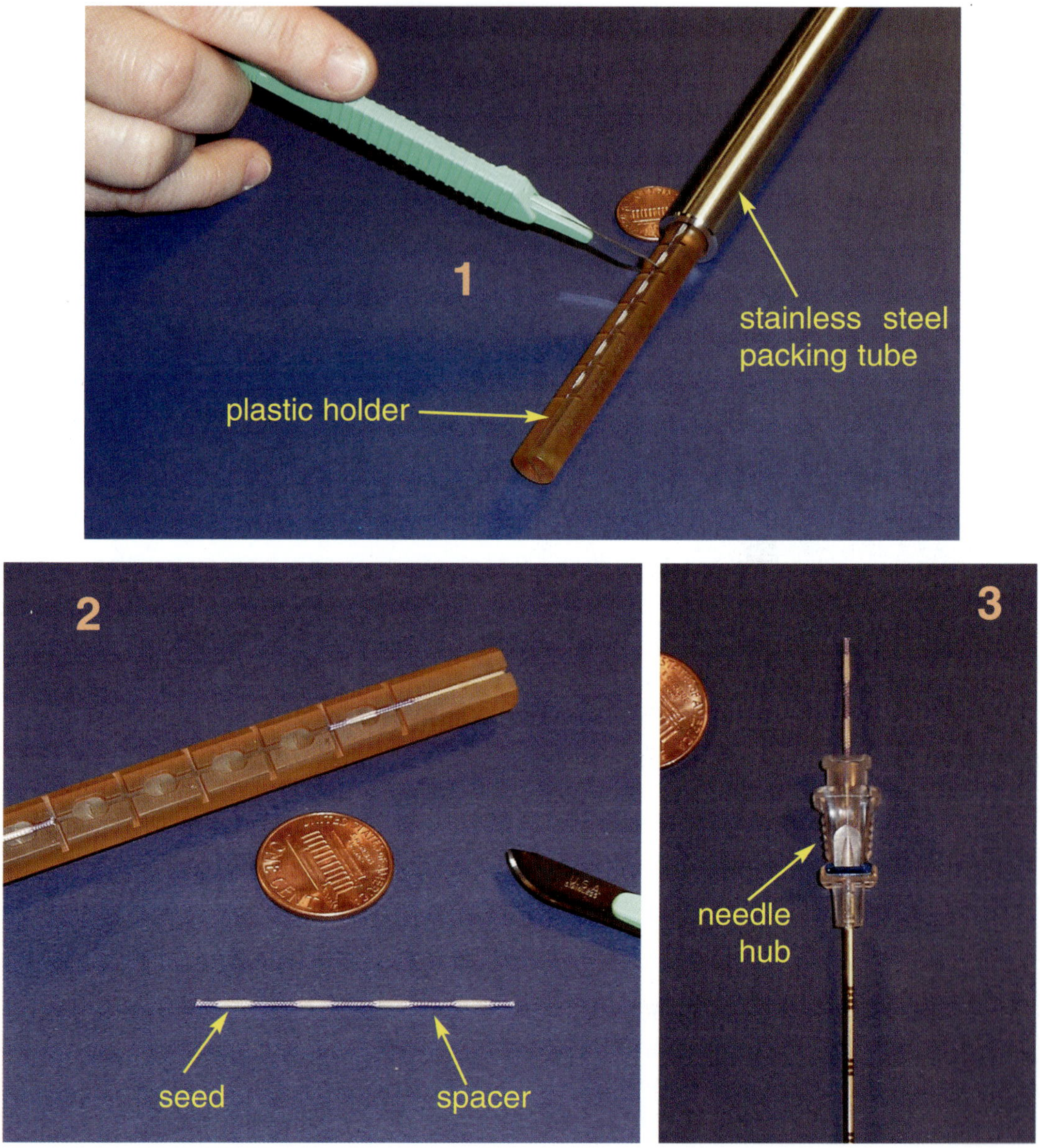

Figure 6-19. Suture-mounted I-125 seeds (RAPID Strand™, Oncura) are shipped inside a plastic spacing jig, which is inside a stainless steel shielding tube. The strand should be cut between the seeds with a razor-sharp blade, and then picked up with tweezers, grasping only the portion that holds a seed.

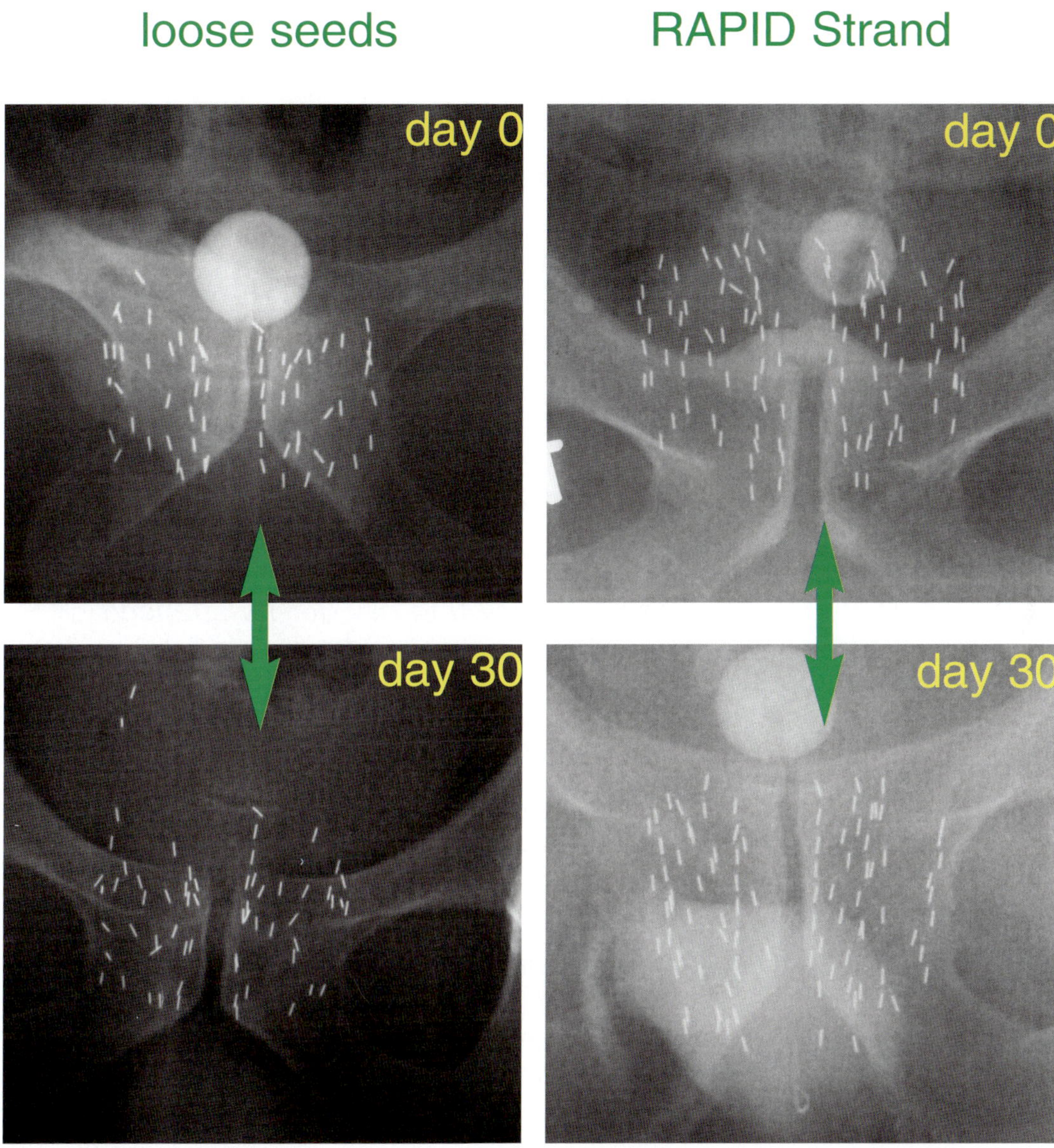

Figure 6-20. Plain frontal view of an implant with loose seeds versus stranded seeds at day 0 (top panels) and day 30 (lower panels). Seed spacing and alignment appears to be better maintained with the stranded product. Seed loss, however, was only slightly improved (see Figure 6-21).

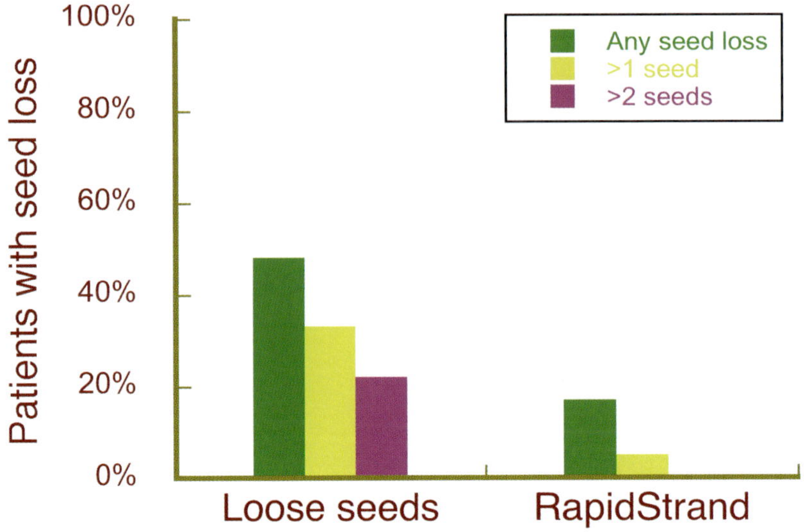

Figure 6-21. Seed loss from day 0 to day 30 for stranded versus loose seeds.

stranded seeds may improve dosimetry for practitioners who do not use a high number of extra-prostatic seeds.(NEDEA) Additionally, stranded seeds should eliminate the occasional case of multiple seeds lost in the early post-implant period (**Figure 6-23**). It would also reduce the already small possibility of cardiac or CNS seed migration.(ZHU. DAVIS)

SO MANY WAYS...

There is a wide variety of seed placement techniques and equipment to carry them out. More manufacturers are getting involved, offering a larger variety of equipment. Some of the new ideas are simply technology-run-amok, making a quick and efficient procedure less so, and with no better final result. Nonetheless, there's still plenty of room for improvement to make the procedure more efficient and less prone to operator error.

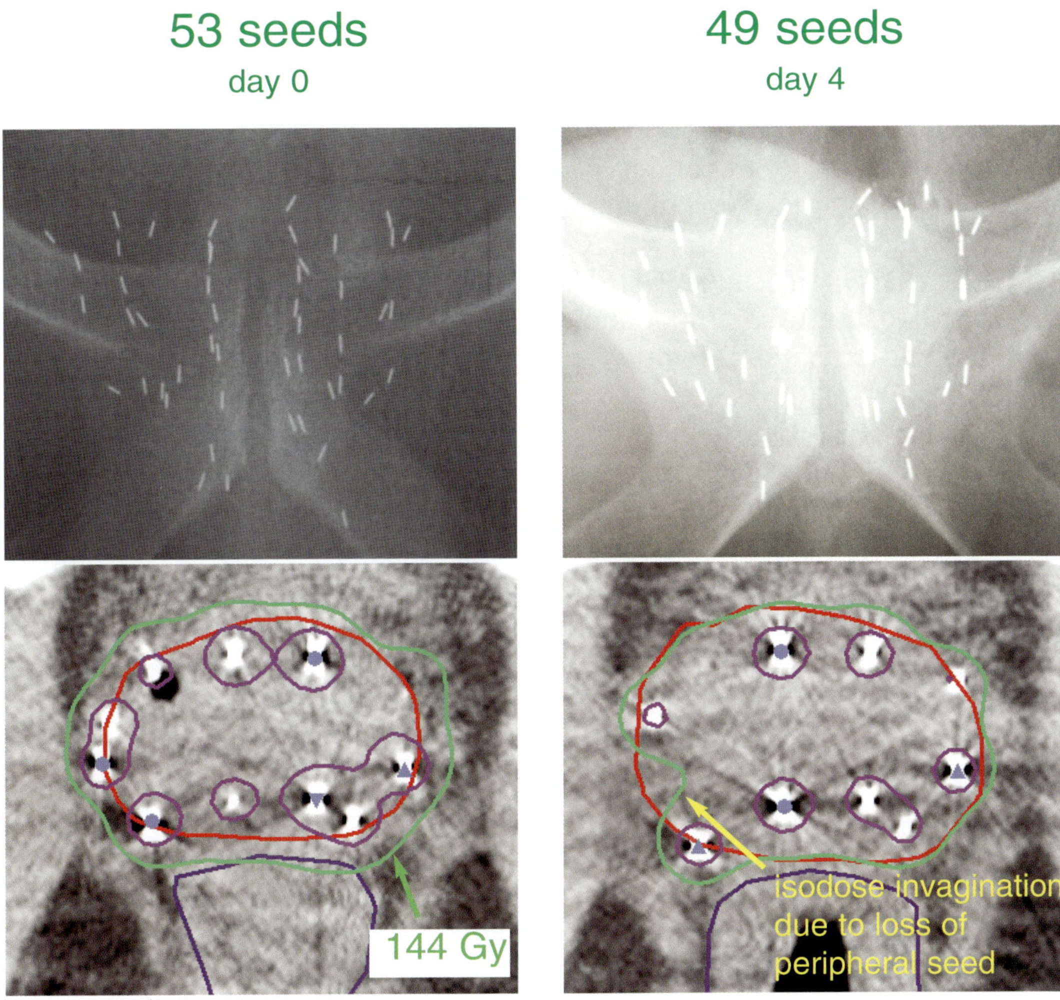

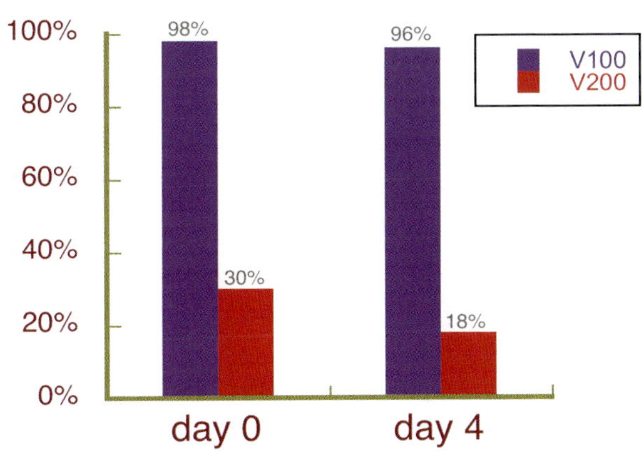

Figure 6.22. Patient with 4 seeds lost in first 24 hours after implant. Note loss of treatment margin on patient's right (yellow arrow), but minimal effect on V100, due to large treatment margins overall. The V200 showed a greater decline, but this has no apparent clinical relevance.

REFERENCES

1. Al-Qaisieh B, Carey B, Ash D, Bottomley. The use of linked seeds eliminates lung embolization following permanent seed implantation for prostate cancer. Int J Rad Oncol Biol Phys 2004; 59:1063-1067.

2. Beyer D, Nath R, Butler W, al e. American Brachytherapy Society recommendations for clinical implementation of NIST-1999 standards for Pd-103 brachytherapy. Int J Rad Oncol Biol Phys 2000; 47:273-275.

3. Bice WS, Prestidge BR, Prete JJ, Dubois DF. Clinical impact of implementing the recommendations of AAPM Task Group 43 on permanent prostate brachytherapy using I-125. Int J Rad Oncol Biol Phys 1998; 40:1237-1241.

4. Butler EB, Scardino PT, Teh BS, al e. The Baylor College of Medicine experience with gold seed implantation. Seminars in Surgical Oncology 1997; 13:406-418.

5. Butler WM, Merrick GS. I-125 Rapid Strand* loading technique. Radiat Oncol Invest 1996; 4:48-49.

6. Davis BJ, Pfeifer EA, Wilson TM, King BF, Eschelman JS, Pisansky TM. Prostate brachytherapy seed migration to the right ventricle found at autopsy following acute cardiac dysrhythmia. J Urol 2000; 164:1661.

7. Dicker AP, Lin C-C, Leeper DB, Waterman FM. Isotope selection for permanent prostate implants? An evaluation of 103-Pd versus 125- based on radiobiological effectiveness and dosimetry. Seminars in Urol Oncol 2000; 18:152-159.

8. Edmundson GK, Yan D, Martinez AA. Intraoperative optimization of needle placement and dwell times for conformal prostate brachytherapy. Int J Rad Oncol Biol Phys 1995; 33:1257-1263.

9. Hedtjarn H, Carlsson GA, Williamson JF. Monte Carlo-aided dosimetry of the Symmetra model 125.S06 125-I, interstitial brachytherapy seed. Med Phys 2000; 27:1076-1085.

10. Herstein A, Wallner K, Merrick G, et al. I-125 versus Pd-103 for low-risk prostate cancer: Long-term morbidity outcomes from a prospective randomized multicenter controlled trial. Cancer J 2005; 11:385-389.

11. Li Z, Palta JR, Fan JJ. Monte Carlo calculations and experimental measurements of dosimetry parameters of a new 103-Pd source. Med Phys 2000; 27:1108-1112.

12. Loening SA. Gold seed implantation in prostate brachytherapy. Seminars in Surgical Oncology 1997; 13:419-424.

13. Luse RW, Blasko J, Grimm P. A method for implementing the American Association of Physicists in Medicine Task Group-43 dosimetry recommendations for I-125 transperineal prostate seed implants on com-

mercial treatment planning systems. Int J Rad Oncol Biol Phys 1997; 37:737-741.

14. Maguire PD, Waterman FM, Dicker AP. Can the cost of permanent prostate implants be reduced? An argument for peripheral loading with higher strength seeds. Techniques in Urology 2000; 6:85-88.

15. Martinez A, Gustafson G, Gonzales J, et al. Dose escalation using conformal high-dose-rate brachytherapy improves outcome in unfavorable prostate cancer. Int J Rad Oncol Biol Phys 2002; 53:316-327.

16. Mate TP, Gottesman JE, Hatton J, al e. High dosed-rate after-loading iridium-192 prostate brachytherapy: feasibility report. Int J Rad Oncol Biol Phys 1998; 41:525-533.

17. Meigooni AS, Sowards K, Soldano M. Dosimetric characteristics of the InterSource-103 palladium brachytherapy source. Med Phys 2000; 27:1093-1100.

18. Nath R, Anderson LL, Luxton G, Weaver KA, Williamson JF, Meigooni AS. Dosimetry of interstitial brachytherapy sources: Recommendations of the AAPM Radiation Therapy Committee Task Group No. 43. Med Phys 1995; 22:209-234.

19. Nath R, Melillo A. Dosimetric characteristics of a double wall 125-I source for interstitial brachytherapy. Med Phys 1993; 20:1475-1483.

20. Nedea E, Wallner K, Reed D, et al. Extra-prostatic seed placement and its effect on seed loss. Cancer Journal (Scientific American) 2005; 11:147-151.

21. Prestidge BR, Prete JJ, Buchholz TA, et al. A survey of current clinical practice of permanent prostate brachytherapy in the United States. Int J Rad Oncol Biol Phys 1998; 40:461-465.

22. Reed D, Wallner K, Merrick G, et al. A prospective randomized comparison of stranded versus loose iodine-125 seeds for prostate brachytherapy. Brachytherapy 2007; in press.

23. Tapen EM, Blasko JC, Grimm PD, al e. Reduction of radioactive seed embolization to the lung following prostate brachytherapy. Int J Rad Oncol Biol Phys 1998; 42:1063-1067.

24. Williamson JF, Coursey BM, DeWerd LA, al e. Recommendations of the American Association of Physicists in Medicine on 103-Pd interstitial source calibration and dosimetry: Implications for dose specification and prescription. Med Phys 2000; 27:634-642.

25. Yu Y, Anderson LL, Li Z, et al. Permanent prostate seed implant brachytherapy: Report of the American Association of Physicists in Medicine Task Group No. 64. Med Phys 1999; 26:2054-2076.

26. Zhu A, Wallner K, Frivold G, Ferry D, Jutzy K, Foster G. Prostate brachytherapy seed migration to the right coronary artery associated with an acute myocardial infarction. Brachytherapy 2006; 5:262-265.

7

Design

Treatment planning, design or pre-implant dosimetry, refer to the determination of how many seeds will be used and where they will be placed. Planning has traditionally been performed a week or more ahead of the implant procedure, but many brachytherapists have switched to intra-operative planning. Whether you choose to do your planning ahead of time or not, the same principles apply.

Despite a rapidly accumulated body of favorable clinical outcomes reports, rational treatment planning guidelines have lagged behind. Until the mid-2000's, treatment planning remained largely a mysterious endeavor, based

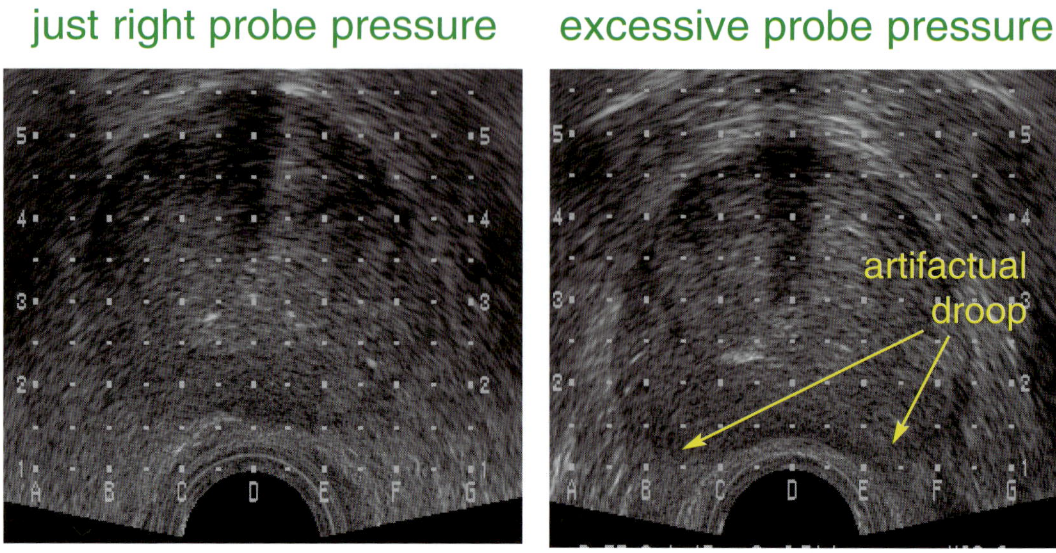

Figure 7-1. Excessive probe pressure deforms the prostatic image. These two mid prostatic images of the same patient were taken with minimal (left) or substantial (right) probe pressure, causing artifactual drooping of the posterior-lateral margins. Note that increased probe pressure also moves the prostate lower on the grid.

more on gut instinct than on a critical look at the relationship between planning parameters and outcomes. Although the stated prescription doses are fairly uniform, there has been substantial variability from one implant team to another in regards to the actual isodose patterns achieved, primarily due to inconsistencies in the use of treatment margins and due to dose inhomogeneity.(MERRICK 05) Fortunately, some key publications have emerged in recent years, better describing and documenting optimal planning guidelines. The best way to avoid problems in your own practice is to understand the differences that exist and the potential pitfalls in comparing nominal doses from one implant team to another.

PLANNING IMAGES

Implants are typically planned from TRUS images taken at 5 mm intervals from the prostatic base through the apex. The patient should be in the lithotomy position, similar to that for the implant procedure itself. It's important that the prostate images are not deformed by excessive probe pres-

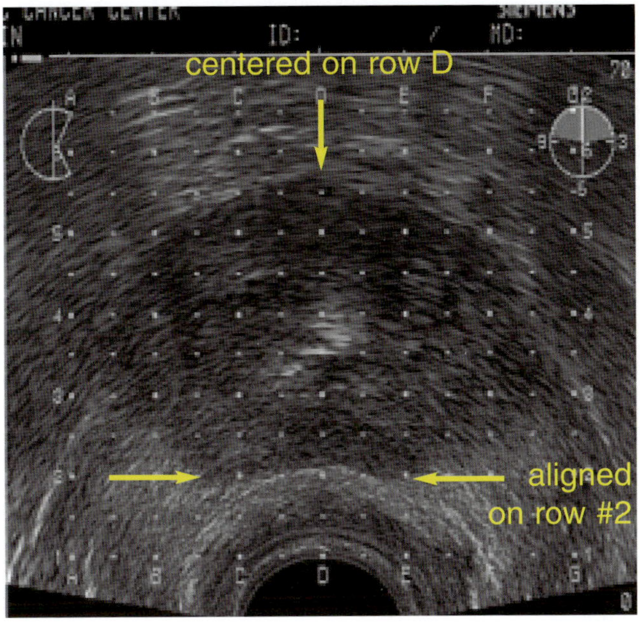

Figure 7-2. You're less likely to make mistakes going from the plan to the operating room if the prostate is consistently centered on the grid, with the back of the gland aligned along the same row for each case.

sure (**Figure 7-1**) and that the prostate remains centered on the grid with the posterior margin aligned along a consistent grid row (**Figure 7-2**).

The most proximal image is considered the *zero plane* or *0.0 plane*. It is located by visualizing the most proximal image or *base*, usually including a portion of the seminal vesicles (**Figure 7-3 and 7-4**). Sagittal imaging can be used to check that your 0.0 plane corresponds to the top of the prostate. Images and seed positions are typically specified by their distance from the zero plane. Going caudally, transverse planes are numbered by their distance (in cm) from the 0 plane (i.e., the *1.0 plane* is 1.0 cm caudal to the 0.0 plane). The most caudal image, or *apex*, typically is indistinct on transverse imaging but can be readily verified on sagittal imaging (**Figure 7-3**).

TARGET DEFINITIONS

ICRU 50 treatment planning definitions were written for external beam treatment planning, but are generally applicable to brachytherapy.(ICRU, HAN) The *gross target volume* (GTV) is the prostate itself, as visualized on the TRUS images. The *clinical target volume* (CTV) is designed to cover the prostate plus peri-prostatic regions of potential microscopic tumor spread. For external beam planning, the *planning target volume* (PTV) includes a margin around the CTV to allow for variability in patient setup and prostatic motion. For prostate brachytherapy, the PTV is not as rele-

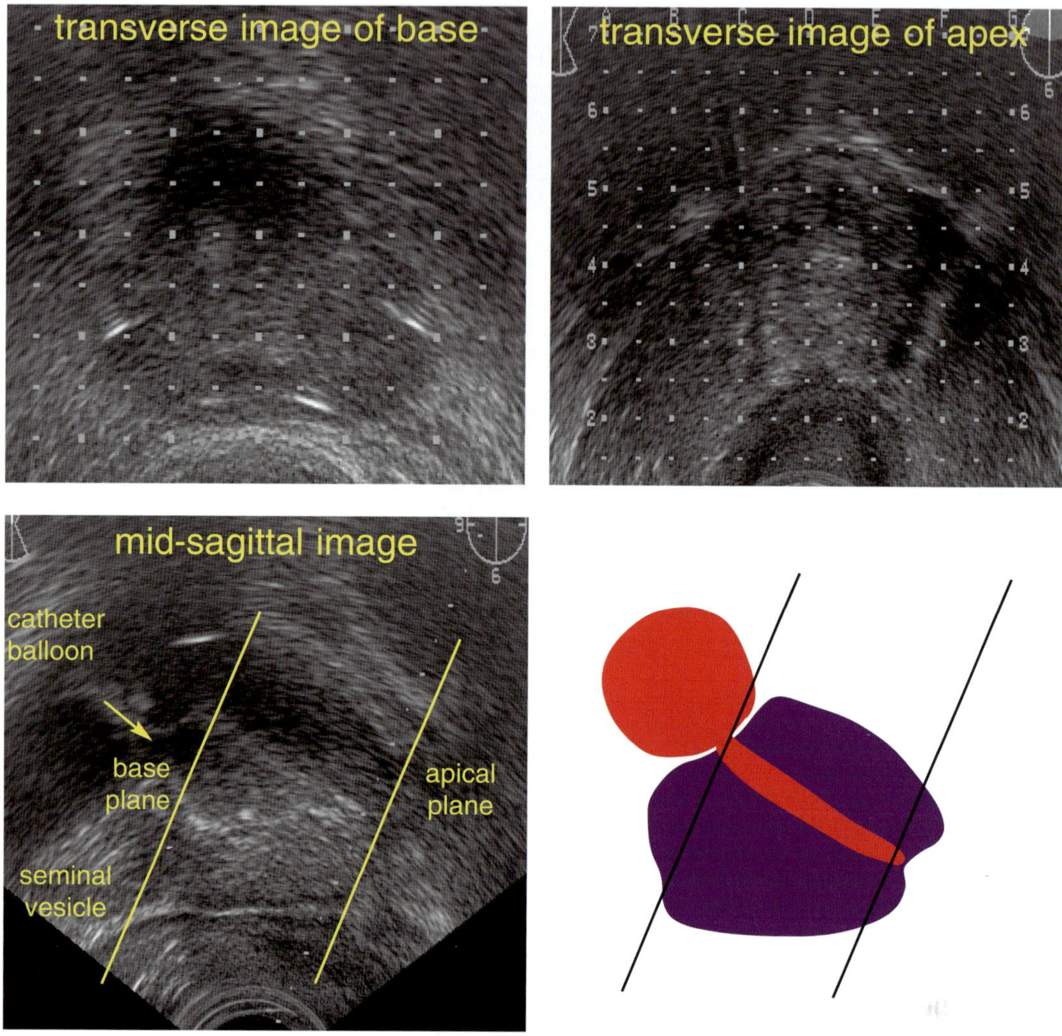

Figure 7-3. Sagittal imaging helps verify the base and apical planes. The transverse images (top) of the base and apex are typically less distinct than those of the mid-prostate. The sagittal view (bottom images) helps confirm the base and apical planes, in part because the continuous prostatic contour can be visually extrapolated from the mid-portion of the prostate. (yellow lines show transverse imaging planes).

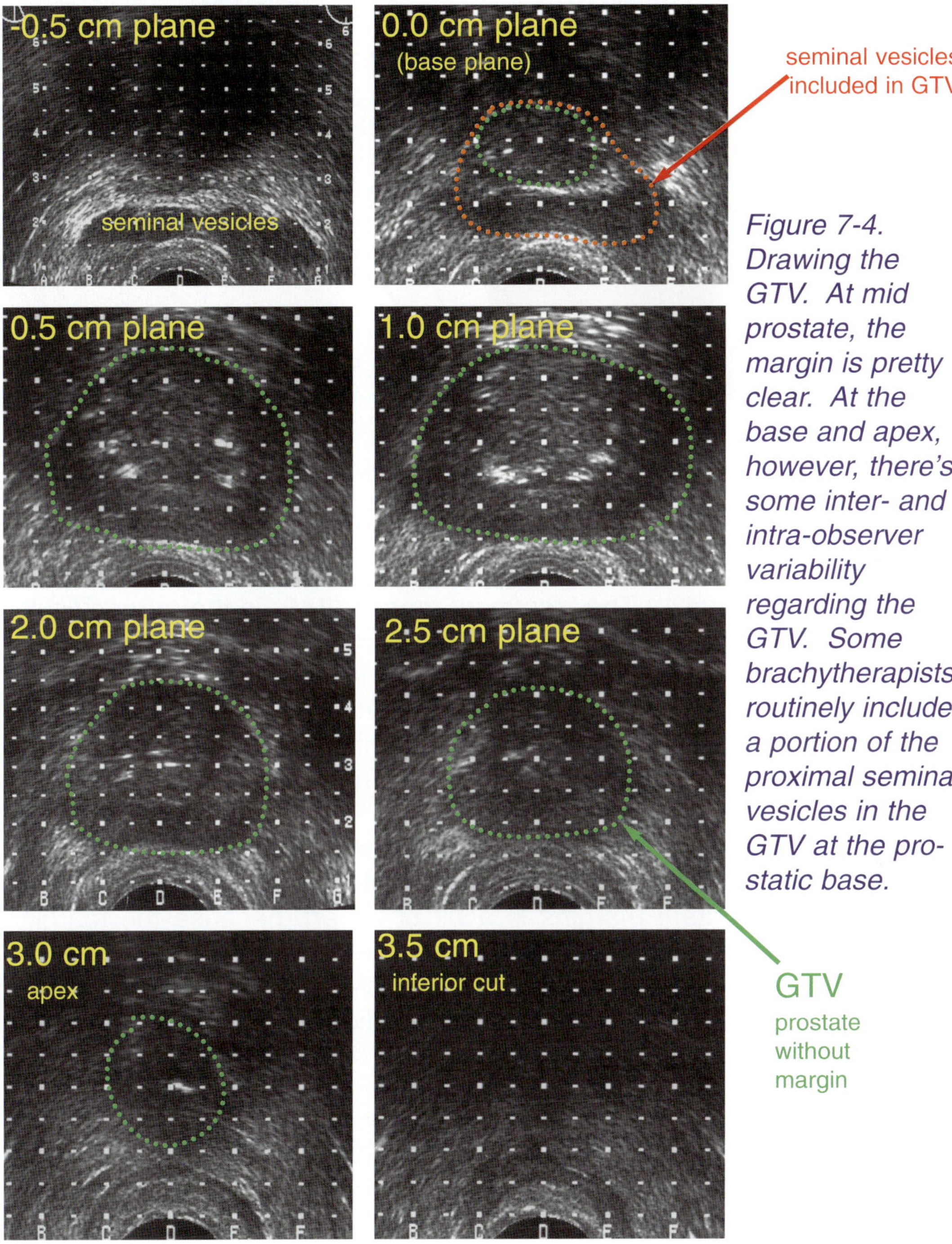

Figure 7-4. Drawing the GTV. At mid prostate, the margin is pretty clear. At the base and apex, however, there's some inter- and intra-observer variability regarding the GTV. Some brachytherapists routinely include a portion of the proximal seminal vesicles in the GTV at the prostatic base.

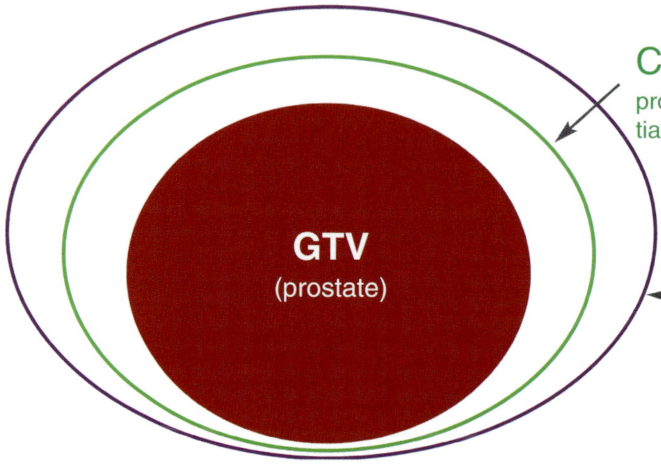

Figure 7-5. Schematic of GTV, CTV, and TV.(ICRU, HAN)

vant, since the prostatic position on the template should not change during the implant procedure. The *treatment margin* (*TM*), is the perpendicular distance between the GTV and the prescription isodose (**Figure 7-5**).(CHOI) The *treated volume* (TV) is that enclosed by the prescription isodose. In contrast to external beam radiation, brachytherapy delivers doses far higher than the prescription dose, due to high dose regions near the implanted seeds and the use of treatment margins.

To start the treatment planning process, the prostatic margin (GTV) is outlined on the TRUS images and transferred into a planning program. Identifying the prostate margins is a bit of an *art*, because the margins appear fuzzy, especially at the apex, where the prostatic tissue blends into the nearly isodense pelvic floor musculature. When in doubt, we err on the side of being generous with margin identification. Fortunately, the posterior prostatic edge is typically sharply defined on TRUS.

MARGIN SIZE

While modern TRUS equipment has made the identification of the GTV fairly simple, there is surprisingly little data regarding the optimum treatment planning margins to add to the GTV. In practice, "a few mm" have typically been added, but the optimal magnitude of the TM has not been rigorously studied. The problem with the arbitrariness of the magnitude of the margins is that the actual dose to the prostate may be far different than the prescription dose, depending on how large a TM is used. Use of min-

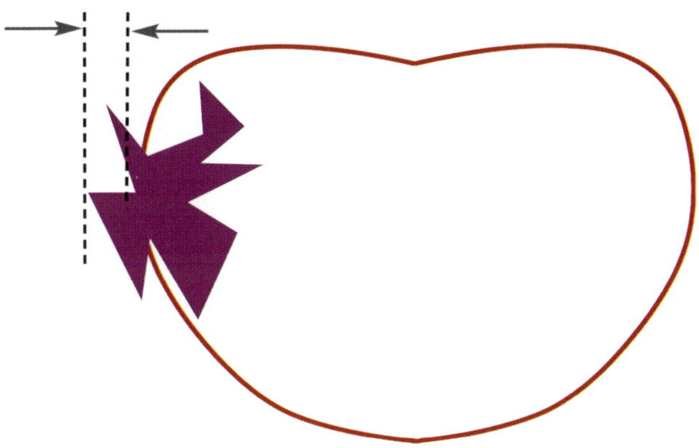

Figure 7-6. Schematic of extra-capsular extension (ECE), measured radially from the prostatic margin. The degree of radial extra-capsular cancer extension is limited to within 3 mm in nearly all patients (see chapter 11).

imal treatment margins probably explained the poor brachytherapy results seen in some series.(D'AMICO) Recent studies regarding the extent of ECE and the effect of implant-related edema on post-implant TMs are bringing us closer to a more rational choice of treatment margins.(HAN, MERRICK 02) Larger margins lead to less edema-related underdosing, and to better cancer-control rates.(MERRICK 00, CHOI)

Extra-capsular cancer extension (ECE)
Ideally, brachytherapy delivers a tumorcidal dose to the prostate, with a sufficient margin to encompass the likely extent of cancer extension beyond the prostatic capsule (ECE) (**Figure 7-6**). Prostatectomy specimen studies revealed that ECE is nearly always within 3 mm of the prostatic edge, so that a post-implant 3 mm TM should suffice to eradicate cancer within the prostate, along with any ECE(**Figure 7-7**).(DAVIS, SOHAYDA)

Pre-implant versus post-implant TMs
In the absence of seed placement errors or implant-related prostate swelling, a planning TM of 3 mm should be sufficient to achieve a post-implant margin of 3 mm. But in order to achieve adequate margins on the *post*-implant prostate, some allowance must be made for seed placement error and implant-related swelling that continues over much of the active life of the isotopes.(WILLINS 98, WATERMAN 98) On average, the prostate volume increases approximately 25% by the completion of the implant proce-

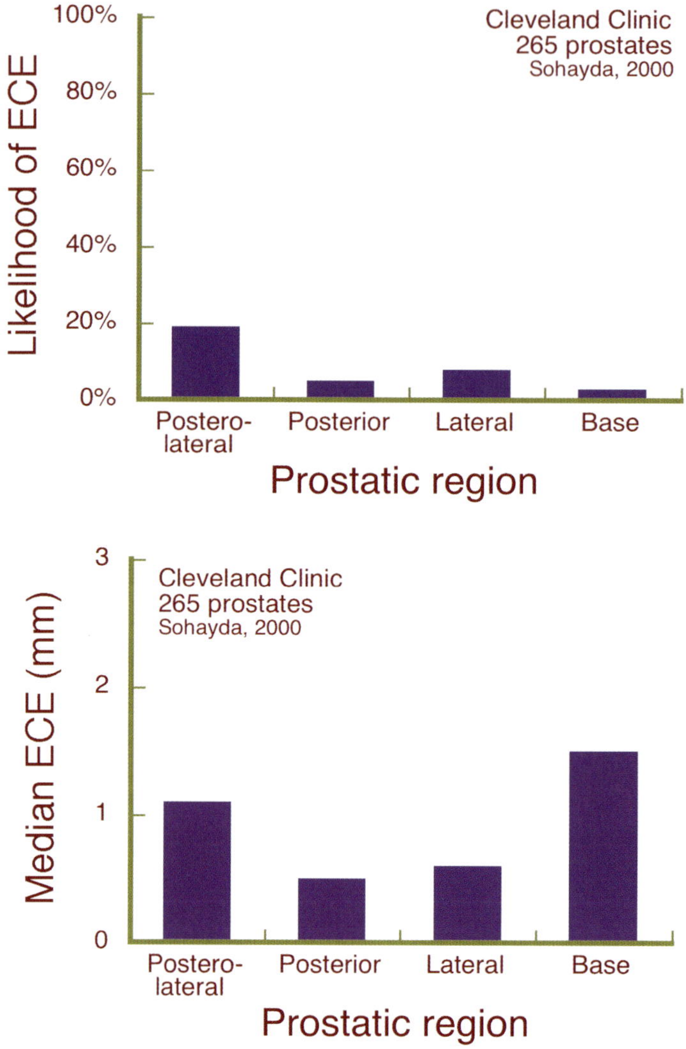

Figure 7-7. The likelihood of ECE and its radial extent vary by the region of the prostate. In this series by Sohayda and colleagues at the Cleveland Clinic, ECE was most common at the posterior-lateral margins, and of greatest radial extent at the base. The apex was not analyzed separately, due to lack of a well-defined capsule in that region.

dure, but with a large degree of variability among patients. Badiozamani and colleagues compared implant-related volume changes with pre-implant clinical parameters, including pre-implant volume, hormonal ablation, and pre-implant external beam radiation in 50 patients.(BADIOZAMANI) In most patients, the greatest size increase was in the anterior-posterior dimension. Changes in the lateral and craniocaudal (length) dimensions were smaller and inconsistent (**Figure 7-8**). And as expected, the degree of post-implant target coverage was less in patients with greater volume increase (**Figure 7-9**). The absolute volume change was similar in patients with small versus large pre-implant prostate volume, but the proportional

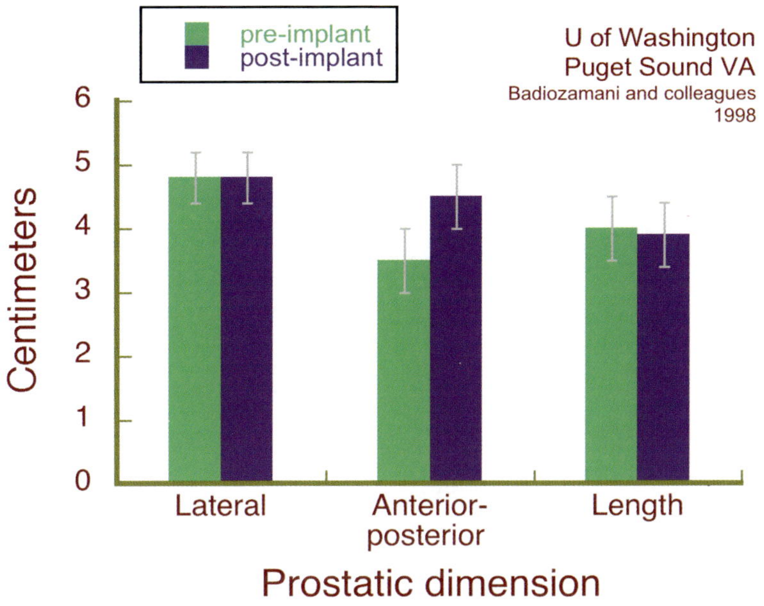

Figure 7-8. Prostatic dimensions before and after implant procedure.

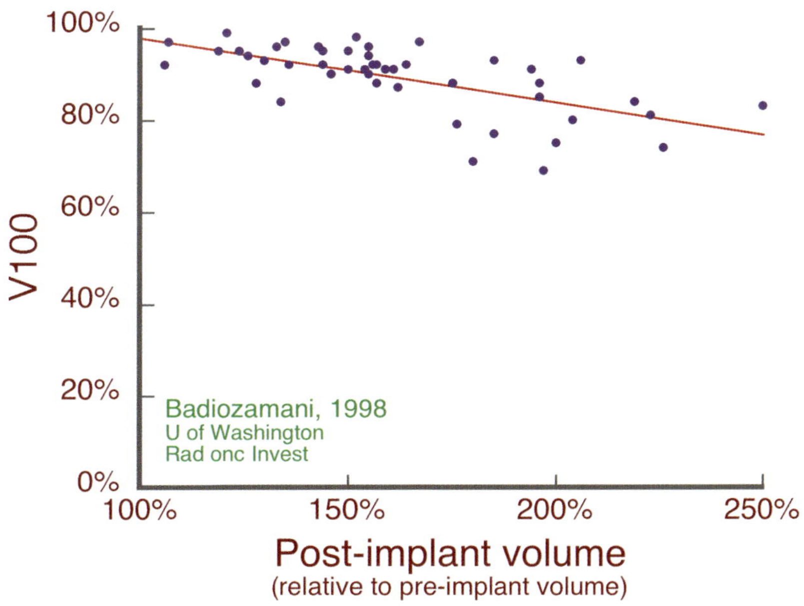

Figure 7-9. Fraction of post-implant target coverage versus degree of procedure-related swelling.

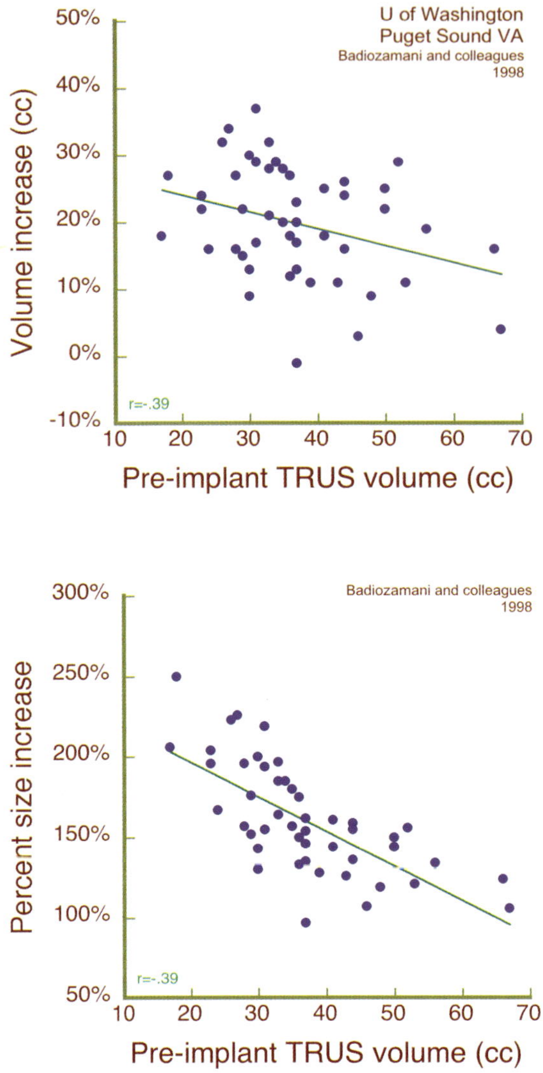

Figure 7-10. Absolute (top panel) and proportional (lower panel) prostate volume increase versus pre-implant TRUS volume.

increase was less in patients with a larger prostate volume (**Figure 7-10**). Because patients with a small pre-implant prostate had proportionately greater volume increase, their post-implant target coverage was generally *lower*, contrary to popular belief. Pre-implant hormonal therapy or supplemental external beam radiation had no consistent effect on post-implant volume changes (**Figure 7-11**).

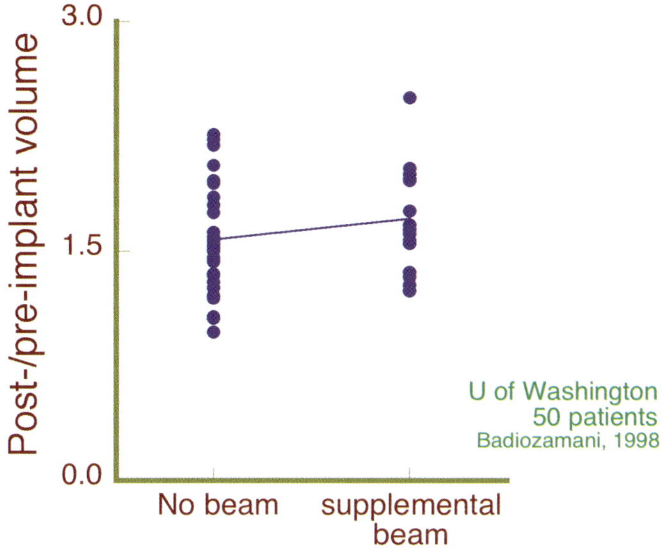

Figure 7-11. Degree of implant-related swelling versus use of pre-implant supplemental external radiation.

In a broad sense, Badiozamani's findings suggest that TMs should be larger for patients with smaller prostate volumes, and should not be influenced by prior hormonal manipulation or external beam radiation. However, no single parameter can accurately predict the degree of swelling for an individual patient. The best solution to the unpredictability of implant-related prostate volume changes is to use generous pre-implant TMs, which minimizes the effect of edema on prostate coverage (**Figures 7-12 and 7-13**).(MERRICK 00)

PROSTATIC REGIONS

Another factor to consider in the choice of pre-implant margins is prostatic cancer regionalization. Cancers occur more frequently in the posterior-lateral regions, where EPE is also more common.(ROSEN, MCNEAL) While it seems logical to use larger treatment margins where EPE is greatest—posterior-laterally and at the base, saturation biopsy studies show a substantial number of anterior cancers, so that TMs should also be generous laterally and anteriorly.(MERRICK 07)

Seminal vesicles

With a typical implant, only the most proximal portion of the seminal vesicle, in the region between the bladder and the prostatic base, receives a

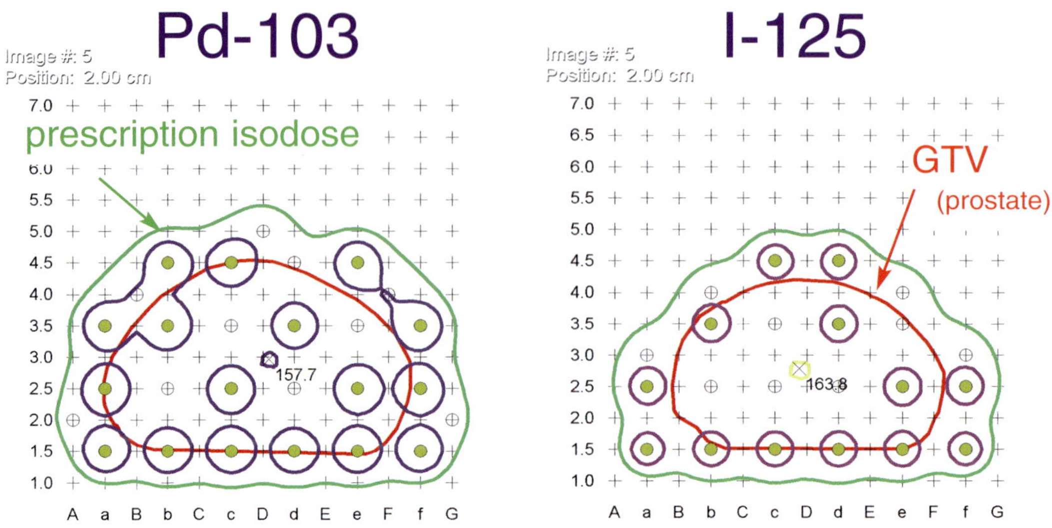

Figure 7-12. Typical mid-prostatic treatment margins used by G. Merrick.

Very important point

The generous treatment margins shown here are needed to achieve the very high cure rates reported by some brachytherapists. (MERRICK 06, DATTOLI 07)

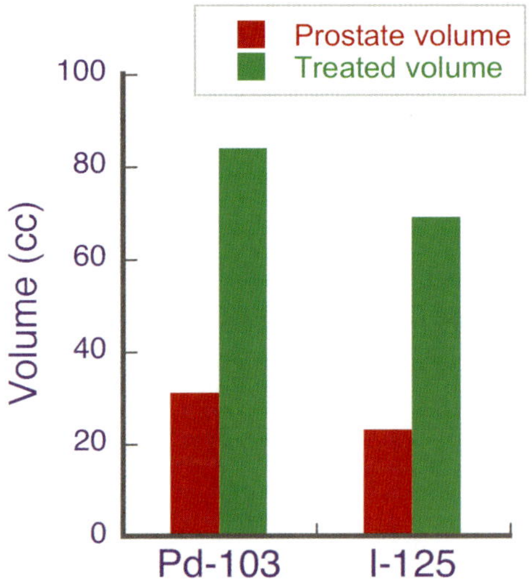

Figure 7-13. GTV versus treated volume for the G Merrick Pd-103 and I-125 plans shown above. Treated volume refers to the total tissue, prostatic and peri-prostatic, that receives the prescripion dose or higher. Note that the treated volume is almost three times as large as the prostate itself!

cancericidal dose (**Figure 7-14**). It's not practical to implant portions of the seminal vesicles that extend cephalad to the base of the prostate, because they move when pushed by a needle tip; seeds deposited in or near the more distal portions of the seminal vesicles tissue tend to bunch up or migrate. Stock and colleagues calculated that seminal vesicle tissue above the top of the prostate typically receives less than 50% of the prescription dose.(STOCK 99) Seminal vesicle biopsies generally target the more cephalad portion of the vesicles, so that finding cancer in such biopsies means that external beam radiation would be needed to achieve cancercidal doses.

Extensive seminal vesicle invasion reaching above the prostate cannot be reliably treated with brachytherapy and may be synonymous with metastatic disease. However, early cases of vesicle invasion, typically limited to the confluence of the vesicles with the vas deferens, would likely be covered with a cancercidal brachytherapy dose.(KESTIN) In drawing the CTV it is, in fact, difficult to separate the seminal vesicles from the posterior prostate and we routinely include the peri-prostatic seminal vesicle within the TV (**Figure 7-4**). Seeds *do* fix properly in the region of the confluence of the seminal vesicles and the ejaculatory ducts, the site of early seminal vesicular cancerous invasion (**Figure 7-15**).(VILLERS) Accordingly, *early* seminal vesicle invasion is probably treatable with brachytherapy, and such patients may be highly curable with an implant alone, in the absence of micrometastases.(STOCK, KESTIN)

Base
In the report by Sohyada and colleagues, radial EPE measurements were largest at the prostatic base, where it seems logical to use larger margins due to a concern for greater ECE, and because the prostatic margins here are less sharply defined on TRUS images.(CROOK 02) The use of more generous margins at the base seems safe, partly because the rectum tends to be further from the prostate at that point.

Mid-prostate
Perhaps smaller TMs can be used at the mid-prostate, because it is sharply visualized and because the rectum appears to limit the geographic posterior ECE extent. However, the authors tend to use greater TMs postero-laterally, where the ECE is greater and where excessive rectal doses are unlikely to occur.

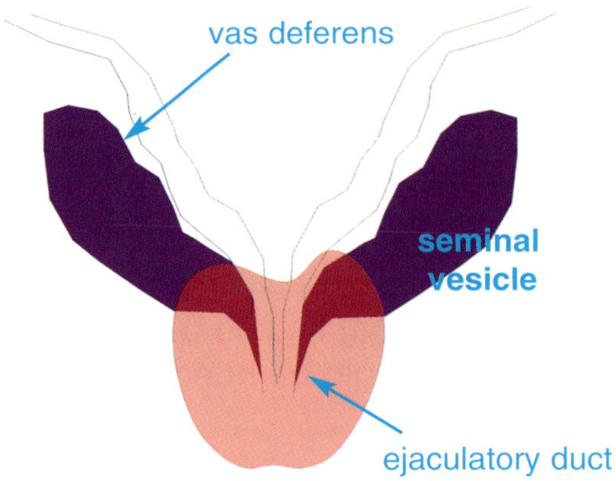

Figure 7-14. Position of seminal vesicles in relation to vas deferens and prostate. That portion of the vesicles most proximal to the prostate is indistinguishable on TRUS from the prostate itself (see Figure 7-15).

Apex
Surgical resection margins are frequently positive at the prostatic apex, in part because tumor can track outside the prostate where the neurovascular bundles pierce the capsule posteriorly.(STAMEY) Because of the risk of tumor extension through the apical region, the apex is drawn generously on the planning images. Extra-prostatic seeds usually "fix" well in the region of the apex, imbedded in the pelvic floor musculature. However, overly aggressive apical treatment margins can lead to a higher risk of urinary incontinence, urethral stricture, sexual impotence, or rectal damage (see Chapters 20-22).

URETHRAL DOSES
Probably the hardest-learned lesson from the early TRUS experience was that of urethral tolerance. In their initial experience, Blasko and colleagues used a homogeneous seed loading pattern, assuming very high urethral tolerance. After several cases of superficial urethral necrosis were seen,

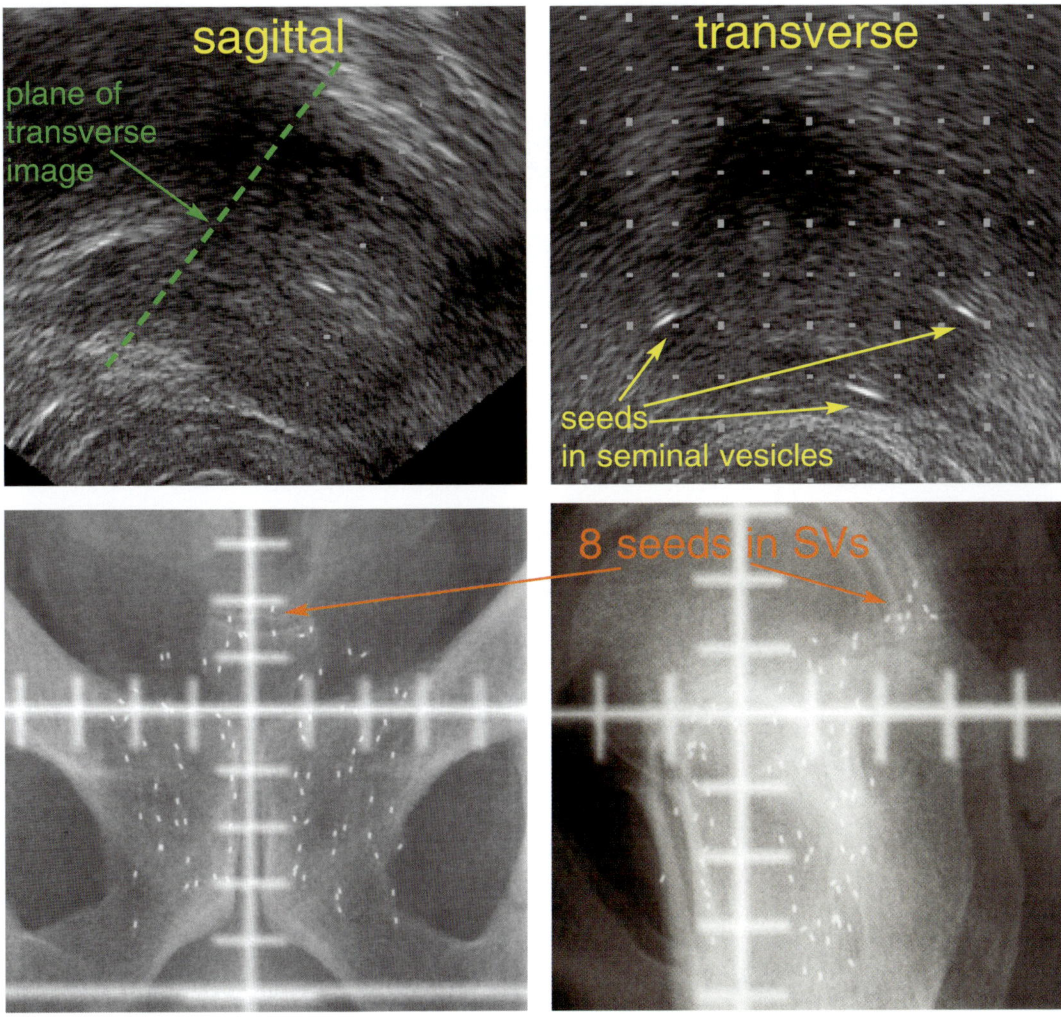

Figure 7-15. A portion of the seminal vesicles are typically included with the prostatic base, so that brachytherapy probably eradicates early vesicle invasion. Some brachytherapists make a conscious effort to place seeds in what appears to be the proximal seminal vesicles. In the upper TRUS images, seeds are visible in seminal vesicle tissue near the prostate. The lower images show plain films of seeds a little further in the seminal vesicles bases.

they switched to peripheral loading (see chapter 15). In 1995, Wallner and colleagues showed that excessive urethral doses were associated with

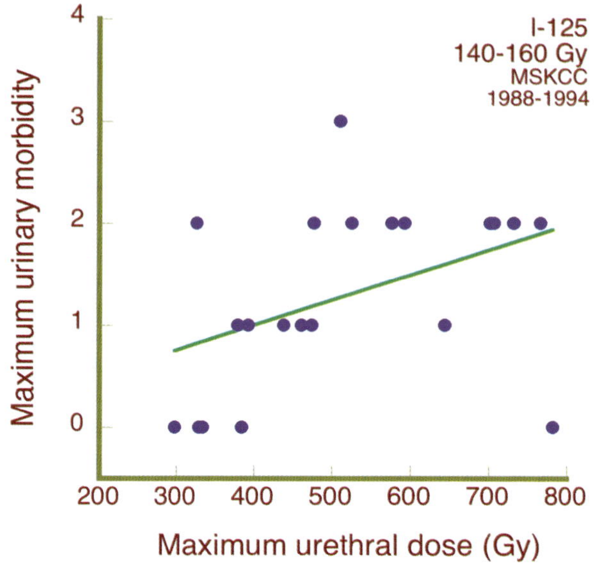

Figure 7-16. RTOG urinary morbidity versus the maximal urethral dose. There was a suggestion of higher morbidity in patients with a higher maximal dose, but with a lot of scatter in the data.(WALLNER 95)

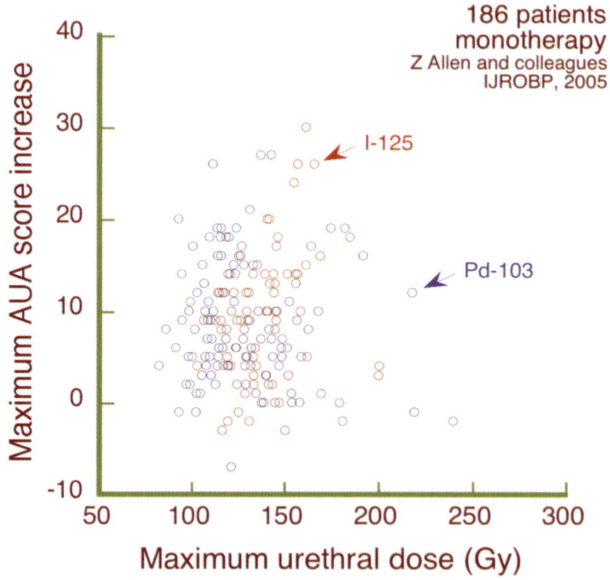

Figure 7-17. With a peripheral loading pattern, the maximal urethral dose is not related to the maximum AUA score increase. (ALLEN)

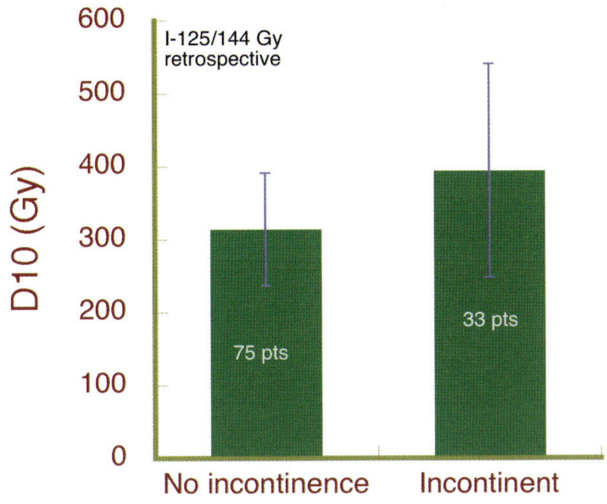

Figure 7-18. Urinary incontrinence versus urethral dose. (MCELVEEN)

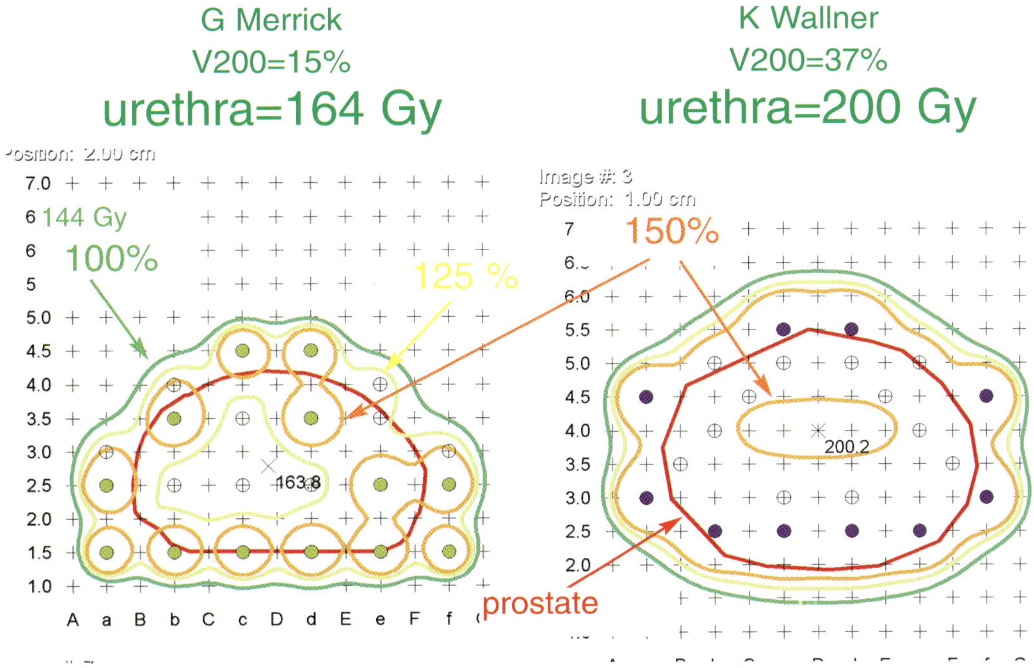

Figure 7-19. Mid-prostate peri-urethral doses for typical 144 Gy I-125 treatment plans by G Merrick or K Wallner. Note that the plans have similar 5-10 mm treatment margins, but that Wallner's V200 and central dose are higher.

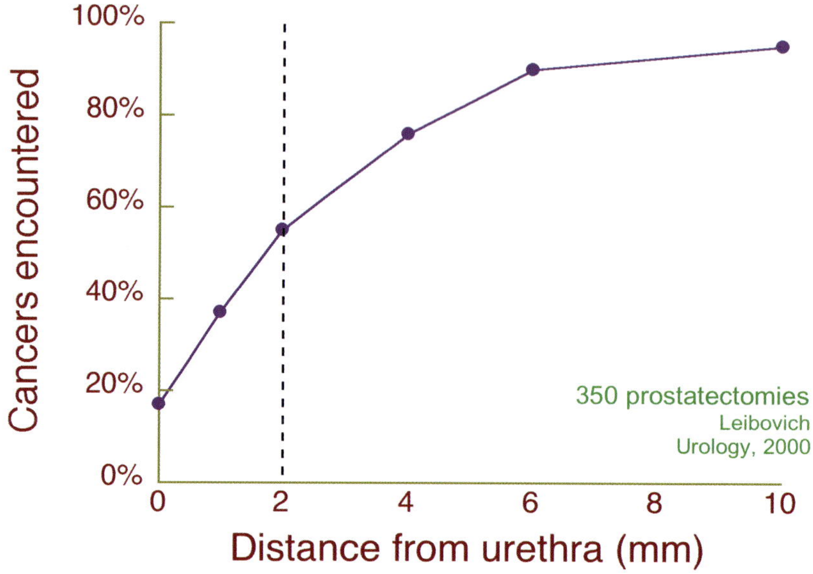

Figure 7-20. Proximity of cancer to the urethra. More than half of cancers are within 2 mm of the urethra. Be careful not to let the peri-urethral doses fall below prescription.

increased urinary morbidity, and recommended that maximal urethral doses be kept below 250% of the prescription dose (**Figure 7-16**).(WALLNER 95)

The correlation between urethral doses and urinary morbidity, first described by Wallner and colleagues, has not been reproduced by others, probably because more recent investigators have consistently used peripheral loading patterns without the extreme central doses characteristic of homogeneous loading patterns. Correlations between urethral dose and morbidity are far less with the less extreme urethral doses seen today(**Figures 7-17 and 7-18**). When doing your treatment planning, a rule of thumb is to keep the urethral dose below 150% of the prescription dose, a goal that is readily met using modified peripheral seed placement patterns (**Figure 7-19**).(MERRICK 00) On the other hand, make sure to keep the urethral dose comfortably *above* the prescription dose, perhaps a minimum of 125% of prescription dose, to allow for the possibility of some seed misplacement and for implant-related prostatic swelling that could bring the

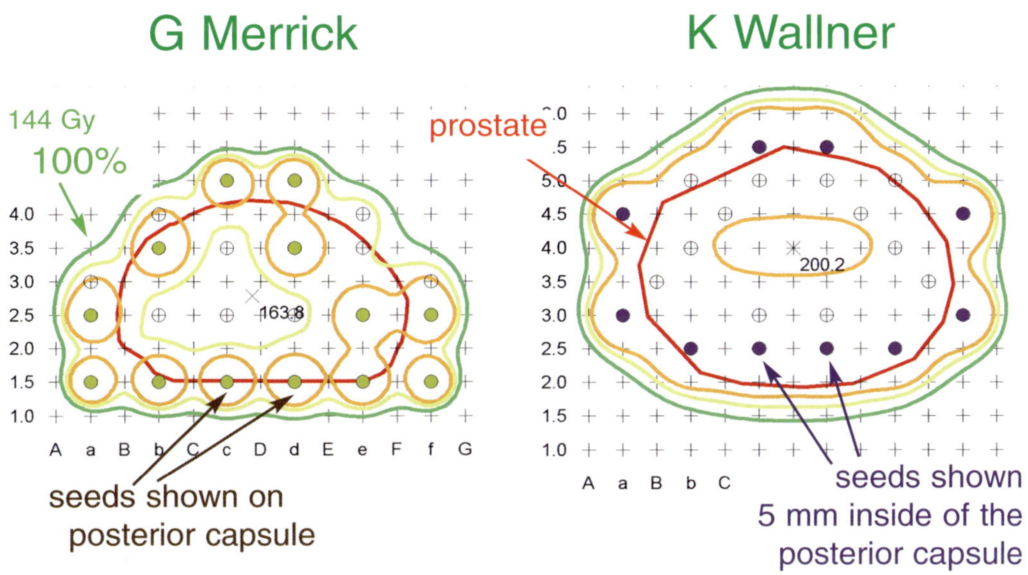

Figure 7-21. These plans show posterior seeds right on posterior prostatic margin (Merrick) or 5 mm inside of the posterior capsule (Wallner). But at the time of implant, the posterior seeds are arbitrarily placed 2-4 mm inside of the capsule by both authors.

central dose below cancericidal levels.(WATERMAN 98, LEIBOVICH) Remember—many cancers are within 2 mm of the urethra (**Figure 7-20**). Don't take "urethral sparing" to the extreme!

> **Very important point**
>
> Do not routinely place seeds at or behind the posterior prostatic margin. Doing so invites excessive R100s.

Some brachytherapists advocate identifying the urethra on the planning images to help avoid placing seeds too near it, but most brachytherapists don't bother. One can assume that it is midline and keep seeds 1 cm or more from the midprostate, because the mid-point dose typically estimates the urethral dose accurately.(WATERMAN 00) If a patient turns out at the time of implant to have a markedly asymmetric urethra, some needle adjustments can be made intra-operatively—typically simply moving one or more needles several mm away from wherever the urethra

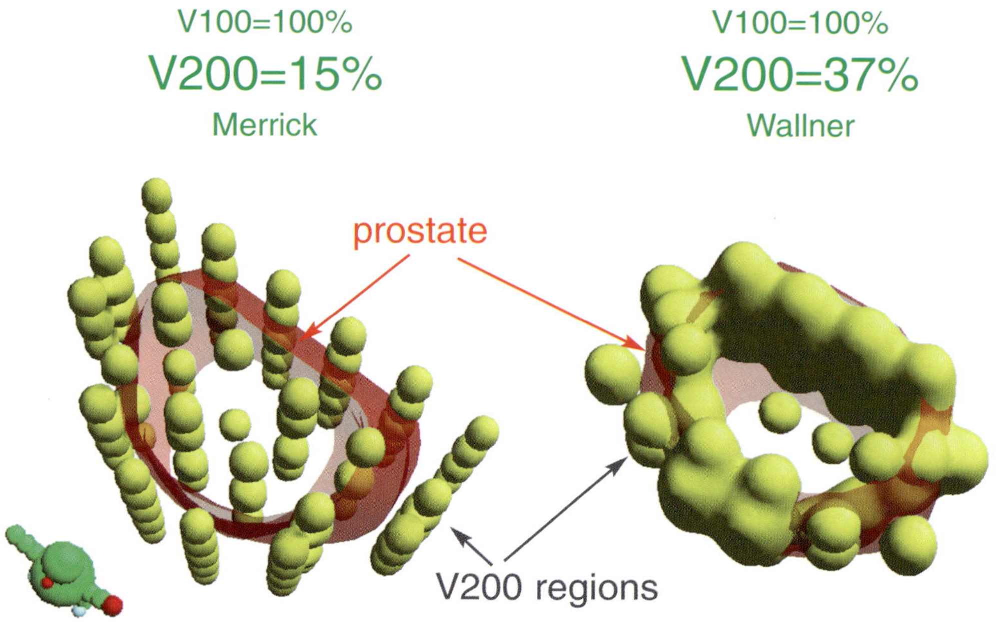

Figure 7-22. Remarkable variability in high dose regions (V200) for implants designed by Merrick versus Wallner, with equal prescription dose coverage (V100=100%). Note that both plans use highly peripheral seed placement with relatively cool central zones. But Wallner's plan has much larger high dose regions at the prostate periphery.

is. This sort of intra-operative adjustment should have no significant effect on the overall prostate coverage.

Rectum

Rectal doses are of substantial concern when designing posterior prostatic coverage. The rectal dose is typically quantified as the R100—the volume of rectum that receives prescription dose or higher. Several investigators have shown that late rectal bleeding is dose related. The general recommendation is to keep the R100 below 1.0 cc (see Chapter 21).(MUELLER, SNYDER)

Going from the treatment plan to the actual seed placement is probably the murkiest part of the treatment plan. Part of the problem is that the commercial programs only allow seed spacing of every 5 mm; finer adjustment of seed location relative to the rectum is not possible. Making the situation even trickier is that the rectum itself is deformed on TRUS images due to probe pressure against it. For these reasons, regardless of what the treatment plan calls for, at the time of implant we typically place the posterior seeds 2-5 mm inside the posterior prostatic margin, generating a posterior treatment margin of 0-3 mm (**Figure 7-21**). Following this policy, posterior prostatic coverage appears sufficient and little of the anterior rectal wall receives the prescription dose or higher. As long as you're careful not to exceed that, oand not to place seeds behind the back edge of the prostate, the chance of serious complications is very small (see chapter 21). It is important to remember, though, that minor errors in seed placement at the time of implantation could substantially increase the final R100. Placing many seeds even one or two mm too posteriorly can be a problem.

HIGH DOSE REGIONS

High dose regions are summarized by acronyms that specify the percent of the prostate covered by a particular dose as a multiple of the prescription dose. For instance, the *V200* refers to the percent of the prostate covered by 200% of the prescription dose.

There has been a wide range of recommended values for high dose regions, with very little clinical correlation for guidance (**Figure 7-22**). Despite a widespread assumption that high dose regions are bad, Jones found no relation between high V200s or V300s and morbidity, as long as the urethral and rectal doses are limited.(JONES) Merrick and colleagues showed a huge variability in planned high dose regions between experienced brachytherapists, most of whom report acceptable morbidity.(MERRICK) High dose regions seem to have no relation to tumor control rates, providing the prostate is covered by the minimal cancercidal dose.(WALLNER 05) Suffice it to say that high dose regions should be minimized only to the degree that doing so does not compromise coverage of the prostate and peri-prostatic region.

TOTAL ACTIVITY

Before the widespread availability of desktop computers and TRUS-based pre-planning, the total activity needed to treat the prostate was determined from standardized tables, based on past clinical experience. The prostatic volume was estimated using three orthogonal dimensions and the total activity was spaced at approximately one cm intervals throughout the prostate.(ANDERSON 76, ANDERSON 91) Most of us now consider the use of

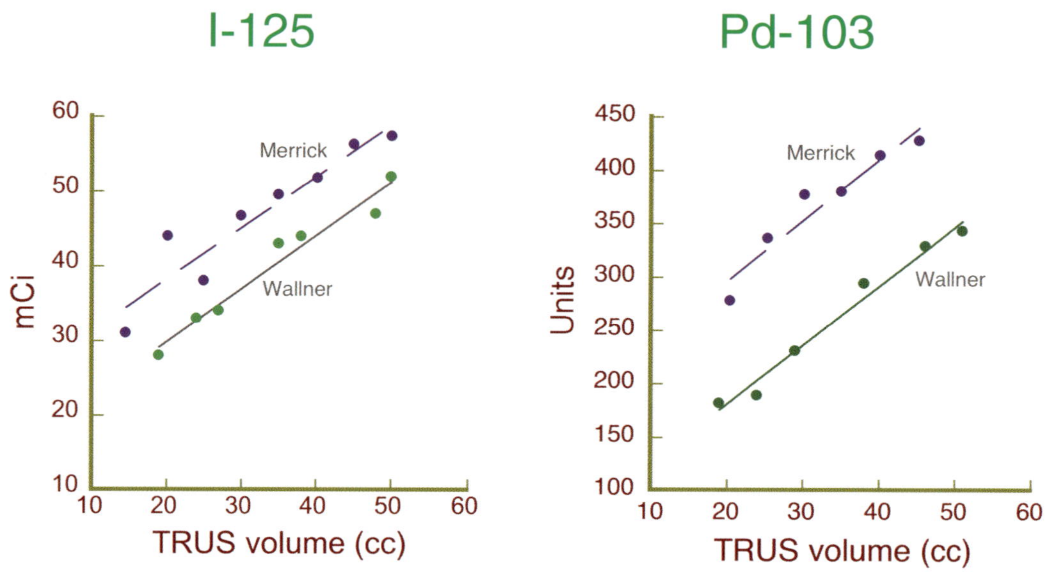

Figure 7-23. Total activity used for I-125 (144 Gy) and Pd-103 (124 Gy) implants by Merrick and Wallner. The scatter and slope of the relationship between prostate volume and total activity will vary, depending on the treatment margins used in the planning process, the degree of peripheral versus homogeneous source placement, and the volume of high dose regions.(mCi and activities are specified according to TG-43 and NIST-99)

standard prostate volume-total activity tables to be Paleolithic-era treatment planning.

Dosimetry for permanent implants is now computerized, and can be closely tailored to an individual patient's prostate. Instead of relying on standard tables, seeds are placed at the prostate periphery to achieve intra-prostate doses and peri-prostatic coverage that is tailored to a particular patient's prostatic volume and shape. After a preliminary seed placement on the computer screen, the target coverage is calculated and seeds are added or deleted interactively to achieve the desired coverage of the entire target periphery.

The total activity needed for an implant increases as the prostate volume increases (**Figure 7-23**). However, the correlation is imperfect because

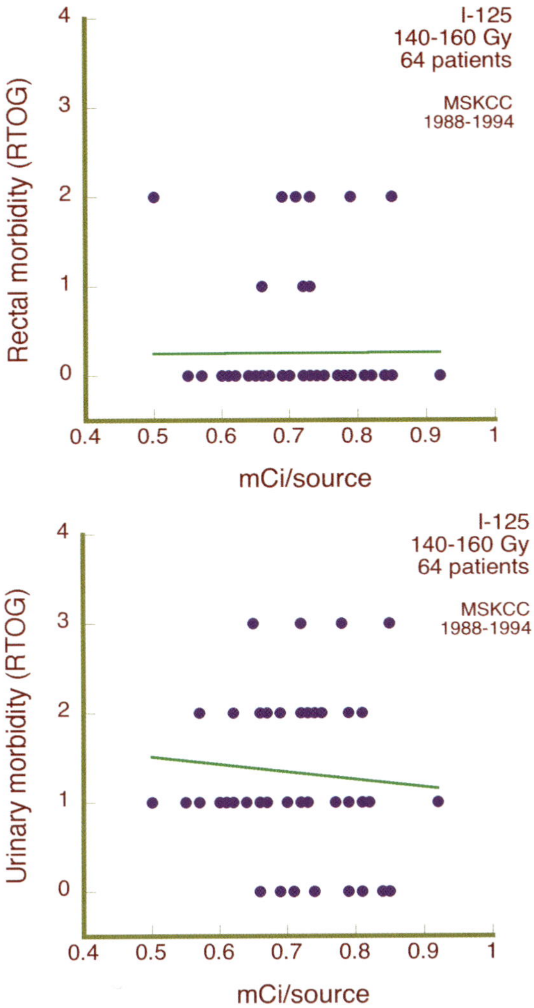

Figure 7-24. There was no relationship between seed strength and the degree of rectal or urethral morbidity following I-125 implantation at MSKCC (140-160 Gy). (RTOG 1=rectal bleeding or minimal urinary symptoms, RTOG 2=rectal ulceration or the need for alpha blockers to relieve urinary symptoms). (WALLNER 95)

the actual activity for a given target volume will depend on the shape of a particular prostate, how much effort is made to minimize the rectal and urethral dose, and how generous the treatment margins are. Adopting the total activity tables of another brachytherapy team should be undertaken with caution. Given the speed and ease with which individualized treatment plans can be custom-generated, volume-activity guidelines are an anachronism.

SEED STRENGTH

A wide variety of seed strengths have been used for prostate brachytherapy, with no clinical evidence of any effect on outcomes. I-125 seeds typ-

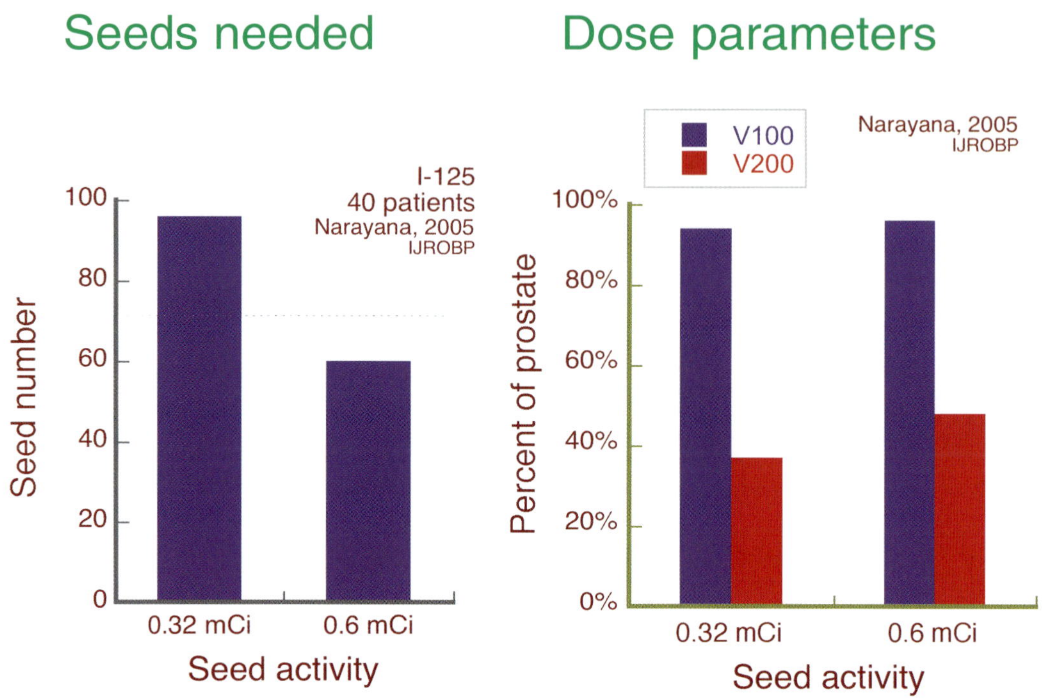

Figure 7-25. V100s, V200s and seed numbers achieved in patient randomized to implantation with lower versus higher activity seeds.(NARAYANA 05) Note that the high dose regions (V200s) are a little higher with higher activity seeds.

ically vary in strength from 0.2 to 0.9 mCi and Pd-103 seeds vary from 2.0 to 4.3 U (NIST-99). Using higher activity seeds reduces the number required.(MAGUIRE) It has been argued that use of high activity seeds could lead to a higher complication rate or less adequate target coverage. Cumes and colleagues analyzed fourteen I-125 patients, concluding that higher activity seeds were more likely to lead to complications.(CUMES) They recommended that individual I-125 seed strength be limited to 0.4 mCi or less. Their data, widely quoted in the early days of ultrasound-based brachytherapy, was scientific garbage. It was derived from patients implanted at Stanford with the retropubic method following recurrence of cancer after external beam radiation or prior retropubic implant. Only seven patients had high activity seeds. Drawing *any* conclusion based on such skimpy data is laughable.

Contrary to the Stanford experience, a detailed analysis of I-125 patients at MSKCC showed no relationship between seed strength and urinary or rectal morbidity (**Figure 7-24**). The MSKCC experience is more convincing than that of Stanford because it is based on many more patients, without previous treatment, and implanted in a fairly uniform fashion. The lack of a relationship between seed strength and morbidity should not be surprising—radiation-related complications result from the dose delivered to significant volumes of sensitive structures, not to the dose delivered in the immediate vicinity of an individual seed.(MUELLER)

One argument for using lower strength seeds is that there may be less likelihood of underdosing if a few seeds are incorrectly placed. With a greater number of lower activity seeds the potential for error is spread out over a greater number of seeds, so that misplacement of a few is of less consequence. This argument has some logical merit. On the other hand are the arguments that fewer, high strength seeds require fewer needle sticks, fewer hot spots around seeds, and fewer seeds near the urethra.

In an effort to better answer the question of optimal seed strength, Narayana and colleagues randomized 40 I-125 patients to implantation with 0.6 mCi versus 0.32 mCi seeds.(NARAYANA 05) They achieved higher V100s using less seeds in patients with greater seed activity (**Figure 7-25**). Most other investigators have concluded that higher activity seeds are superior.(SLOBODA, D'SOUZA, BEAULIEU)

Regardless of the seed strength you use, it is a good idea to keep it low enough to require at least 40 or 50 seeds for an implant. Using less than 40 seeds for an implant seems to place too much emphasis on each seed, such that the loss of two or three could substantially decrease final coverage.

SEED SPACING

There is no evidence that any particular lateral or longitudinal spacing is advantageous. Ultrasound templates are constructed with 5.0 mm spacing between needles. Some brachytherapists prefer to maintain a minimum 5.0 mm end-to-end spacing between seeds, but there is no evidence that end-to-end placement has any detrimental effect. It's where the *isodoses* are, not the seed separation *per se*, that determines outcome.

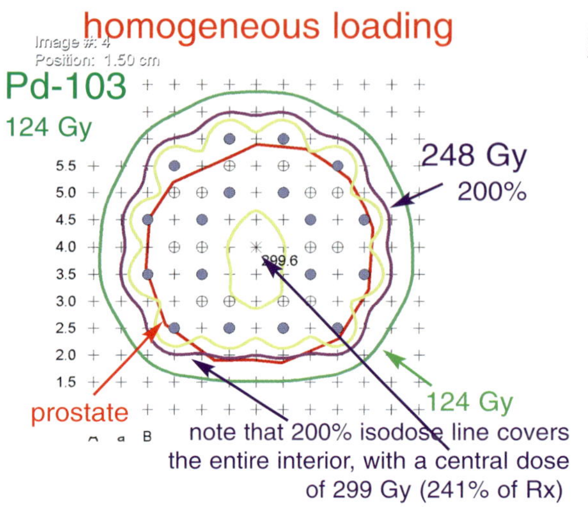

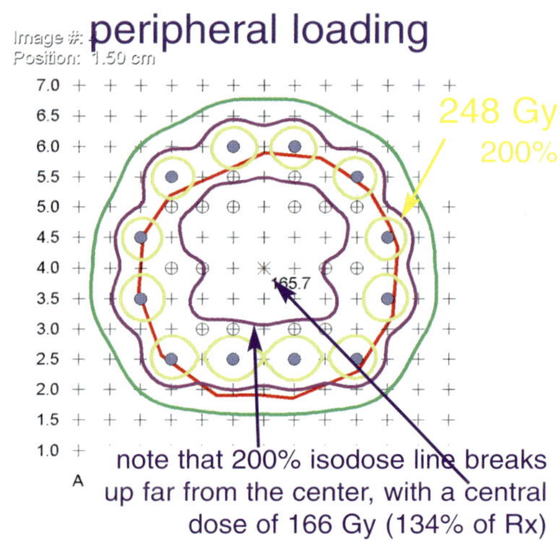

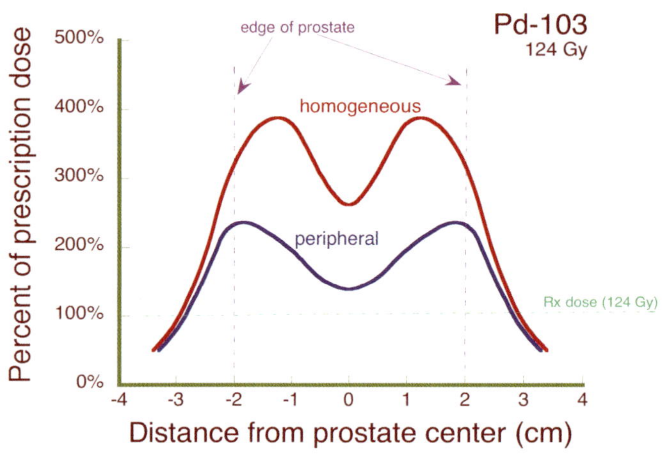

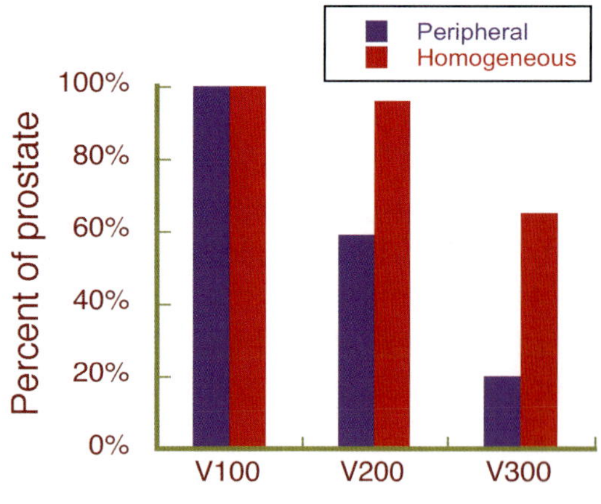

Figure 7-26. Homogenous versus peripheral loading patterns for Pd-103. The homogeneous pattern (top left) achieves the intended 5 mm TM using 108 1.9 mCi sources, but with central doses almost four times the prescription dose (left). By removing 26 sources from the center of the prostate, the central doses are decreased to about twice the prescription dose, with very little effect on the treatment margin. The most striking difference between the two placement patterns is the larger high dose regions within the prostate (bottom left).

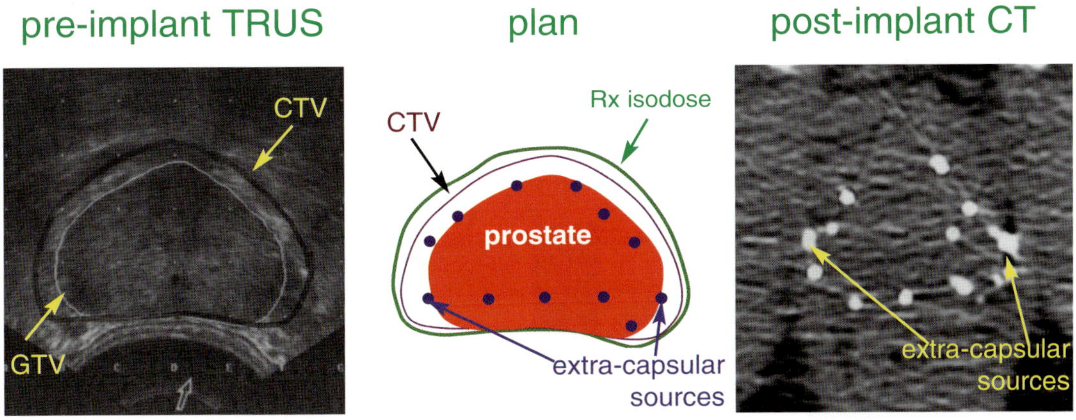

Figure 7-27. M. Dattoli and G Merrick have long advocated placing sources 1–5 mm outside of the prostatic capsule to achieve wide treatment margins.(DATTOLI, MERRICK 00)

TARGETING THE TUMOR

Prostatic carcinoma is multifocal in 50% to 80% of cases, so that the entire prostate should be treated to the prescription dose.(MCNEAL, MERRICK 07) It has been suggested that more activity be placed where tumor is known to exist and there is a certain degree of common sense to doing so. Advances in radiographic imaging could allow targeting of specific tumor sites within the prostate, but we're not there yet.(ZAIDER) In practice, brachytherapists commonly place several extra seeds "ad hoc" in known tumor-bearing areas at the time of the procedure. This practice is generally safe, but it's probably best to keep extra seeds away from the urethra and rectum.

HOMOGENEOUS VERSUS PERIPHERAL LOADING

Seeds can be distributed in a regular pattern throughout the prostate or kept toward the periphery. While a homogeneous pattern is conceptually appealing, it leads to excessive urethral doses, easily exceeding 400% of the prescription dose and leading to increased urinary morbidity.(WALLNER 95)

Limiting seeds to the periphery, the prostatic margins can be treated adequately, without excessive central doses (**Figures 7-26**).(NARAYANA) *Pure* peripheral loading is not practical because with larger prostates, especially, the central portion of the gland may be under-dosed if *all* seeds were at the periphery. In fact, the current norm is neither pure peripheral nor pure

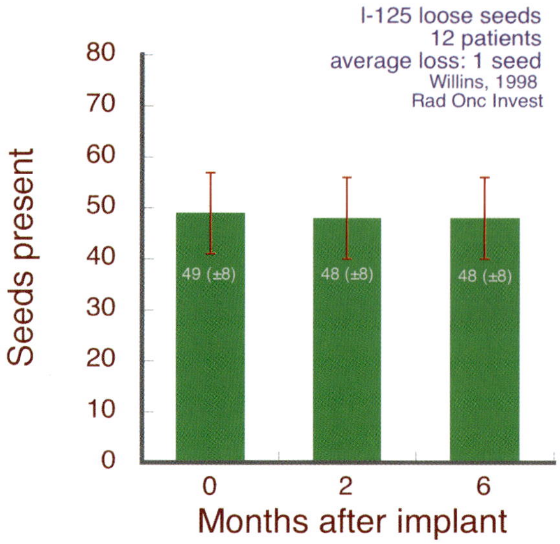

Figure 7-28. Seeds remaining at two and six months after implantation. (WILLINS 98)

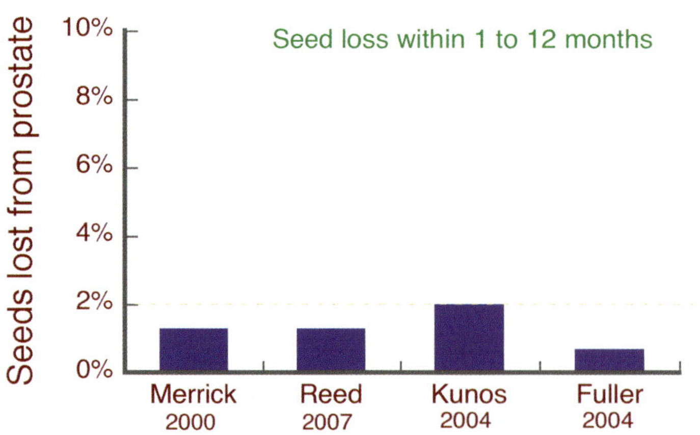

Figure 7-29. Percent of implanted seeds lost from the prostate and peri-prostatic region, from 1 to 12 months after implantation. Note that less than 1 in 50 seeds typically are lost.

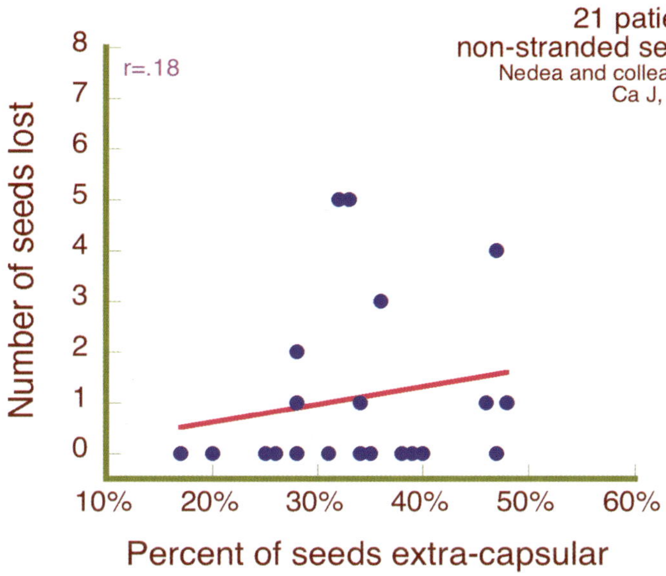

Figure 7-30. There is minimal relationship between the number of extra-prostate seeds and the number lost.

homogenous loading, but a *modified peripheral loading.*(MERRICK 00) With modified peripheral loading the central dose is kept below 150-200% of the prescription dose, minimizing the likelihood of urinary morbidity.

EXTRA-PROSTATIC SEEDS

One of most contentious seed placement issues is the use of extra-prostatic seeds. Many brachytherapists refrain from placing seeds outside of the prostate, because there has long been a perception that extra-prostatic seeds were likely to migrate to the retroperitoneum or lungs. While a small number of seeds do wind up in the pulmonary vasculature, extra-prostatic seeds generally do *not* migrate, a phenomenon that has been extensively documented (**Figures 7-27 through 7-29**).(MERRICK 00, WILLINS 98, NEDEA)

Nedea and colleagues did a meticulous analysis of seed loss from the day of implantation and at 30 days post-implant, using serial CT and MR images to quantify the number of extra-prostatic seeds placed versus the number of seeds lost. Even with 35% of seeds placed extra-capsularly, less than 5% were lost between day 0 and day 30.(NEDEA) There was no

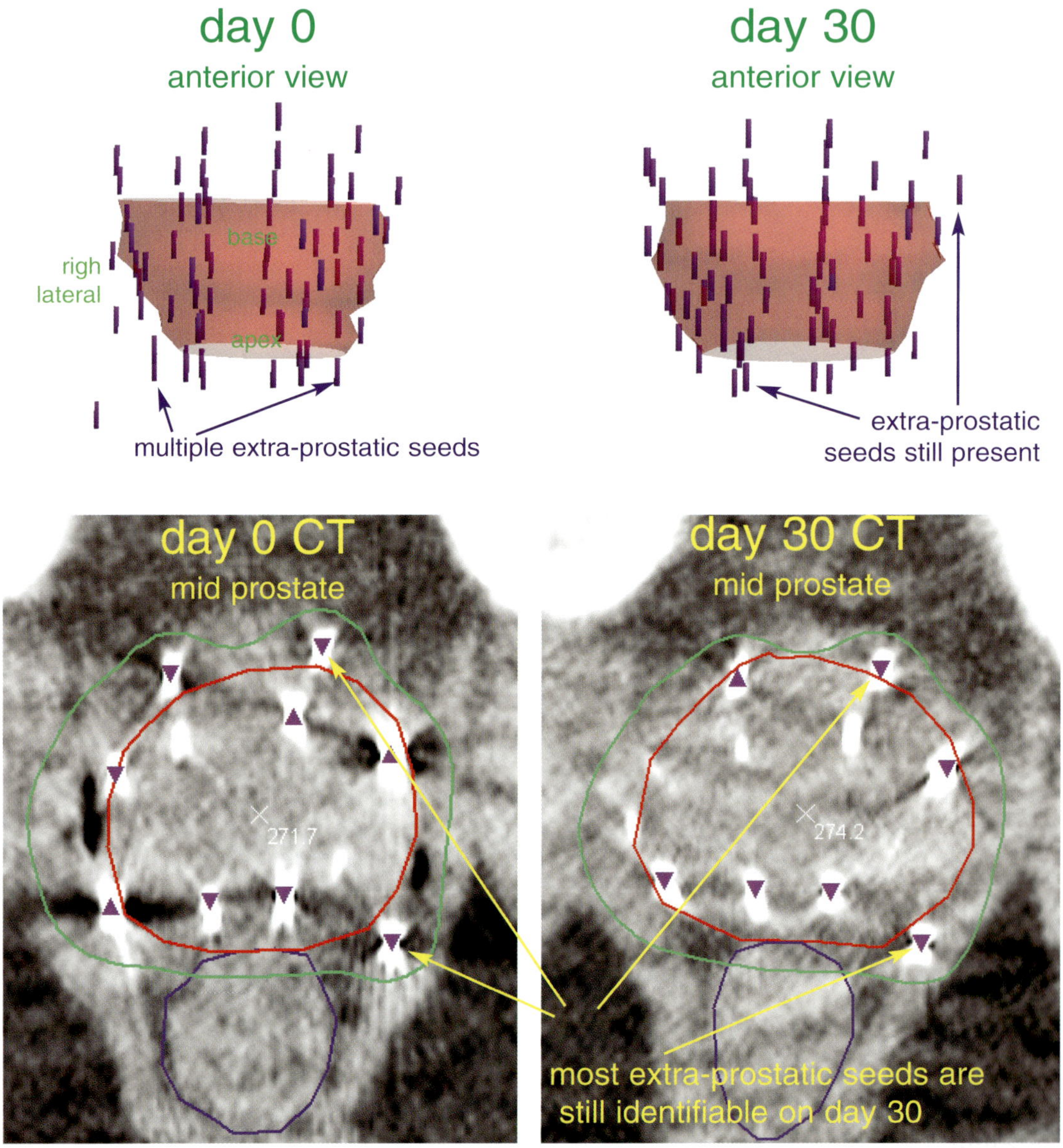

Figure 7-31. Representative case from Nedea and colleagues, showing 3-D views (top), and mid-prostatic CT images on day 0 and day 30. This patient had 33 extra-prostatic seeds (48% of 69 total seeds) and a V100 of 100% on day 0. He lost one seed between day 0 and day 30.

relationship between the number of seeds lost and the percent of seeds that were placed extra-capsularly (**Figures 7-30 and 7-31**). Apparently, seeds are well imbedded in the peri-prostatic tissue, whether it is the pelvic floor musculature near the apex, or the peri-prostatic connective tissue and muscle.

The rationale for placing seeds outside is that the extra-prostatic coverage can be extended, keeping urethral doses within acceptable limits. A brief perusal of plans later in this chapter shows that the prescription isodose is typically 4–5 mm outside of the most peripheral seeds of the implant, so that achieving a 5 mm treatment margin around the prostate requires seeds at (or outside of) the edge of the prostate. Davis and colleagues showed that maximal ECE may be treatable without the use of extra-prostatic seeds, but many brachytherapists use them routinely.(DAVIS 00).

SEED PLACEMENT MADE EASY

Okay, okay. Take a break. Yes, there is a bewildering maze of treatment planning minutiae with a lot of yet-to-be-resolved issues. But in routine practice, as we now know it, treatment planning is actually a quick and easy procedure. With computer-based planning, seed placement can be quickly optimized to minimize the central dose, while achieving the prescription dose at the prostatic periphery. And while one could spend endless hours agonizing over a millimeter or two here or there, such agonizing isn't really called for, since we don't know precisely where the treatment margins *should* be.

While there are no hard and fast rules for seed placement, some general rules of thumb can help keep things simple. First, keep the right and left sides of the prostate symmetric. Second, avoid placing seeds near the urethra. Third, when possible, avoid needles with less than three seeds, to minimize the number of needles required.

Seeds should be placed first around the periphery, at 1.0 cm spacing and keeping within 2–5 mm from the prostatic margin. Seeds at the periphery alone often will not give adequate coverage of the entire volume. So additional seeds are then placed more centrally and/or peripherally until adequate target coverage is achieved, with acceptable central doses.

Although there are commercially available automatic seed placement programs, with modern treatment planning systems the process can be com-summary list of each needle

VariSeed: Needle Loading Report [Page 1]

VA Puget Sound · 567 · 1 · 9/29/2006 1:43:46 PM

Name: **1GMexample, Richard** PID: **05-531** Dept. ID:	Study: **0.414 mCi I-125** Variation: **KW modified** Images: **9** Template: **Siemens Alternate**	Source: **I-125 (6711) [NIST 99]** Comment: Sources: **87** Anisotropy: **Factors (Point Model)** Source Activity: **0.526 U [0.414 mCi]**
Procedure Date: **10/11/2005**	Prescription Dose: **144.0 Gy**	Total Activity: **45.762 U [36.033 mCi]**

template face shows where each needle to to be inserted on actual template

	Needle Number	Retraction (cm)	Hole Location	Number Seeds
	1	0.00	c4.5	5
	2	0.00	d4.5	5
	3	0.50	b4.0	4
	4	0.50	e4.0	4
●	*5*	*0.00*	*b3.5*	*3*
●	*6*	*0.00*	*c3.5*	*4*
●	*7*	*0.00*	*d3.5*	*3*
●	*8*	*0.00*	*e3.5*	*4*
	9	0.50	a3.0	3
	10	0.50	f3.0	3
	11	0.00	a2.5	4
●	*12*	*0.00*	*b2.5*	*4*
●	*13*	*0.00*	*c2.5*	*2*
●	*14*	*0.00*	*d2.5*	*4*
●	*15*	*0.00*	*e2.5*	*3*
	16	0.00	f2.5	4
	17	0.00	a1.5	4
	18	0.00	b1.5	5
	19	0.00	c1.5	5
	20	0.00	d1.5	5
	21	0.00	e1.5	5
	22	0.00	f1.5	4

● = *Special loading*

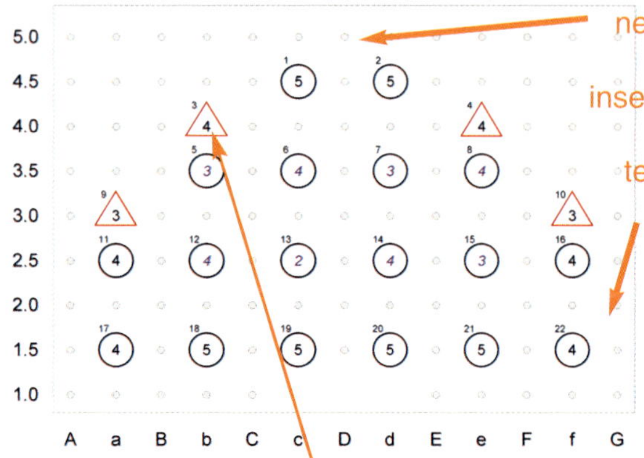

Retraction Legend					
Plane 0	Plane 1	Plane 2	Plane 3	Plane 4	Special
0.00 cm	0.50 cm	1.00 cm	1.50 cm	2.00 cm	Other
○	△	□	◇	▽	○

shapes represent retraction plane for first seed in the needle

Number of Needles	Seeds per needle
1	2
5	3
10	4
6	5

Plan Summary	
Total Activity [U]	45.76
Total Activity [mCi]	36.03
Total Needles	22
Total Seeds	87
Extra Seeds	
Total Seeds to Order	

dosimetrist and physician signature lines

Study Created by ________________________

Study Approved by ________________________

VariSeed 7.1 (Build 2780) fff3 a34b 9bc2 df9f 0330 2980 1a

Figure 7-32a. Print-out of needle loading for an I-125 plan used by G. Merrick.

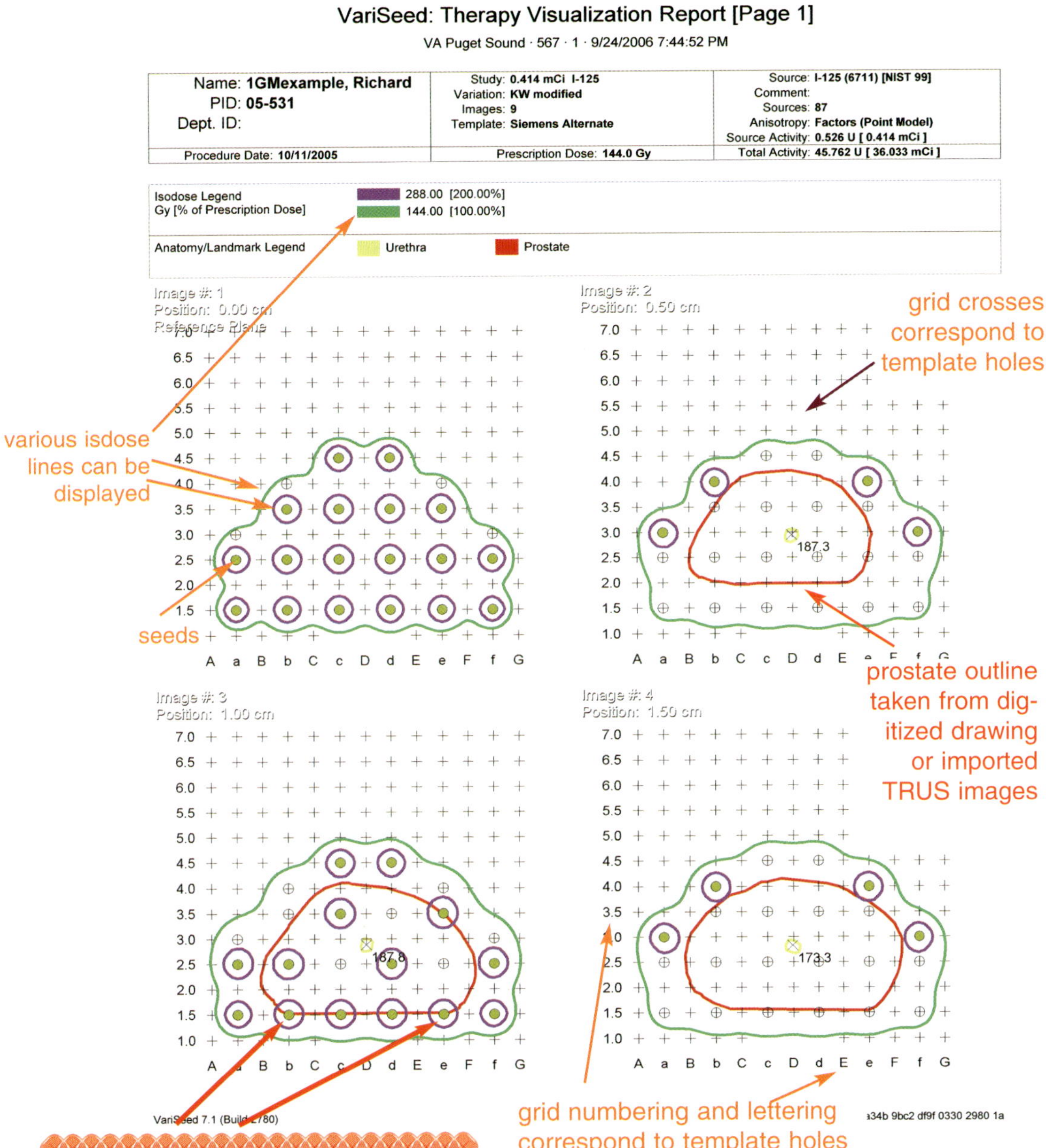

Very important point

Remember! These posterior seeds are moved 2-3 mm inside of the prostate at the time of the procedure.

Figure 7-32b. Print-out of source placement within each TRUS plane.

VariSeed: Needle Loading Report [Page 2]

VA Puget Sound · 567 · 1 · 10/4/2006 2:41:03 PM

Name: **1GMexample, Richard** PID: **05-531** Dept. ID:	Study: **0.414 mCi I-125** Variation: **KW modified** Images: **9** Template: **Siemens Alternate**	Source: **I-125 (6711) [NIST 99]** Comment: Sources: **87** Anisotropy: **Factors (Point Model)** Source Activity: **0.526 U [0.414 mCi]**
Procedure Date: **10/11/2005**	Prescription Dose: **144.0 Gy**	Total Activity: **45.762 U [36.033 mCi]**

Needle Number	Retraction (cm)	Hole Location	Number Seeds
1	0.00	c4.5	5
2	0.00	d4.5	5
3	0.50	b4.0	4
4	0.50	e4.0	4
● *5*	*0.00*	*b3.5*	*3*
● *6*	*0.00*	*c3.5*	*4*
● *7*	*0.00*	*d3.5*	*3*
● *8*	*0.00*	*e3.5*	*4*
9	0.50	a3.0	3
10	0.50	f3.0	3
11	0.00	a2.5	4
● *12*	*0.00*	*b2.5*	*4*
● *13*	*0.00*	*c2.5*	*2*
● *14*	*0.00*	*d2.5*	*4*
● *15*	*0.00*	*e2.5*	*3*
16	0.00	f2.5	4
17	0.00	a1.5	4
18	0.00	b1.5	5
19	0.00	c1.5	5
20	0.00	d1.5	5
21	0.00	e1.5	5
22	0.00	f1.5	4

● = *Special loading*

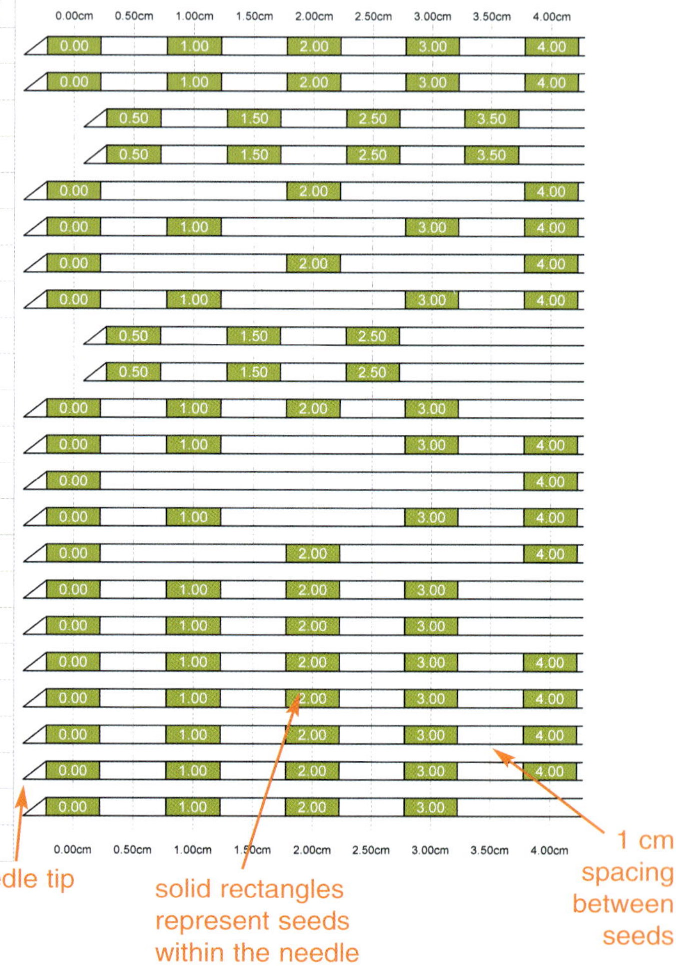

VariSeed 7.1 (Build 2780)

fff3 a34b 9bc2 df9f 0330 2980 1a

Figure 7-32c. Print-out of individual needle loading. This is used for pre-loading needles, or to visualize seed spacing to be accomplished via the Mick Applicator.

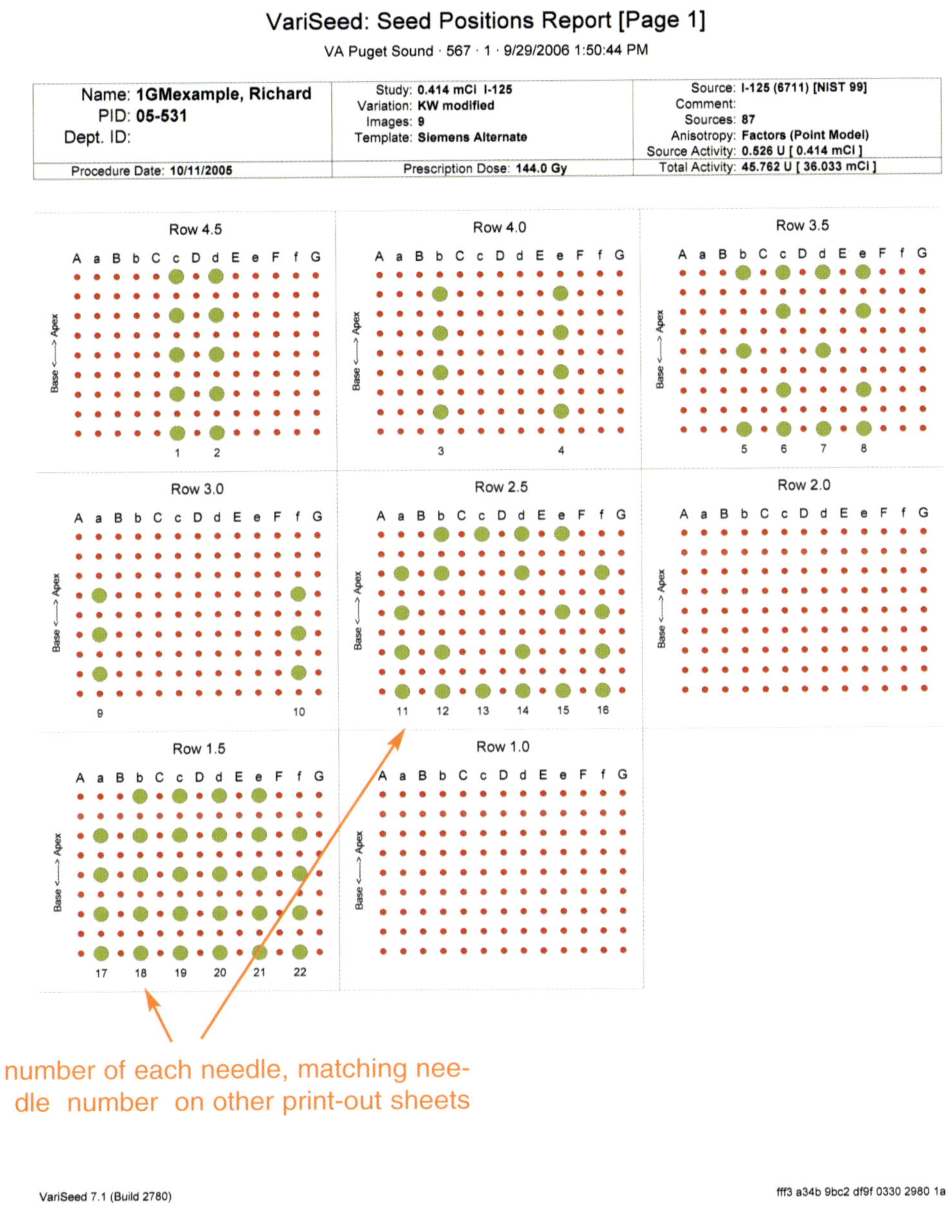

Figure 7-32d. Print-out of top view of seed positioning within each needle.

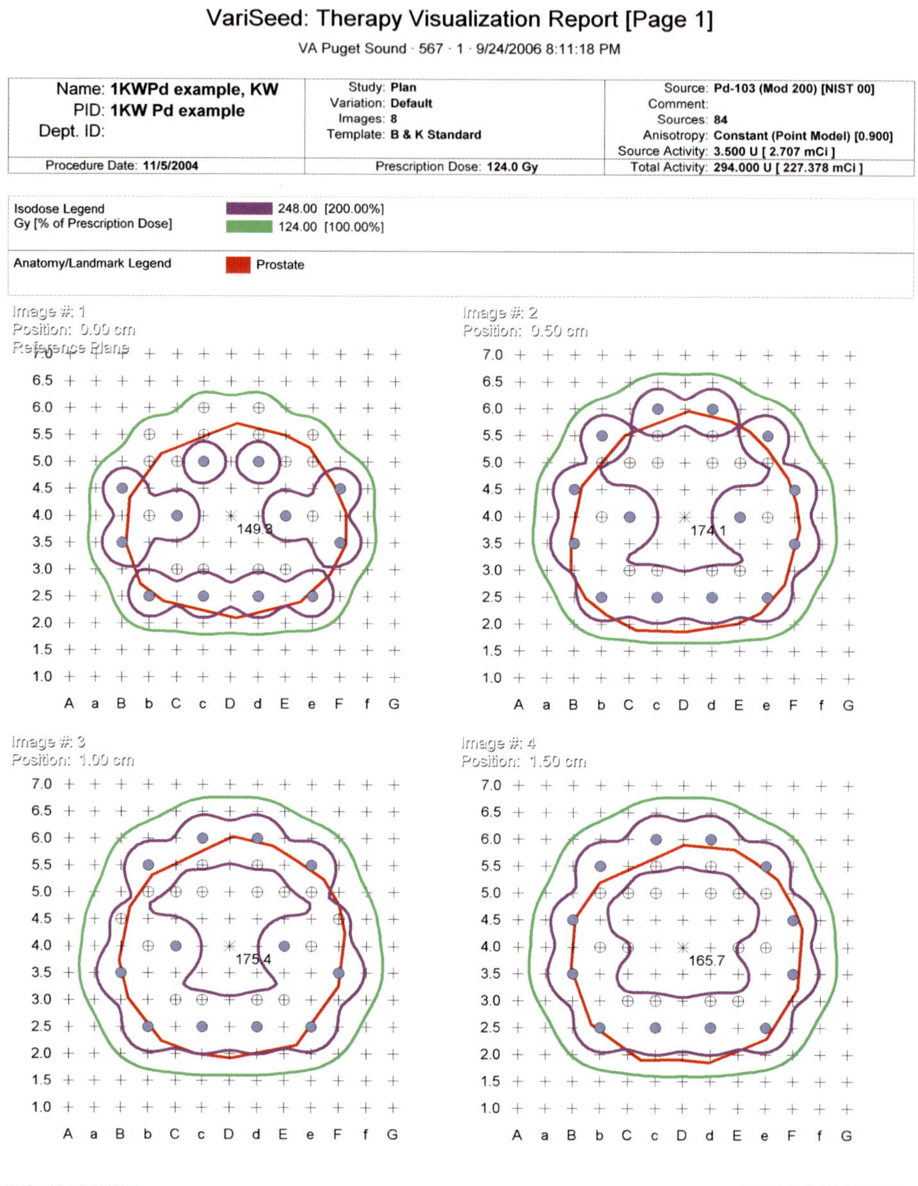

Figure 7-33. Example of Pd-103 monotherapy by K. Wallner. Note similar TMs but larger V200 regions than that used by G. Merrick.

VariSeed: Therapy Visualization Report [Page 2]

VA Puget Sound · 567 · 1 · 9/24/2006 8:14:48 PM

Name: **1KWPd example, KW** PID: **1KW Pd example** Dept. ID:	Study: **Plan** Variation: **Default** Images: **8** Template: **B & K Standard**	Source: **Pd-103 (Mod 200) [NIST 00]** Comment: Sources: **84** Anisotropy: **Constant (Point Model) [0.900]** Source Activity: **3.500 U [2.707 mCi]**
Procedure Date: **11/5/2004**	Prescription Dose: **124.0 Gy**	Total Activity: **294.000 U [227.378 mCi]**

Isodose Legend Gy [% of Prescription Dose]	248.00 [200.00%] 124.00 [100.00%]
Anatomy/Landmark Legend	Prostate

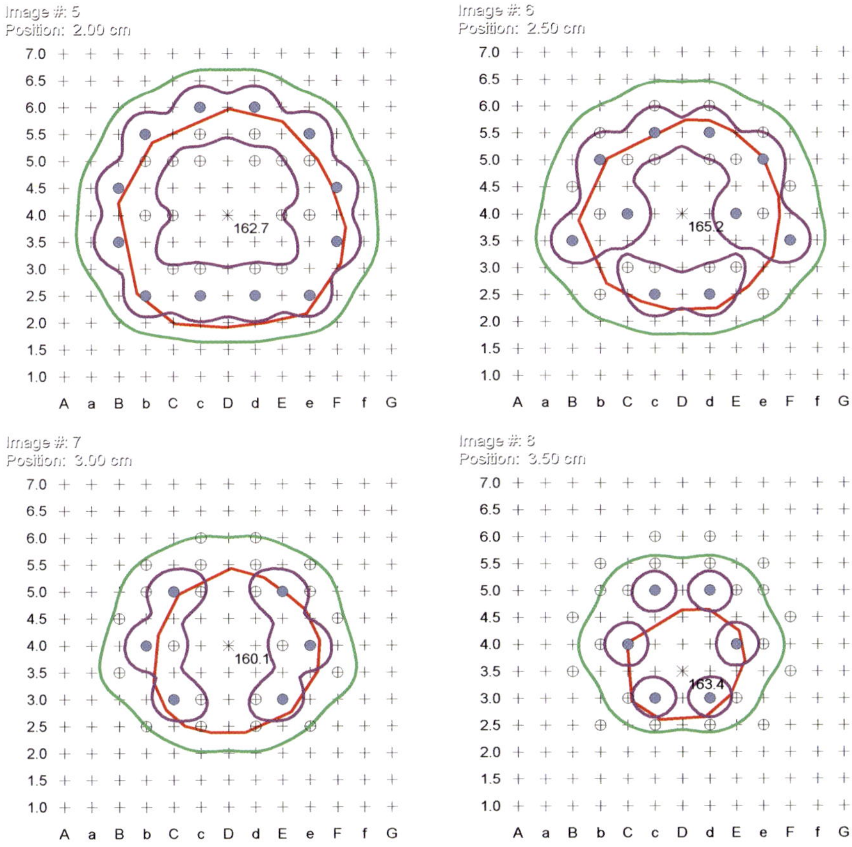

VariSeed 7.1 (Build 2780) fff3 a34b 9bc2 df9f 0330 2980 1a

Figure 7-33 continued.

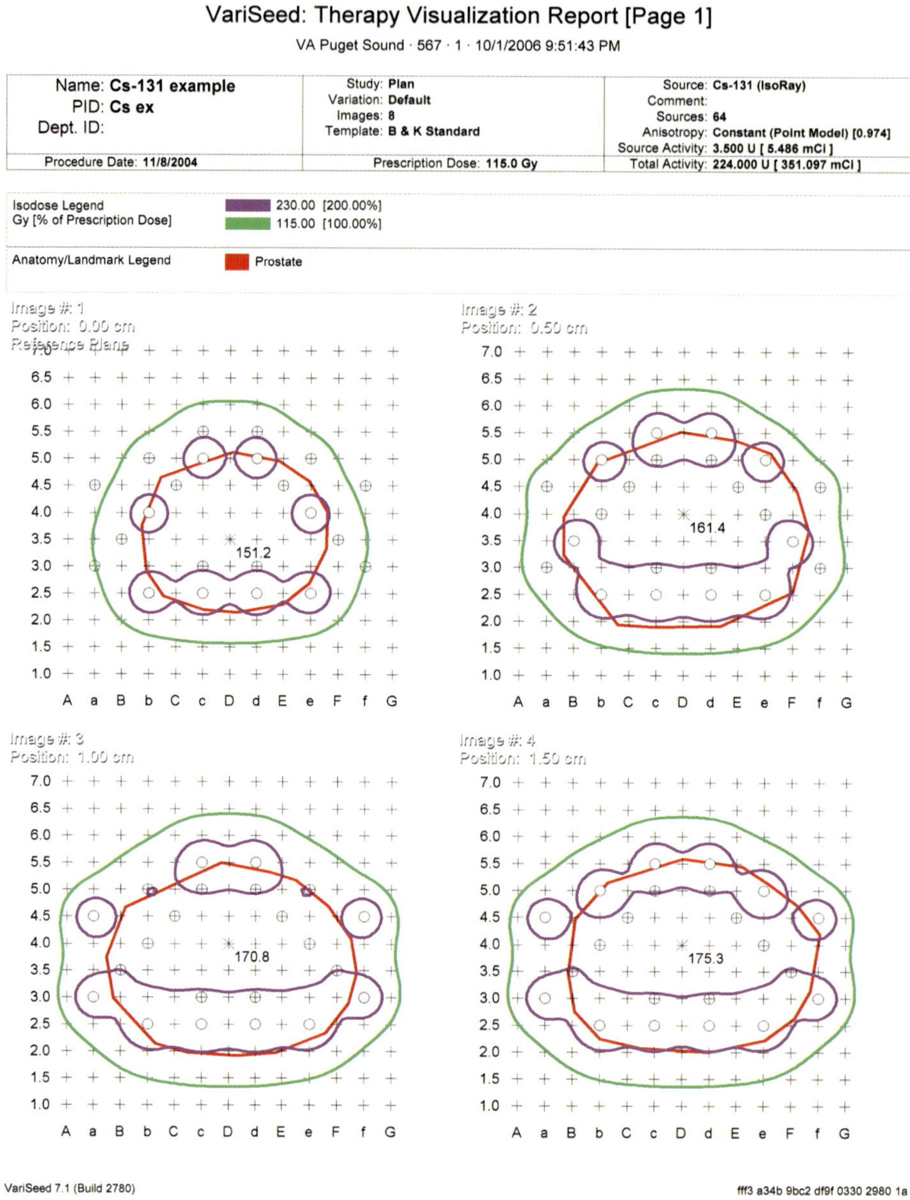

Figure 7-34. Example of Cs-103 monotherapy by K. Wallner.

VariSeed: Therapy Visualization Report [Page 2]

VA Puget Sound · 567 · 1 · 10/1/2006 9:55:10 PM

Name: **Cs-131 example** PID: **Cs ex** Dept. ID:	Study: **Plan** Variation: **Default** Images: **8** Template: **B & K Standard**	Source: **Cs-131 (IsoRay)** Comment: Sources: **64** Anisotropy: **Constant (Point Model) [0.974]** Source Activity: **3.500 U [5.486 mCi]**
Procedure Date: **11/8/2004**	Prescription Dose: **115.0 Gy**	Total Activity: **224.000 U [351.097 mCi]**

Isodose Legend Gy [% of Prescription Dose]	230.00 [200.00%] 115.00 [100.00%]
Anatomy/Landmark Legend	Prostate

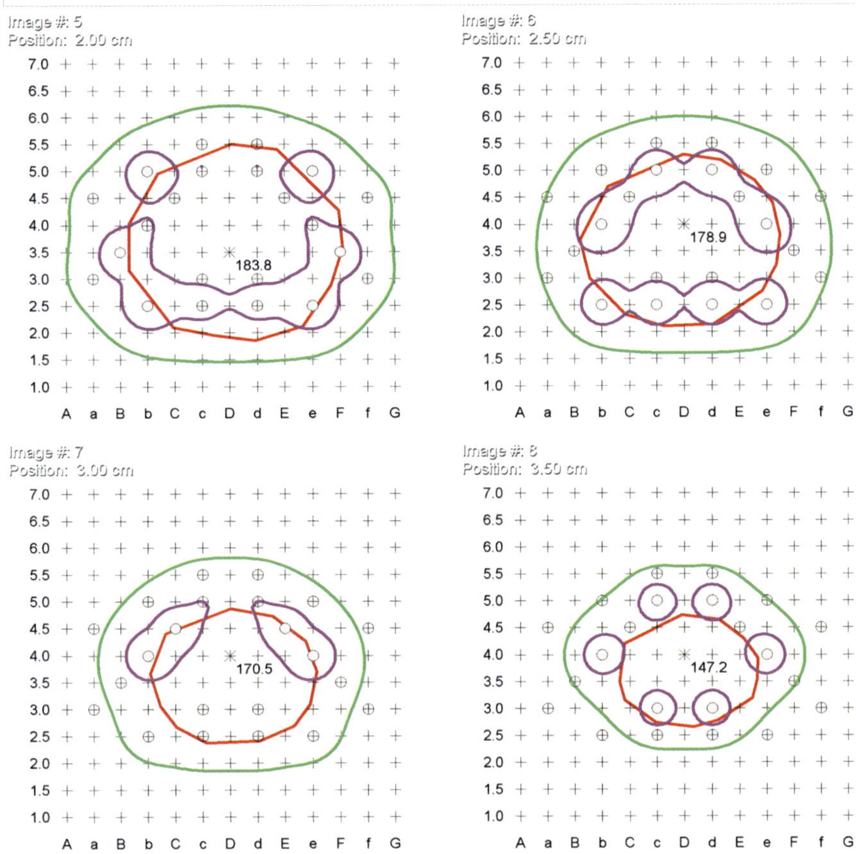

VariSeed 7.1 (Build 2780)

fff3 a34b 9bc2 df9f 0330 2980 1a

Figure 7-34 continued.

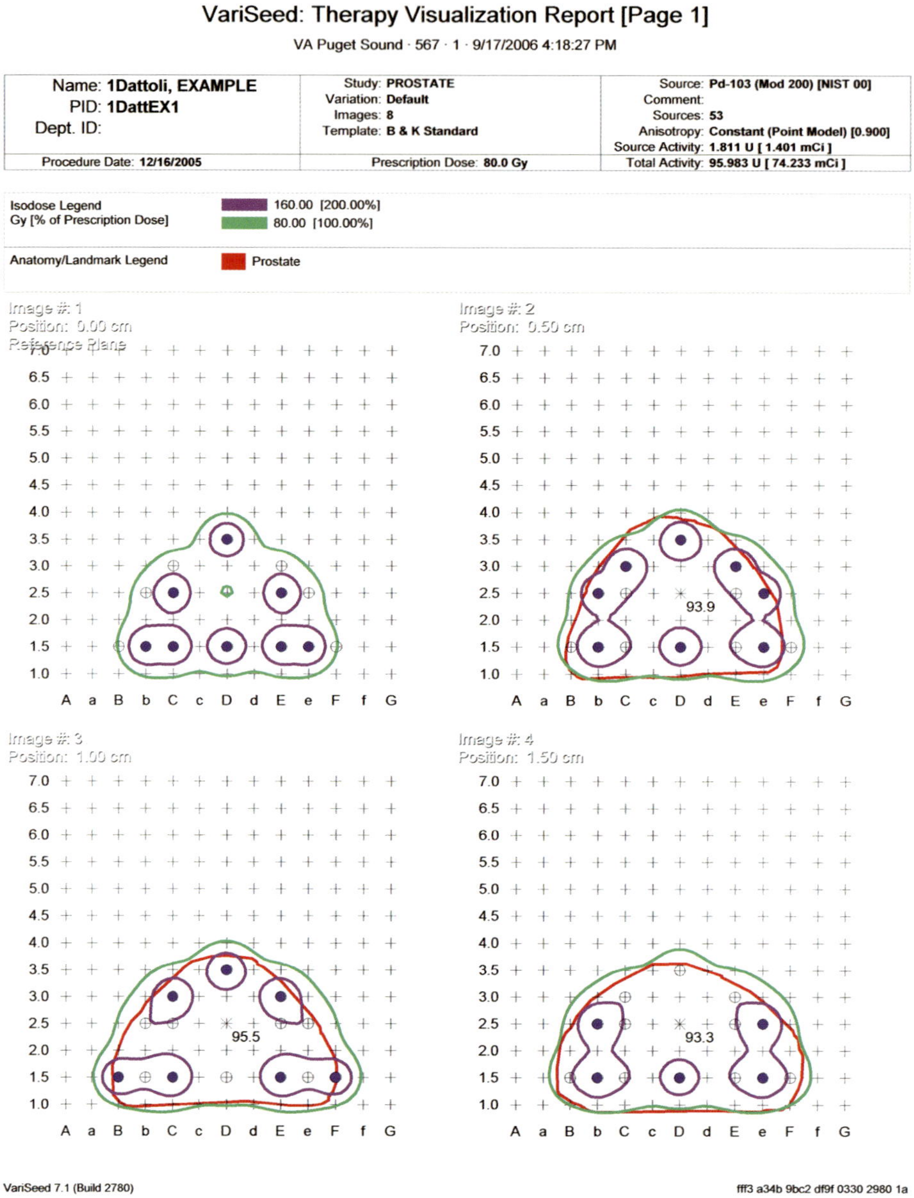

Figure 7-35. Example 80 Gy Pd-103 boost by M. Dattoli. Note slightly smaller TMs and larger V200 regions than that used by G. Merrick. Also note the placement of seeds superior to identifiable prostate.

VariSeed: Therapy Visualization Report [Page 2]

VA Puget Sound · 567 · 1 · 9/18/2006 10:10:43 PM

Name: **1Dattoli, EXAMPLE** PID: **1DattEX1** Dept. ID:	Study: **PROSTATE** Variation: **Default** Images: **8** Template: **B & K Standard**	Source: **Pd-103 (Mod 200) [NIST 00]** Comment: Sources: **53** Anisotropy: **Constant (Point Model) [0.900]** Source Activity: **1.811 U [1.401 mCi]**
Procedure Date: **12/16/2005**	Prescription Dose: **80.0 Gy**	Total Activity: **95.983 U [74.233 mCi]**

Isodose Legend Gy [% of Prescription Dose]	160.00 [200.00%] 80.00 [100.00%]
Anatomy/Landmark Legend	Prostate

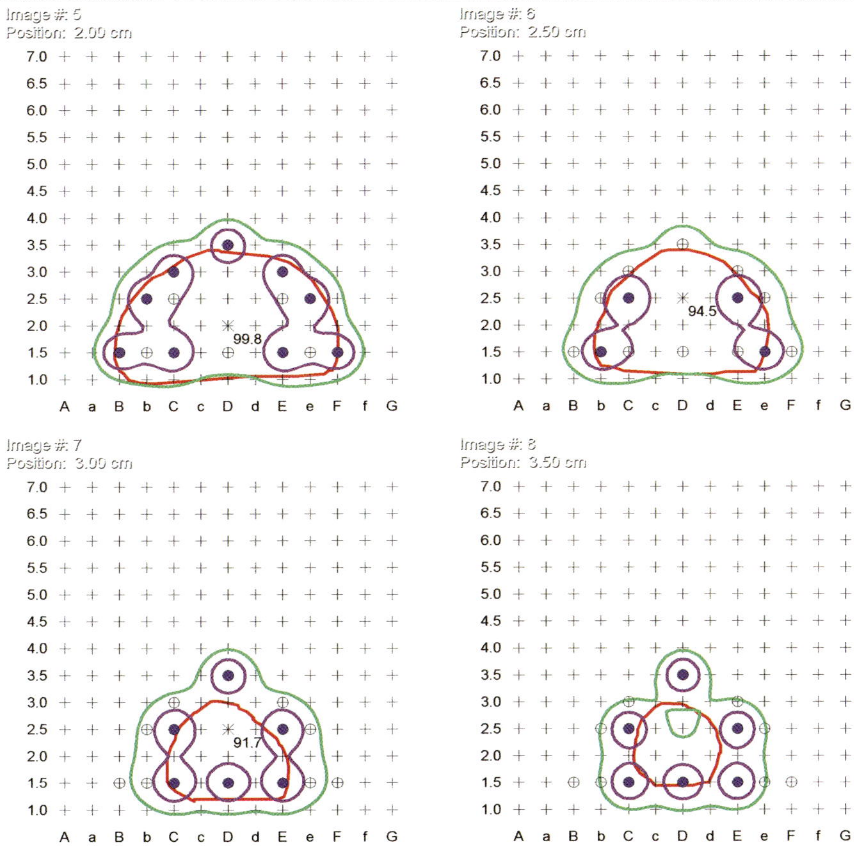

VariSeed 7.1 (Build 2780) fff3 a34b 9bc2 df9f 0330 2980 1a

Figure 7-35. continued.

VariSeed: Therapy Visualization Report [Page 1]

VA Puget Sound · 567 · 1 · 9/28/2006 3:46:06 PM

Name: PID: **531-62-0507** Dept. ID:	Study: **PREPLAN I-125/ PRIMARY** Variation: **Default** Images: **10** Template: **Siemens Alternate**	Source: **I-125 (6711) [NIST 99]** Comment: Sources: **122** Anisotropy: **Factors (Point Model)** Source Activity: **0.419 U [0.330 mCi]**
Procedure Date: **9/13/2006**	Prescription Dose: **145.0 Gy**	Total Activity: **51.118 U [40.250 mCi]**

Isodose Legend Gy [% of Prescription Dose]	290.00 [200.00%] 145.00 [100.00%]
Anatomy/Landmark Legend	Prostate · Rectum · Urethra · Trigone

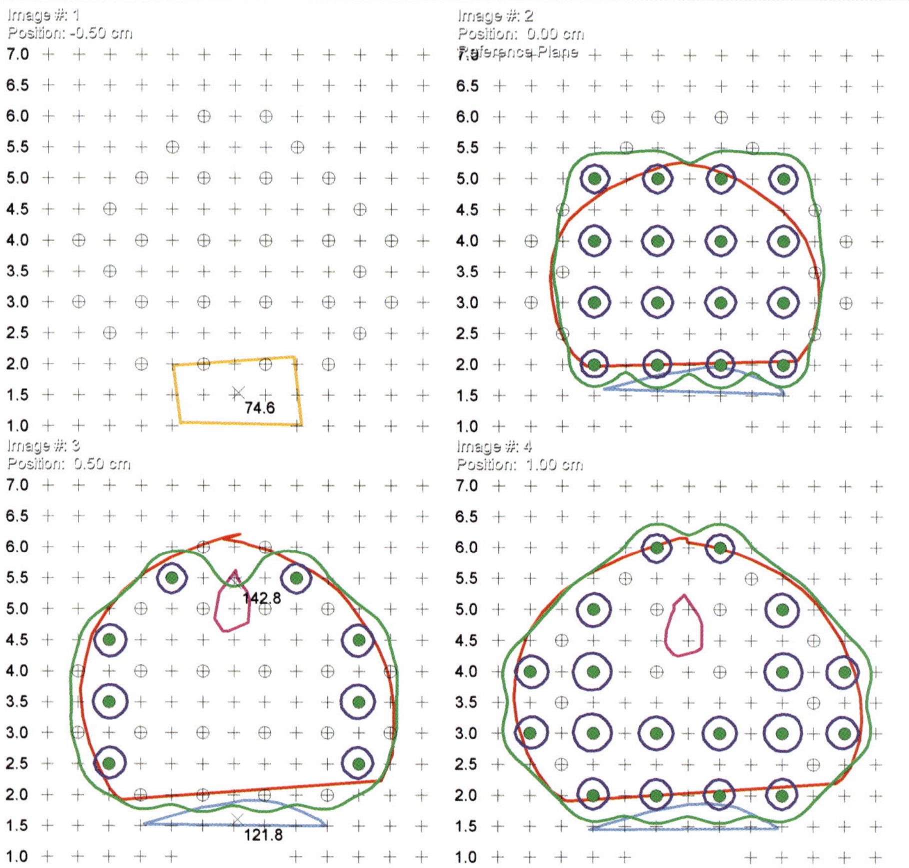

VariSeed 7.1 (Build 2780)

fff3 a34b 9bc2 df9f 0330 2980 1a

Figure 7-36. Example of I-125 monotherapy by J Blasko.

Isodose Legend Gy [% of Prescription Dose]	290.00 [200.00%] 145.00 [100.00%]			
Anatomy/Landmark Legend	Prostate	Rectum	Urethra	Trigone

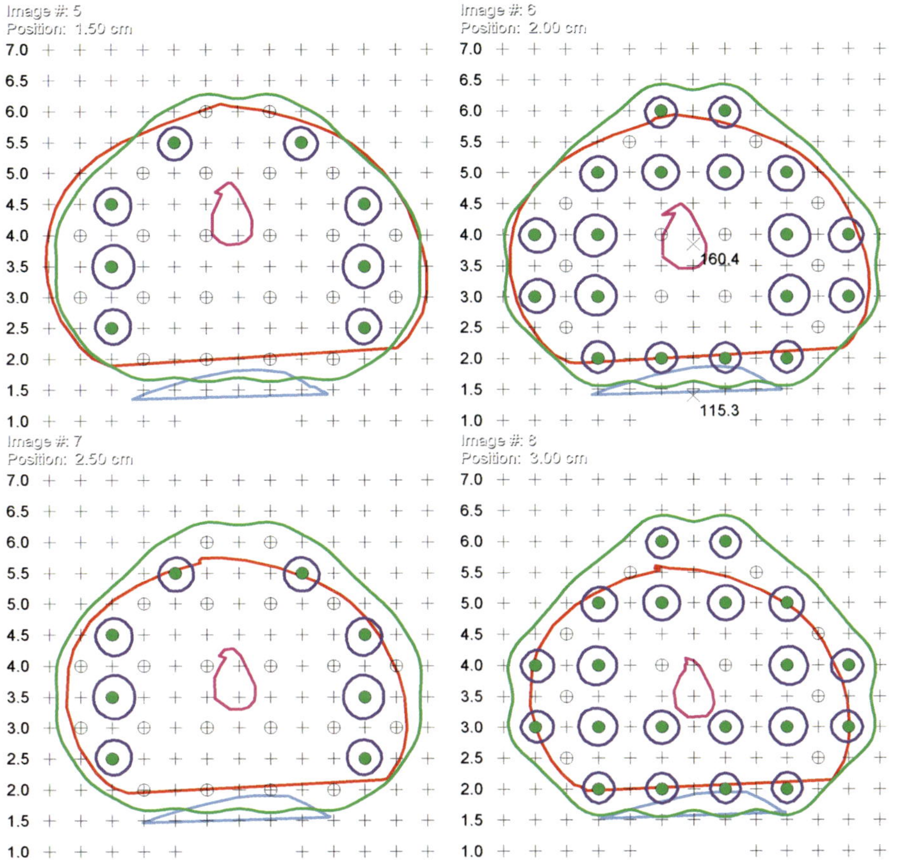

VariSeed 7.1 (Build 2780)

fff3 a34b 9bc2 df9f 0330 2980 1a

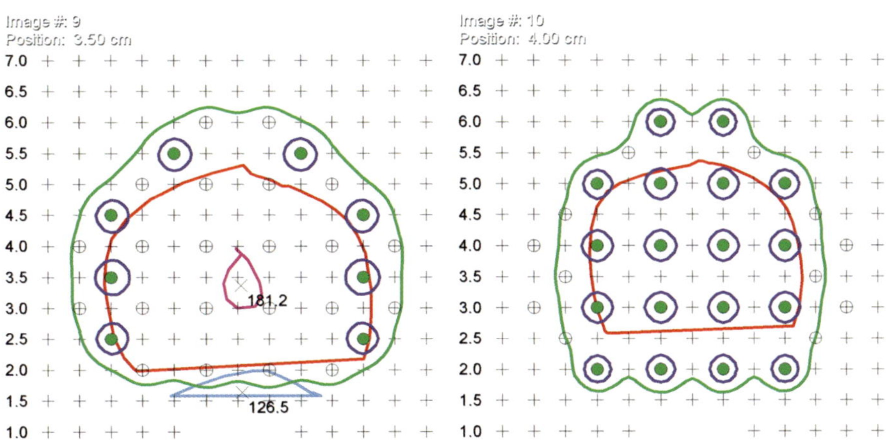

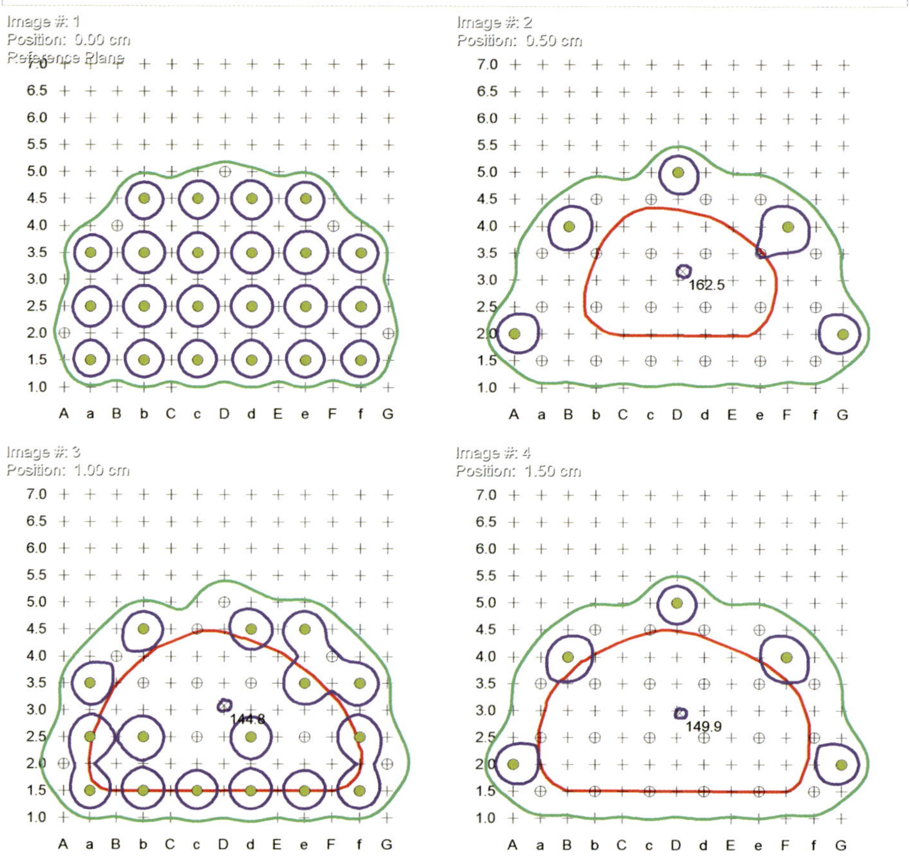

VariSeed: Therapy Visualization Report [Page 1]

VA Puget Sound · 567 · 1 · 11/4/2006 6:20:22 PM

Name: **1GM ex Pd, Sample** PID: **1GM ex Pd** Dept. ID:	Study: **3.150 U Pd-103** Variation: **31cc TRUS, 57 cc PTV** Images: **9** Template: **Siemens Alternate**	Source: **Pd-103 (Mod 200) [NIST 00]** Comment: Sources: **99** Anisotropy: **Factors (Point Model)** Source Activity: **3.150 U [2.436 mCi]**
Procedure Date: **10/23/2006**	Prescription Dose: **125.0 Gy**	Total Activity: **311.850 U [241.183 mCi]**

Isodose Legend
Gy [% of Prescription Dose]
250.00 [200.00%]
125.00 [100.00%]

Anatomy/Landmark Legend
Urethra
Prostate

VariSeed 7.1 (Build 2780)

fff3 a34b 9bc2 df9f 0330 2980 1a

Figure 7-37. Example of Pd-103 monotherapy by G. Merrick.

Procedure Date: **10/23/2006**	Prescription Dose: **125.0 Gy**	Source Activity: **3.150 U [2.436 mCi]** Total Activity: **311.850 U [241.183 mCi]**

Isodose Legend Gy [% of Prescription Dose]	250.00 [200.00%] 125.00 [100.00%]	
Anatomy/Landmark Legend	Urethra	Prostate

Image #: 5
Position: 2.00 cm

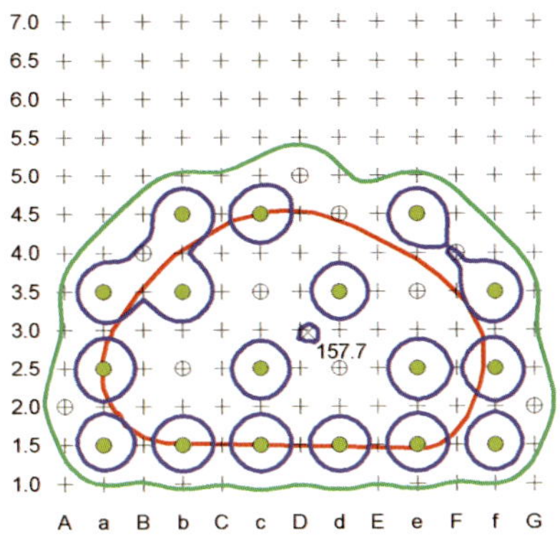

Image #: 6
Position: 2.50 cm

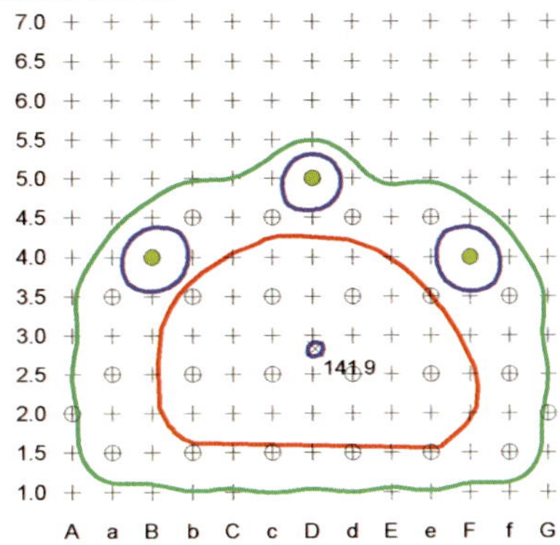

Image #: 7
Position: 3.00 cm

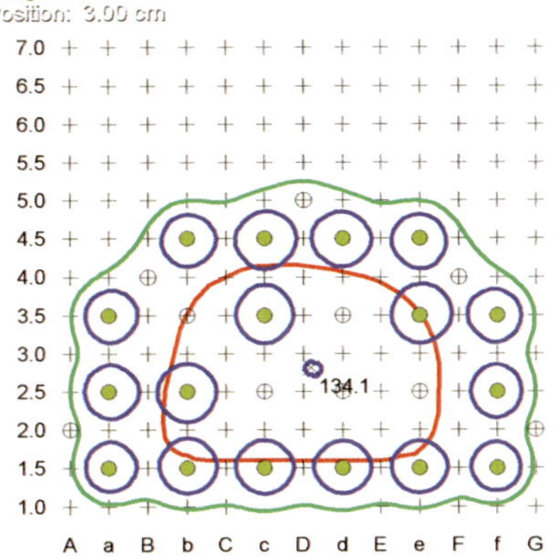

Image #: 8
Position: 3.50 cm

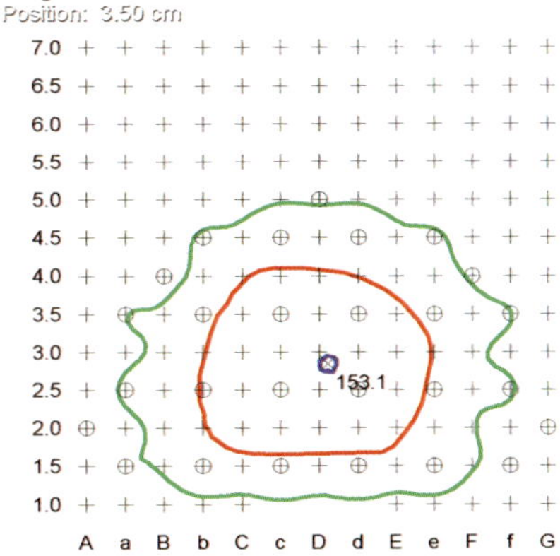

Image #: 9
Position: 4.00 cm

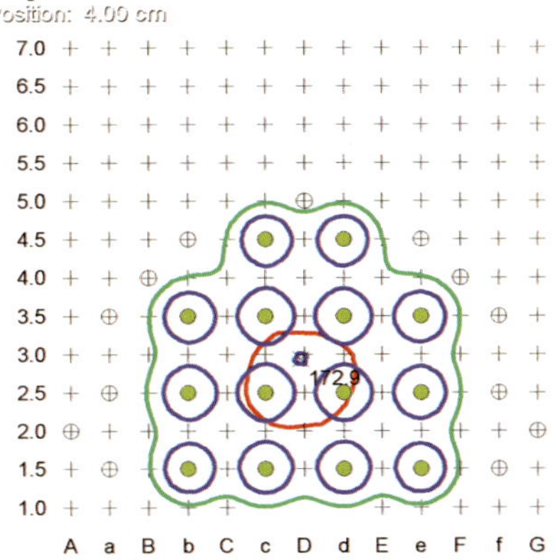

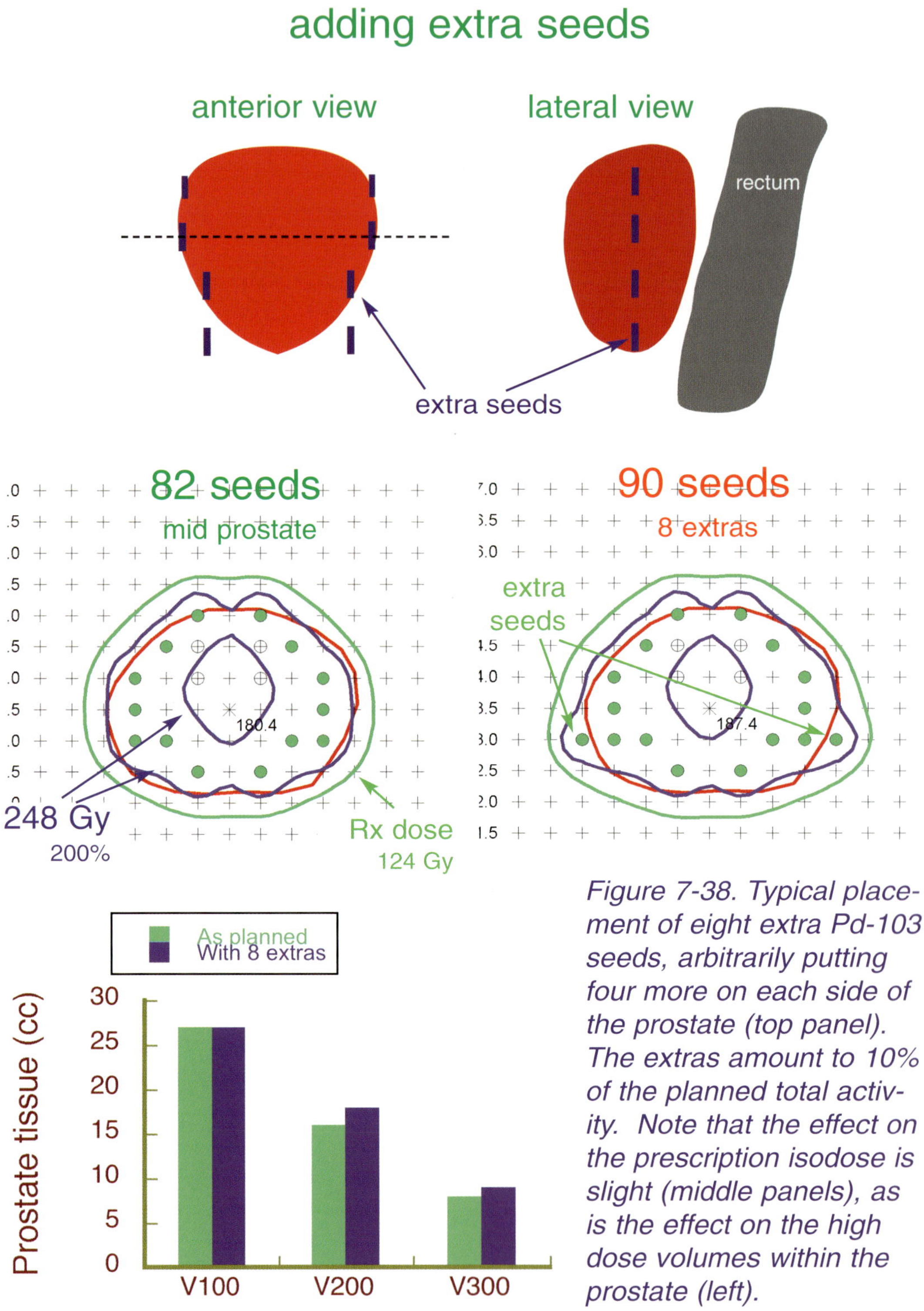

Figure 7-38. Typical placement of eight extra Pd-103 seeds, arbitrarily putting four more on each side of the prostate (top panel). The extras amount to 10% of the planned total activity. Note that the effect on the prescription isodose is slight (middle panels), as is the effect on the high dose volumes within the prostate (left).

pleted by trial and error within a few minutes by an experienced dosimetrist, adding or moving seeds until optimal peripheral coverage is achieved. When you are done with your design, the treatment planning programs can generate a summary of the plan to be used as a guide in the operating room (**Figure 7-32 a-d**)

Figures 7-33 through 7-37 show typical treatment plans used by each of the authors of this textbook. It is a good idea to peruse these examples as the kind of things we do. Merrick and colleagues published a valuable, detailed accounting of their own treatment planning technique.(MERRICK 00) While some of our colleagues would quibble over the examples, remember that all four authors of this text have published their long-term outcomes, which appear very favorable. We notice that most who criticize our methods have never actually published their own tumor control or morbidity rates. Your plans don't need to look the same as those shown here. Remember, even following the guidelines described in the preceding pages, there's room to be creative!

EXTRAS

For better or worse, it's common practice to add extra seeds at the time of implant, beyond what is called for in the computer-generated plan. Extra seeds are typically added to areas where biopsies are known to be positive, or to regions where seed placement appear sub-optimal, based on intra-operative TRUS or fluoroscopic images. Adding seeds ad hoc is a somewhat risky practice that could lead to excessive urethral or rectal doses. If you choose to do so, it is prudent to place extras laterally, to minimize additional radiation to the urethra and the rectum.

If you're going to add extras, keep in mind that the typical six to eight extras amount to 5–10% of the total seeds, modestly increasing the high dose volumes (**Figure 7-38**).

The days of arbitrary extras are probably numbered. There is considerable interest in the development of intra-operative, post-implant dosimetry. Real-time evaluation would make the use of additional seeds to boost inadequately implanted regions a more rational endeavor.

HORMONAL DOWNSIZING

Androgen deprivation typically reduces the prostate volume by approximately 25% to 50%.(SHEARER, ZELEFSKY, FORMAN, MERRICK 05) When pre-

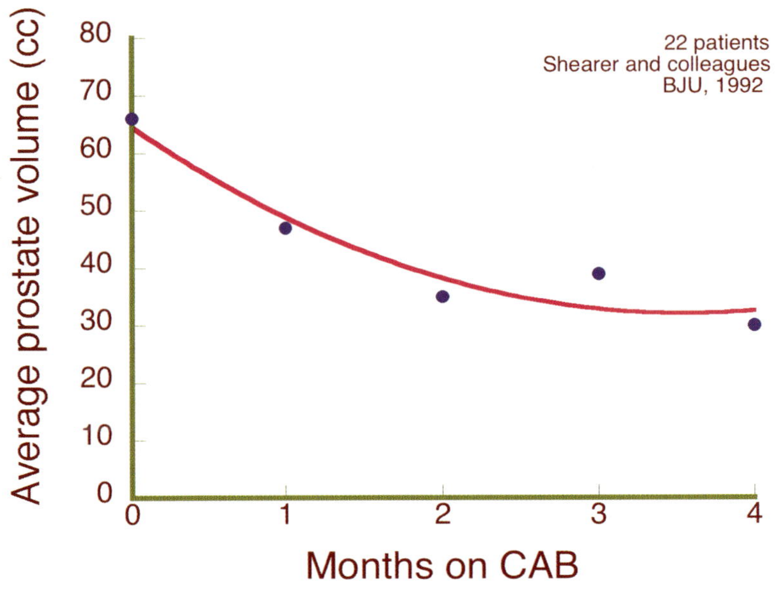

Figure 7-39. Prostate volume reduction after initiating androgen blockade. The volume reduction slows at two months, although the time course varies substantially from patient to patient.

treatment androgen deprivation is used, dosimetry should be based on the reduced prostate volume. Sufficient time should be given to allow near maximal shrinkage before obtaining the planning images. Most of the shrinkage occurs in the first two months of androgen deprivation (**Figure 7-39**).

PRE-PLANNING VERSUS INTRA-OPERATIVE PLANNING

Stone, Stock and DeWyngaart were quick to develop intra-operative TRUS-based planning, without use of pre-planning images. The prostate size was estimated from pre-implant office TRUS, and the approximate number of seeds needed is determined from a nomogram. At the time of the procedure, two-thirds of the activity is placed at the prostatic periphery, and the remainder in the interior of the gland. Satisfactory dosimetry is achievable with their method.(STONE) More recently, faster treatment-planning systems allow true intra-operative planning based on intra-operative image capture, and many people are getting into the act.(MESSING, ZELEFSKY 00, GEWANTER, BEYER)

Table 7-1. Pre-operative versus intra-operative planning

	Intra-operative	Pre-operative
Pros	Better tailored to image(?)	Less OR time Easier seed management More time to evaluate plans
Cons	Increase OR time -20-30 mins added Need extra seeds -10-20 additional	Need meticulous pre-implant TRUS study

Intra-operative planning has its pros and cons (**Table 7-1**). Probably the most touted advantage is better matching of the planning images with what is actually used, circumventing the potential problem of a discrepancy between the pre-planning versus the intra-operative images. While this could be a legitimate advantage, in experienced hands we find that such discrepancies are minimal and likely inconsequential. Reports of improved results with one technique over the other likely reflect inadequate brachytherapy skills, rather than a true advantage to either method.

Probably the most appealing aspect of pre-planning is the increased time available to evaluate the plan, and make minor changes beforehand.

From a purely practical standpoint, intra-operative planning has some substantial *dis*advantages. It can increase operating time by 20–30 minutes or more, and requires a greater degree of physics support intra-operatively. Additionally, it requires extra seeds on hand, in case the intra-operative plan calls for more seeds than was estimated. The bottom line—there are many ways to do transperineal implants, and good results are more dependent on the skill and experience of the brachytherapy team than on the particular planning method.

VARIABILITY IN TREATMENT PLANNING

While there are a number of studies now regarding treatment parameter optimization, there are still many issues left to be defined. There is little question that generous treatment margins and high V100s lead to greater

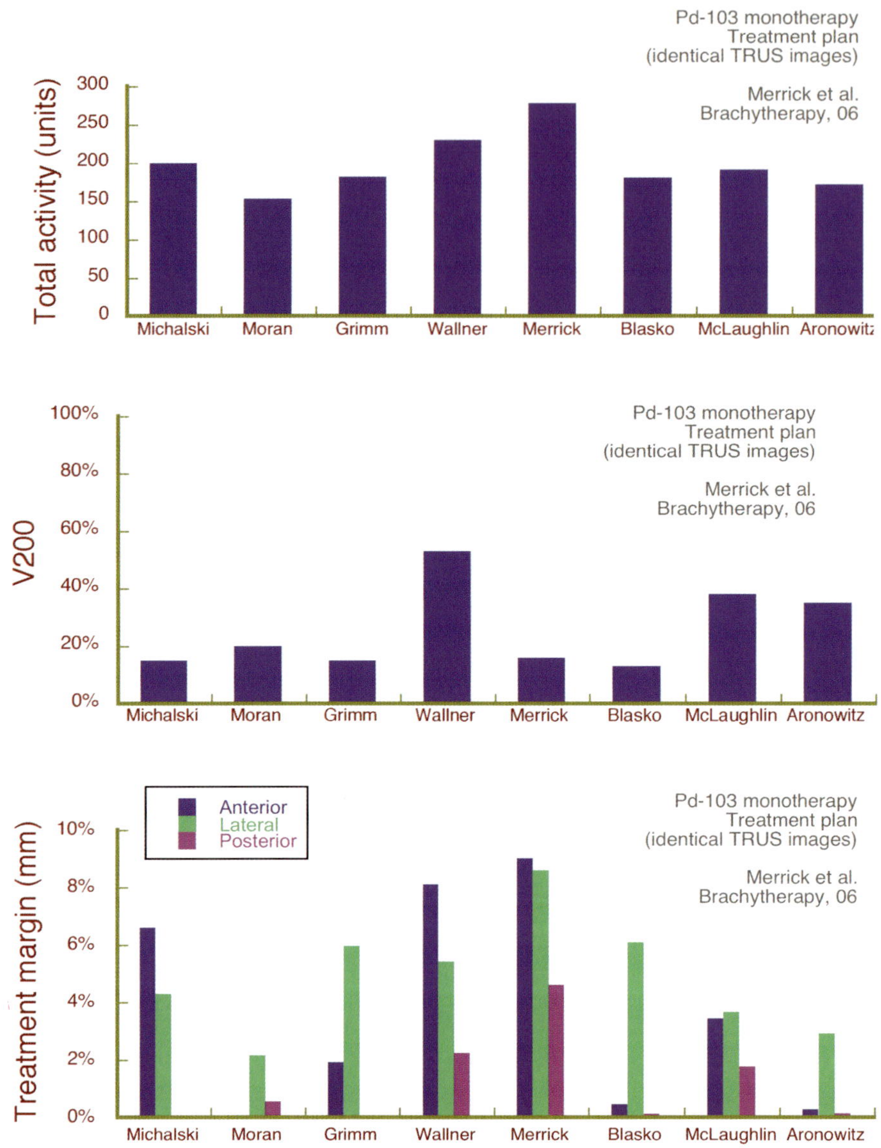

Figure 7-40. Identical set of TRUS images were used by various experts to design what for each participant was an ideal plan. These experienced practitioners varied markedly in what they considered ideal coverage and acceptable high dose regions. The point here is that there is a wide range in what "experts" consider an ideal plan.

Table 7-2. Implant boost treatment schemes used by various groups.

Investigator	1st modality	EBRT dose	Isotope	Imp dose	Time between
Blasko	EBRT	45 Gy	Pd-103	90 Gy	2-6 wks
Wallner (1997)	EBRT	50 Gy	Pd-103	60 Gy	2-4 wks
Wallner (1999)	EBRT	20 Gy	Pd-103	115 Gy	1-5 days
Dattoli	EBRT	41 Gy	Pd-103	80 Gy	2-6 wks
	EBRT	20 Gy			0-1 week
Critz	Implant	45 Gy	I-125	80 Gy	3-6 wks
Stone/Stock	Implant	60 Gy	Pd-103	80-90 Gy	8 wks

cure rates.(CHOI, POTTERS, STOCK, WALLNER 05, ORIO) It has also been shown that the rectal dose must be limited to decrease the likelihood of proctitis. On the other hand, there appears to be little clinical importance to seed strength or high dose regions within the prostate (V200s and V300s). The lack of clear clinical sequelae of some treatment planning specifics has allowed a great deal of variability in treatment planning strategies between practitioners. To show the potential for variability even among seasoned practitioners, Merrick and colleagues sent a pre-implant TRUS study to eight brachytherapists and asked them to produce a plan in accordance with their customary practice. The eight plans were then compared in regards to planning parameters including seed number, total activity and V200 and V300 regions. The only thing in common was complete coverage of the prostate (V100 of 100%). Even among these like-minded experts, there was substantial variability in other parameters (**Figure 7-40**). Even more surprisingly, this high degree of variability likely has minimal effect on outcomes, providing rectal doses are kept within recommended limits. Given the lack of adverse sequelae despite great variability in high dose regions and urethral doses, we suspect that these variabilities between practitioners will persist well into the future.

DOSE DE-ESCALATION

Given the remarkably high cure rates in capable brachytherapy hands, and increasing knowledge of desirable minimal and maximal doses, the time is ripe to explore the possibility of decreasing the prescription doses.

Based on accumulated knowledge regarding the radiation dose needed to eradicate cancer, Merrick, Wallner and colleagues have initiated prospective, randomized trials testing the effect of a lowered radiation prescription dose on the cure and complication rates.

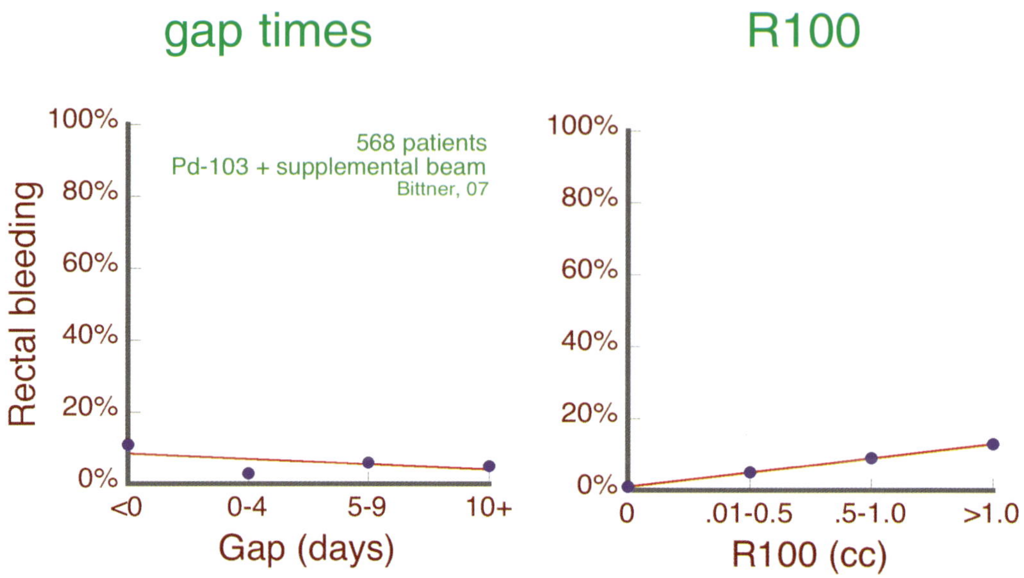

Figure 7-41. The likelihood of rectal bleeding had little relation to gap time between beam and implant (left panel). In contrast, rectal bleeding was directly related to the R100 from the implant (right panel). Based on this data, gap times are minimized.

A total of 2,000 low-risk patients are being randomized to a prescription dose of 124 Gy versus 100 Gy. The primary endpoint will be biochemical tumor control. At current accrual rates, the full complement of 2,000 patients should be enrolled by 2010.

COMBINING BEAM RADIATION AND BRACHYTHERAPY

The use of supplemental beam radiation with prostate brachytherapy has been widely practiced since the days of low dose rate Ir-192 (see Chapter 13). Combining brachytherapy with beam radiation presents a number of additional treatment design choices. There are many possible combinations of brachytherapy and supplemental radiation—the sequencing, radionuclides, and doses can all be varied. While there is no lack of opinions as to how modalities should be combined, little data is available to support one scheme versus another.

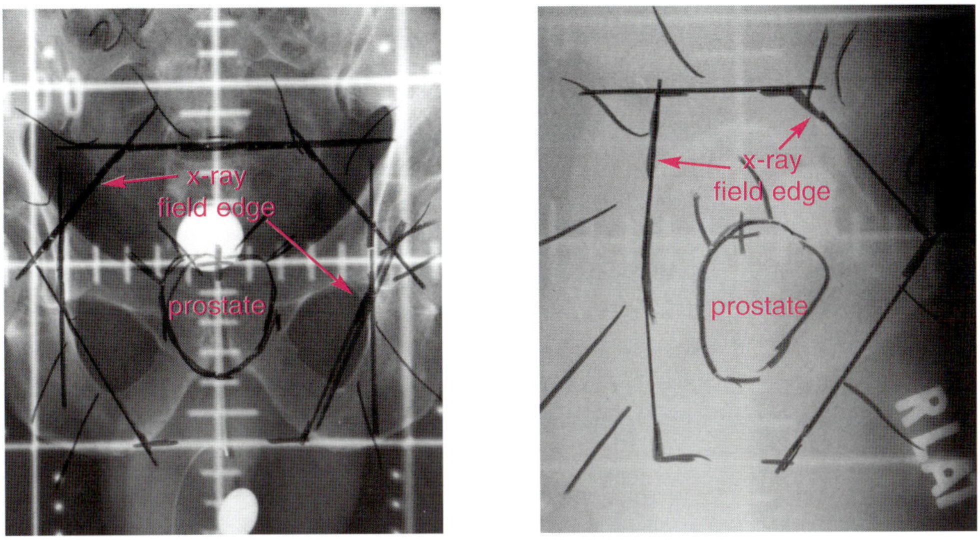

Figure 7-42. Typical anterior and lateral fields used for supplemental external beam radiation. No studies have been done regarding optimal beam field sizes in the setting of brachytherapy plus beam radiation.

Sequencing

Theoretical arguments can be made for using either radiation sequencing scheme: beam first or implant first. In the absence of solid data that one is better than the other, pre-implant external beam has generally been favored. But if properly carried out, both sequences appear effective, with a very small likelihood of serious complications (**Table 7-2**).(CRITZ, BLASKO, DATTOLI)

There is some concern that doing the implant first could lead to a higher incidence of rectal complications, in part because patients still are receiving some implant radiation while the beam radiation is being delivered. In an early European report, patients who were implanted first had a very high incidence of rectal complications.(IVERSEN) However, in addition to doing the implant first, the investigators gave large fractions of beam radiation (2.5 Gy per day to the whole pelvis) and a *full* dose I-125 implant. Delivering full doses with both radiation modalities, rather than their sequencing was more likely the cause of the elevated rectal risk.

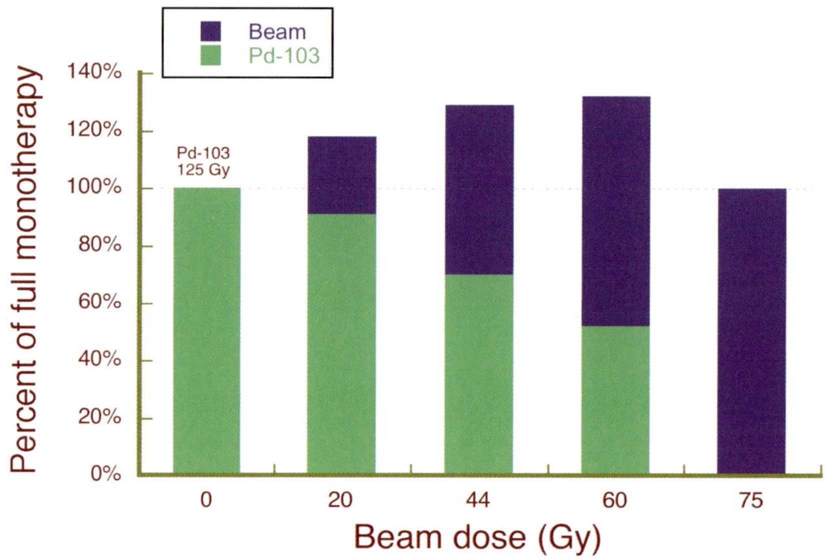

Figure 7-43. Total doses, expressed as percent of monotherapy dose, with various combinations of beam radiation and brachytherapy, estimated by assuming that equivalent full monotherapy doses for Pd-103 and beam radiation are 115 Gy and 75 Gy, respectively.

Gap time

The time interval between implant and external radiation varied from two to eight weeks in earlier published studies(**Table 7-2**). Bittner and colleagues have shown that shorter gap times are safe and equally effective. (corriveau, BITTNER) Rectal bleeding was related to the R100s, and independent of the gap times (**Figure 7-41**). Accordingly, it seems reasonable to shorten the gap times to enhance patient convenience and possibly increase effectiveness.

Field sizes

Limited external beam radiation fields are the norm, typically designed to cover the prostate and base of the seminal vesicles, with a 2 cm margin (reduced to 1 cm margin posteriorly) (**Figures 7-42**). Whole pelvic radiation, designed to cover the pelvic lymph nodes, has limited clinical justification.(ROACH)

Doses

A wide variety of implant and beam radiation dose combinations can be used (**Table 7-2**). When combined with beam radiation, implant doses are generally dropped to about 50% to 80% of monotherapy doses, ranging from 90–120 Gy with I-125 and 60–113 Gy with Pd-103 (**Figure 7-43**). Caution should be used when extrapolating combined brachytherapy and beam doses between institutions, due to differences in high dose volumes and treatment margins (see above).

External beam doses of 20–60 Gy have all been used extensively, with no clear evidence of superiority of one dose scheme over another. Prospective randomized trials are bringing some logic to the subject.(see Chapter 13).

Radionuclides

The optimal isotope to combine with beam radiation has not been clearly established. The majority of favorable, published series have used Pd-103, but there are also encouraging reports of I-125 combined with supplemental external radiation.(CRITZ)

THE ART OF PROSTATE BRACHYTHERAPY

This chapter, more than any other, points out the technical inconsistencies among brachytherapists. *Art* is a euphemism for the insufficiency of scientific evidence regarding optimal brachytherapy design. Much of the variability is due to personal bias. Fortunately, there is an array of good quality prospective studies that should enhance the art of brachytherapy with good quality clinical science. In the meantime, there are lots of ways to get an effective implant—just because the methodology is not standardized doesn't mean that prostate brachytherapy doesn't work well. Remember, despite the multitude of uncertainties in brachytherapy treatment planning and the widely varying treatment schemes, the clinical results are very favorable in most hands. Nevertheless, it's important to understand the nuances of implant design to maximize cure rates and minimize complications in your own practice.

REFERENCES

1. Allen Z, Merrick G, Butler E, et al. Detailed urethral dosimetry in the evaluation of prostate brachytherapy-related urinary morbidity. Int J Rad Oncol Biol Phys 2005; 62:981-987.

2. Anderson LL. Spacing nomograph for interstitial implants of I-125 seeds. Med Phys 1976; 3:48-51.
3. Anderson LL. Brachytherapy planning and evaluation. Endo/Hyper Oncol 1991; 7:139-146.
4. Badiozamani K, Wallner K, Sutlief S, Ellis W, Blasko J, Russell K. Anticipating prostatic volume changes due to prostate brachytherapy. Radiat Oncol Invest 1999; 7:360-364.
5. Beaulieu L, Archambault L, Aubin M, Oral E, Taschereau R, Pouliot J. The robustness of dose ditributions to displacement and migration of I-125 permanent seed implants over a wide range of seed number, activity, and designs. Int J Rad Oncol Biol Phys 2004; 58:1298-1308.
6. Beyer DC, Shapiro RH, Puente F. Real-time optimized intraoperative dosimetry for prostate brachytherapy: A pilot study. Int J Radiat Oncol Biolo Phys 2000; 48:1583-1589.
7. Bittner N, Wallner K, Merrick G, et al. Time gap between Pd-103 prostate brachytherapy and supplemental beam radiation versus morbidity and the likelihood of cure
. submitted 2007.
8. Blasko JC, Grimm PD, Sylvester JE, Cavanagh W. The role of external beam radiotherapy with I-125/Pd-103 brachytherapy for prostate carcinoma. Radiother and Oncol 2000; 57:273-278.
9. Choi S, Wallner KE, Merrick G, Butler W. Treatment margins predict biochemical outcomes after prostate brachytherapy. Cancer Journal (Scientific American) 2004; 10:175-180.
10. Corriveau J, Wallner K, Merrick G, et al. Morbidity effect of the time gap between supplemental beam radiation and Pd-103 prostate brachytherapy. Brachytherapy 2003; 2:108-113.
11. Critz F. Summary of simultaneous irradiation for prostate cancer. Urology 2004; 64:633-636.
12. Crook J, Milosevic M, Catton P, et al. Interobserver variation in postimplant computed tomography contouring affects quality assessment of prostate brachytherapy. Brachytherapy 2002; 1:66-73.
13. Cumes DM, Goffinet DR, Martinez A, Stamey TA. Complications of 125-Iodine implantation and pelvic lymphadenectomy for prostatic cancer with special reference to patients who had failed external beam therapy as their initial mode of therapy. J Urol 1981; 126:620-622.
14. D'Amico AV, Whittington R, Malkowicz SB, al e. Biochemical outcome after radical prostatectomy, external beam radiation therapy, or interstitial radiation therapy for clinically localized prostate cancer. JAMA 1998; 280:969-974.

15. D'Souza W, Meyer R. Dose homogeneity as a funcion of source activity in optimized I-125 prosrtate implant treatment plans. Int J Rad Oncol Biol Phys 2001; 51:1120-1130.
16. Dattoli M, Wallner K, True L, Cash J, Sorace R. Long-term prostate cancer control using Palladium-103 brachytherapy and external beam radiotherapy in patients with a high likelihood of extracapsular cancer extension. Urology 2007; 69:334-337.
17. Dattoli MJ, Wallner KE, Sorace R, Ting J. Planned extracapsular seed placement using palladium-103 for prostate brachytherapy. JBI 2000; 16:35-43.
18. Davis BJ, Haddock MG, Wilson TM, al e. Treatment of extraprostatic cancer in clinically organ-confined prostate cancer by permanent intersititial brachytherapy: Is extraprostatic seed placement necessary? Techniques in Urology 2000; 6:70-77.
19. Davis BJ, Pisansky TM, Wilson TM, et al. The radial distance of extraprostatic extension of prostate carcinoma: implications for prostate brachytherapy. Cancer 1999; 85:2630-2637.
20. Forman JD, Kumar R, Haas G, Montie J. Neoadjuvant hormonal downsizing of localized carcinoma of the prostate: Effects on the volume of normal tissue irradiation. Ca Invest 1995; 13:8-15.
21. Fuller D, Koziol J, Feng A. Prostate brachytherapy seed migration and dosimetry: analysis of stranded sources and other potential predictive factors. Brachytherapy 2004; 2004:10-19.
22. Han B, Wallner K, Aggarwal S, Armstrong J, Sutlief S. Treatment margins for prostate brachytherapy. Seminars in Urol Oncol 2000; 18:137-141.
23. ICRU. Prescribing, recording, and reporting photon beam therapy. ICRU Report 50 1993:1-8.
24. Iversen P, Nielsen L, Bak M, et al. Ultrasonically guided 125Iodine seed implantation with external radiation in management of localized prostatic carcinoma. Urol 1989; 34:181-186.
25. Jones S, Wallner K, Merrick G, Cavanagh W, Butler W. Clinical correlates of high brachytherapy dose regions within the prostate. Int J Rad Oncol Biol Phys 2002; 53:328-333.
26. Kestin L, Goldstein N, Vicini F, Yan D, Korman H, Martinez A. Treatment of prostate cancer with radiotherapy: should the entire seminal vesicles be included in the the clinical target volume? Int J Rad Oncol Biol Phys 2002; 54:686-697.

27. Kunos C, Resnick M, Kinsella T, Ellis RJ. Migration of implanted free radioactive seeds for adenocarcinoma of the prostate using a Mick applicator. Brachytherapy 2004; 3:71-77.
28. Leibovich BC, Blute ML, Bostwick DG, Wilson TM, al e. Proximity of prostate cancer to the urethra: Implications for minimally invasive ablative therapies. Urol 2000; 56:726-729.
29. Maguire PD, Waterman FM, Dicker AP. Can the cost of permanent prostate implants be reduced? An argument for peripheral loading with higher strength seeds. Techniques in Urology 2000; 6:85-88.
30. McElveen TL, Waterman FM, Kim H, Dicker AP. Factors predicting for urinary incontinence after prostate brachytherapy. Int J Rad Oncol Biol Phys 2004; 59:1395-1404.
31. McNeal JE, Price HM, Redwine EA, Freiha FS, Stamey TA. Stage A Versus Stage B Adenocarcinoma of the Prostate: Morphological Comparison and Biological Significance. J Urol 1988; 139:61-65.
32. Merrick G, Butler E, Wallner K, et al. Variability of prostate brachytherapy preimplant dosimetry: A multi-institutional analysis. Brachytherapy 2005; 4:241-251.
33. Merrick G, Butler W, Wallner K, Galbreath R, Allen Z, Kurko BS. Efficacy of neoadjuvant bicalutamide and dutasteride as a cytoreductive regimen before prostate brachytherapy. Urology 2006; 68:116-120.
34. Merrick G, Gutman s, Andreini H, et al. Prostate cancer distribution in patients diagnosed by transperineal template-guided saturation biopsy. European Urology 2007.
35. Merrick G, Wallner K, Butler W, et al. Brachytherapy in men aged ″54 years with clinically localized prostate cancer. BJU International 2006; 98:324-328.
36. Merrick GS, Butler WM. Modified uniform seed loading for prostate brachytherapy: rationale, design, and evaluation. Techniques in Urology 2000; 6:78-84.
37. Merrick GS, Butler WM, Dorsey AT, Lief JH, Benson ML. Seed fixity in the prostate/periprostatic region following brachytherapy. Int J Rad Oncol Biol Phys 2000; 46:215-220.
38. Messing EM, Zhang JBY, Rubens DJ, al e. Intraoperative optimized inverse planning for prostate brachytherapy: early experience. Int J Rad Oncol Biol Phys 1999; 44:801-808.
39. Mueller A, Wallner K, Merrick G, Cavanagh W, Butler W. Peri-rectal seeds as a risk factor for prostate brachytherapy-related rectal bleeding. Int J Rad Oncol Biol Phys 2004; 59:1047-1052.

40. Narayana V, Roberson PL, Winfield RJ, Kessler ML. Optimal placement of radioisotopes for permanent prostate implants. Radiol 1996; 199:457-460.

41. Narayana V, Troyer S, Evans V, Winfield R, Roberson P, McLaughlin P. Randomized trial of high- and low-source strength 125-I prostate seed implants. Int J Rad Oncol Biol Phys 2005; 61:44-51.

42. Nedea E, Wallner K, Reed D, et al. Extra-prostatic seed placement and its effect on seed loss. Cancer Journal (Scientific American) 2005; 11:147-151.

43. Orio P, Wallner K, Merrick G, et al. Dosimetric parameters as predictive factors for biochemical control in patients with higher risk prostate cancer treated with Pd-103 and supplemental beam radiation. Int J Rad Oncol Biol Phys 2007; 67:342-346.

44. Potters L, Cao Y, Calugaru E, Torre T, Fearn P, Wang X. A comprehensive review of CT-based dosimetry parameters and biochemical control in patients treated with permanent prostate brachytherapy. Int J Rad Oncol Biol Phys 2001; 50:605-614.

45. Reed D, Wallner K, Merrick G, et al. A prospective randomized comparison of stranded versus loose iodine-125 seeds for prostate brachytherapy. Brachytherapy 2007; in press.

46. Roach M, DeSilva M, Lawton C, Uhl V, Machtay M, Seider M. Phase III triall comparing whole pelvic versus prostate-only radiotherapy and neoadjuvant versus adjuvant combined adndrogen suppression: Radiation Therapy Oncology Group 9413. J Clin Oncol 2003; 21:1904-1911.

47. Rosen MA, Goldstone L, Lapin S, Wheeler T, Scardino PT. Frequency and location of extracapsular extension and positive surgical margins in radical prostatectomy specimens. J Urol 1992; 148:331-337.

48. Shearer RJ, Davies JH, Gelister JSK, Dearnaley DP. Hormonal cytoreduction and radiotherapy for carcinoma of the prostate. Br J Urol 1992; 69:521-524.

49. Sloboda R, Pedersen J, Halperin R. Is there a preferred strength for regularly spaced 125-I seeds in inverse-planned prostate implant? Int J Rad Oncol Biol Phys 2003; 55:234-244.

50. Snyder KM, Stock RG, Hong SM, Lo YC, Stone NN. Defining the risk of developing grade 2 proctitis following 125-I prostate brachytherapy using a rectal dose-volume histogram analysis. Int J Rad Oncol Biol Phys 2001; 50:335-341.

51. Sohayda C, Kupelian PA, Levin JS, Klein EA. Extent of extracapsular extension in localized prostate cancer. Urol 2000; 55:382-386.

52. Stamey TA, Villers AA, McNeal JE, Link PC, Freiha FS. Positive surgical margins at radical prostatectomy: importance of the apical dissection. J Urol 1990; 143:1166-1173.
53. Stock RG, Lo Y, Gaildon M, Stone NN. Does prostate brachytherapy treat the seminal vesicles: A dose-volume histogram analysis of seminal vesicles in patients undergoing combined Pd-103 prostate implantation and external beam irradiation. Int J Rad Oncol Biol Phys 1999; 45:385-389.
54. Stock RG, Stone NN, Cesaaretti J, Rosenstein B. Biologically effective dose values for prostate brachytherrapy: Effects on PSA failure and posttreatment biopsy results. Int J Rad Oncol Biol Phys 2006; 64:527-533.
55. Stone NN, Stock RG, DeWyngaert JK, Tabert A. Prostate brachytherapy: Improvements in prostate volume measurements and dose distribution using interactive ultrasound guided implantation and three-dimensional dosimetry. Radiat Oncol Invest 1995; 3:185-195.
56. Tran A, Wallner K, Merrick G, Seeberger J, Armstrong J, Mueller A. Rectal fistulas following prostate brachytherapy. Int J Rad Oncol Biol Phys 2005; 63:150-154.
57. Villers A, McNeal JE, Redwine EA, Freiha FS. The role of perineural space invasion in the local spread of prostatic adenocarcinoma. J Urol 1989; 142:763-768.
58. Wallner K, Merrick G, Sutlief S, True L, Butler E. High-dose regions versus likelihood of cure after prostate brachytherapy. Int J Rad Oncol Biol Phys 2005; 62:170-174.
59. Wallner K, Merrick G, True L, Sutlief S, Cavanagh W, Butler W. I-125 versus Pd-103 for low risk prostate cancer: Preliminary biochemical outcomes from a prospective randomized mulitcenter trial. Int J Rad Oncol Biol Phys 2003; 57:1297-1303.
60. Wallner KE, Roy J, Harrison L. Dosimetry guidelines to minimize urethral and rectal morbidity following transperineal I-125 prostate brachytherapy. Int J Radiat Oncol Biol Phys 1995; 32:465-471.
61. Waterman FM, Dicker AP. Determination of the urethral dose in prostate brachytherapy when the urethra cannot be visualized in the postimplant CT scan. Med Phys 2000; 27:448-451.
62. Waterman FM, Yue N, Corn BW, Dicker AP. Edema associated with I-125 or Pd-103 prostate brachytherapy and its impact on post-implant dosimetry: an analysis based on serial CT acquistion. Int J Rad Oncol Biol Phys 1998; 41:1069-1077.
63. Willins J, Wallner KE. Time-dependent changes in CT-based dosimetry of I-125 prostate brachytherapy. Radiat Oncol Invest 1998; 6:157-160.

64. Zaider M, Zelefsky MJ, Lee EK, al e. Treatment planning for prostate implants using magnetic-resonance sprectroscopy imaging. Int J Rad Oncol Biol Phys 2000; 47:1085-1096.
65. Zelefsky MJ, Leibel SA, Burman CM, Kutcher GJ. Neoadjuvant hormonal therapy improves the therapeutic ratio in patients with bulky prostatic cancer treated with three-dimensional conformal radiation therapy. Int J Radiat Oncol Biol Phys 1994; 29:755-761.
66. Zelefsky MJ, Yamada Y, Cohen G, al e. Postimplantation dosimetric analysis of permanent transperineal prostate implantation: improved dose distributions with an intraoperative computer-optimized conformal planning technique. Int J Rad Oncol Biol Phys 2000; 48:601-608.

8

Patient Preparation

Proper patient preparation should facilitate the implant procedure and decrease the risk of post-operative morbidity. There is a wide variety of preparatory practices, with little data to support one policy over another. The following is a summary of various policies, all of which seem acceptable. Some are more practical than others.

BOWEL PREPARATION

The rectum should be clear of feces to facilitate proper TRUS imaging. Lower GI clearing may also decrease the risk of infection should the rectum inadvertently be pierced. A variety of enemas, diets, and laxative

Table 8-1. Lower GI clearing protocols.

	Diet	Enema	Laxative
Blasko	low fiber (24 hr) NPO after midnight	night before & AM of implant	none
Dattoli	NPO after midnight (liquid breakfast for evening cases)	night before (2) & AM (2) of implant	none
Wallner	Light breakfast	none	none

cocktails can be used, all with an 80 to 90% likelihood of success (**Table 8-1**).(POUND) Some regimens are more onerous than others. Given the lack of any apparent difference, it seems wise to use the least expensive, least uncomfortable, and most patient-friendly regimen. We have abandoned the use of laxatives, as they too often lead to intra-operative diarrheal disasters. An early morning enema is usually sufficient. If feces obscures the TRUS image, intra-operative rectal lavage with a large bore tube is a practical (but unpleasant) solution.

INFECTION CONTROL

In the late 1800s, post-operative infection rates fell from nearly 100% to less than 5%, primarily due to adoption of hand-washing and clothing changes. Since that time, a large number of additional antiseptic procedures to cleanse tissue and maneuvers to sterilize surgical accesories have been introduced, without much further reduction in the infection rate. Prostate brachytherapy offers a good sampling of ritualistic infection control practices based on modern medical mysticism.

Shaving

Several investigators have reported a *higher* likelihood of infection if the skin is shaved prior to surgery, probably resulting from microscopic skin breaks.(SEROPIAN, BIRD) Considering that perineal skin or subcutaneous infection after transperineal prostate brachytherapy appears to be very, very rare, and that shaving may actually *increase* the likelihood of infection, it's a practice that should be avoided.

Cleansing

Whether or not the skin is shaved, it should be cleansed with an antiseptic. There is no substantial difference between commonly used skin cleansers regarding their antimicrobial effect.(RITTER) Alcohol (70%) is as effective as any other cleanser, but may cause skin irritation. Free iodine (tincture) is no longer used, due to its tendency to cause skin irritation. Povodine-complexed iodine (10% povodine-iodine solution, Betadine™) is less likely to irritate the skin—it works as well as tincture of iodine and reactions to it are rare.

Antibiotics

In general, prophylactic antibiotics are prescribed far more frequently than is justified by the medical literature.(DURACK) Data to support their use for transperineal implantation are scarce. Two randomized trials have shown that prophylactic antibiotics can decrease the incidence of bacteriuria or bacteremia following transrectal *biopsy*.(RUEBUSH, CRAWFORD) However, no significant decrease in clinically recognized sepsis or urinary infection was shown. Apparently, patients with post-surgical bacteriuria or bacteremia nearly always clear bacteria with natural defenses.

No randomized trials have tested the benefit of routine antibiotics for transperineal biopsy or implantation. In a non-randomized retrospective trial, Packer and colleagues found no benefit to antibiotic use in patients with a documented negative urine culture prior to transperineal biopsy.(PACKER) Although investigators have been unable to find good data to justify routine use of prophylactic antibiotics, their inclusion is standard (**Table 8-2**).(WALLNER, DICKER) Routine pre-implant urinary cultures do not seem necessary.

Timing

If prophylactic antibiotics are used, they should be given within one hour pre-operatively, so that they are present at the time of the procedure. They should then be effective against the most likely contaminants—presumably E. Coli and Enterococcus faecalis.

BLOOD WORK AND CHEST X-RAYS

Considering the minimally invasive nature of transperineal brachytherapy and the rarity of intra-operative complications, routine pre-operative complete blood counts (CBC) or blood clotting tests (PT/PTT) are probably unnecessary in otherwise healthy patients. Similarly, routine electrolytes,

Table 8-2. Antibiotic regimens used by the authors (actual charges to the patient may be higher than those listed)

	Antibiotic(s)	Dose	Timing	Cost ($US)
Blasko	levofloxacin	500 mg IV	immediately prior	$48
	ciprofloxacin	250 mg	bid x 3 days	$25
Dattoli	levofloxacin	500 mg IV	immediately prior	$48
	500 mg	bid x 7 days		$55
Merrick	levofloxacin	500 mg IV	immediately prior	$48
	ciprofloxacin	500 mg PO	bid x 7 days	$55
Wallner	levofloxacin	500 mg POx1	immediately prior	$8

liver function tests, or pre-operative chest X-rays, in otherwise healthy patients without specific indications, are probably unnecessary.(SCHEIN)

ANTI-COAGULANTS

Traditionally, aspirin and nonsteroidal anti-inflammatory agents (NSAID) are stopped one week prior to the implant procedure, and Coumadin (warfarin) should be stopped three days prior.(KEARON) These policies are probably overly cautious considering the rarity of bleeding complications with needle biopsies, even when patients have recently taken NSAIDs.(HERGET)

DVT PROPHYLAXIS

Patients are in the lithotomy position for approximately one to two hours for the implant procedure, and could be at risk for deep venous thrombosis (DVT) or symptomatic thromboembolism. Presumably the risk is very low, and prophylactic measures are not routinely used in these typically otherwise healthy patients. Compression stockings could be used. Prophylactic heparin (6,000 units SubQ immediately prior to the procedure) may be warranted in patients with past history of thrombosis, or other predisposing condition.

OBESE PATIENTS

Obese patients are generally more likely to experience adverse post-operative events, including thromboembolism and heart failure.(MITSUYAMA) No excess risk of complications has been reported specifically for transperineal implantation of morbidly obese patients, so that any risk of serious complications is probably very low.(MERRICK, ROCKHILL)

STERILE BARRIERS

Like prophylactic antibiotics, sterile barriers are used far more than warranted by objective data. It seems sensical that liberal use of sterile gowns or drapes would decrease the likelihood of infectious complications, but this has never been shown. Disposable sterile barriers are unnecessary and wasteful, but often mandated by zealous infection control committees. Considering that transperineal implantation is a minimally invasive procedure, and that the skin is cleansed immediately pre-operatively, routine use of gowns is more decorative than medically beneficial.

Sterile leg and pelvic drapes are another common, but highly questionable, anti-infection practice. Drapes can actually *increase* the infection rate by trapping bacteria on the warm, moist surface under the barrier.(LEWIS, ALEXANDER) The routine use of sterile drapes might be justified as a way to define and preserve a sterile field, but should not be necessary in experienced hands.

Face masks have never been shown to decrease the risk of peri-operative infection for any surgical procedure. In a large, randomized Swedish trial, masks did not decrease the infectious rate for open operations.(TUNEVALL)

ANESTHESIA

Spinal (epidural), general, or local anesthesia can be used. Of 262 orthopedic patients randomized to general or spinal anesthesia at Cornell University Medical College, there was no safety advantage from either a cardiac or cognitive standpoint.(WILLIAMS-RUSSO) The primary advantage of general anesthesia is quick induction. Patients may recover bladder function more quickly with general rather than spinal anesthesia. Spinal anesthesia may prevent perineal discomfort in the immediate post-operative period. Local anesthesia, with or without conscious sedation, is an alternative to spinal or general, and probably cuts down the risk of anesthesia-related problems (see Chapter 9).

PROPHYLACTIC CORTICOSTEROIDS

Approximately 2% to 10% of patients develop post-implant urinary retention, requiring temporary catheter drainage (see chapter 12). Prophylactic corticosteroids might decrease the likelihood of post-operative urinary retention by reducing post-implant tissue swelling. Corticosteroids are rou-

Table 8-3. Dexamethasone schedule used by M. Dattoli.

- •10 mg IV intra-operative
- •4 mg IV at 8 PM
- •4 mg IV at 6 AM
- •discharge with 1-2 week taper schedule

tinely given by M. Dattoli (**Table 8-3**), but they are not currently widely prescribed. One retrospective study supported the use of dexamethsone. (SACCO) Although the concept is appealing, prospective trials have shown no benefit in terms of prostate swelling or urinary retention (MERRICK 00, CARLSON)

ALPHA BLOCKERS

Alpha blockers are widely accepted as standard post-implant therapy for radiation prostatitis (**Figure 8-1**).(MERRICK, ZELEFSKY) Their use pre-implant is more controversial. Merrick and colleagues showed in a retrospective analysis that patients who received prophylactic alpha-blockers had less AUA score elevation and quicker return to pre-implant status compared to patients who were started on alpha blockers only when required for substantial obstructive symptoms.(MERRICK) In contrast, Elshaikh and colleagues, in a prospective randomized study, showed only minimal benefit to prophylactic versus as-needed institution of medication.(ELSHAIKH) The minimal benefit shown by Elshaikh and colleagues seems way out-of-line with retrospective analysis of non-randomized patients, and with the present authors' clinical impression that patients are highly benefitted by their use. More randomized trials are warranted.

HOSPITALIZATION

The vast majority of implants are performed on an outpatient basis, with consistently low peri-operative complications.(HAN, BENOIT) Without data to the contrary, it is hard to justify routine overnight hospitalization. Patients occasionally request to be hospitalized, in case they develop a post-operative problem. Such hospitalization, in the absence of extenuating circumstances, should be discouraged. For the vast majority of patients, it's expensive and unnecessary, and might increase the likelihood of hospital-acquired infection.

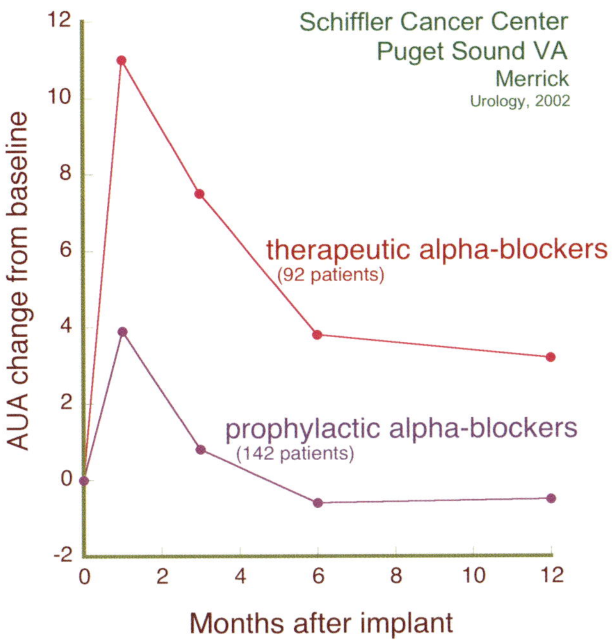

Figure 8-1. Change in AUA scores after brachytherapy in patients who did or did not receive prophylactic alpha-blockers. This was a retrospective analysis of patients randomized between I-125 and Pd-103. The use of alpha-blockers was not specified in the trial methodology.(MERRICK 02)

An alternative to the cost of overnight hospitalization that still provides the patient an extra sense of security is "23-hour hospitalization," whereby patients are observed overnight but spared the full charge of an overnight hospitalization. M. Dattoli has used 23-hour hospitalization routinely. The urinary catheter is removed at 4:00 AM to allow a voiding trial before discharge.

INFORMING PATIENTS

What and how much to tell patients beforehand is largely a matter of personal practice. We have learned a few things the hard way. Patients commonly get the impression from the news media or overly zealous brachytherapists that side effects with brachytherapy are minimal. When considered in comparison to radical prostatectomy, that is likely true. Nevertheless, there is still some risk of acute urinary retention, and a very high likelihood of longer-term (but usually temporary) radiation-related prostatitis. It is prudent to warn patients about these probabilities, if only to allay their concerns as they go through their recovery period (**Table 8-4**).

The possibility of post-operative fever and bleeding should be mentioned. Patients should be warned that they have a 2–10% likelihood of requiring a catheter to relieve urinary retention in the first few weeks following the

Table 8-4. Informed patients—a general list of temporary side effects that patients should be told about beforehand.

- substantial urinary frequency, urgency,slowness, and burning immediately afterward, subsiding over next 24 hours and then returning for 6–24 months
- abnormal bowel function for at least a couple of days
- intermittent gross hematuria for several days, and sometimes later
- 5–10% chance of needing a urinary catheter, for one day or longer
- 2–10% risk of intermittent, painless rectal bleeding (spontaneous healing)

procedure, and that a very small percentage of patients require catheterization for much longer. Patients should expect to have burning with urination, frequent daytime urination, a significant degree of urinary urgency, and perhaps a very slow stream, especially during the night. The potential use of alpha blockers to alleviate radiation-related urinary symptoms for three months or longer should be mentioned.

Patients should be told that they may experience frequent bowel movements, loose stools, and some rectal urgency for several months after implantation. Rectal symptoms usually resolve within six to twelve months of the procedure, usually earlier than the urinary symptoms.(MERRICK 03) We tell patients that the risk of permanent urinary incontinence or serious rectal bleeding or ulceration has been very low in most reported series.

Considering that many patients choose brachytherapy because of their hope to maintain potency, it's a good idea to explicitly warn sexually active patients that they are likely to experience pain with orgasm for several months, and that they are likely to have less ejaculate volume.(MERRICK 01 AND 03) They should also be warned that a small proportion of patients are impotent immediately after the procedure, with some chance that they will improve with time. Although there's no evidence that sexual abstinence is necessary, it seems prudent to use a condom for one week following the procedure.

Most importantly, patients should be reminded to call sooner rather than later if they experience symptoms in excess or different from what they have been told. It's much better, for instance, to juggle a patient's alpha-

Table 8-5. Informed patients—a written list of potential complications that patients could be told about beforehand.

Potential complications from prostate seed implants
temporary use of tube (catheter) in penis to allow urination (1 out of 20 patients)
permanent urine leakage, requiring pads (1 out of 20 patients)
permanent impotence (loss of erections) and/or loss of semen (1 out of 2 patients)
radiation burn to rectum, requiring major surgery (1 out of 500 patients)
movement of seeds to the heart or brain, causing serious damage (1 out of 2,000)
movement of seeds to the lungs, with no known damage (1 out of 4)

I have read these potential complications and have had a chance to clarify my questions
Patient Initials: X__________

blocker dose over a few weeks, rather than to hear first about his urinary obstruction from the emergency room staff at 4:00 AM.

In addition to expected side effects that patients should be warned about to prepare them to cope with their recovery, it is a good idea to supply a written list of potential complications as part of informed consent. **Table 8-5** summarizes the potential complications given to patients at the Puget Sound Veterans Hospital.

REFERENCES

1. Benoit RM, Naslund MJ, Cohen JK. Complications after prostate brachytherapy in the Medicare population. Urol 2000; 55:91-96.
2. Bird BJ, Chrisp DB, Scrimgeour G. Extensive pre-operative shaving: a costly exercise. N Z Med J 1984; 97:727-729.
3. Carlson T, Ciezki J, Elshaikh M, et al. The role of prophylactic tamsulosin ± dexamethasone in patients undergoing prostate I-125 seed implants for prostate carcinoma. A randomized bouble-blind study. Int J Rad Oncol Biol Phys 2004; 60(suppl):S269.
4. Crawford ED, Haynes AL, Story MW, Borden TA. Prevention of urinary tract infection and sepsis following transrectal prostatic biopsy. J Urol 1982; 127:449-451.
5. Dicker AP, Figura AT, Waterman FM, al e. Is there a role for antibiotic prophylaxis in transperineal interstitial permanent prostate brachytherapy? Techniques in Urology 2000; 6:104-108.

6. Durack DT. Prevention of infective endocarditis. NEJM 1995; 332:38-44.
7. Elshaikh M, Ulchaker J, Reddy C, et al. Prophylactic tamsulosin (Flomax) in patients undergoing prostate I-125 brachytherapy for prostate carcinoma: Final report of a double-blind placebo-controlled randomized study. Int J Rad Oncol Biol Phys 2005; 62:164-169.
8. Han BH, Demel KC, Wallner KE, Young L. Patient reported short-term complications after prostate brachytherapy. J Urol 2001; (in press).
9. Herget EJ, Saliken JC, Donnely BJ, Gray RR, Wiseman D, Brunet G. Transrectal ultrasound-guided biopsy of the prostate: Relation between ASA use and bleeding complications. Can Assoc Radiol 1999; 50:173-176.
10. Kearon C, Hirsh J. Management of anticoagulation before and after elective surgery. NEJM 1997; 336:1506-1511.
11. Merrick G, Butler W, Wallner K, et al. Permanent prostate brachytherapy-induced morbidity in patients with grade II and III obesity. Urol 2002; 60:104-108.
12. Merrick G, Wallner K, Butler W. Sexual dysfunction after prostate brachytherapy. Oncol 2003; 17:52-62.
13. Merrick GS, Butler WM, Dorsey AT, al e. Influence of prophylactic dexamethasone on edema following prostate brachytherapy. Techniques in Urology 2000; 6:117-122.
14. Merrick GS, Butler WM, Wallner K, Hines AL, Allen Z. Late rectal function after prostate brachytherapy. Int J Rad Oncol Biol Phys 2003; 57:42-48.
15. Merrick GS, Butler WM, Wallner KE, Lief JH, Galbreath RW. Prophylactive versus therapeutic alpha blockers following permanent prostate brachytherapy. Urol 2002; 60:650-655.
16. Merrick GS, Wallner KE, Butler WM, Lief JH, Sutlief S. Short-term sexual function after prostate brachytherapy. Radiat Oncol Invest 2001; 96:313-319.
17. Mitsuyama H, Wallner K, Merrick G. Treatment of prostate cancer in obese patients. Oncol 2006; 20:1191-1197.
18. Packer MG, Russo P, Fair WR. Prophylactic antibiotics and foley catheter use in transperineal needle biopsy of the prostate. J Urol 1984; 131:687-689.
19. Pound DC. Flexible sigmoidoscopy: Techniques and utilization. Baltimore: Williams & Wilkins, 1990.
20. Ritter MA, French MLV, Eitzen HE. The antimicrobial effectiveness of operative-site preparative agents: a microbiological and clinical study. J Bone Joint Surg 1980; 62A:826.

21. Rockhill J, Wallner K, Hoffman C, Hummel S, Arthurs S. Prostate brachytherapy in massively obese patients. Brachytherapy 2002; 1:54-60.
22. Ruebush TK, McConville JH, Calia FM. A double-blind study of timethoprim-sulfamethoxazole prophylaxis in patients having transrectal needle biopsy of the prostate. J Urol 1979; 122:492-494.
23. Sacco D, Daller M, Grocela J, Babayan R, Zietman A. Corticosteroid use after prostate brachytherapy reduces the risk of acute urinary retention. BJU International 2002; 91:345-349.
24. Seropian R, Reynolds BM. Wound infections after preoperative depilatory versus razor preparation. AM J Surg 1997; 121:251-254.
25. Wallner KE, Roy J, Harrison L. Low risk of perioperative infection without prophylactic antibiotics for transperineal prostate brachytherapy. Int J Radiat Oncol Biol Phys 1996; 36:681-683.
26. Williams-Russo P, Sharrock NE, Mattis S, Szatrowski TP. Cognitive effects after epidural vs general anesthesia in older adults. JAMA 1995; 274:44-50.
27. Zelefsky MJ, Ginor R, Fuks Z, Leibel SA. Efficacy of selective alpha-1 blocker therapy in the treatment of acute urinary symptoms during radiotherapy for localized prostate cancer. Int J Rad Oncol Biol Phys 1999; 45:567-570.

9

Local anesthesia

Traditionally, prostate brachytherapy has been performed under spinal (epidural) or general anesthesia. In the early days of TRUS-based transperineal implants, Haaken Ragde considered performing the procedure under local anesthesia in the outpatient setting, but did not pursue the policy. Roy wrote about using conscious sedation, but did so in a full OR with an anesthesiologist present.(ROY) It was not until 1998 that Wallner and colleagues re-examined the use of local anesthesia. They did so due to a pressing demand for procedure time at the Veterans Hospital in Seattle. Patient safety, efficiency and cost savings are compelling advantages to local anesthesia.

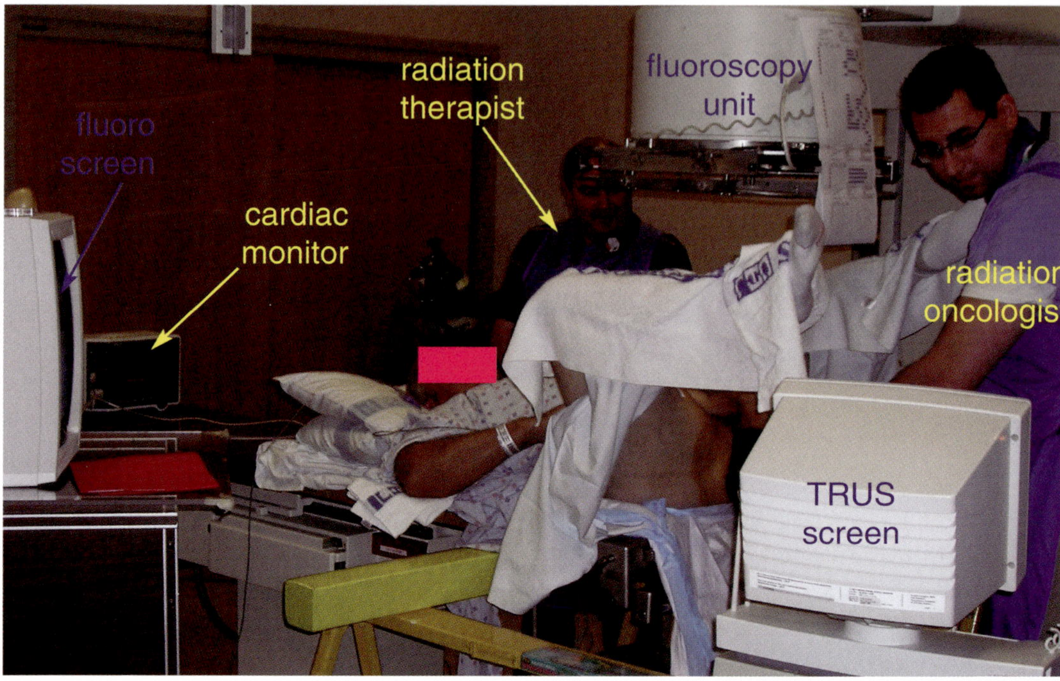

Figure 9-1. Patient is fully awake for their implant procedure in the simulator suite in the Veterans Affairs Puget Sound Health Care System.

When Wallner first proposed using local anesthesia alone, there was a great deal of skepticism from colleagues. However, he reasoned that performing an implant is less invasive than a prostate biopsy, since no tissue is taken with the former, and should require little or no anesthesia, as is customary for biopsies. The possibility of patient movement was also brought up, but turned out to be a non-issue.

LOCAL ANESTHESIA METHODOLOGY

Local anesthesia has been used almost exclusively for the last 2,000+ brachytherapy patients at the Puget Sound VA and at Group Health Cooperative.(WALLNER 99) Several summaries have been published over the past 10 years, but we continue to institute minor changes to our procedure to make it more efficient and easier for patients. The following is our current procedure summary:

Patient selection
Very, very few patients are excluded from local anesthesia. An occasional patient declines local anesthesia, usually because he simply does not want to be aware of the procedure being performed. Such patients typically prefer general anesthesia over local or spinal.

Pre-procedure interview
At the time of initial consultation, a brief pre-operative interview is conducted by the brachytherapist, noting medications and previous medical history. We typically ask the patient how he tolerated the biopsy, to give some indication as to his likely level of procedural tolerance.

Positioning
The patient is positioned supine on the simulator suite in the radiation oncology department. A urinary catheter is inserted. An intravenous line is *not* routinely inserted. He is then placed in the lithotomy position, using stirrups attached to the simulator table (**Figure 9-1**).

Lidocaine injection
All parenteral lidocaine is given in a 0.5% solution with epinephrine (1:100,000) and bicarbonate (**Table 9-1**). The injections are done with a series of increasingly longer and thinner needles, in four stages (**Figure 9-2**).

To start, a 5-8 cm patch of perineal skin is anesthetized by local infiltration of 10 cc of 1% lidocaine, using a 25 gauge 1.5-inch needle (**Figure 9-3, top left**). Immediately following injection into the skin, the underlying subcuta-

Table 9-1. Sandra Arthur's Lidocaine mix (as of 8/2006)
5 cc 1% Lidocaine (with epinephrine 1:100,000)
4 cc 9% NaCl
1 cc 8.4% NaHCO3
10 cc syringe

neous tissue is anesthetized by injecting 15 cc lidocaine solution with approximately eight passes of the same 25-gauge 1.5-inch needle, going perpendicular to the skin surface (**Figure 9-3, top right**).

The transrectal ultrasound (TRUS) probe is then inserted and positioned to reproduce the planning images (**Figure 9-4**). A 3.5-inch 22-gauge spinal needle is inserted into the peripheral planned needle tracks, using TRUS to pick the insertion points on the grid (**Figure 9.3 bottom left**). The tip of a 3.5 inch needle will generally barely reach the apex of the prostate.

For the final phase of injection, a 7.0 inch 22-gauge spinal needle is inserted through the same template positions and advanced to the prostatic base. A 3.5-inch spinal needle is used to introduce the 7.0 inch 22 gauge needle, and prevent excessive deviation within the tissue (**Figure 9-3**). We typically check on fluoro when approaching the pubic arch. We advance the needle slowly in the vicinity of the arch, so as not to cause undue pain if the needle touches the arch (**Figure 9-5**). Some re-positioning of the probe may be needed to circumvent pubic arch interference. A small volume of solution is injected during insertion and a greater volume is injected in the intra-prostatic track as the needle is slowly withdrawn, for a total volume of 5 to 15 cc for this 4th phase of lidocaine injections (**Figure 9-2, right**). At this point in the procedure, the total dose of lidocaine injected is approximately 200 to 300 mg (**Figure 9-6**). The total dose of lidocaine, for the entire procedure, is generally limited to 500 mg.

SEED INSERTION AFTER LIDOCAINE INFILTRATION

When using a Mick® Applicator, only one or two needles are inserted and loaded at a time, to avoid bouncing the prostate against inserted needle tips. During the implant procedure, additional lidocaine solution is injected into one or more needle tracks if the patient experiences substantial discomfort.

LARGE PROSTATES

Large prostate glands have not posed a particular problem in completing the procedure, any more than they do with general anesthesia. Local anesthesia, as described here, still allows for maneuvering to avoid pubic arch interference. Surprisingly, the pubic bone itself is not particularly pain sensitive, although we make an effort not to hit it with a needle tip (**Figure 9-5**).

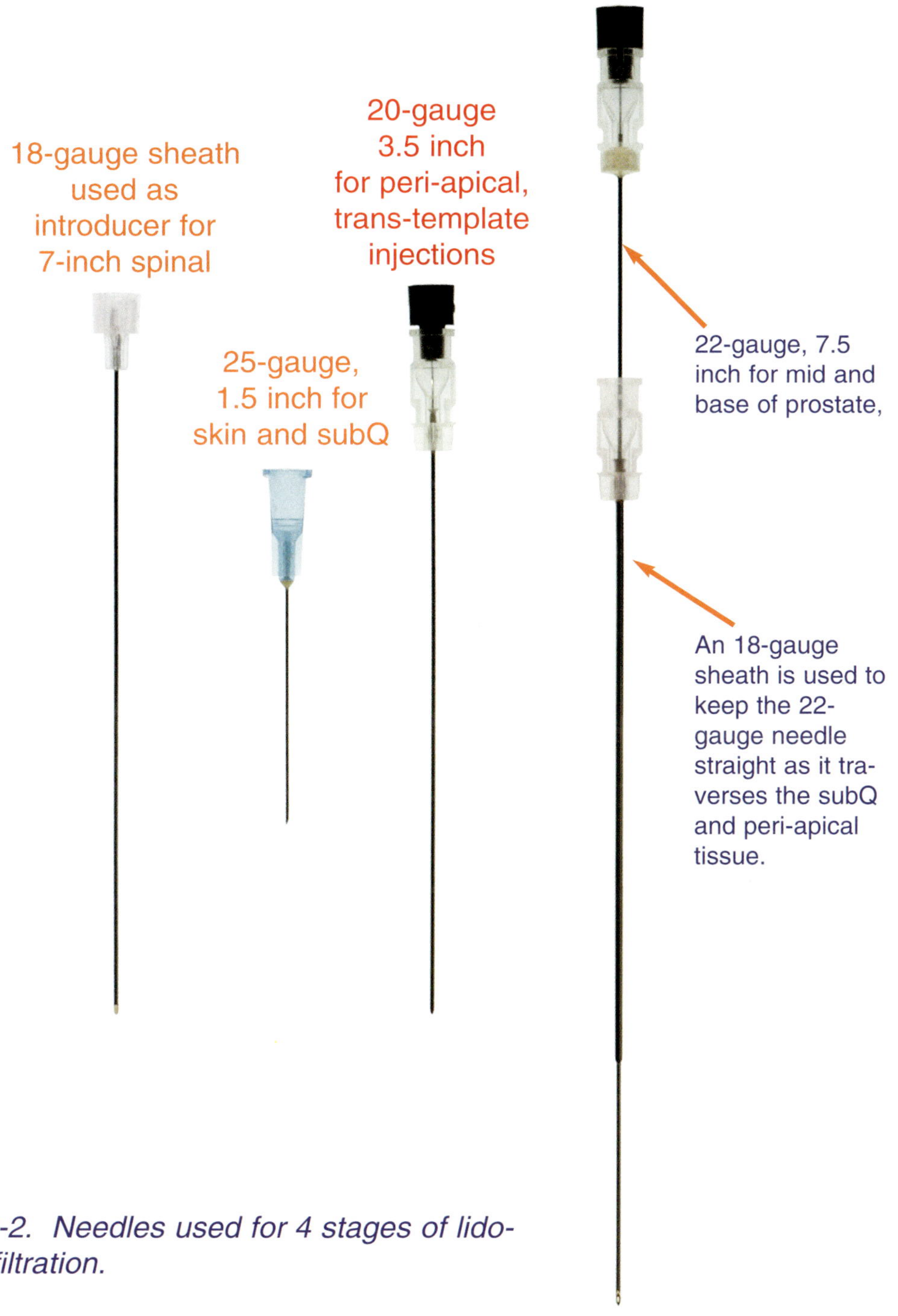

Figure 9-2. Needles used for 4 stages of lidocaine infiltration.

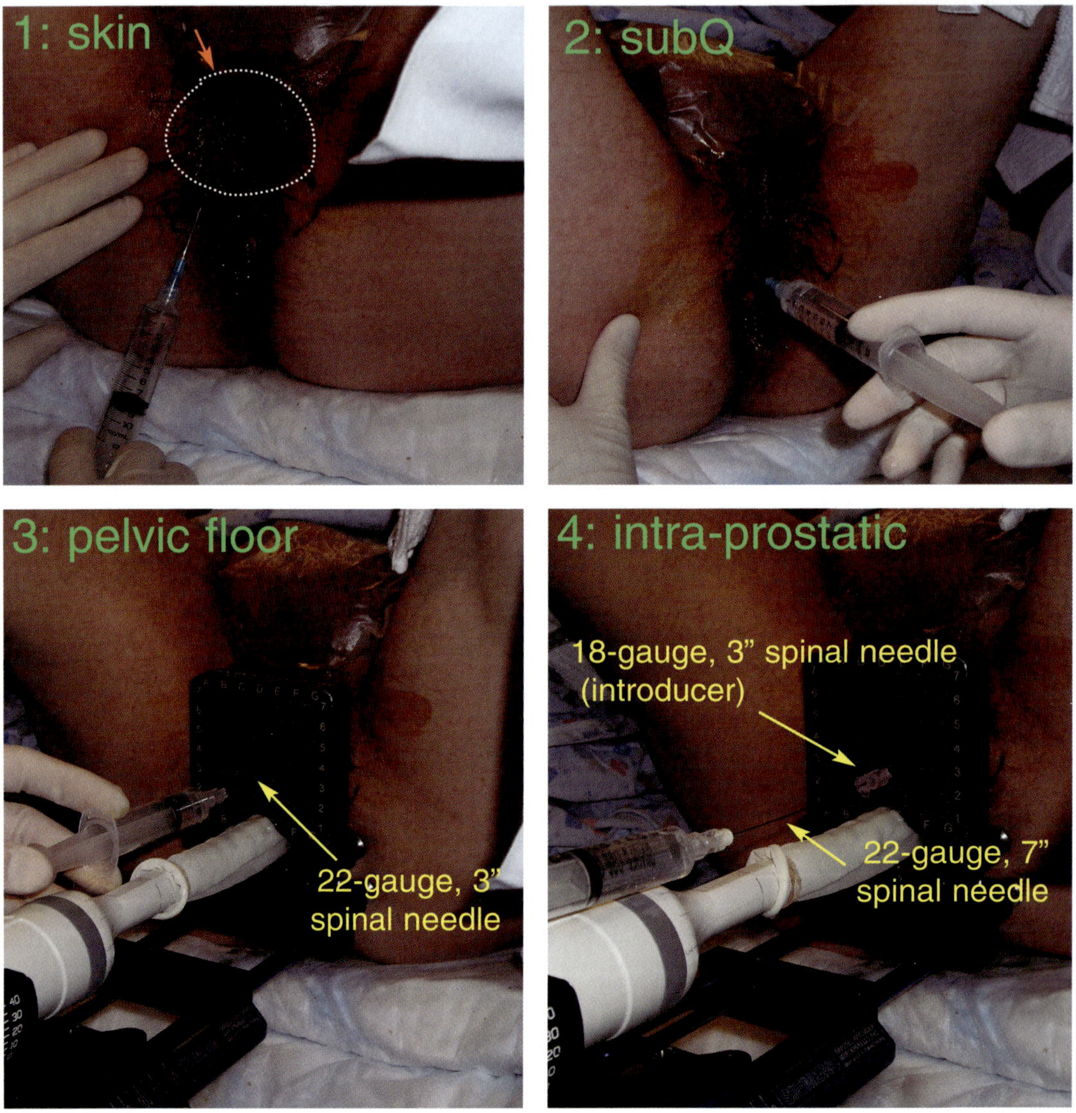

Figure 9-3. Injection of lidocaine into perineal skin, subcutaneous, pelvic floor musculature/peri-apical prostatic region and more prostatic tissue (right). The deeper injections are done with a 7-inch 22-gauge spinal needle, through the TRUS template to monitor position within the prostate.

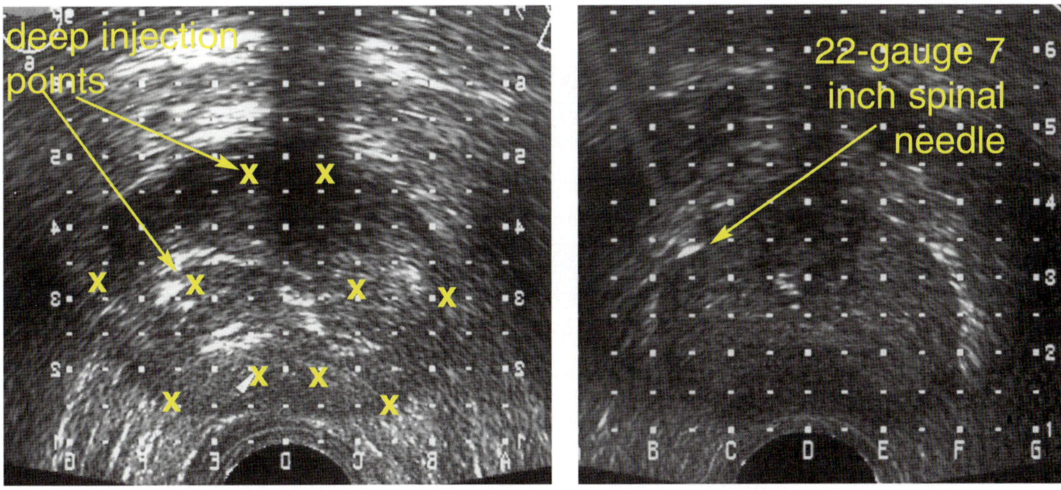

Figure 9-4. *lidocaine injection points (yellow x's) for peri-apical- and prostatic sites. Patients tend to be most difficult to anesthetize along the neurovascular bundles and anterior to the rectum.*

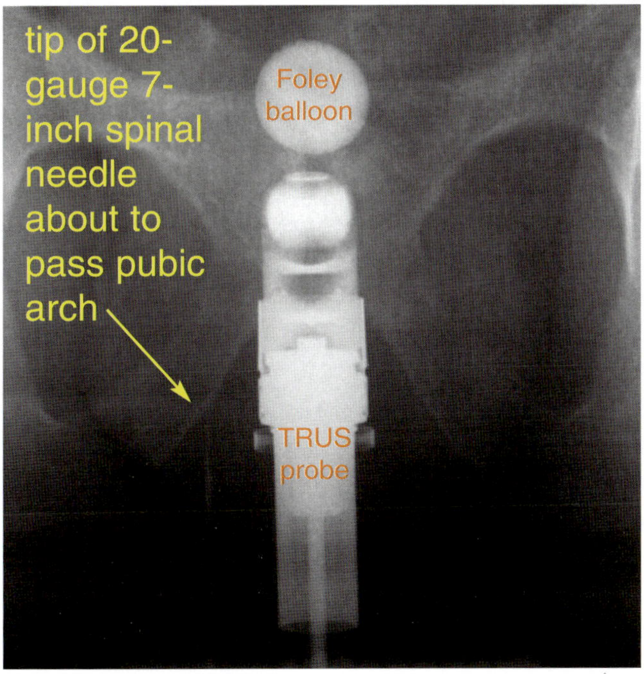

Figure 9-5. Fluoroscopy can be used to alert you when a needle tip is about to pass the pubic arch.

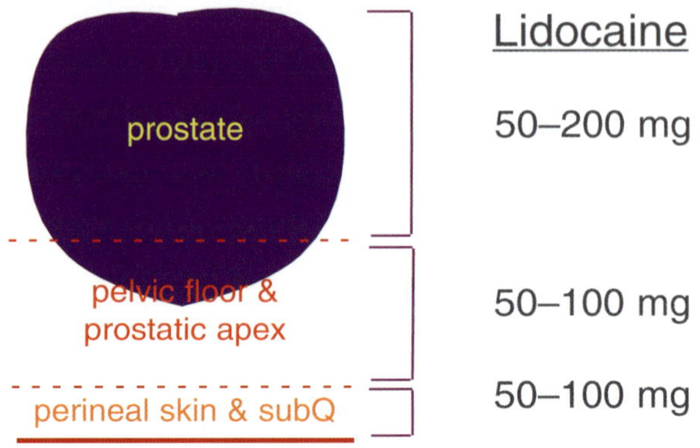

Figure 9-6. Approximate amounts of lidocaine injected into various areas. Other strategies, like injecting into the neurovascular bundles, may be helpful.(NASH)

RECOVERY PERIOD

At the completion of the seed placement, the TRUS probe is removed and plain orthogonal pelvic radiographs taken with the catheter in place. The patient is helped off the simulator table and walks across the hall for his post-implant CT scan. He is then given 30-60 minutes to get dressed, have a snack, and review discharge instructions. Patients are discharged home about one or two hours after completing the implant. They are allowed to drive themselves home, provided that no oral or IV sedation was given.

SEDATION

In addition to local lidocaine infiltration, we have used a variety of sedation techniques over the last three years, including oral agents (benzodiazepines), conscious sedation with midazolam/fentanyl and nitrous oxide (laughing gas). After the first few hundred patients, we have abandoned the routine use of sedation, and currently rely on local lidocaine infiltration alone. From experience, we came to the conclusion that local lidocaine is the primary mode of pain control, and that patient anxiety is best allayed with personal contact and communication during the procedure. In cases of excessive apprehension, various oral or intravenous agents could be given.

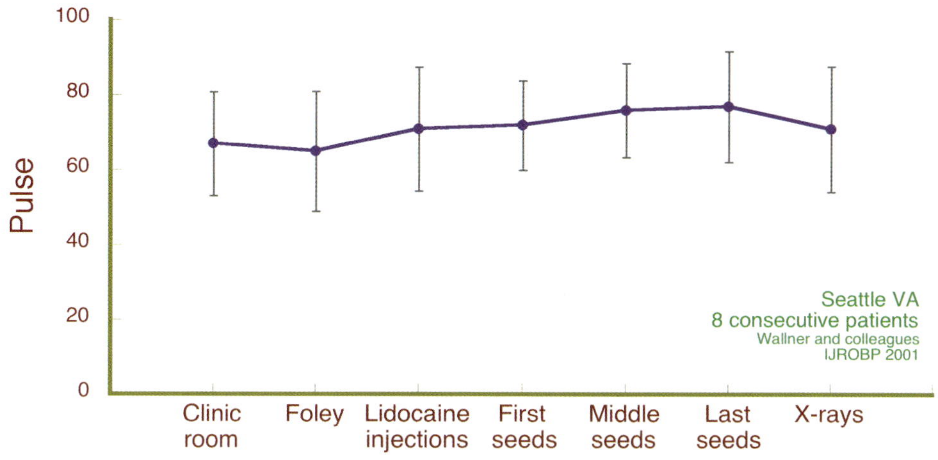

Figure 9-7. Patients' pulse during journey from pre-implant clinic room through Foley catheter insertion, lidocaine injections, seed insertion and final x-rays taken after completion of seed placement.(WALLNER)

PATIENT ACCEPTANCE

Patients tolerate brachytherapy under local anesthesia surprisingly well. Their heart rate and diastolic blood pressure usually show minimal changes, consistent with mild discomfort (**Figures 9-7**). Serum lidocaine levels are typically low.(WALLNER)

As of December 2007, nearly 3,000 patients have received implants under local anesthesia at the Seattle VA or Group Health Cooperative. In all but a few cases, the implant was completed as planned at the first try, with no deviation in needle or seed number due to patient intolerance. However, there was a substantial learning curve, and the procedure has become easier with increasing experience.

To evaluate patients' comfort level early in our experience, patients were interviewed by telephone and asked to rate their pain with the prostate biopsy versus their prostate implant on a scale of 0 to 10. Of 58 patients interviewed at a median of six months since an implant, the median biopsy pain score was 4.5 and the median implant pain score was 3.0 (**Figure 9-8**). There was no correlation between the two scores, nor have we found a

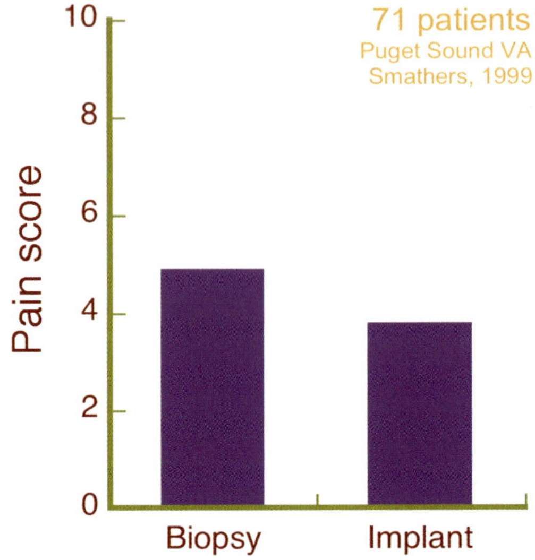

Figure 9-8. Average patient-reported pain scores related to their prostate biopsy versus implant procedure.(SMATHERS)

correlation between the number of needles or the prostate size and the implant pain score.(SMATHERS) Five of the 58 patients (9%) interviewed by Smathers and colleagues stated that they would have preferred to have the procedure under general anesthesia.(SMATHERS) In a more recent patient tolerance study, patients reported similar degrees of pain with their biopssies, and the various steps of their implant procedures (**Figure 9-9**).(MUELLER)

The fact that patients typically rate their implant procedure-related pain as similar or *less* than their prostate biopsy pain, should allay any ethical concerns about switching to local anesthesia. While a small percentage of patients stated in retrospect that they would have preferred general over local anesthesia, it is also common for patients to express relief over not needing general or spinal anesthesia. Local anesthesia may entail more discomfort with the procedure itself than would be experienced with spinal or general anesthesia, but it offers patients the advantages of a lower risk of anesthesia-related complications, and a more rapid return to normal function.

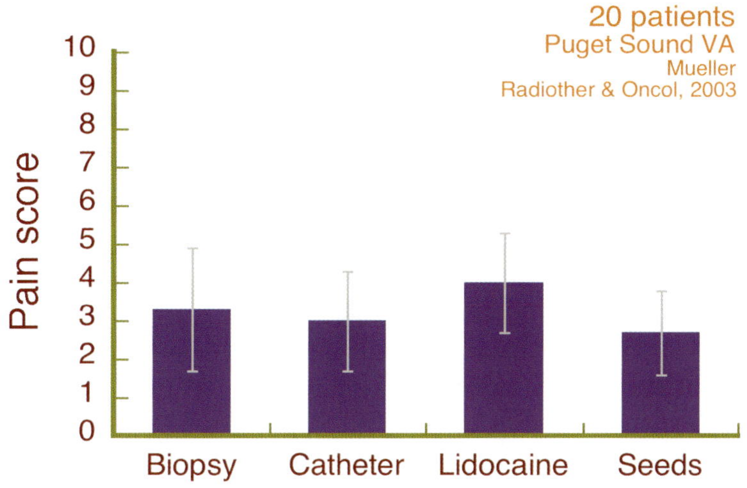

Figure 9-9. Patient-reported pain with various steps of their implant procedure, queried immediately at completion of the procedure.

In addition to a high degree of patient satisfaction, performing implants under local anesthesia allows for phenomenal logistical and cost advantages. Moving the procedure from an operating room or cystoscopy suite avoids the scheduling difficulties of a busy operating room, and slashes operating and recovery room costs.

That's not to say that performing implants with local anesthesia is without its problems. There's no question that patients are more likely to move, requiring some adjustments in positioning of the TRUS probe. But with an easily adjustable TRUS stand, this has not been a big problem. It is also important to point out that patients exhibit an amazingly varied discomfort level with the procedural steps (**Figure 9-10**). Predicting how a given patient will tolerate the procedure is not easy. Even sophisticated psychologic testing did not help us identify the occasional patient who would have trouble tolerating brachytherapy without sedation.(SIMPSON)

STAFFING
At the Puget Sound VA, the staff in attendance include the brachytherapist, a dosimetrist and one radiation therapist. No anesthesiologist is present for the implant procedure. Lidocaine injections are generally done by the

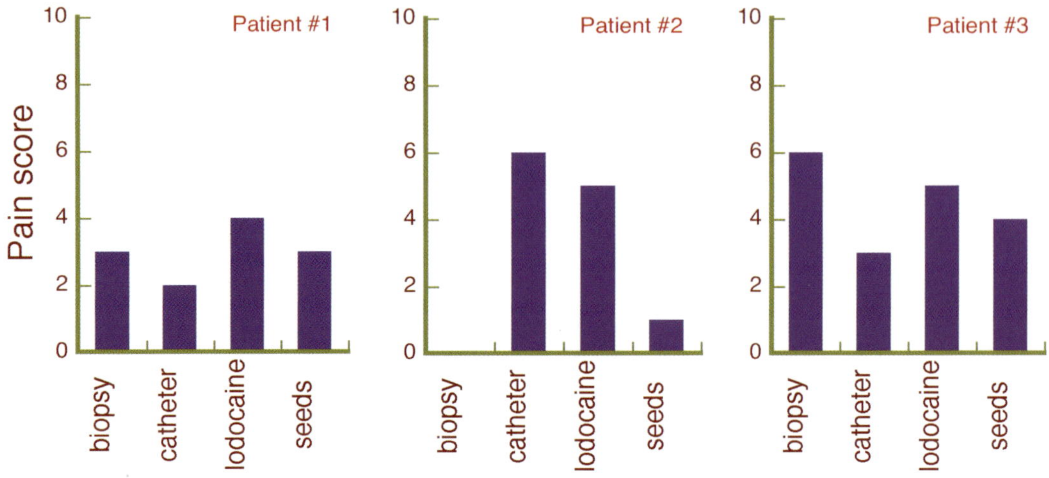

Figure 9-10. Individual patients' response to pain from their biopsy versus catheterization, lidocaine instillation or seed insertion. The point here is that patients respond very differently to different components.(MUELLER)

brachytherapist, but could be done by a nurse practitioner or physician assistant.

Patient tolerance is partly dependent on the attitude of the staff. The procedure is facilitated by light-hearted rapport between the patient and staff.

PROCEDURE TIME

In experienced hands, about 10-15 minutes is needed to complete the lidocaine infiltration process. Once the lidocaine infiltration is completed, placing seeds typically requires another 20-30 minutes, depending on the implant technique (**Figure 9-11**).

REFERENCES

1. Mueller A, Wallner K, Corriveau J, Arthurs S, Gwinn M, Sutlief S. A reappraisal of local anesthesia for prostate brachytherapy. Radiother and Oncol 2003; 67:309-312.

2. Nash PA, Bruce JE, Indudhara R, Shinohara K. Transrectal ultrasound guided prostatic nerve blockade eases systematic needle biopsy of the prostate. J Urol 1996; 155:607-609.

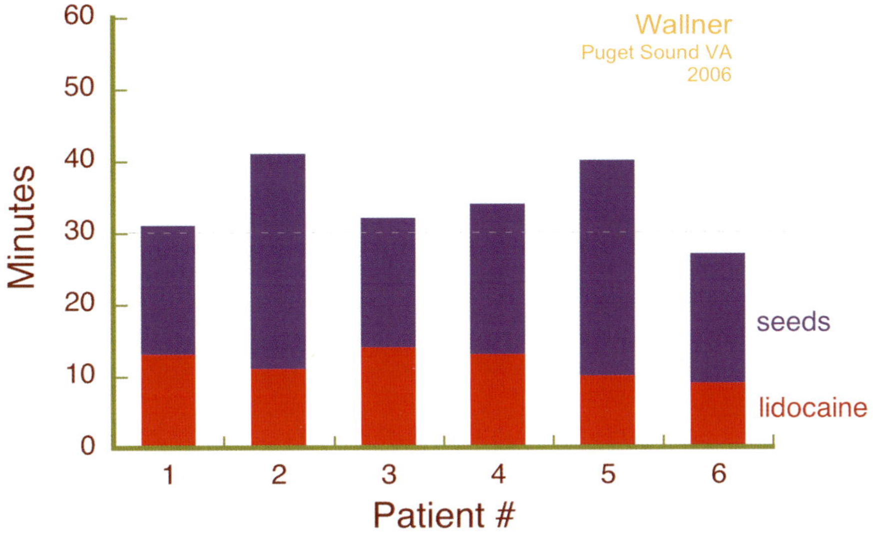

Figure 9-11. Time taken for lidocaine injections and seed implantation for 6 consecutive patients treated by K Wallner. Total time in brachytherapy suite is longer, due to patient set-up and radiation safety check times.

3. Roy J, Pouliot J, Taschereau R. Permanent transperineal prostate implants performed under local anesthesia. Int J Rad Oncol Biol Phys 1998; 42(suppl):296.

4. Simpson C, Wallner K, Sanchez D, et al. Patient anxiety and tolerance of prostate brachytherapy under local anesthesia. JBI 2001; 17:77-81.

5. Smathers S, Wallner K, Simpson C, Roof J. Patient perception of local anesthesia for prostate brachytherapy. Seminars in Urol Oncol 2000; 18:142-146.

6. Wallner KE, Simpson C, Roof J, Arthurs S, Korssjoen T, Sutlief S. Local anesthesia for prostate brachytherapy. Int J Rad Oncol Biol Phys 1999; 45:401-406.

10

Technique

One of the more remarkable things about prostate brachytherapy is the variety of ways to do a good implant. A good result is not as much dependent on which technique you use, but rather how careful and proficient you are with the methods you choose. In this chapter, we'll walk through the implant procedure from start to finish, describing a variety of methods for each step. Take your pick. If you're new to brachytherapy, don't assume that what's here is best for you—do your own reading and then visit with other brachytherapists to decide which techniques best fit your practice setting. If you're a rigid, arrogant, old brachytherapist already set in your ways, consider trying some of the technical variations described

Lithotomy   Extended lithotomy

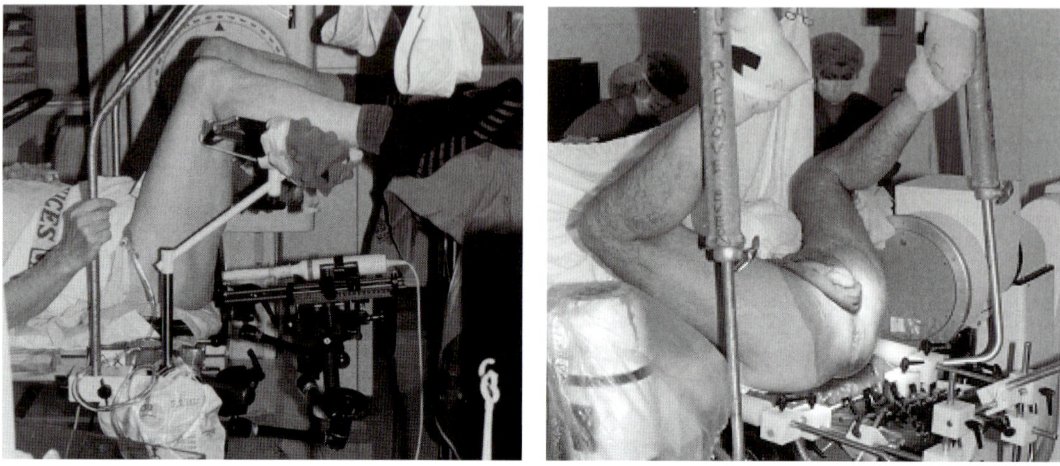

Figure 10-1. Patient positioning. Keep the pelvis square. More extended lithotomy (right) helps avoid pubic arch interference, but be careful to orient the probe such that the prostate lines up on the grid as it did for the planning images (see Figure 10-16).

here. Often, there are more efficient or downright better ways than what you're accustomed to, partly because the equipment keeps getting better.

PATIENT POSITIONING

After induction of anesthesia, place the patient in the lithotomy position (**Figure 10-1**). Try to reproduce the positioning of the planning scan, realizing that there will always be minor differences. The legs should be symmetrically rotated and extended at the hips and at the knees to avoid rotating the pelvis on the head-to-toe axis. Step back when you think you're done setting up and make sure the patient is as squarely lined up as possible, in the middle of the table. The perineum should be at the very end of the table to allow room to maneuver the ultrasound probe.

The extended lithotomy position helps to avoid pubic arch interference by tilting the pelvis back, moving the pubic bones away from the anterior surface of the prostate. This can be achieved by adjusting the leg stirrups or by pulling the patient's pelvis toward the end of the table, without changing the position of the stirrups. Some brachytherapists place patients in the extended position at the time of initial setup, while others start with the

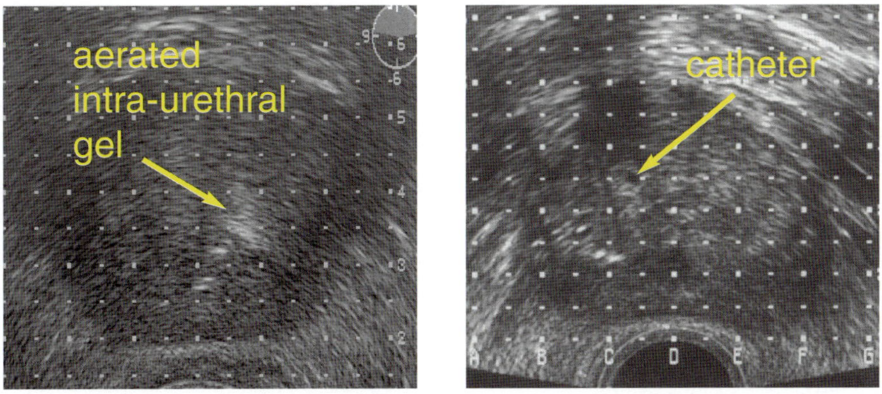

Figure 10-2. Some patients have a remarkably asymmetric urethra. The patient on the left has aerated intra-urethral gel. The patient on the right has a catheter in place.

femurs at 90 degrees to the floor, and move to the extended lithotomy position only if pubic arch interference calls for it.

A good set of stirrups can really make your life easier. Rigid boots, which are easy to adjust and minimize the likelihood that a patient's legs shift position, are probably best.

URETHRAL VISUALIZATION

There's no shortage of opinions as to how (or even *if*) the urethra should be visualized during the procedure. Most brachytherapists use some technique to visualize the urethra during the procedure, primarily to make sure that seeds are not placed inside it. The biggest problem with intraurethral seeds is that they'll be expelled and won't contribute to the dose as planned. Admittedly, most patients' urethras are midline, and simply avoiding seed placement in the prostate midline is enough to keep out of the urethra. But some patients have a markedly asymmetric urethra and its visualization really helps (**Figure 10-2**).

A catheter is the simplest, most reliable way to visualize the urethra and bladder neck. Their downside is that they produce a large ultrasound void (**Figure 10-3**). There is some concern that having a catheter in place during the procedure will lead to urethral tears if the urethral lining gets caught between an advancing needle tip and the catheter. This doesn't seem to be the case, since many brachytherapists use a catheter routinely and per-

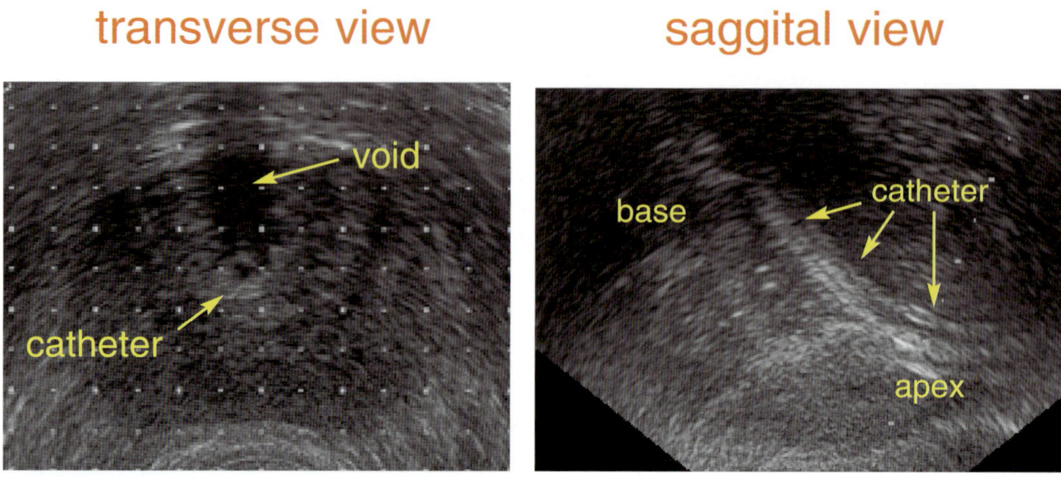

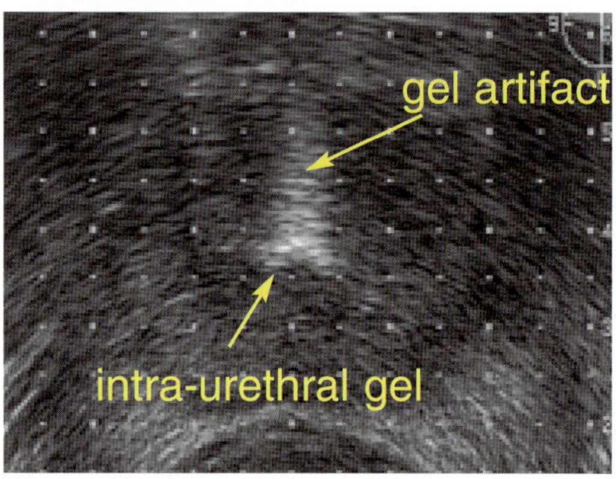

Figure 10-3. Top panels show transverse and sagittal TRUS images with a Foley catheter in place and an ultrasound void behind it. The left panel shows a transverse image with aerated intra-urethral gel, with substantial artifact behind it.

sistent post-implant gross urethral bleeding is unusual. Concern has also been raised that a catheter might deform the prostate, altering the seed placement. Not so. The prostate is a very firm gland—a soft, flexible catheter won't change its shape substantially.

An advantage of a catheter is that the balloon marks the prostatic base on fluoroscopy, so long as the balloon is snug against it (**Figure 10-4**). Place some traction on the catheter to make sure that the balloon is pulled against the prostate, but don't overdo it so that you displace the prostate caudally.

As an alternative to keeping a catheter in during the procedure, M. Dattoli uses one prior to starting the implant, placing 50 cc of 100% Renografin™ into the bladder, and taking a lateral fluoroscopic view. The image is held on the second fluoroscopy screen throughout the implant procedure, to

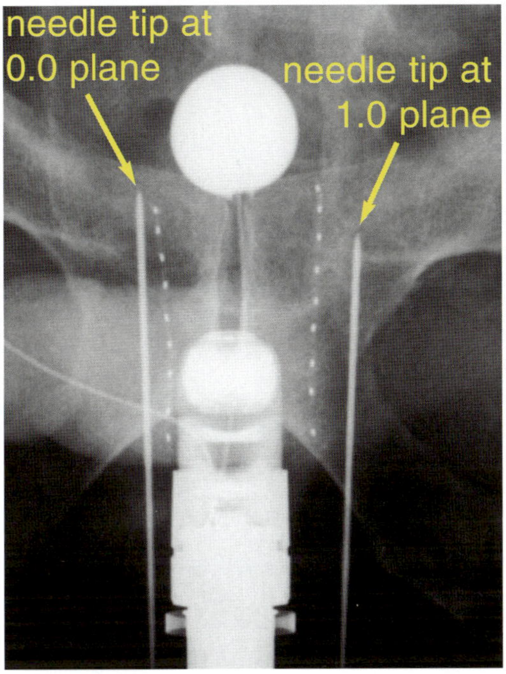

Figure 10-4. The catheter balloon is a simple marker of the prostatic base. Positioning the needle tip at the lower edge of the balloon on fluoroscopy is one way to check that you're at the 0.0 plane (assuming a normally shaped prostate).

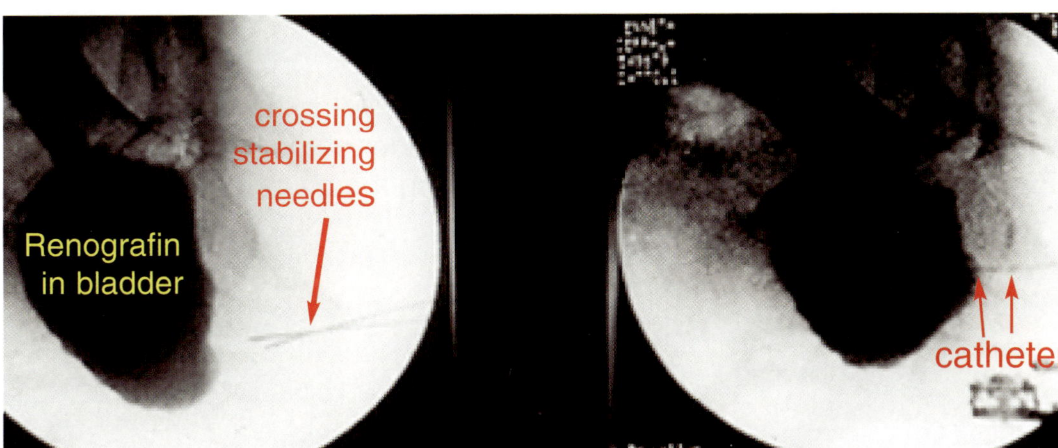

Figure 10-5. Fluoroscopy screens during procedure by M. Dattoli. On the right is the pre-procedure view with a urinary catheter in place (arrows) and 50 ml Renografin™ in the bladder. The right-sided image is kept during the procedure, to help identify the urethra. The left-sided screen is used during the procedure to help monitor needle and seed placement. Note posterior crossing stabilization needles on the left screen.

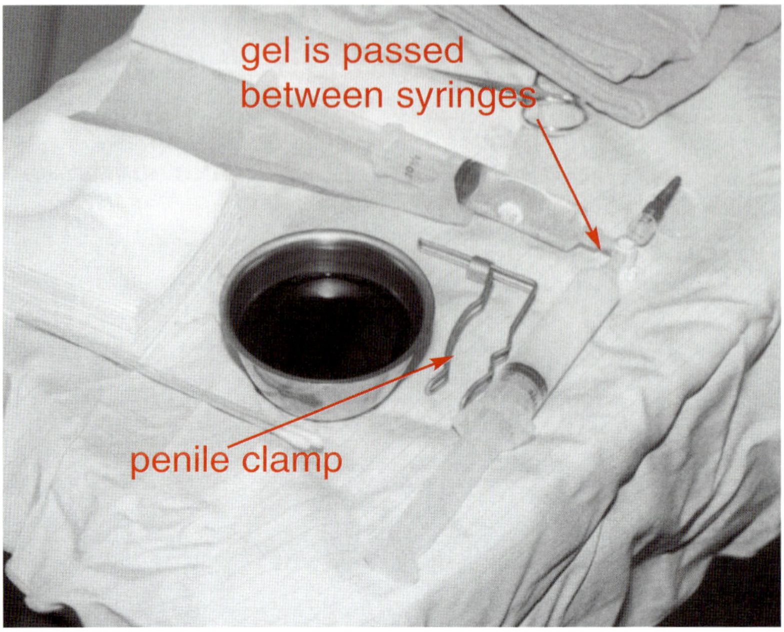

Figure 10-6. Gel is aerated by repeatedly passing it between syringes through a stopcock. Once instilled, a penile clamp is applied to keep the gel from leaking out.

serve as a reference as to where the urethra is. After the reference image is taken the catheter is removed for the remainder of the implant procedure (**Figure 10-5**). Dye is left in the bladder during the procedure to help visu-

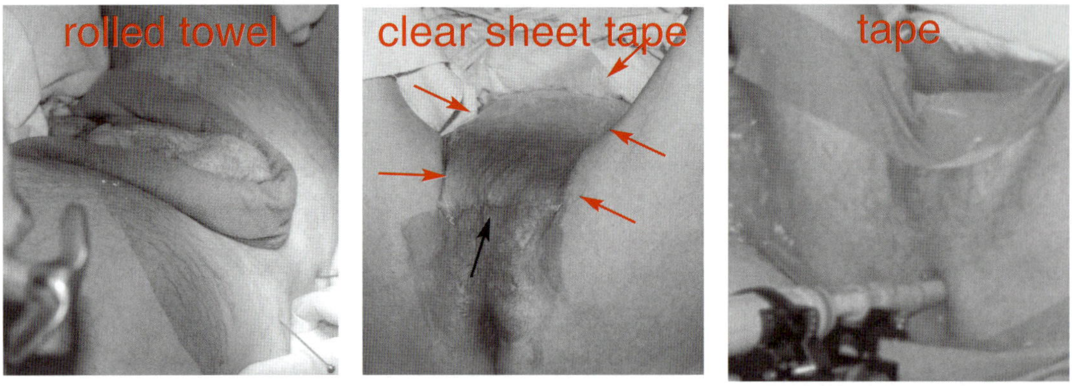

Figure 10-7. Scrotal solutions. A rolled surgical towel or tape are usually sufficient to keep the testicles out of the perineal field.

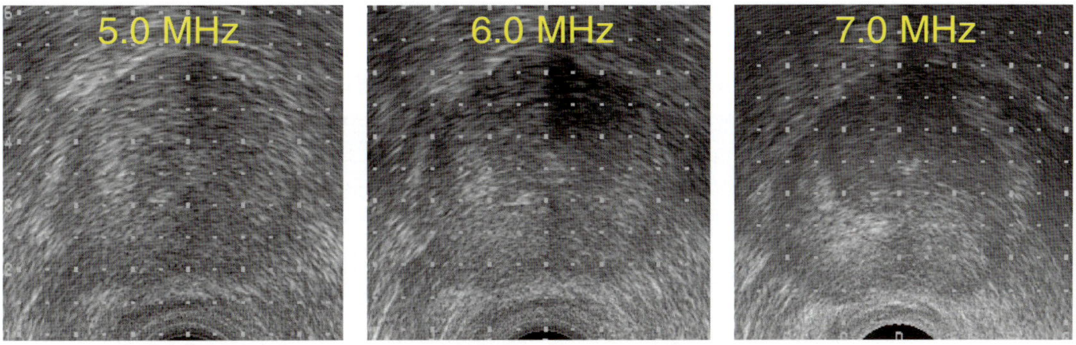

Figure 10-8. Various TRUS frequencies—6.0 MHz typically gives the best overall tissue contrast, but the differences aren't huge.

alize the interface between bladder and prostate on lateral or anterior fluoroscopy.

Another popular urethral visualization technique is installation of aerated gel (**Figure 10-3**). Sterile water-soluble lubricating jelly or ultrasound gel is passed back and forth between two syringes until it turns milky white. It is then instilled through the urethra using a 20 cc syringe with a catheter tip. A penile clamp keeps it from leaking out (**Figure 10-6**).(SYLVESTER) During the procedure, the gel will often not be visible on some TRUS slices, but can be milked into view by pressing on the anterior pelvic wall.

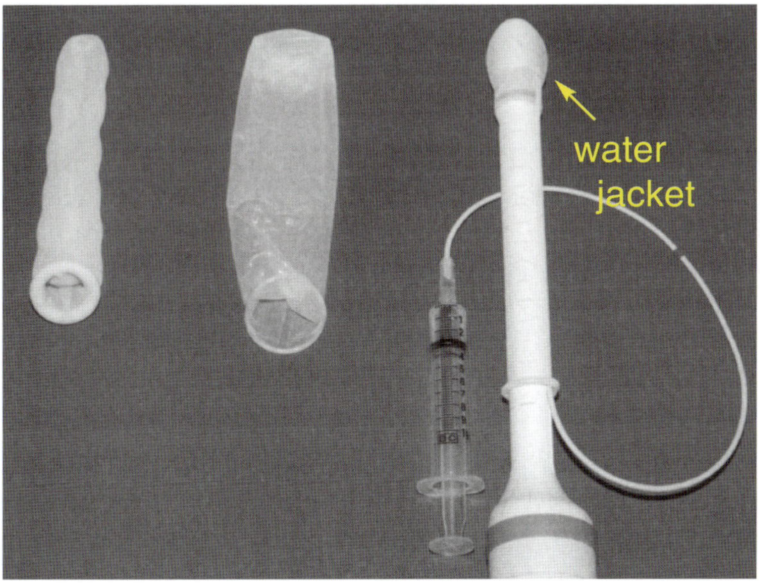

Figure 10-9. A variety of probe covers are available. We're not convinced that they make much difference in image quality, despite wide differences in price.

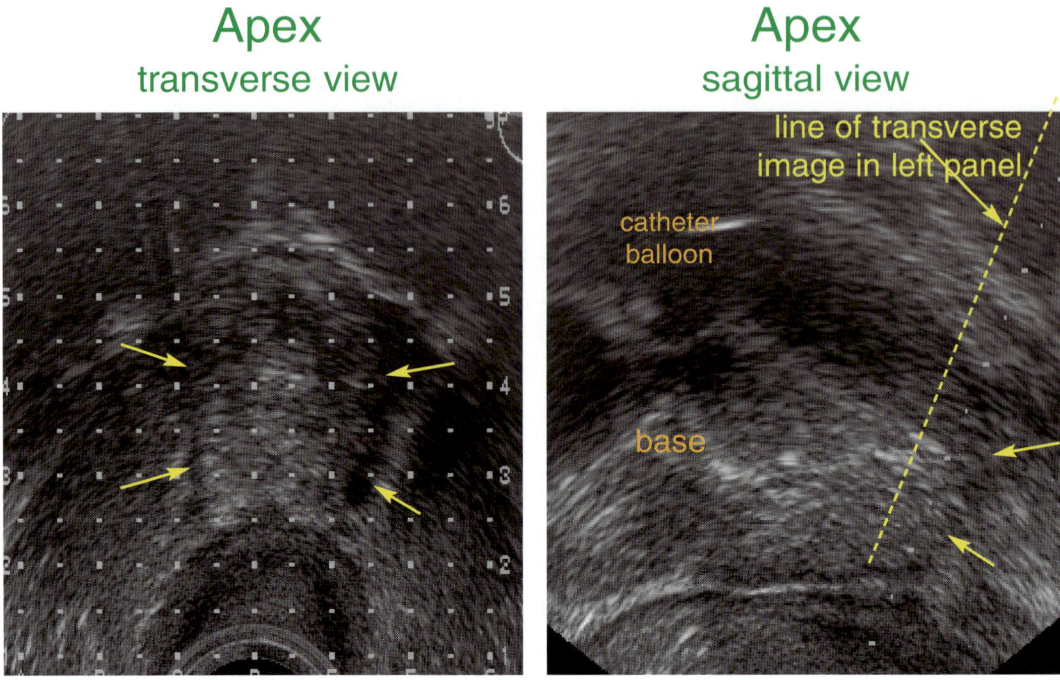

Figure 10-10. The transverse image on the left shows poor visualization of the prostatic apex (yellow arrows) because it blends in with the tissue-equivalent pelvic floor. The sagittal view (right) offers a clearer view of the apical margins, in part because the continuous prostatic contour can be visually extrapolated from more proximal portions of the prostate.

Scrotum

The scrotum should be kept away from the perineum. It can be held up to the abdominal wall with tape or a rolled up, wet cloth towel (**Figure 10-7**). Using towel clips to fasten the scrotal skin against the anterior abdominal wall adds unnecessary trauma to the procedure.

TRUS probe

Current TRUS probes are remarkably durable and easy to set up. Frequencies of 5.0, 6.0 and 7.0 MHz are standard. Higher frequencies give better tissue visualization closer to the probe. It comes down to personal preference (**Figure 10-8**).

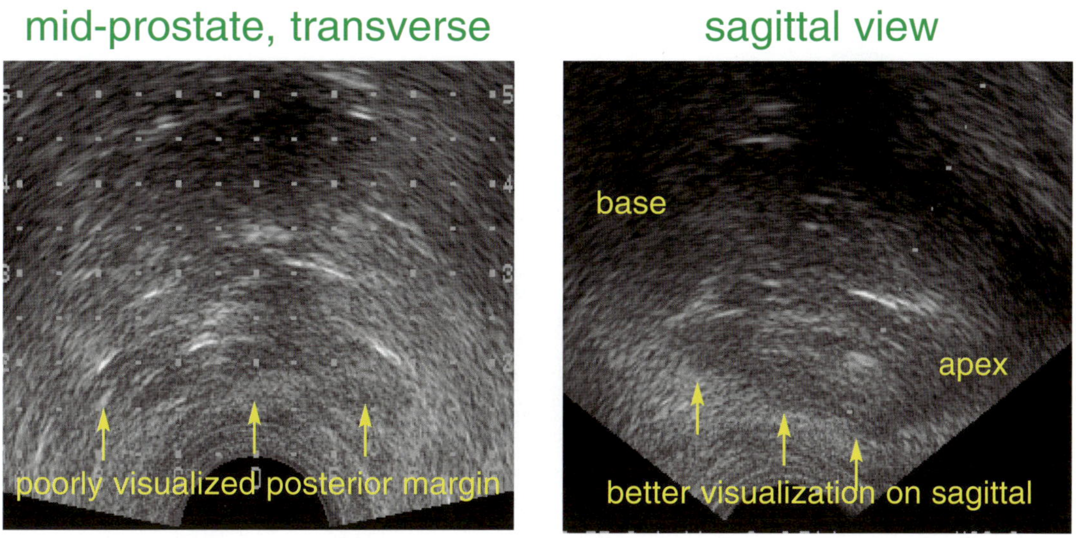

Figure 10-11. Transverse and sagittal images with seeds in place. The posterior rectal wall (arrows) may become obscured toward the end of the case, and it can usually be better seen on sagittal imaging (right).

Probe covers

The probe should be covered generously with lubricant. Water-soluble gel seems to be as good as specially-designated "ultrasound gel." Most brachytherapists use at least one probe cover, primarily to keep the probe clean. A variety of covers can be used, with no obvious advantage of one over the other (**Figure 10-9**). The more sophisticated covers include a water bag that can be filled from a syringe reservoir, allegedly improving coupling between the probe and the rectal wall. An outer condom can be used, but may interfere with image quality. Use ample lubricant between inner and outer condoms.

While implants can be done well with transverse imaging alone, sagittal imaging helps visualize the prostatic base and apex and verify proper needle location and depth (**Figure 10-10**). The sagittal view can help prevent drawing seeds into the urogenital diaphragm and penile bulb. Biplane probes, capable of transverse and sagittal imaging, are now standard. There's a wide variability in the degree to which sagittal imaging is used. It's not essential, but it's good to have it available.

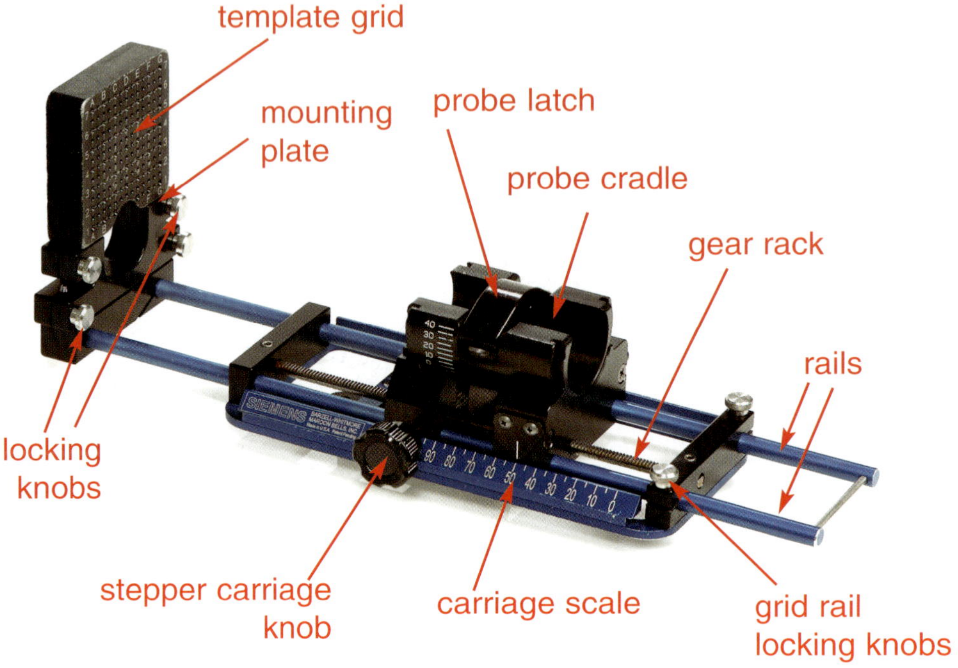

Figure 10-12. The stepping unit allows movement of the TRUS probe at 5 mm increments.

Some brachytherapists use sagittal imaging in lieu of fluoroscopy to check that seeds are not pulled distally with the receding needle tip. Sagittal imaging is especially valuable toward the end of a case, when seed artifact can obscure the prostatic-rectal interface on transverse view (**Figure 10-11**).

Stepping unit and stabilizer
The TRUS probe is held in a *stepping unit*, allowing it to be moved caudal or cephalad at 0.5 cm intervals. The unit should hold the probe steady, without obstructing access to the perineum (**Figure 10-12**). Set the carriage in the middle of its range before inserting the probe, to allow maximal range of useful motion.

The stepping unit is supported by a *stabilizing stand*, either table-mounted or floor-mounted (**Figures 10-13 and 10-14**). The principle advantage of a table-mounted stand is that it moves with the table if the table position is

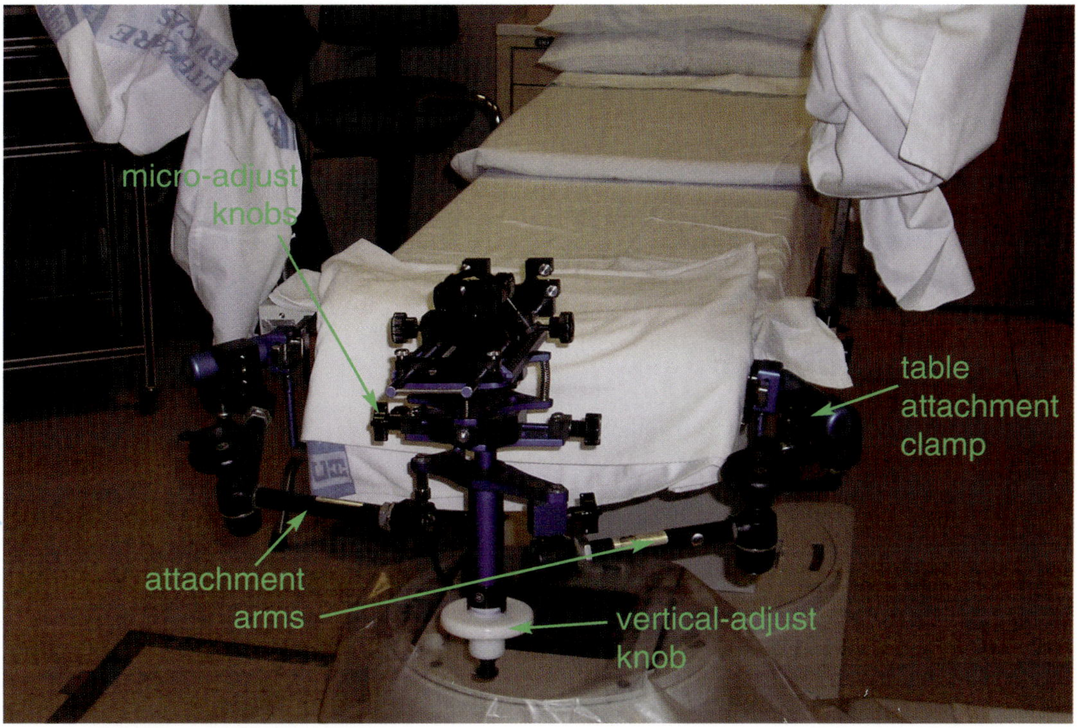

Figure 10-13. Stepping unit mounted to an older model table-mounted stabilizer.

changed during the case. Table-mounted stands are typically lighter and more portable.

A stable, but easily adjustable stepping unit (and stand) can make the difference between a pleasant versus a frustrating implant experience. Even under anesthesia patients commonly move. Sometimes you'll have to make adjustments intra-operatively for pubic arch interference. A variety of units are available, ranging in price from $12,000–$20,000. Your choice could be the most important equipment decision you'll make. Ask for advice from experienced colleagues *before* you buy.

PROBE POSITIONING

A quick digital rectal exam to check the bowl prep is a good idea. To begin imaging the prostate, place the probe tip against the anus, and press gently until the sphincter gives way. The probe should advance easily and the prostate will come into view. Make gross probe adjustments by moving the

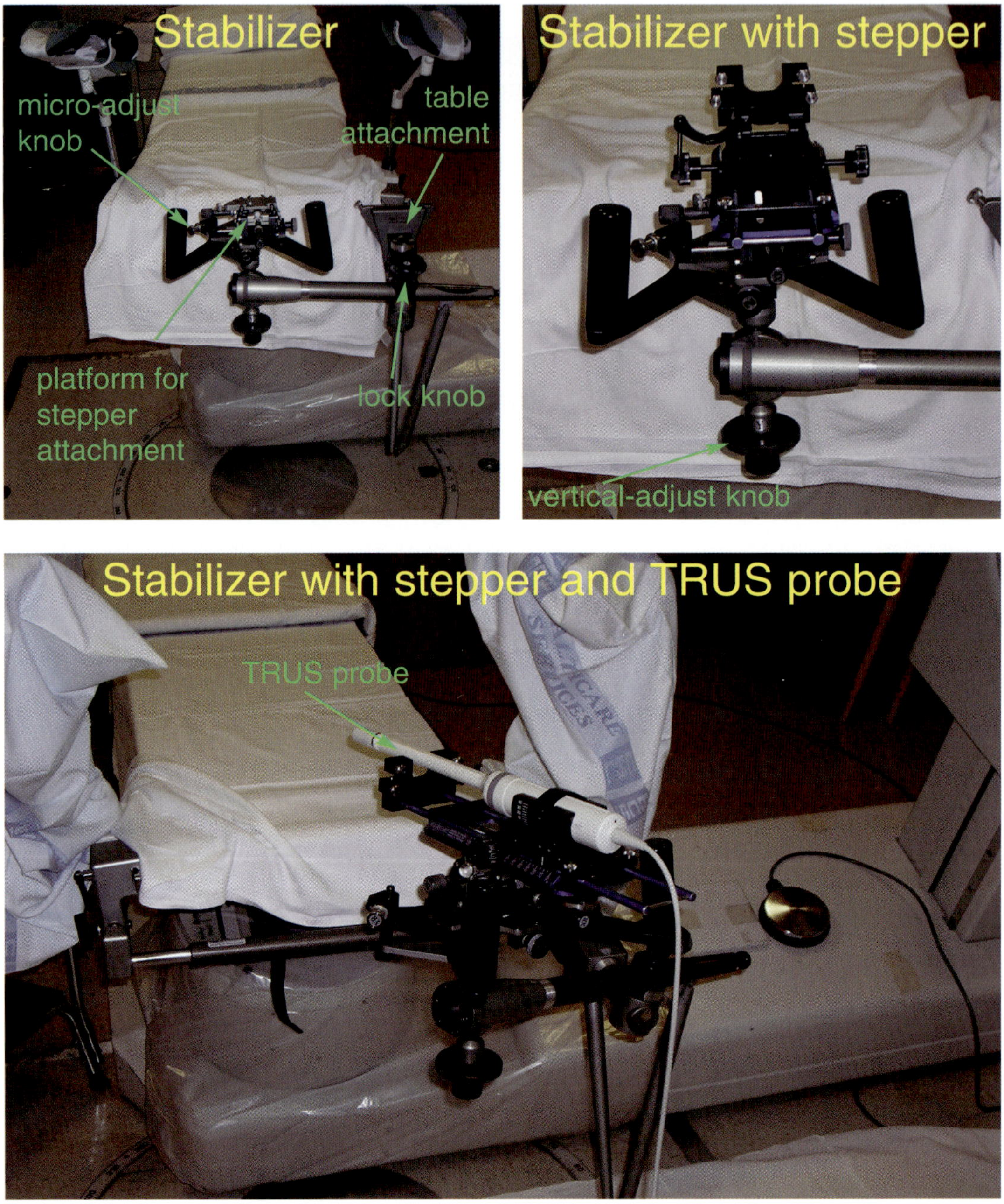

Figure 10-14. Single-arm table-mounted stabilizer. This model has a quick-adjust universal joint that makes for easy, quick changes.

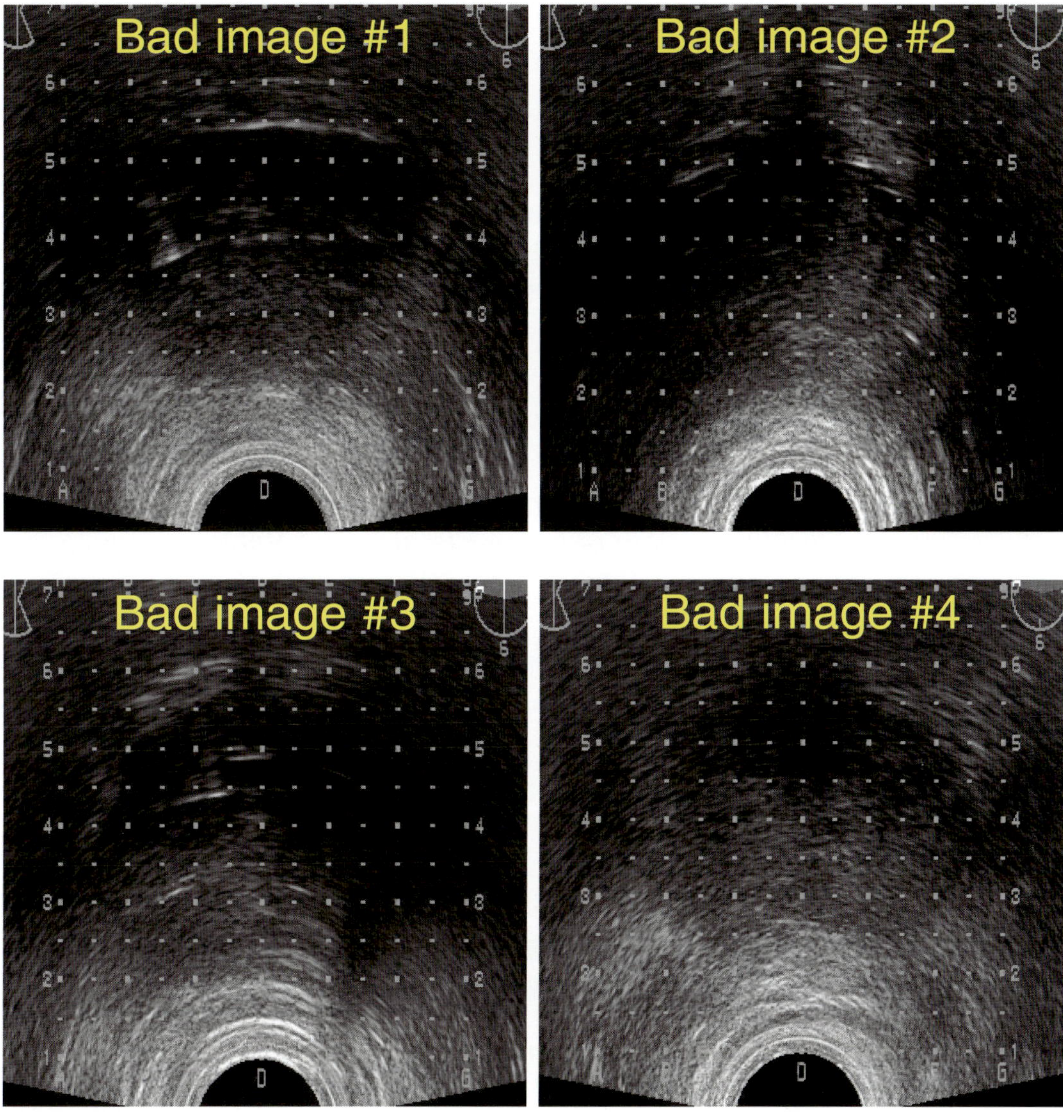

Figure 10-15. Poor images like these can result from inadequate probe pressure against the anterior rectal wall, or by gas, mucous, or feces. Passing the probe in and out of the rectum, or increasing the probe pressure against the rectal wall will usually improve the image. It's always possible to do better than this! Don't proceed until you have a sharp image, even if it means starting over again with a new probe cover.

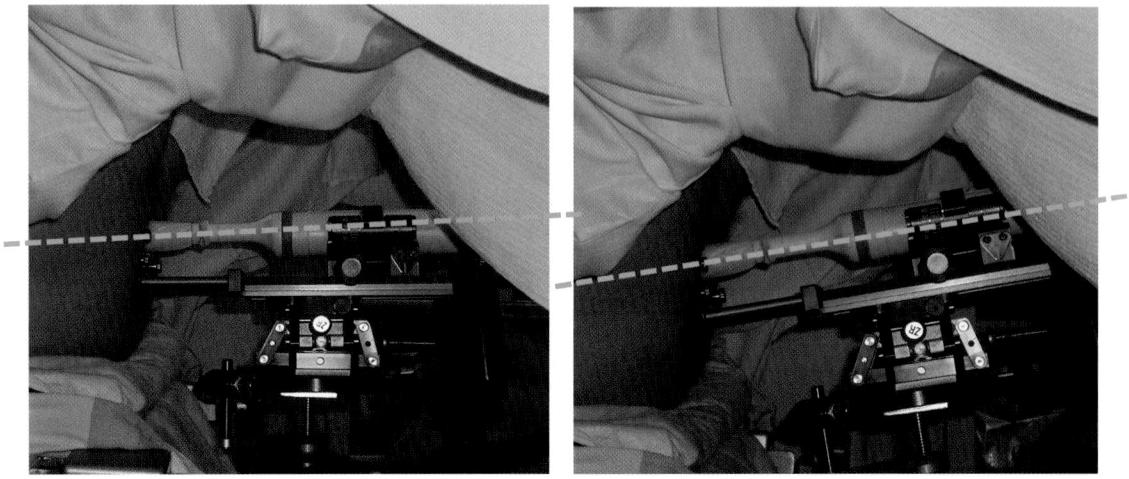

Figure 10-16. The TRUS probe tip is typically angled slightly toward the floor. Both of these tilts are acceptable.

stand itself. Make small changes with the fine adjusters on the stepping unit/stand. If the image is not clear, move the probe in and out to clear gas from the interface between the probe and the anterior rectal wall (**Figure 10-15**). If unsuccessful, completely withdraw and reinsert the probe. If gas or fecal artifact persists, an intra-operative enema using a 30 French red rubber catheter attached to a large syringe will usually clear things.

RECREATE THE PREPLANNING IMAGES

Before placing needles, make sure that the imaging planes match those for the planning images. The images often do not match *exactly*, due in part to daily changes in the prostate shape and volume, or to technical factors. But they should be very close. Use common sense. Don't get too crazy about a couple of millimeters difference between the planning images and those at the time of the procedure. After all, the entire prostate volume will be unpredictably up to 100% larger by the time you're finished with the implant (see Chapter 11).

The probe tip should be angled slightly toward the floor (**Figure 10-16**). The precise angle doesn't make as much difference as you might think, because the prostate tends to follow the angle of the probe. The simplest

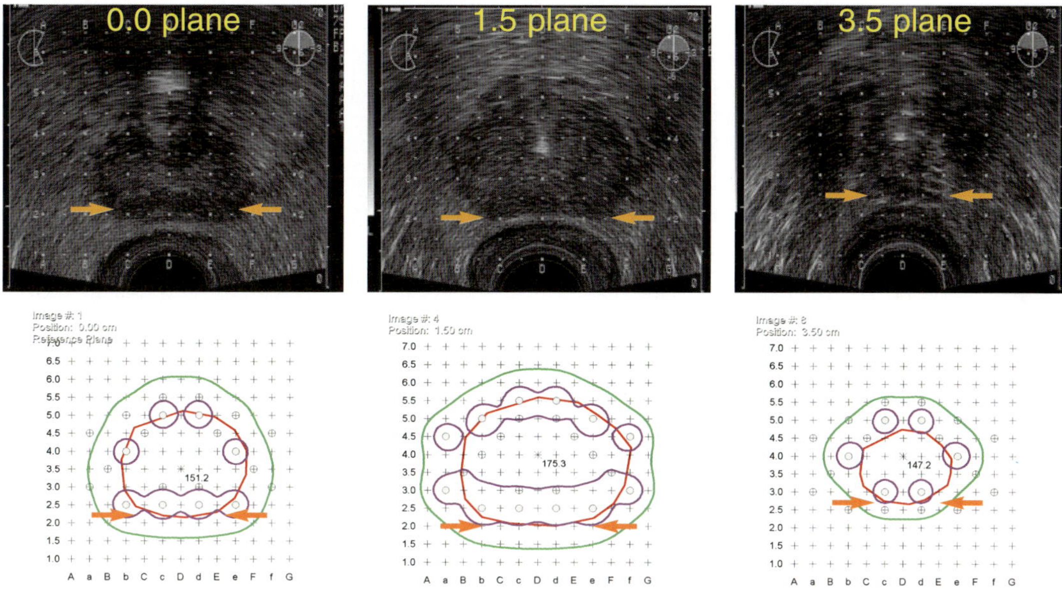

Figure 10-17. Make sure that the posterior prostatic margin aligns on the template the way that it did on the planning images. The prostate should be midline on the screen, typically with the urethra on the middle coordinate. In this case, the posterior prostate is aligned on the 2.0 template row.

way to get the prostate lined up properly on the grid is to make sure that the posterior margin of the mid-prostate is lined up on the template as it was on the planning images, and then to check that the base and apex also match the plan (**Figure 10-17**). To get it "perfect" you may need to tilt the probe slightly in various directions. As long as the back of the prostate aligns properly, slight differences in the anterior margin are probably clinically unimportant.(MCNEAL, ROSEN)

Once you think you've got it right, it's a good idea to step back and look at the probe's position, making sure that it is not grossly skewed in relation to the pelvic bones, increasing the chance of pubic arch interference on one side.

Probe pressure

Gentle probe pressure against the prostate allows good coupling with the tissue, but too much pressure distorts the image, leading to artifactual flattening of the prostate (**Figure 10-18**). In the extreme, "dog ear" artifacts

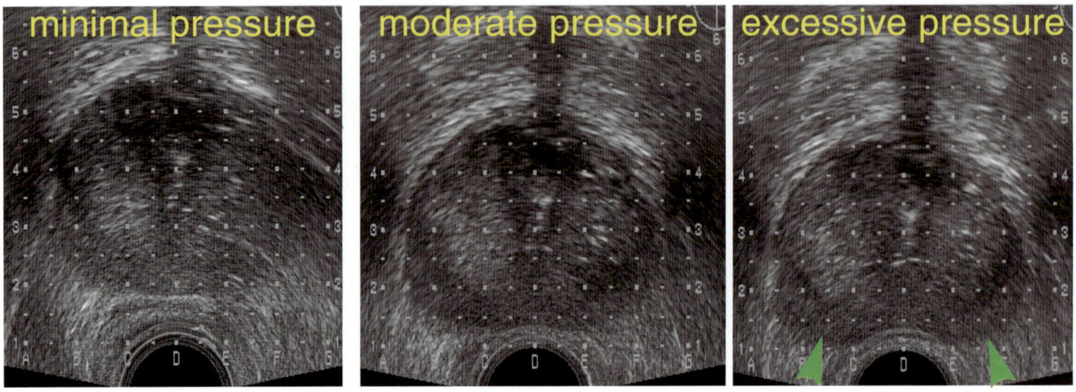

Figure 10-18. Excessive probe pressure deforms the image. These midprostatic images of the same patient were taken with minimal, moderate, and excessive probe pressure, causing artifactual "drooping" of the posterior-lateral margins (arrowheads).

are produced. Considering that the prostate tissue is a very firm organ, these deformities are not due to actual prostatic deformation, but to image artifact. Get rid of them by easing off a little on the probe pressure.

Determine the zero plane

Once the probe is positioned so that the TRUS images match those of the pre-plan, you need to determine the depth at which seed loading will start. The 0.0 plane, at the bladder/prostate interface, should match the corresponding plane of the planning images. The 0.0 plane can be best appreciated by ratcheting the probe through the junction of the seminal vesicles, bladder and prostatic base. It can also be verified on sagittal imaging (**Figure 10-19**). (But remember that when using the Mick Applicator®, the seed will be inserted beyond the tip of the needle, so that you should retract your needle tip 4–5 mm before ejecting a seed at the 0.0 plane.)

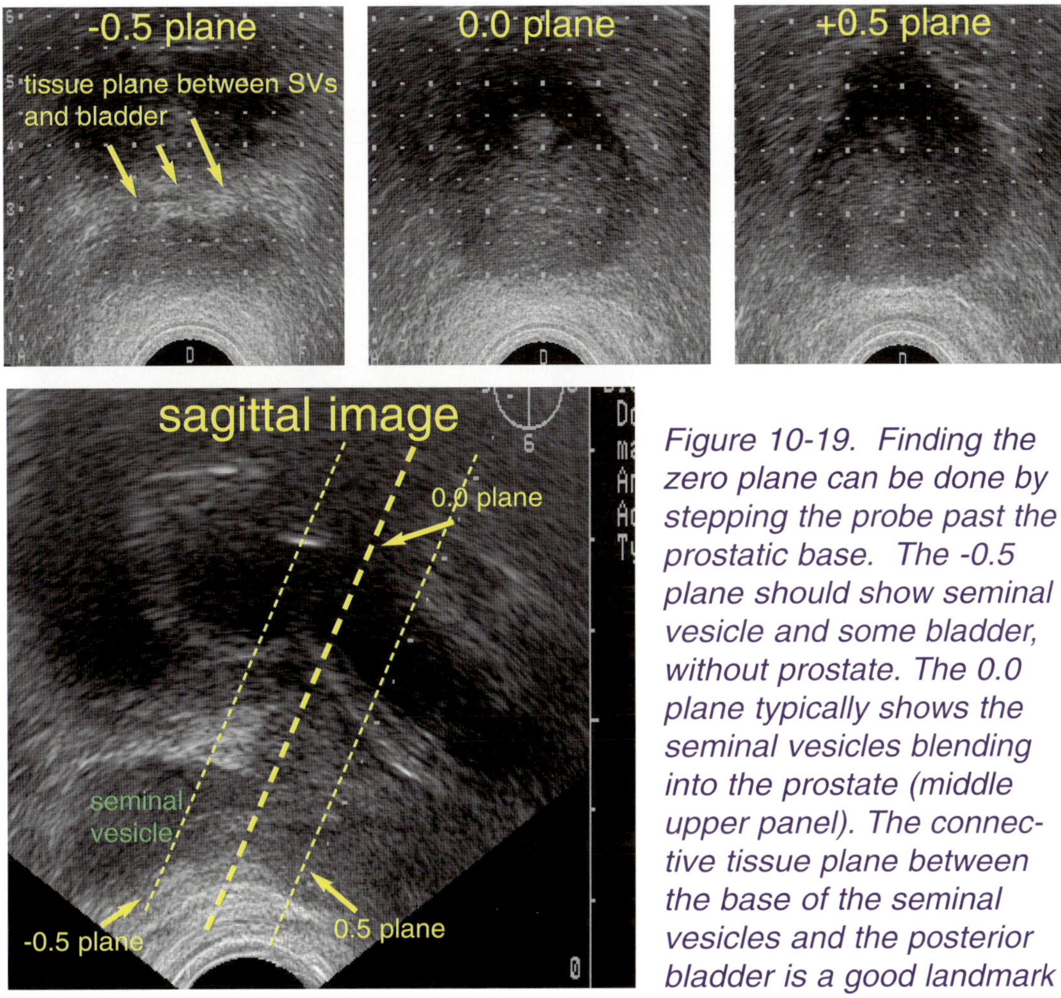

Figure 10-19. Finding the zero plane can be done by stepping the probe past the prostatic base. The -0.5 plane should show seminal vesicle and some bladder, without prostate. The 0.0 plane typically shows the seminal vesicles blending into the prostate (middle upper panel). The connective tissue plane between the base of the seminal vesicles and the posterior bladder is a good landmark to identify the plane above the prostatic base (-0.5). The sagittal image (left) is another good way to verify that you are at the base.

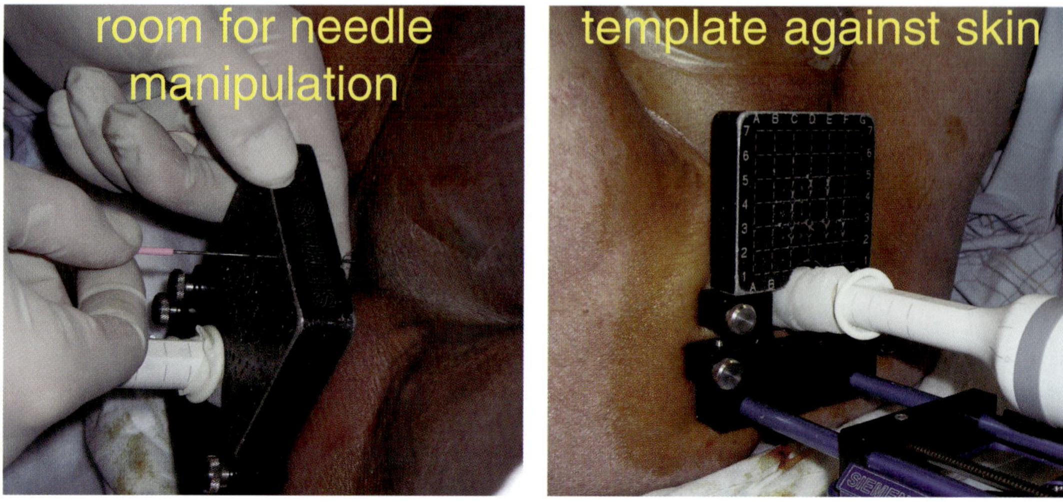

Figure 10-20. Placing the needle-guide template 1-2 cm from perineal skin (left) allows room for finger pressure to alter needle trajectory.

NEEDLE GUIDE TEMPLATE

Once you're satisfied with the image quality and prostatic positioning on the screen grid, mount the needle-guide template on the stepping unit, near the perineum. Some brachytherapists leave 1–2 cm of space between the skin and the template, to allow for manual adjustment of the needle direction (**Figure 10-20**).

Needle insertion

Once TRUS probe positioning is set, needles are inserted through the template holes and through the perineal skin. If the skin is caught tangentially, it's difficult to pierce it—retract the needle, and pull the skin taught and reinsert. To pierce thicker skin, the needle should be pressed firmly against the skin surface and then advanced with a sudden, controlled thrust. Once through the skin, quick advancement will minimize needle deviations. But be careful—a rapid thrust of the tip against the pubic arch can give you a bent (or even broken) needle.

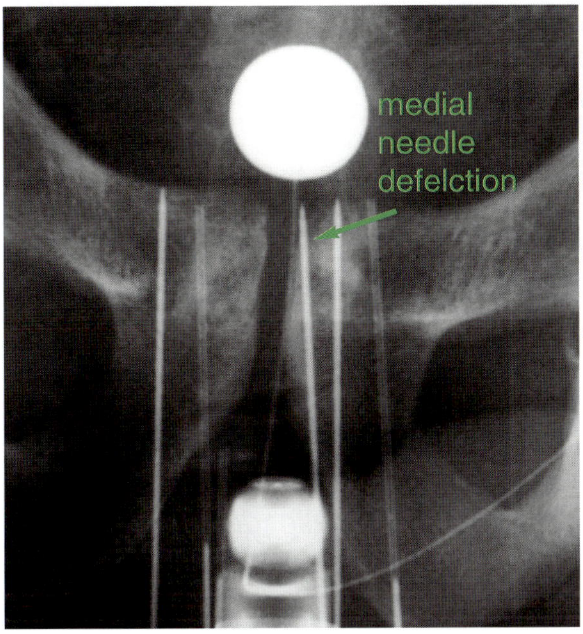

Figure 10-21. Needle deflection is usually obvious on fluoroscopy. In this patient, the most anterior needle has deflected medially as it brushed against the pubic arch. This deflection will cause the needle tip to appear at a more medial template coordinate than intended.

Needle deflection
Needles can be deflected by the skin, by the tissue planes, or by the pubic bones. Deflection will cause the needle to appear in some spot on the TRUS image other than that predicted by the template insertion coordinate. When in doubt, deflection is usually obvious on fluoroscopy (**Figure 10-21**). If it occurs, the needle should be withdrawn several centimeters, and re-inserted. If it's a peripheral needle, make sure you're not grazing the inner surface of the pubic bone. Twisting the needle during insertion may help get it through the offending tissue plane with less deflection. If deflection still occurs, withdraw the needle and check that it's straight!

Visualizing needles
Once multiple needles and seeds have been inserted, image degradation typically occurs (**Figure 10-22**). Degradation may be lessened by inserting and loading the more anterior needles first and proceeding to the more posterior needles. When in doubt, you can usually verify a needle's proper

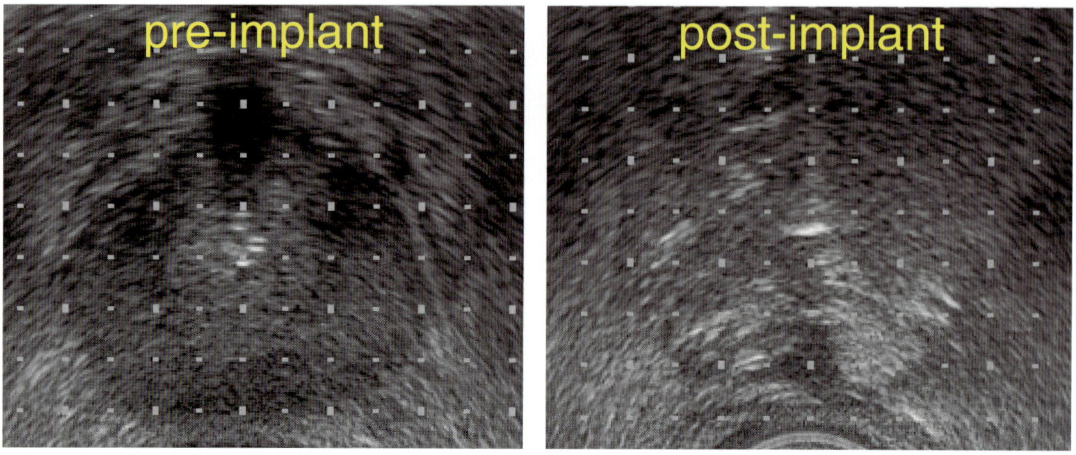

Figure 10-22. The prostate image, needles, and seeds may be markedly obscured toward the end of a case, due to seed artifact, bleeding, and edema.

positioning on TRUS images more proximal to the template (caudal to the prostatic apex), where the image is not obscured by seeds.

Needle depth

Determining the depth of the needle is as important to proper seed placement as is correct positioning in the transverse images. The simplest way to verify proper depth is to insert the needle while viewing the plane to which it is to be inserted, and stopping when you see the needle tip reach that plane. A second way is to view the insertion with fluoroscopy, with the zero plane being at the lower edge of the catheter balloon. If the needle tip is at the base of the prostate, the tip of the needle should be within 2–4 mm of the inferior edge of the balloon (**Figure 10-4**). A third is to measure how many centimeters of the needle should be distal to the template when the needle is inserted to its proper depth (**Figure 10-23**). These methods can be combined to give extra confidence. And if still in doubt as to the proper insertion depth, sagittal imaging can be very helpful (**Figure 10-24**).

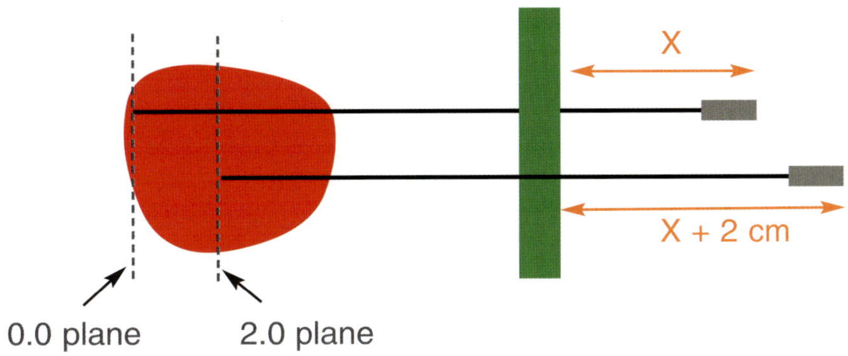

checking needle tip depth

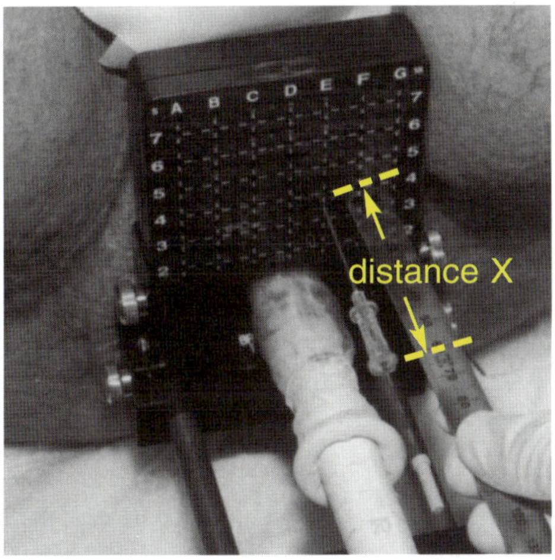

checking source/spacer number

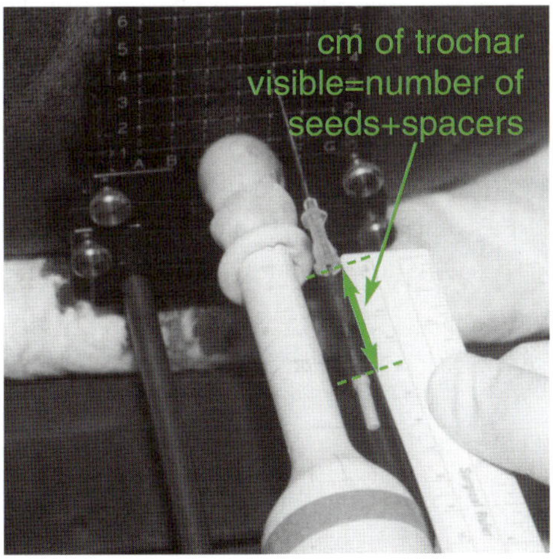

Figure 10-23. Needle depth can be checked by measuring how much is sticking out of the template when the needle is inserted to its proper depth. At the start of the case, the distance X is determined, with the needle tip at the 0.0 plane (top panel). All other hub measurements should be related to that of the zero plane. For instance, if the needle tip is supposed to be at the 2.0 plane for the first seed, the template-to-hub distance should be X+2. This is a quick and effective way to verify proper needle depth, but make sure to check that you're still setup to your zero plane throughout the procedure because the zero plane can shift relative to the stepper as the prostate swells or the patient moves slightly. The middle panel shows the hub measurement being made intra-operatively, to verify depth of the needle tip. The lowest panel shows a check of the number of sources/spacers loaded inside the needle, by measuring how much trocar is sticking out of the sheath.

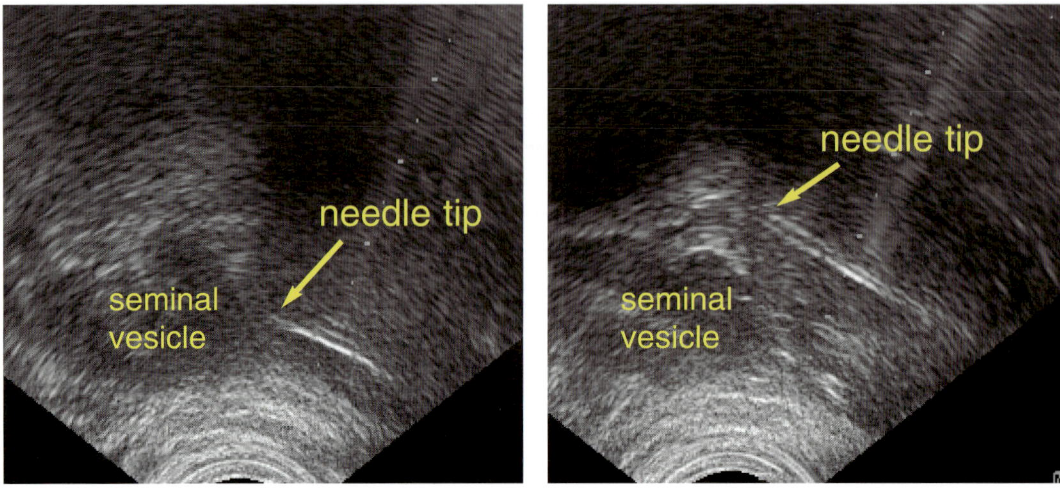

Figure 10-24. Needle depth can be checked on sagittal TRUS, but frequent switching between the transverse and sagittal views can become tedious.

PIERCING THE URETHRA

Even with a catheter in place, the urethra is probably pierced commonly in the course of an implant procedure. Although there is no evidence that piercing it increases acute or chronic morbidity, it seems prudent to minimize doing so.

PERI-RECTAL SEEDS

Using a posterior treatment margin of 3–5 mm, there should be minimal risk of serious rectal complications (see chapters 7 and 11). However, while serious rectal complications have been infrequent in modern implant series, there is a consistent 5% to 10% incidence of proctitis, typically with self-limited rectal bleeding (see Chapter 21). One technical maneuver that may contribute to proctitis is the temptation to place seeds nearer the posterior prostatic margin than called for in the treatment plan. We note this tendency among ourselves and others, with the intention of adding "a little extra margin" for potential extraprostatic extension. Be careful—doing so may increase the likelihood of rectal morbidity (**Figure 10-25**).

PROSTATE MOTION

The prostate can be highly mobile, even when it's not being stuck by needles and shoved by an ultrasound probe. The potential for prostate positioning changes has been well documented in the external beam radiation

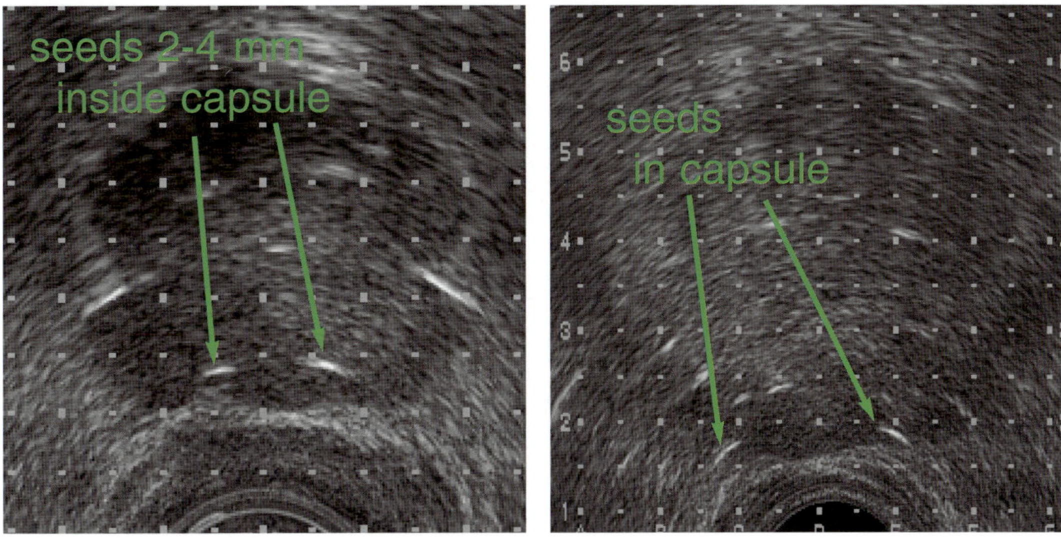

Figure 10-25. Be careful about putting seeds closer to the posterior prostatic margin than called for. In the patient on the left, seeds were properly placed 4 mm inside the capsule. In the patient on the right, seeds were shifted back a couple mm, to just inside the capsule. We generally keep the seeds 2-5 mm inside of the posterior prostatic margin.

literature.(LATTANZI) The primary motion, in the absence of needle insertion, is in the anterior-posterior direction. During needle insertion, fluoroscopy commonly shows lateral and cephalad motion of up to 1.0 cm, possibly leading to seed misplacements (**Figures 10-26 through 10–28**). Anterior displacement occurs when posteriorly placed needles strike the posterior surface tangentially. Presumably, the prostate can also twist around its longitudinal axis, though the degree of twisting has not been documented. These motions can easily be viewed fluoroscopically, looking at the change in position of the catheter balloon and any seeds that have already been implanted (**Figure 10-26**).

Prostate mobility varies substantially from patient to patient, presumably due to differences in periprostatic fat, periprostatic veins, looseness of the pelvic tissues, or changes in the general muscle tone of the organ.

Prostatic motion is something that you need to be aware of and make adjustments for, but that you don't necessarily need to stop. If you prefer,

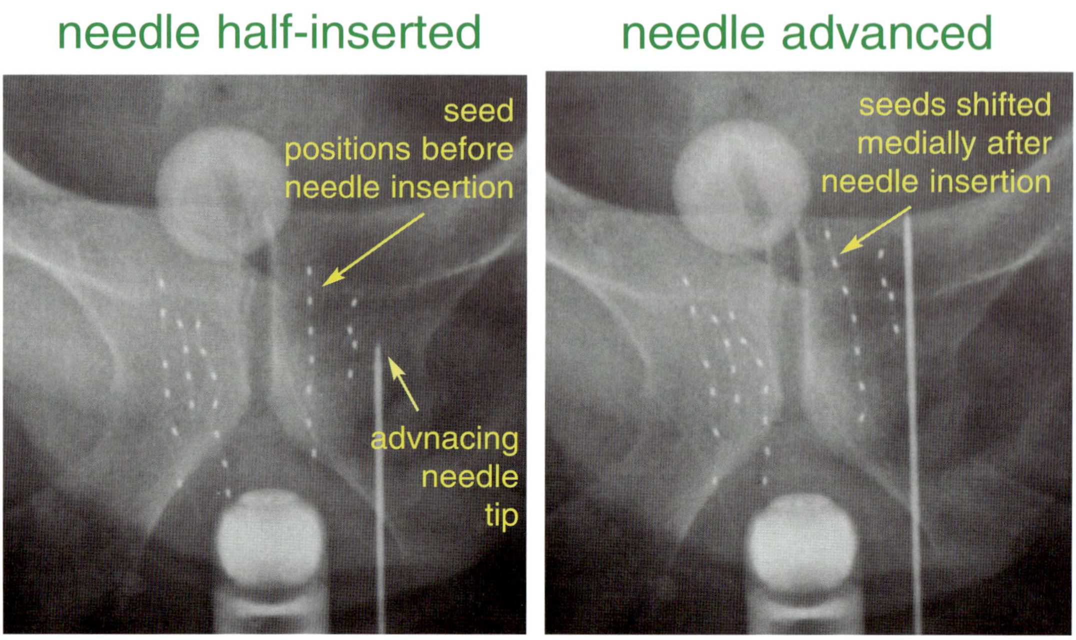

Figure 10-26. Prostate motion as the needle is inserted can be seen fluoroscopically, from changes in the position of prev iously placed seeds.

several methods help to limit prostate motion, but none are completely effective. Tissue-gripping needles hold the prostate and decrease motion along the needle tracks. Commercially available needles are inserted on each side of the prostate, with retractable hooks to grip the tissue once inserted (**Figure 10-29**). Their clinical benefit is a matter of some dispute.(TASCHEREAU)

Another method to decrease prostate motion is insertion of two crossing needles through the posterior aspect of the prostate (**Figure 10-30**).(DATTOLI) Crossing needles limit prostate motion, by anchoring in the pelvic floor musculature at an angle. This works fairly well, but it's still important to pay attention to the prostate position during the implant procedure.

A simpler alternative to transperineal crossing needles is to insert a single central needle through the posterior peripheral zone and leave it there

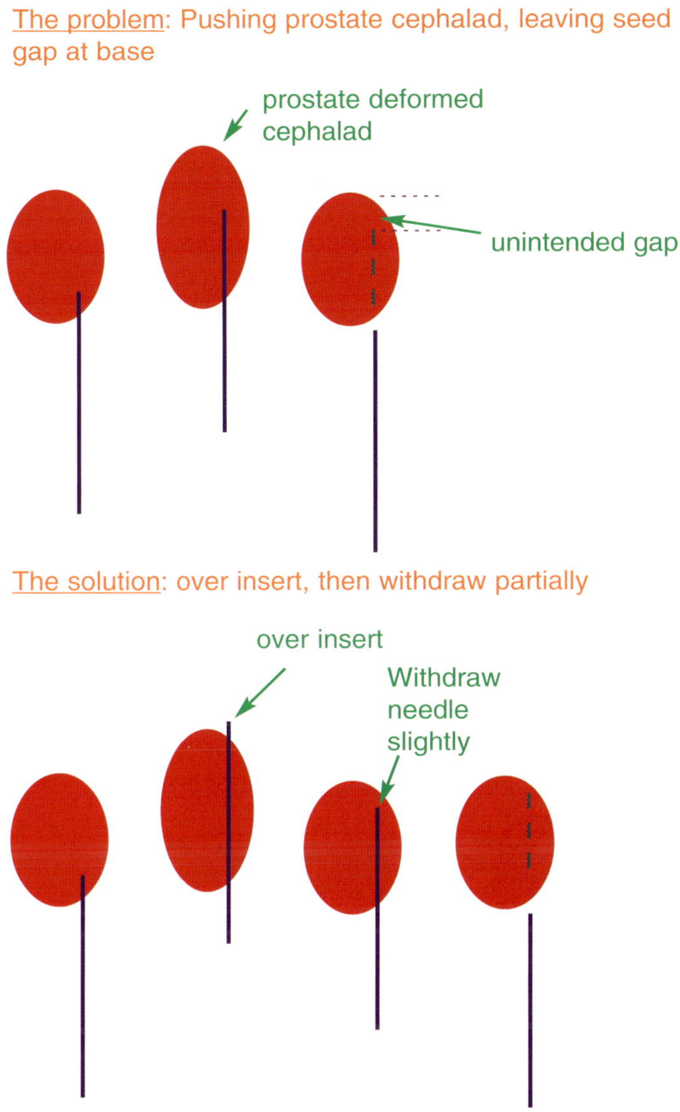

Figure 10-27. Prostate motion can lead to unintended gaps between the prostatic base and the sources, due to superior displacement of the prostate during needle insertion. This is a prime source of really bad mistakes (see Chapter 25). The answer is to over insert the needle, then withdraw it back into the prostate before placing the sources (lower panel).

The problem: The advancing needle tips the prostate medially, leaving seeds too lateral

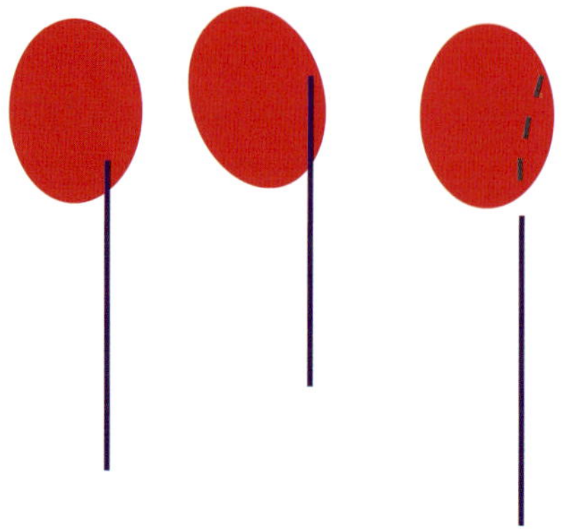

Figure 10-28. Prostate motion can lead to unintended lateral seed placement, due to medial displacement of the prostate during needle insertion. One fix is to insert the needle with a more rapid motion, minimizing displacement of the prostate (lower panel).

The solution: insert the needle more rapidly, to decrease displacement of the prostate. Also, use intra-operative fluoroscopy to monitor for excessive prostate motion.

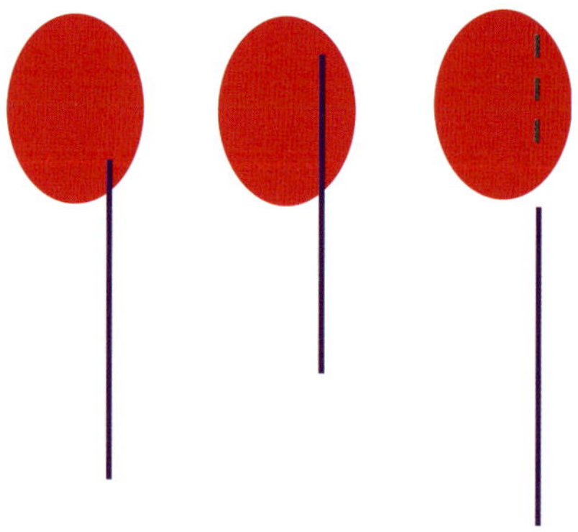

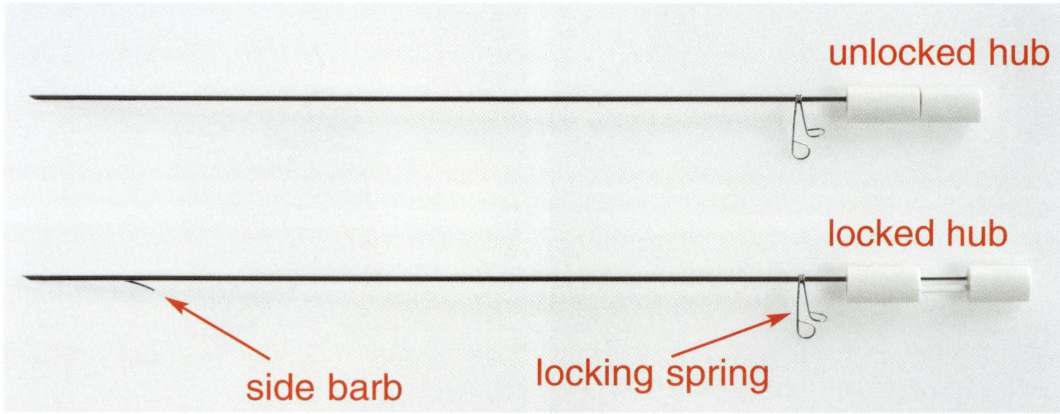

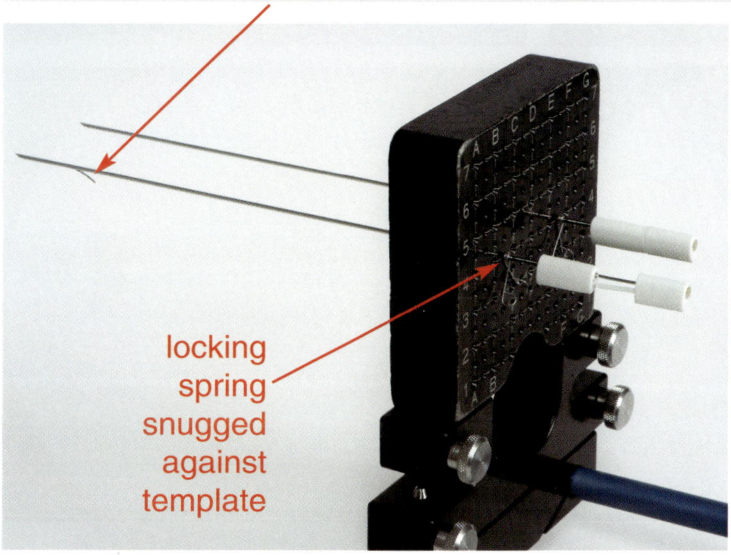

Figure 10-29. Two stabilizing needles can be inserted into the prostate to limit motion. Their side barbs are maintained in the "out" position by locking the hub. The locking springs steady the needle in the template.

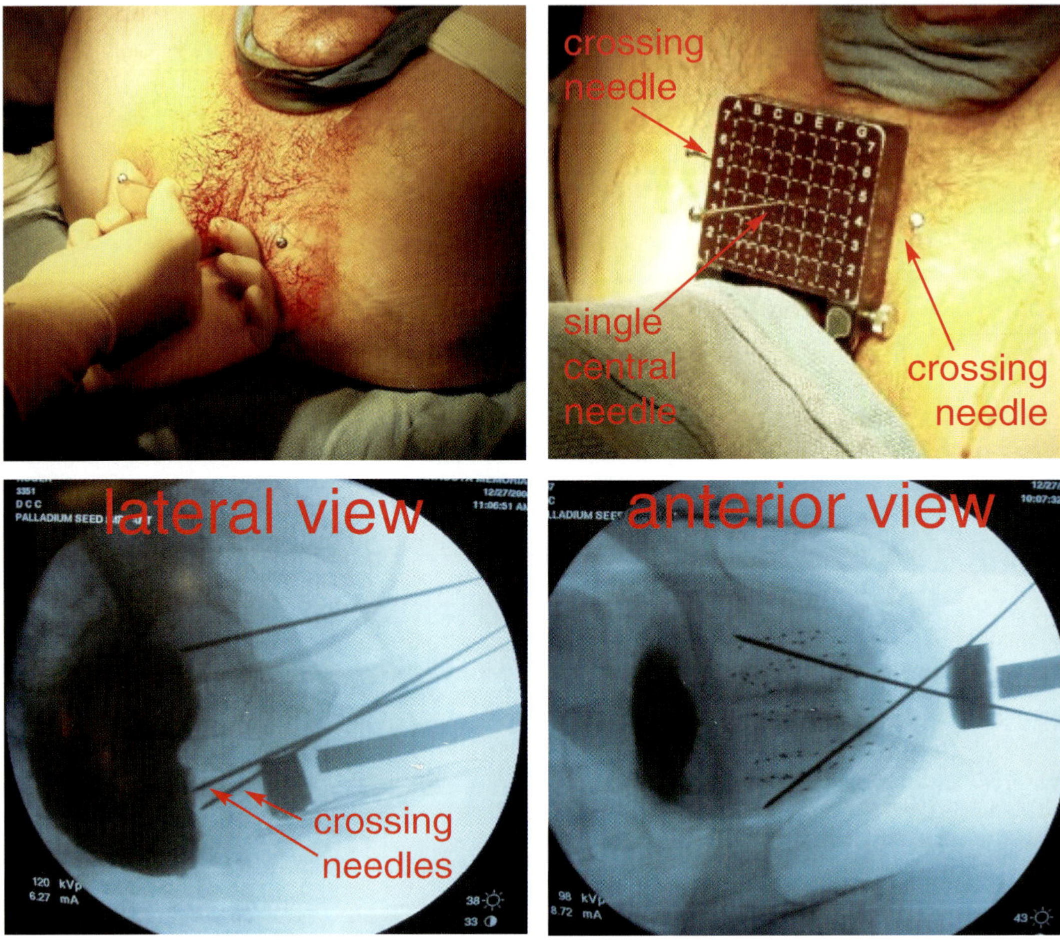

Figure 10-30. Placement of crossing needles to limit prostate motion.(DATTOLI)

throughout the procedure. It will limit torquing, but not cranio-caudal motion.

DEPOSITING SEEDS

Placement of seeds can be done with a variety of tools and techniques (see chapter 5). Regardless of technique, there are ways that errant seeds can occur. They can wind up in unusual places via the retroperitoneal space, veins, or bladder (**Figure 10-30**).

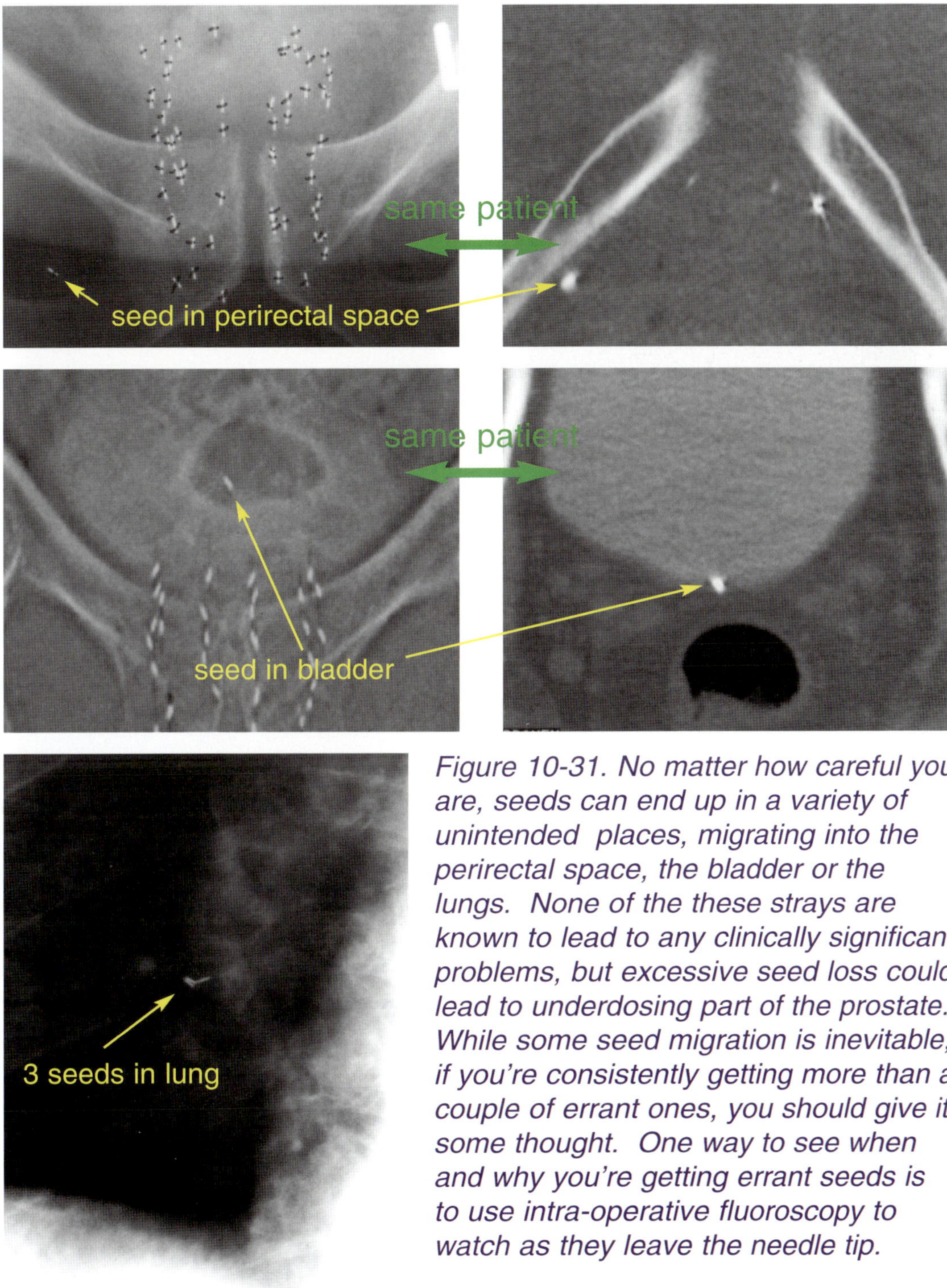

Figure 10-31. No matter how careful you are, seeds can end up in a variety of unintended places, migrating into the perirectal space, the bladder or the lungs. None of the these strays are known to lead to any clinically significant problems, but excessive seed loss could lead to underdosing part of the prostate. While some seed migration is inevitable, if you're consistently getting more than a couple of errant ones, you should give it some thought. One way to see when and why you're getting errant seeds is to use intra-operative fluoroscopy to watch as they leave the needle tip.

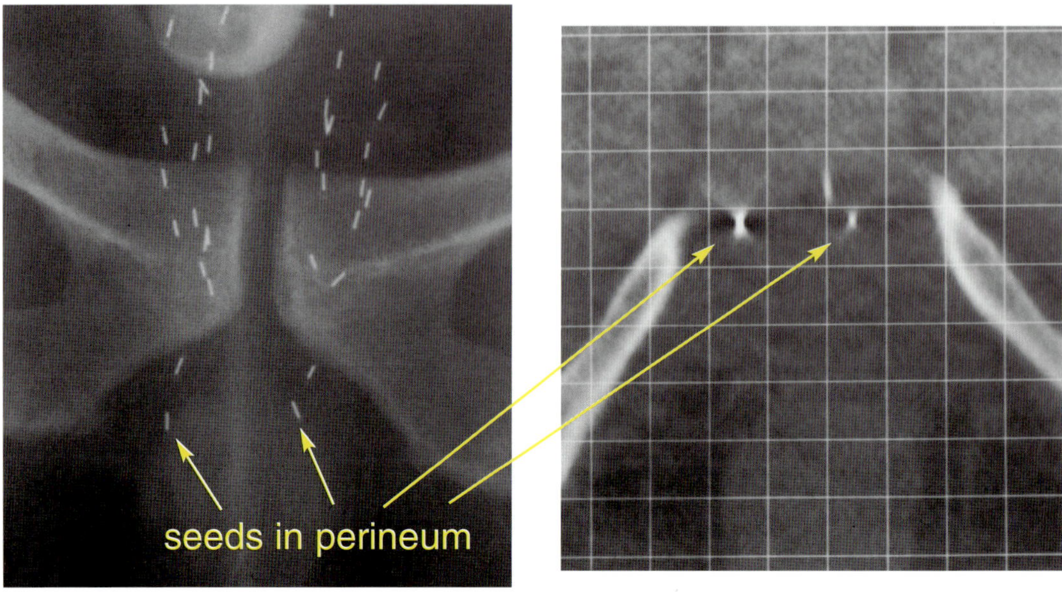

Figure 10-32. Misplaced perineal seeds seen on anterior fluoroscopy and corresponding CT image. Seeds can be pulled down into the perineum as you withdraw the needles.

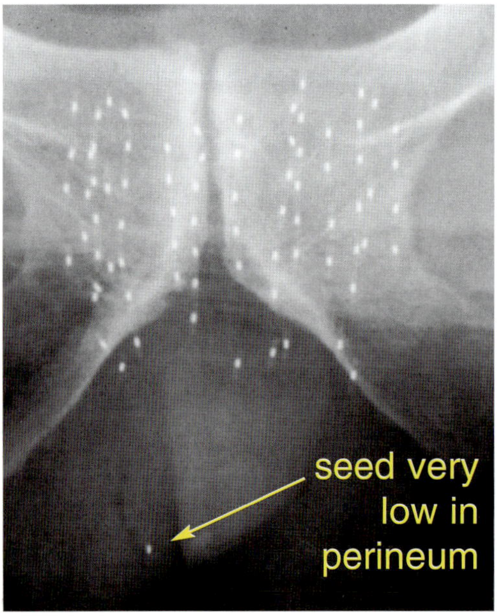

Figure 10-33. Example of seed pulled far down into the perineum as the needle tip was withdrawn. This kind of stray than can be caught and minimized, if fluoroscopy is used during the procedure.

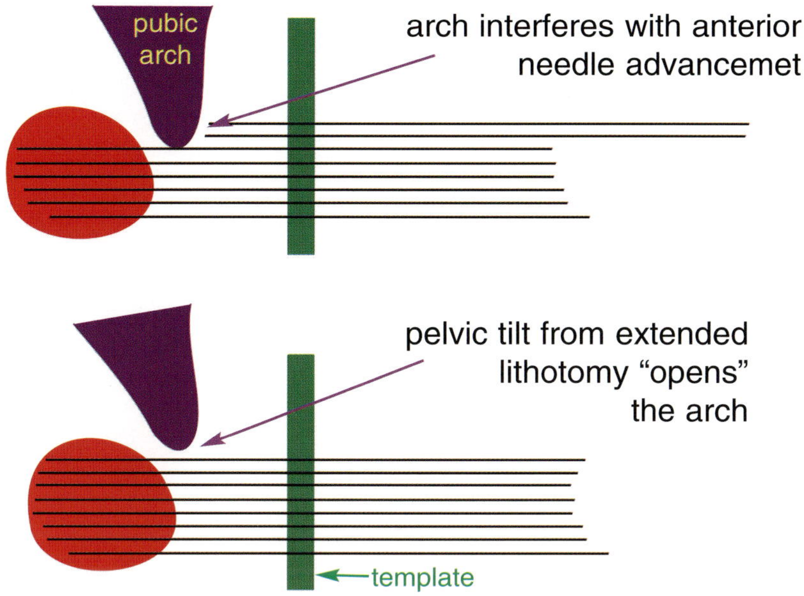

Figure 10-34. By moving to the extended lithotomy position, the pubic arch is drawn back, allowing more room for anterior-lateral needles to clear the pubic bones.

One of the most common problems is seed sliding along the track as a needle is withdrawn (**Figures 10-31 and 32**). This is apparently a vacuum phenomenon and can be largely avoided by moving needles slowly. Watching the seeds under fluoroscopy during needle withdrawal is a good way to guard against misplacement, because you can usually see when seeds are not staying put after they've left the needle tip. Sometimes, seed displacement can be corrected with judicious re-insertion or retraction of the needles, watching under fluoroscopy.

PUBIC ARCH INTERFERENCE

The most anterior and lateral needles may strike the pubic bones, preventing advancement or causing medial deflection. Fortunately, pubic arch interference (PAI) can usually be readily circumvented by one or more maneuvers that alter the needle path in relation to the pubic arch.

The simplest way to circumvent pubic arch interference is to change the patient to a more extended lithotomy position, either by moving the stirrups cephalad or by sliding the buttocks farther down the table (keeping the stir-

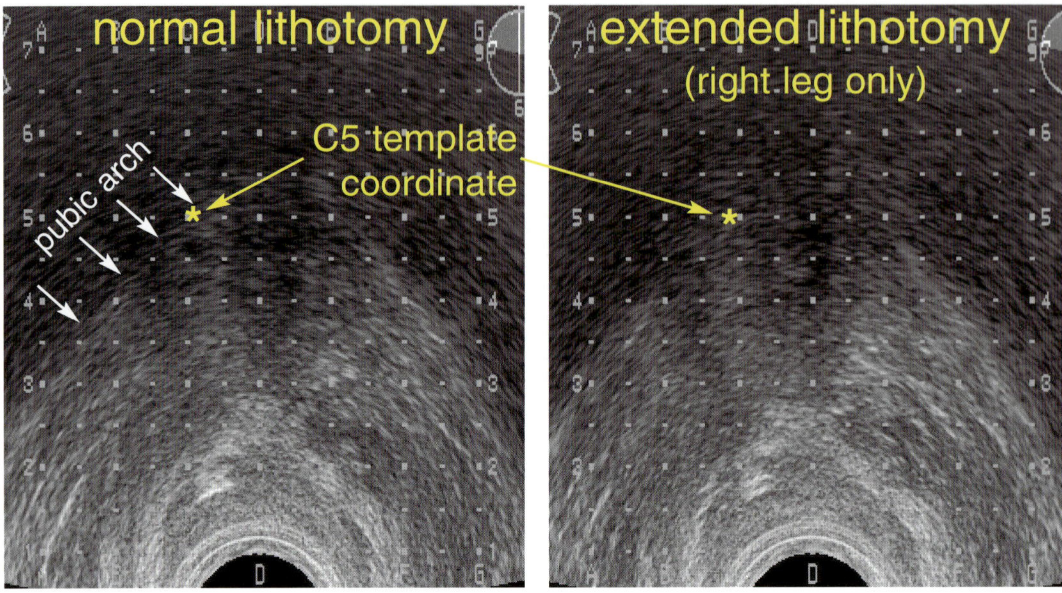

Figure 10-35. Pubic arch interference can be reduced by extending the patient's lithotomy position. In this case, the pubic arch obstructed needle insertion at the C5 template position. By flexing the patient's right hip, the right side of the pubic arch moved away from the TRUS probe, allowing access to the C5 position. A word of caution: if you change a patient's leg positioning during the case, check that the prostate still aligns properly on the grid.

rups in the same place). Extending the lithotomy position rotates the pubic arch superiorly, allowing more room under it (**Figures 10-34 and 35**). The spatial relationship between the pubic arch and prostate and its alteration with pelvic rotation and needle angle have been elegantly illustrated by Tincher and colleagues.(TINCHER)

Changing the probe angulation or depressing the probe away from the prostate to get needles under the pubic arch is the quickest, easiest way to circumvent arch interference (**Figure 10-36**). But you need to keep in mind that such maneuvers will simultaneously change the relationship of the probe to the prostate, shifting its alignment on the template grid. Be sure to check the prostate's grid positioning each time you alter the probe's position.

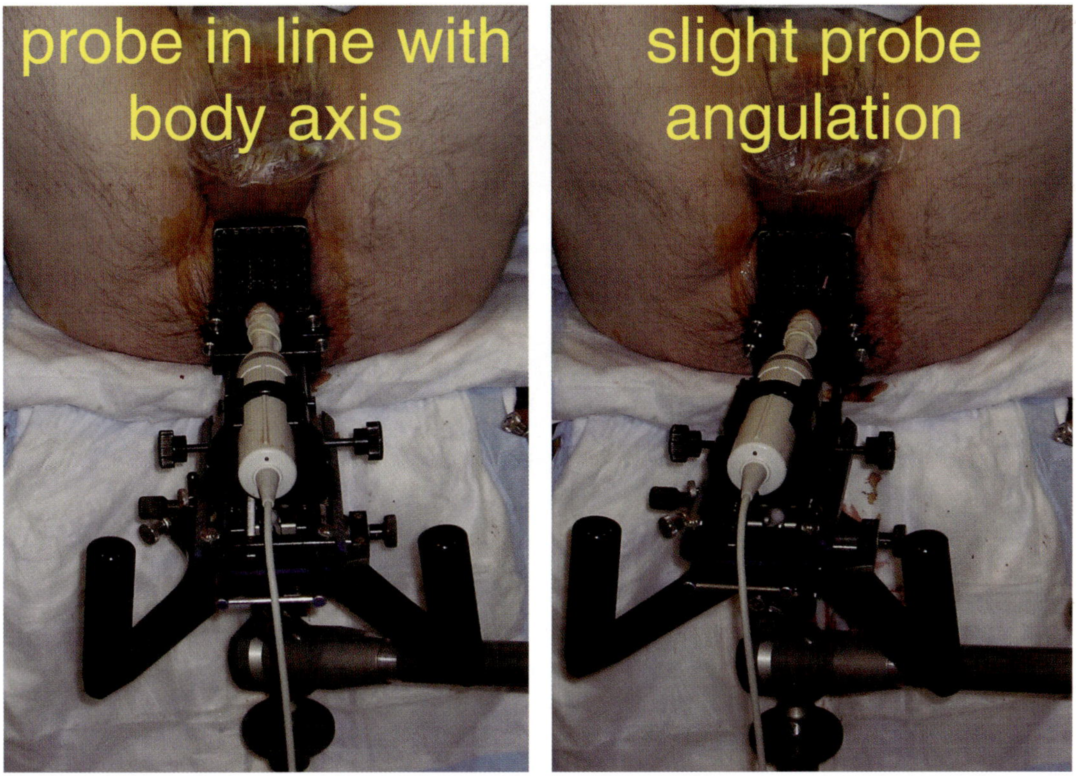

Figure 10-36. A few degrees of probe angulation is usually enough to circumvent arch interference. But be careful—the prostate will move laterally on the grid when you angle the probe. Make sure to re-align the prostate right to left after changing the probe angulation.

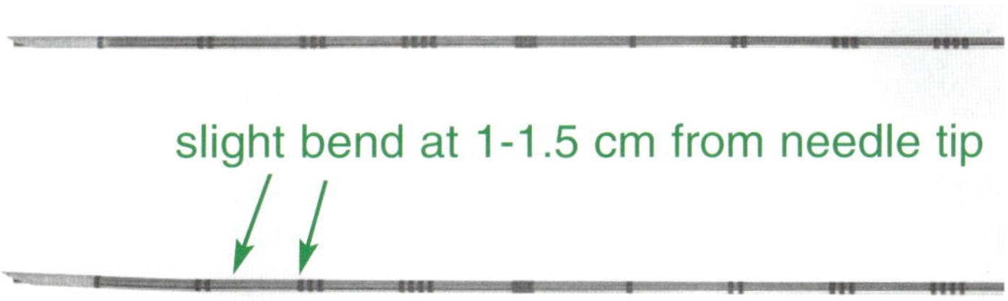

Figure 10-37. Slightly bending a needle tip will cause the needle to veer in the direction of the bend, helping to steer it by the pubic arch.

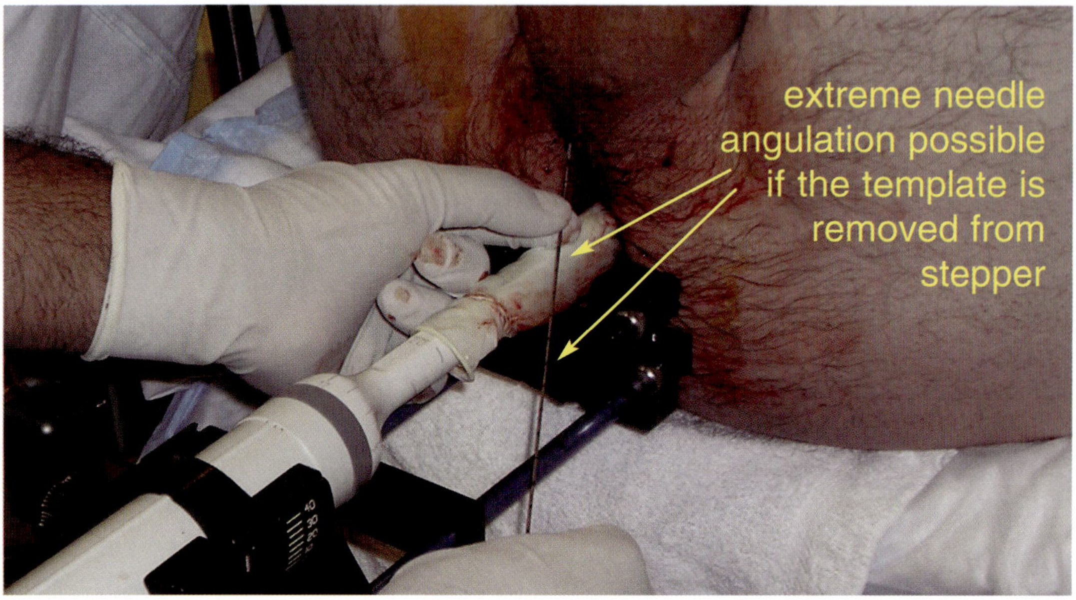

Figure 10-38. Removing the TRUS template allows freehand needle insertion, affording extraordinary angling to get past severe arch interference. We don't do this one very often, but it almost always works in patients with a large degree of arch interference.

A third way to circumvent pubic arch interference is to bend the needle tip slightly, 2.0 to 4.0 cm from the tip (**Figure 10-37**). Insert it 0.5 or 1.0 cm medial and posterior to the intended template position with the tip pointed away from the arch and insert the tip just past the arch. Then rotate the needle 180 degrees, and continue inserting. The bend will force the needle to veer away from the probe after passing the arch, often allowing the tip to reach a tissue point that would have been shielded by the pubic arch. This technique requires some finesse. And even with finesse, it often requires several passes of the needle. In addition to introducing some uncertainty in the grid location of the seeds (since the needle is not completely perpendicular to the template), the technique increases tissue trauma and may, in fact, have been a contributing factor to the high post-implant urinary retention rates seen during an early period at the University of Washington.(WANG)

If you're faced with an extreme case of pubic arch interference, it is possible to remove the TRUS template, and to place seeds by hand, using

TRUS or anterior and lateral fluoroscopy to check for proper positioning in relation to the other seeds or to the Foley catheter (**Figure 10-38**). This is the least desirable option, because it doesn't control for the needle trajectory relative to the template.

POST-PROCEDURE CYSTOSCOPY

Post-implant cystourethroscopy has been practiced as a way to remove intravesicle or intraurethral radioactive seed or blood clots. However, in experienced hands, errant seeds in the bladder or urethra are unusual. And when seeds do enter the bladder, they are readily identified fluoroscopically and simply pass once the urinary catheter is removed. Post-implant blood clots generally pass spontaneously. However, M. Dattoli leaves a 3-way catheter in place for several hours of saline drainage, to minimize the possibility of clot retention. Routine pre- or post-implant cystoscopy serves only to increase the patient's bill, subjecting him to an unnecessary procedure.(GRAY, YAP, STONE)

LOTS OF CHOICES

As we said at the beginning of this chapter, there are a lot of ways to do a good implant. Keep an open mind and look at your many options. Figure out what works best for you, given your own dexterity, practice setting, and the skill level of your team.

REFERENCES

1. Dattoli M, Wallner K. A simple method to stabilize the prostate during transperineal prostate brachytherapy. Int J Rad Oncol Biol Phys 1997; 38:341-342.

2. Gray G, Wallner K, Roof J, Corman J. Cystourethroscopic findings before and after prostate brachytherapy. Techniques in Urology 2000; 6:109-111.

3. Lattanzi J, McNeely S, Hanlon A, Das I, Schultheiss TE, Hanks GE. Daily CT localization for correcting portal errors in the treatment of prostate cancer. Int J Rad Oncol Biol Phys 1998; 41:1079-1086.

4. Stone NN, Stock RG. Dynamic cystography can replace cystoscopy following prostate seed implantation. Techniques in Urology 2000; 6:112-116.

5. Sylvester J, Grimm P, Blasko J, et al. Urethral visualization during transperineal interstitial brachytherapy for early stage prostate cancer. JBI 2000; 16:145-150.

6. Taschereau R, Pouliet J, Roy J, Tremblay D. Seed misplacement and stabilizing needles in transperineal permanent prostate implants. Radiother Oncol 2000; 55:59-63.
7. Tincher SA, Kim RY, Ezekiel MP, al e. Effects of pelvic rotation and needle angle on pubic arch interference during transperineal prostate implants. Int J Rad Oncol Biol Phys 2000; 47:361-363.
8. Yap J, Wallner K, Gray G. Cystourethroscopic findings and long-term urinary function after prostate brachytherapy. JBI 2000; 16:257-262.

11

Implant evaluation

Post-implant evaluation, or *dosimetry*, is a key part of prostate brachytherapy for several reasons (**Table 11-1**). First, it is the cornerstone of quality assurance—it provides a reasonably precise, objective evaluation of your result. Second, post-implant dosimetry is the best way to close the learning loop—it tells you how good (or bad) your technique is. Third, dosimetry is *the* legal document regarding the procedure. Taking pains to dictate a lengthy, detailed operative note isn't so important. But seed strength, number and position are vitaly important—considerably more so than the details of how you put them there. If a patient develops a serious complication and turns to the courts, the first thing that the

Table 11-1. Why postimplant dosimetry is important.

- Quality assurance
- Closes the learning loop
- Legal document
- Patient interest

lawyers (his *and* yours) will want is the post-implant dosimetry, especially the CT scans. If the dosimetry looks bad, you've got a serious problem, no matter how smoothly you thought things went in the operating room.

One more reason to do post-implant dosimetry is that patients frequently ask about it. With patients' do-it-yourself approach and medical savvy, many will have already read extensively about brachytherapy (some will even have read this book!). Patients may ask about their "DVH" or may even want to *see* their post-implant CT scan and dosimetric calculations. You'll look better if you have something to show them—otherwise they would rightly conclude that you're not interested in the quality of your work.

As data emerge regarding the clinical relevance of some basic dose parameters, prostate brachytherapy is becoming better standardized. We still have a lot of work to do in order to understand what constitutes a good implant as opposed to a bad implant. But we're getting there.

CRUDE INDICES

In the days of retropubic implants and in the early days of TRUS-guided implants, total activity and matched peripheral dose (MPD) were the standard criteria for evaluating implant quality. Both are crude indices, at best.

The simplest way to describe an implant is to state the total amount of radioactivity implanted—a very crude quality indicator because it gives no information regarding the spatial relationship between dose and the prostate. If the activity implanted is in the usual range, it doesn't mean much. However, the total amount implanted can be telling if it is far from the norm. If very low, it would be likely that the prostate was not covered adequately. If very high, the prostatic or normal tissue doses could be excessive.

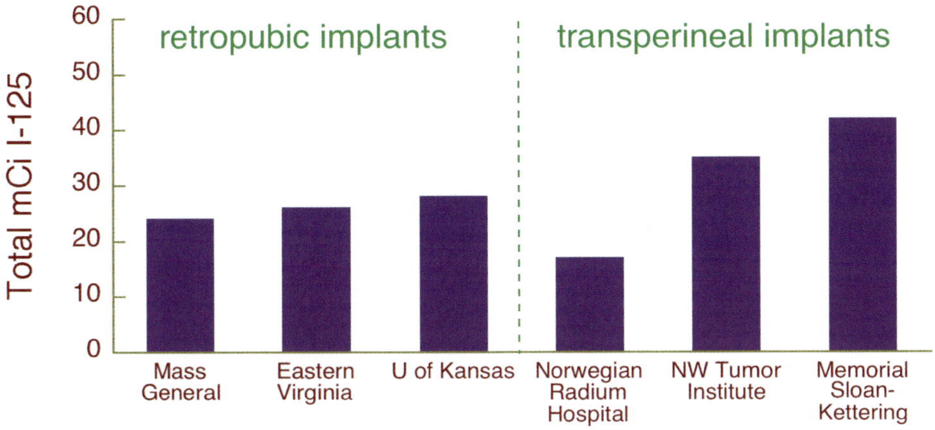

Figure 11-1. Average total activity used for retropubic and early transperineal implants. Clinical results from the Norwegian Radium Hospital were abysmal—a very low amount of I-125 was used, and there was apparently no quality assurance system in place. With such low amounts of activity, the target coverage would almost certainly have been poor.(WAEHRE, DELANEY, REDDY)

The total activity used for prostate brachytherapy has increased over the years. Current amounts are approximately double what was used for retropubic implants in the 1970s (**Figure 11-1**). The higher activites used in transperineal series partly reflects more accurate determination of prostate volume and shape with TRUS imaging, and a better match of isodose lines to the prostate periphery.

The matched peripheral dose (MPD) (not to be confused with mPD, the minimum tumor dose) is an ingenious concept that was devised by Lowell Anderson before wide availability of CT-based dosimetry.(ANDERSON) The MPD is the dose for which the isodose contour volume equals the volume of an ellipsoid having the same orthogonal dimensions as the target volume. To calculate the MPD, seed position is reproduced in three dimensions using orthogonal or stereo-shift films. Dose to a lattice of points throughout the implant volume is determined by summing the contribution from each seed using computerized dose look-up tables. Several isodoses and their corresponding volumes are graphed. The MPD, corresponding to

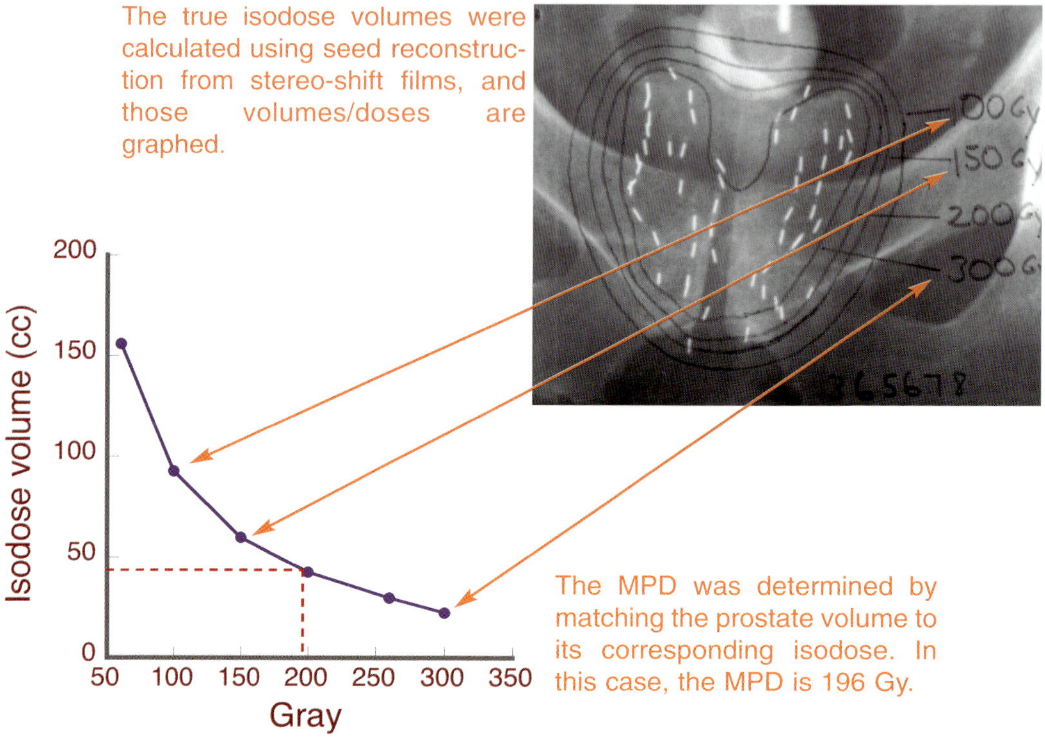

Figure 11-2. Schematic illustration of the MPD calculation. The volumes encompassed by several isodose lines are graphed against the isodose levels. The dose to the approximation of the prostatic volume is taken from the graph, going from the y-axis to the x-axis. The target volume was estimated from orthogonal dimensions, or determined from planar reconstruction of CT, TRUS, or MR images.

the ellipsoidal volume estimation (y-axis), is taken from the x-axis of the graph (**Figure 11-2**). The MPD isodose line can be drawn in relation to the seeds, on the original set of radiographs. Points outside of the MPD volume receive less than the MPD dose. While the actual isodose volumes, calculated from seed positions on orthogonal films, are accurate the problem with MPD calculations is that without CT-derived prostate definition, you can't accurately match the isodose volumes with the prostate margin.

Because MPD calculations use orthogonal dimensions to estimate the prostatic size (and shape), the MPD is an approximation of the dose to an

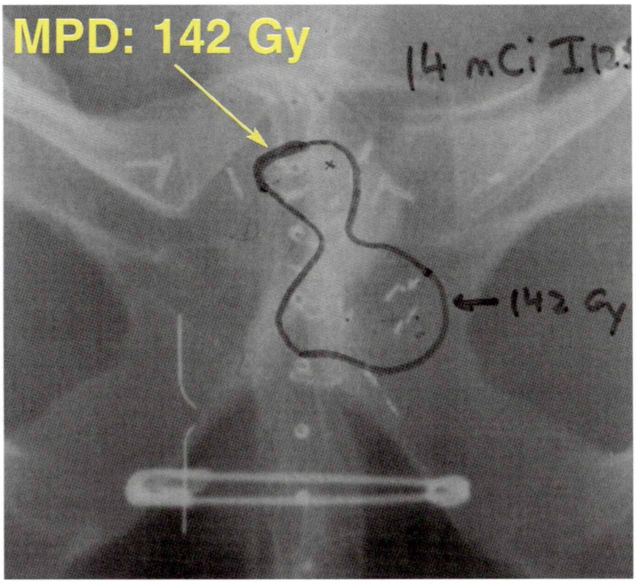

Figure 11-3. Anterior view of a 1980 retropubic implant, for which the calculated matched peripheral dose is 142 Gy. While the MPD is close to the prescription dose of 150 Gy, it's obvious that this was an awful implant. The 142 Gy isodose line could not possibly match the prostatic margins. But judging from the MPD alone, the implant was a good one!

approximation of the prostate volume—it does not accurately reflect the true dose to the prostate. This limitation of the MPD in defining an adequate implant is obvious by looking at the MPD of a 1980 retropubic implant from MSKCC (**Figure 11-3**).

Despite the inherent inaccuracy of the MPD calculation, some correlation between higher MPDs and local control rates has been reported.(FUKS) While suggesting that the MPD is a valid concept, the data upon which thsi correlation is based are very suspect, being based on vague definitions of local failure. More important, the quality of the retropubic implants on which it is based was so poor by today's standards that such data are of historical interest only. The introduction of CT-based dosimetry made the MPD concept obsolete. It has no place in modern dosimetry.

IMAGING MODALITIES

To perform meaningful dosimetry, both the seeds and the prostatic margins must be identified. The choices for post-implant imaging include TRUS, CT, and MR, each with distinct qualities (**Figure 11-4**). CT currently is the most practical dosimetric imaging modality. Its principle advantages are wide availability and easy seed identification. But CT images are only so-so for visualizing the prostatic margins. Unfortunately, typical images are not nearly as nice as the ones that make it to the cover of a textbook

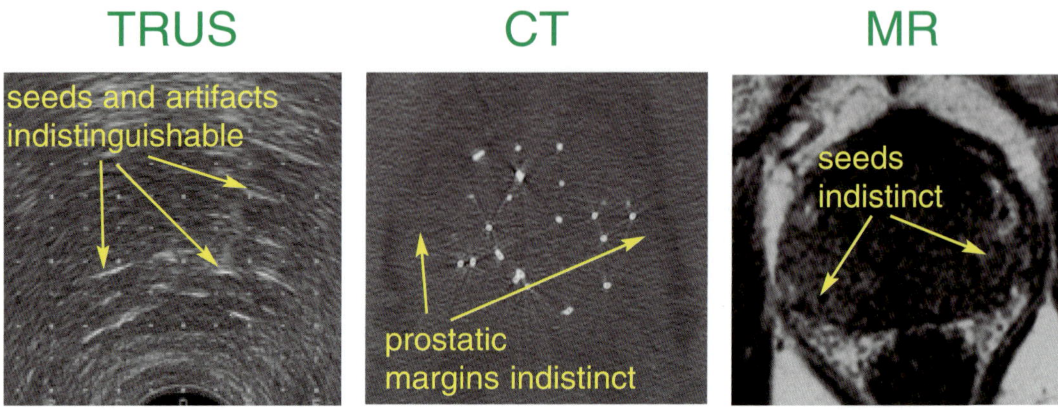

Figure 11-4. TRUS, CT, and MR each have their advantages and disadvantages as post-implant imaging modalities. (DUBOIS, AMDUR)

(**Figure 11-5**). In reality, the prostatic margins are indistinct, especially near the prostatic base and apex.(CROOK, HAN 03)

MR and TRUS are potential alternative to CT-based dosimetry. Compared to CT, MR typically offers better visualization of the prostatic margins, but far less distinct seed identification. Despite some claims that two sets of MR images can identify seeds well, MR alone for dosimetric evaluation is not good.(AMDUR) Image fusion between MR and CT could optimize seed location and prostatic margin definition, but such an approach makes post-implant dosimetry more cumbersome, with no demonstrable clinical benefit. A switch to MR as the standard is unlikely, due partly to its higher cost, and mostly to the fact that it is unlikely to enhance clinical outcomes.

Real-time TRUS could be the most practical post-implant imaging modality, since it is readily available intra-operatively. The biggest problem with TRUS is that accurate identification of individual seeds is not possible with the modality as we now know it.(HAN 03) Another problem with TRUS as an imaging modality for implant evaluation is image degradation that typically occurs once a large number of seeds are implanted (**Figure 11-6**).

With technologic improvements, the future may bring a melding of modalities, or replacement of CT by TRUS or MR. But in the meantime, CT remains the standard of care for implant evaluation. The remainder of this chapter will focus on CT-based dosimetry.

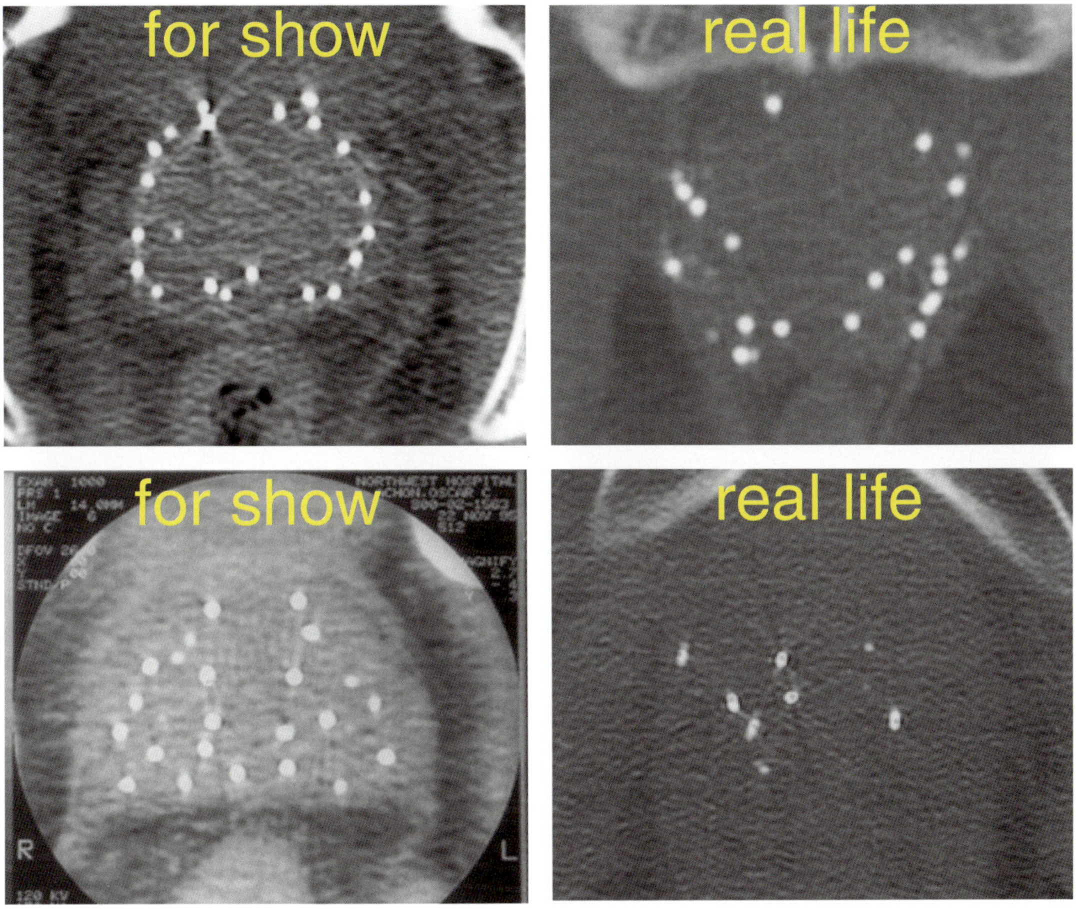

Figure 11-5. Fantasy versus reality. The CT images on the left are particularly nice ones, the kind that are typically shown in books! Unfortunately, the prostatic margins and seeds frequently look more like the ones on the right. Note how indistinct the margins are near the prostatic apex, seen in the lower right panel.

CASUAL INSPECTION

The first step in implant analysis is to take a minute to peruse the post-implant images. If the scan was done in the immediate post-implant period, there may be air in or around the prostate (**Figure 11-7**). Air is typically at the prostate periphery, and should not substantially affect the determination of prostatic coverage.

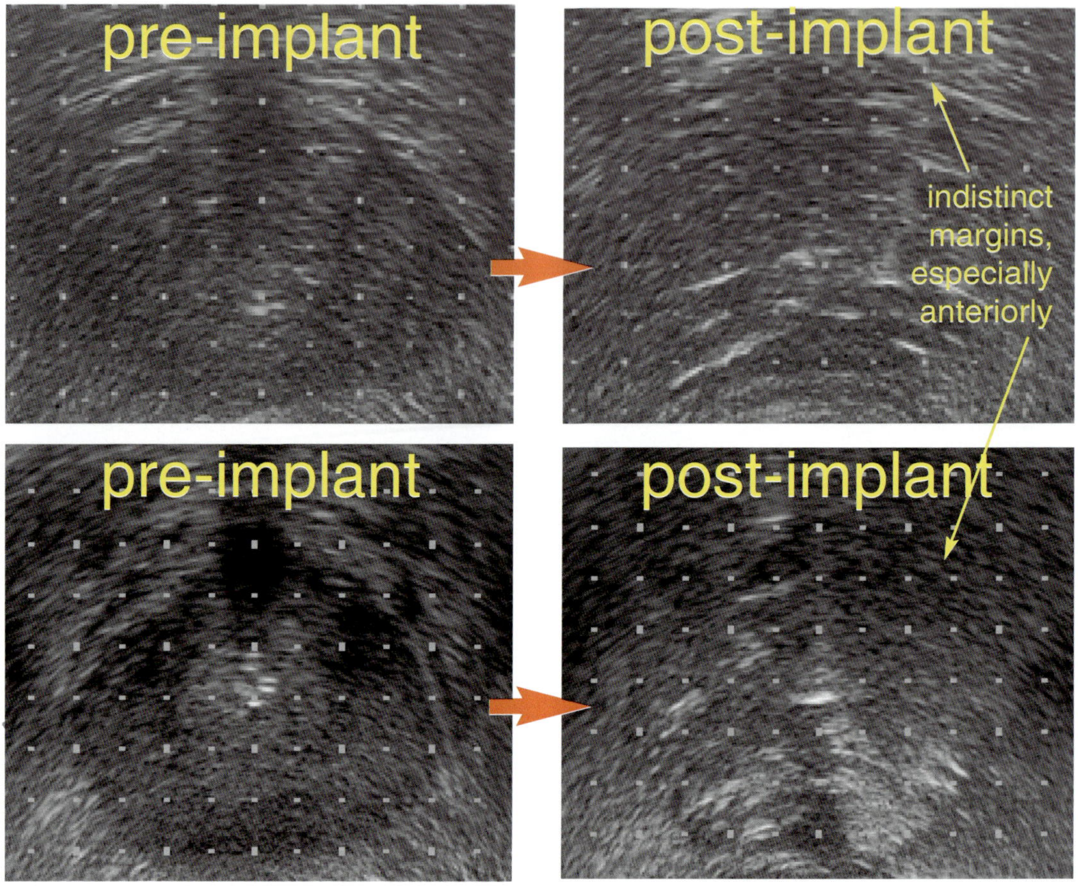

Figure 11-6. Pre- and post-implant TRUS images. Seed placement tends to obscure the prostatic margin. The post-implant margin visibility varies substantially from patient-to-patient, and at different levels in the same patient. These examples are fairly typical of what you'll see.

Simple visual inspection of a post-implant CT scan is an important way to evaluate what you've done in the operating room. You may see, for instance, that you've placed seeds too close to the urethra or rectum (**Figure 11-8**).

Isodose overlays
The best way to assess an implant is visual inspection of the isodoses overlaid on cross sections of the prostate (**Figure 11-9**). Despite the emphasis on dosimetric parameters, looking at the overlays remains the

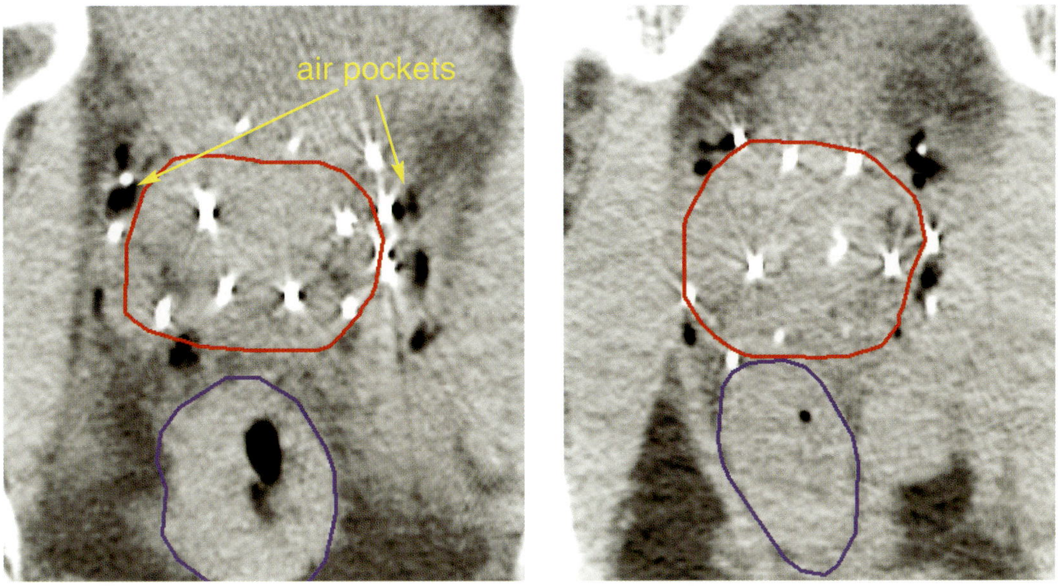

Figure 11-7. Examples of air around prostate immediataely following implant procedure. This can interfere with what is already a sometimes difficult job of outlining the prostate.

best way to evaluate the dose distribution. That's because dose parameters like *D90* or *V100* don't take into account the geography of the isodose lines or the cancer. Consider the case of a patient's whose only site of cancer was his left apex. He could have an an implant with an acceptable V100 of 85% (see below), but with the 15% cold tissue including his left apex. In his case, a V100 of 85% could hide the fact that his cancer was not covered with a cancercidal dose.

QUANTIFYING TARGET COVERAGE

While isodose overlays are the best way to evaluate an individual patient's implant, analyzing groups of patients regarding the dose-related clinical effects requires summary dosimetric indices. The *dose-volume histogram* (DVH) graphs the percent of the target covered versus increasing doses (see **Figures 11-9 and 11-10**). A nearly endless variety of indices can be taken from the DVH to summarize implant quality. Probably the simplest of the DVH-derived indices to conceptualize is the V100, the percent of the post-implant prostate volume covered by the prescription dose (**Table 11-2**). Roy and colleagues were the first to use post-implant CTs to calculate

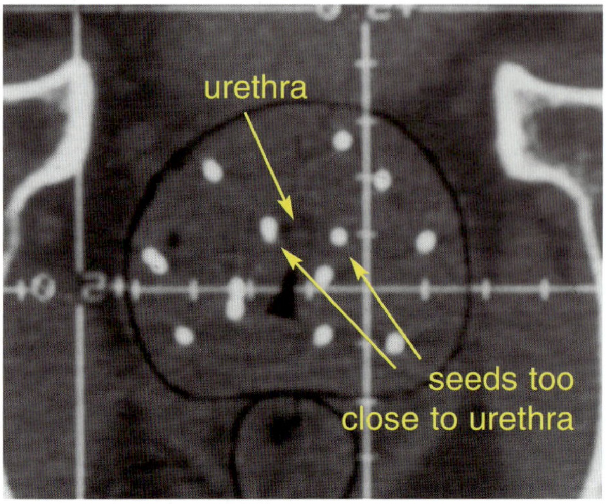

Figure 11-8. Casual inspection of a post-implant CT scan is enough to appreciate some problems. In this image, excessive periurethral seeds are obvious.

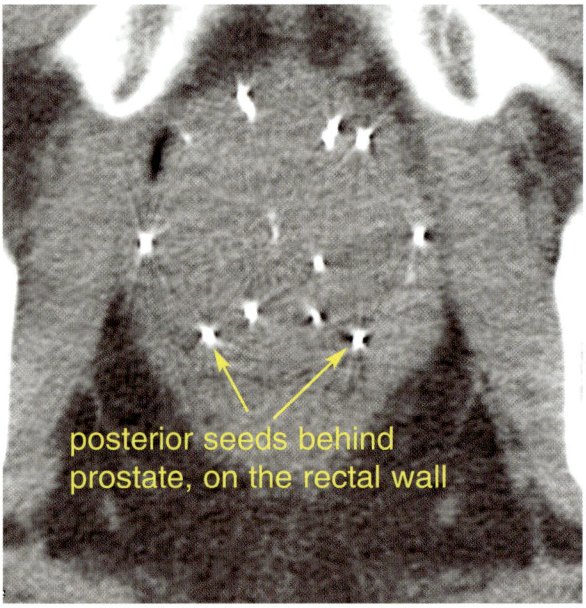

In this example, it's obvious that seeds were mistakenly placed too posteriorly, on the rectal wall. This kind of mistake does not require sophisticated dosimetric evaluation to see—a quick look at the CT is enough!

Table 11-2. Some indices used to quantify implant quality.

V100:	The percentage of the prostate volume that receives the prescription dose or higher
V200:	The percentage of the prostate volume that receives more than twice the prescription dose
V300:	The percentage of the prostate volume that receives more than three times the prescription dose
D90:	The minimum dose that covers 90% of the prostate volume
Dmin:	The minimum dose delivered to any part of the prostate

V100s.(ROY) A second common way to summarize coverage is the D90, defined as the minimum dose that covers 90% of the prostate.(STOCK)

DOSE RESPONSE STUDIES
Several investigators have correlated dosimetric parameters with PSA-based freedom from cancer relapse and showed that tumor control is better with higher prostate doses (**Figures 11-11 through 11-14**). Most clinical series are plagued by the fact the lower dose implants tended to be done earlier in the cohort studied, so that inferior implants are more likely to have time to fail, leading to artifactual bias in favor of their PSA-based cancer control calculations.(VICINI) Still, most investigators have shown better cancer control with better coverage of the prostate. That makes sense!

The D90 and V100 are closely correlated, and both are commonly used in clinical practice (**Figures 11-15 through 11-17**). The principle advantage of the V100 is that it's easier to conceptualize. In fact, all parameters tend to be higher in patients with biochemical control (**Figures 11-18 and 11-19**). The optimal dosimetric parameters for clinical practice remain a subject of investigation.(HERSTEIN) The minimum prostatic dose (Dmin) is not a good summary parameter because it is too sensitive to minor variations in seed placement or target definitions.(ROY)

HOT SPOTS
Due to the nature of brachytherapy whereby tissue adjacent to the seeds receives extremely high doses, a substantial amount of prostate gets *far*

A pretty good implant

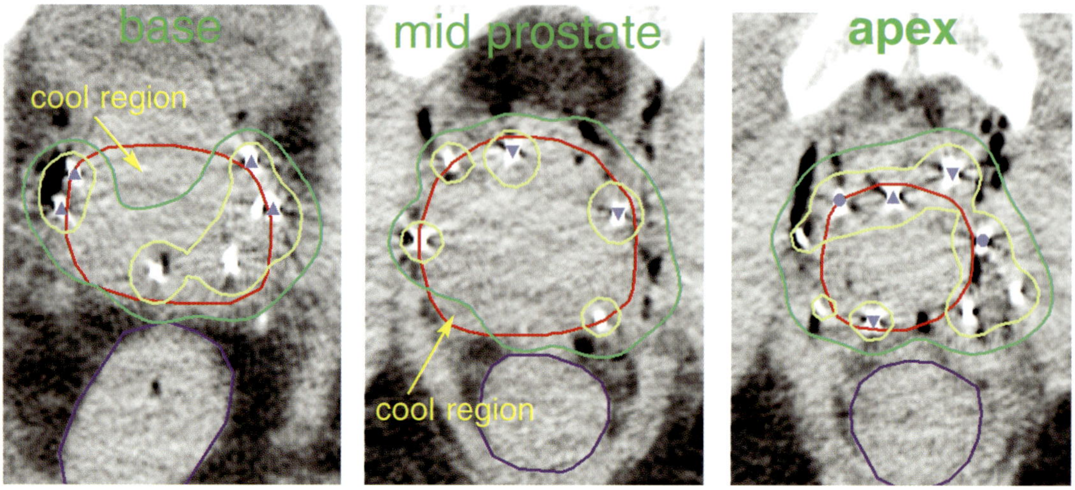

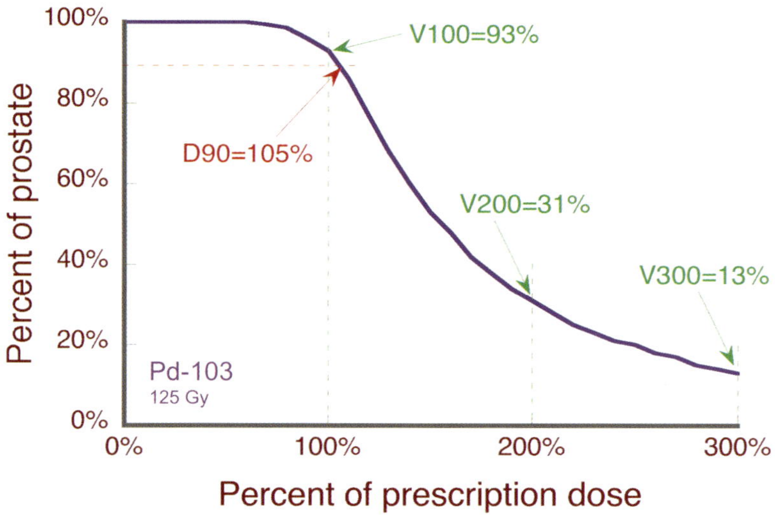

Figure 11-9. CT-based evaluation of a 124 Gy Pd-103 implant. This patient had 93% coverage of the post-implant CT-defined prostate volume. Cold spots are at the anterior base and right posterior-lateral corner. Various dosimetric parameters can be taken from the DVH.

A near-perfect implant

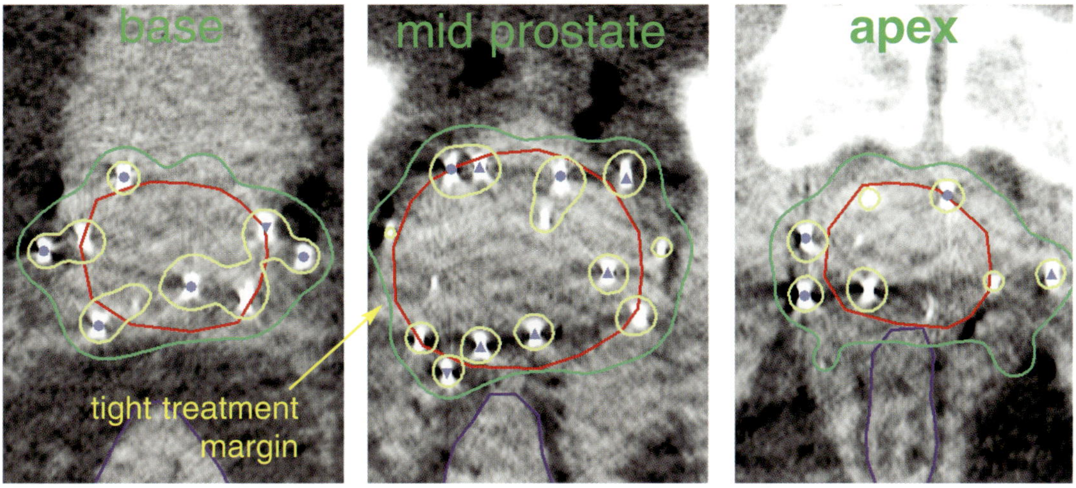

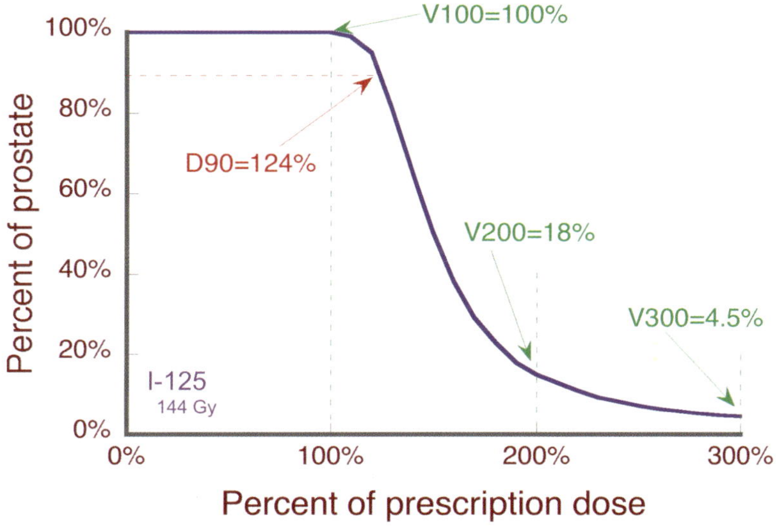

Figure 11-10. CT-based evaluation of a 144 Gy I-125 implant. This patient had 100% coverage of the post-implant CT-defined prostate volume. The only real criticism is the slightly tight treatment margin at the right mid portion (top middle panel).

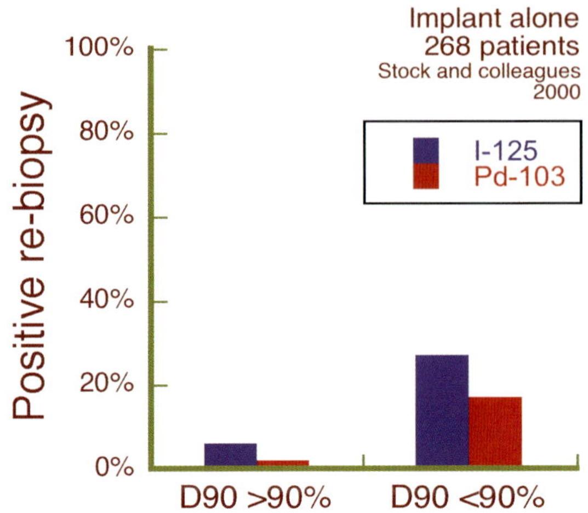

Figure 11-11. Post-implant negative biopsy rates (upper panel) and biochemical control (lower panel) increase with higher D90s. These are important landmark studies, but with substantial caveats (see text).

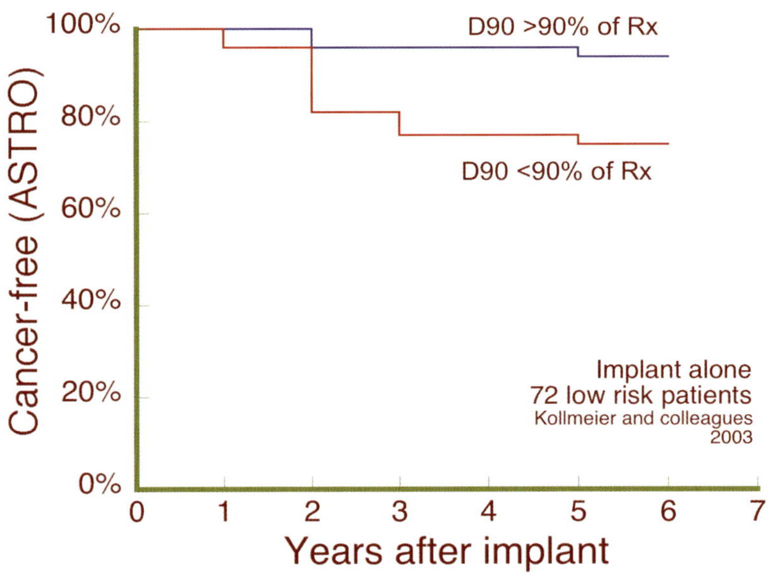

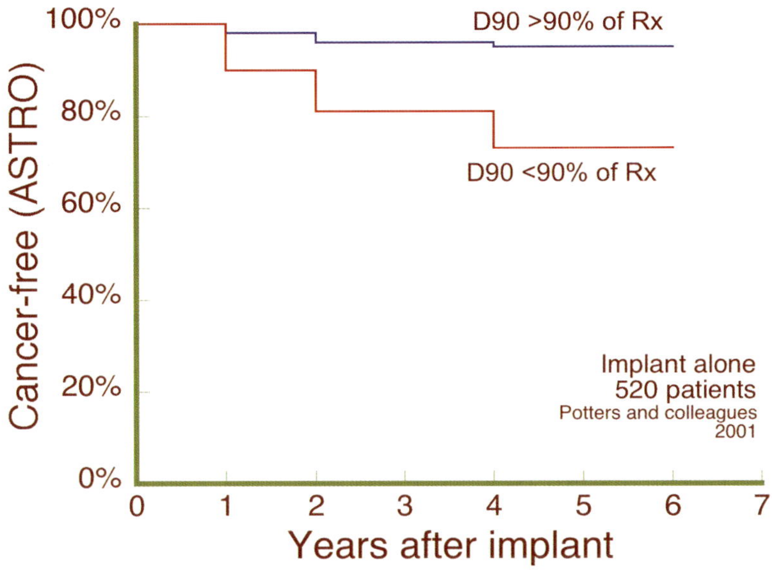

Figure 11-12. Dose response for I-125 or Pd-103 monotherapy.

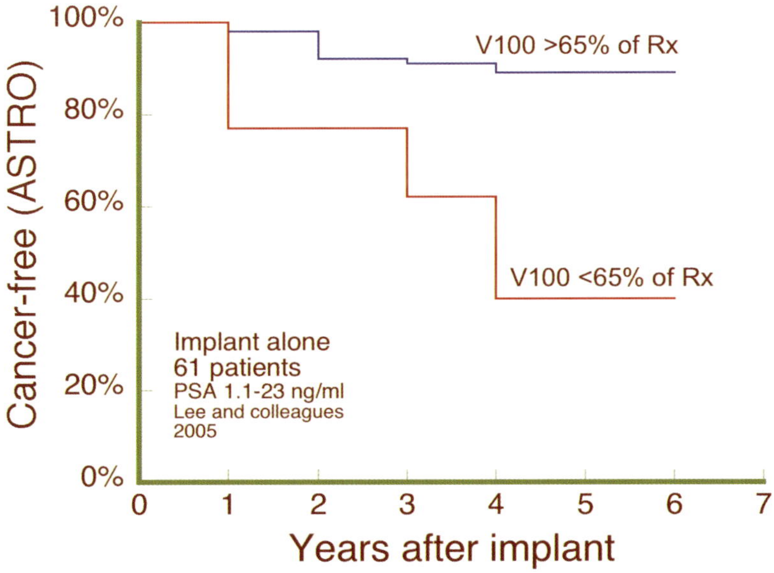

Figure 11-13. Dose response for I-125 or Pd-103 monotherapy.

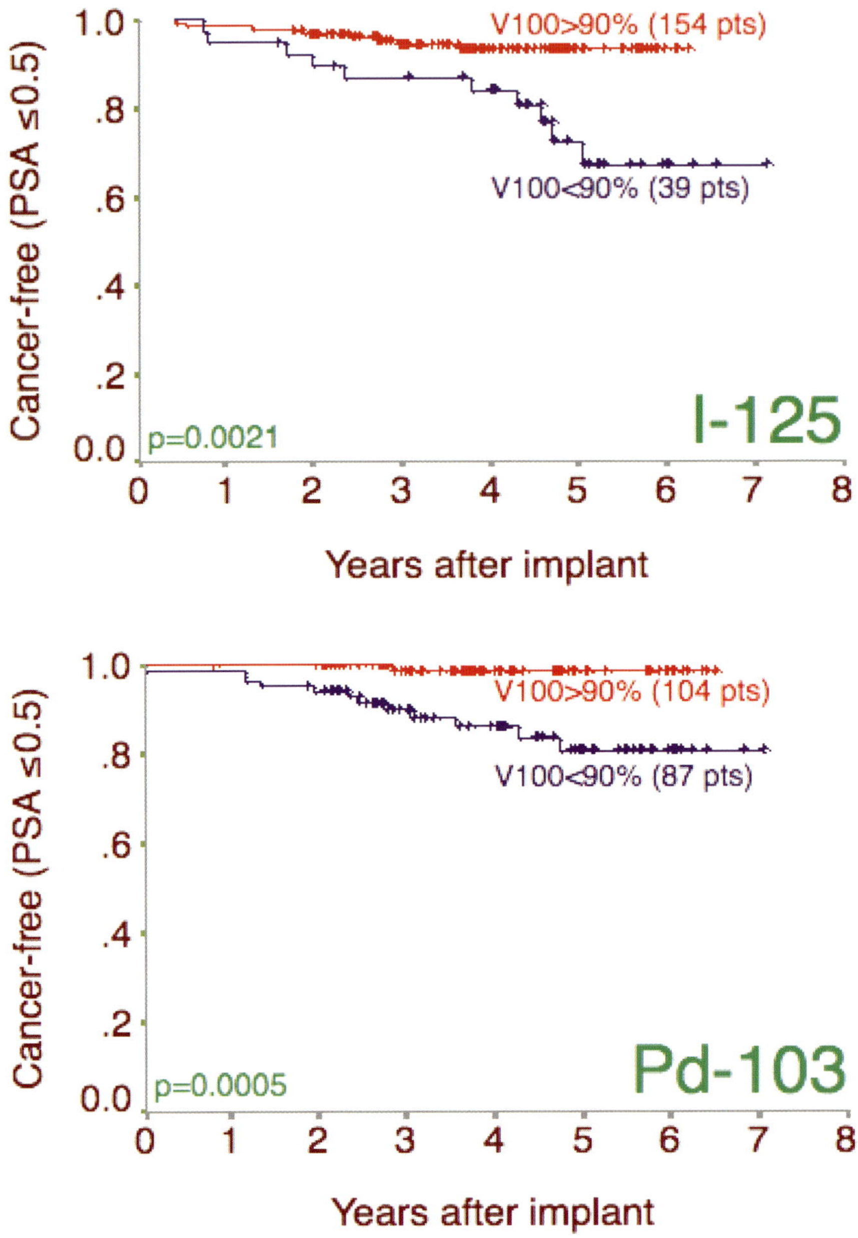

Figure 11-14. Freedom from biochemical failure for I-125 or Pd-103 with a V100 of greater or less than 90%, for patients randomized to I-125 or Pd-103 monotherapy.(WALLNER 03)

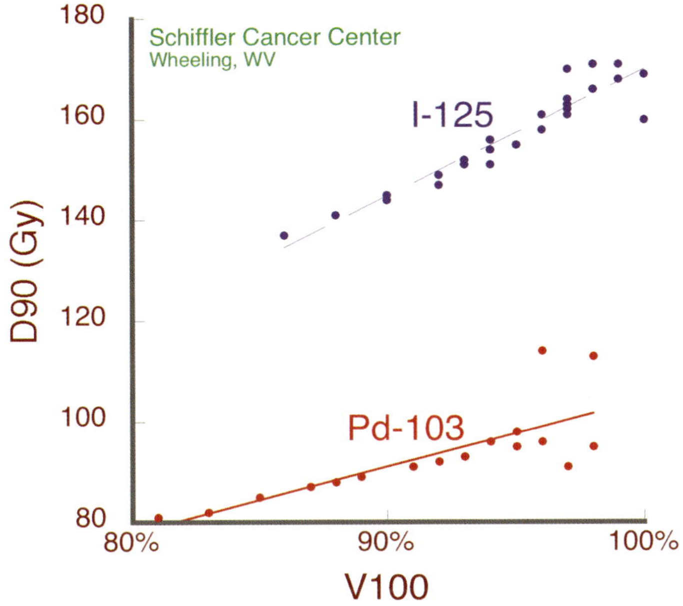

Figure 11-15. There is a very tight correlation between D90 and V100, so that the choice of one or the other probably doesn't make much difference. (MERRICK 99)

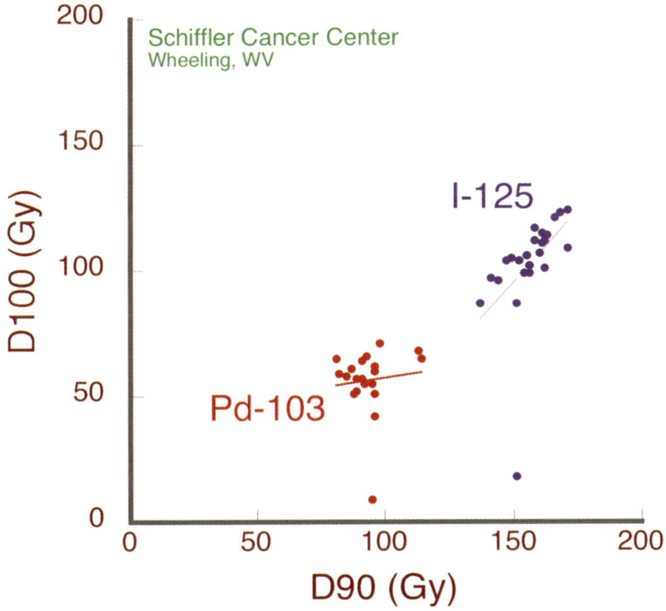

There's much less correlation between the D90 and V100, and other parameters that are highly affected by small high or low dose regions, like the D100. (MERRICK 99)

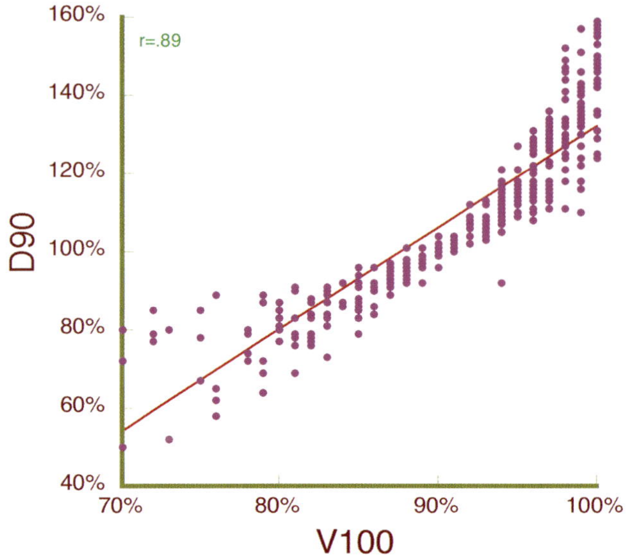

Figure 11-16. There is a fairly tight correlation between D90 and V100, so that the choice of one or the other probably doesn't make much difference. (MERRICK 99)

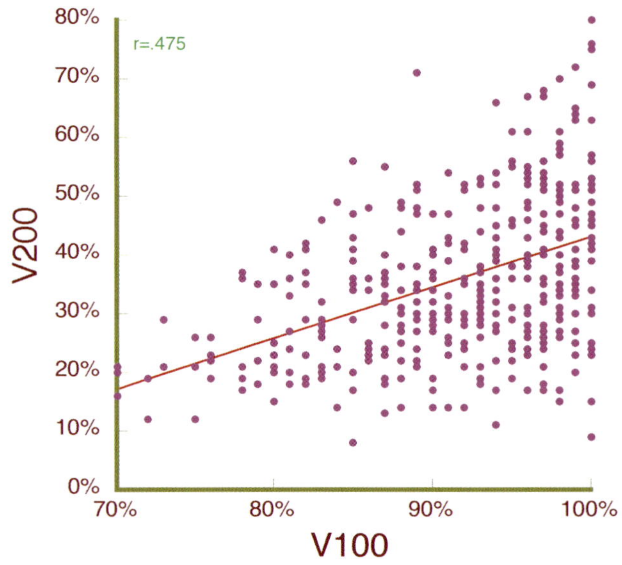

There's little correlation correlation between V100 and V200. (MERRICK 99)

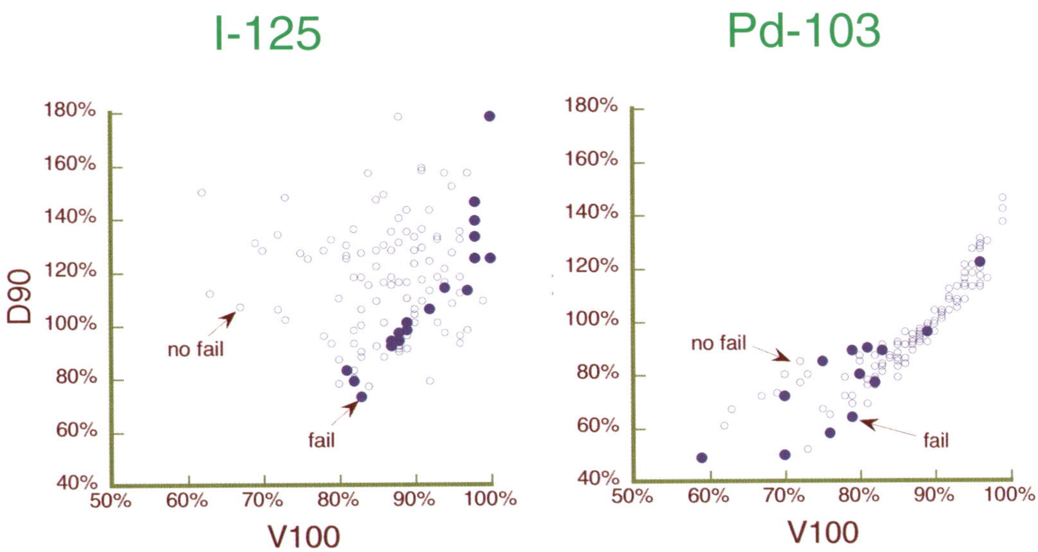

Figure 11-17. Scatter plots of V100s and D90s for patients with or without biochemical failure. Includes only patients treated at the Puget Sound VA and the University of Washington.(WALLNER 03)

greater than the prescription dose (**Figures 11-20 and 11-21**). The prescription dose is the *minimum* desired, while tissue close to the seeds receive doses far in excess of that.

The clinical significance of hot spots is unclear. High-dose regions encompassing the urethra or rectum increase the chance of morbidity, but it appears that excessive dose to the parenchyma itself carry little significance. Based on the fact that serious complications (incontinence, rectal ulcers, or parenchymal necrosis) are unusual, parenchymal hot spots are probably not all that important, at least with the peripheral loading patterns that are now standard.(JONES) High-dose regions do not appear to influence tumor control rates, when controlled for coverage by the prescription dose.(LING, WALLNER)

PROBLEMS WITH CT-BASED DOSIMETRY

The introduction of CT-based dosimetry was a milestone in modern prostate brachytherapy.(WILLINS) But CT has its shortcomings, the most

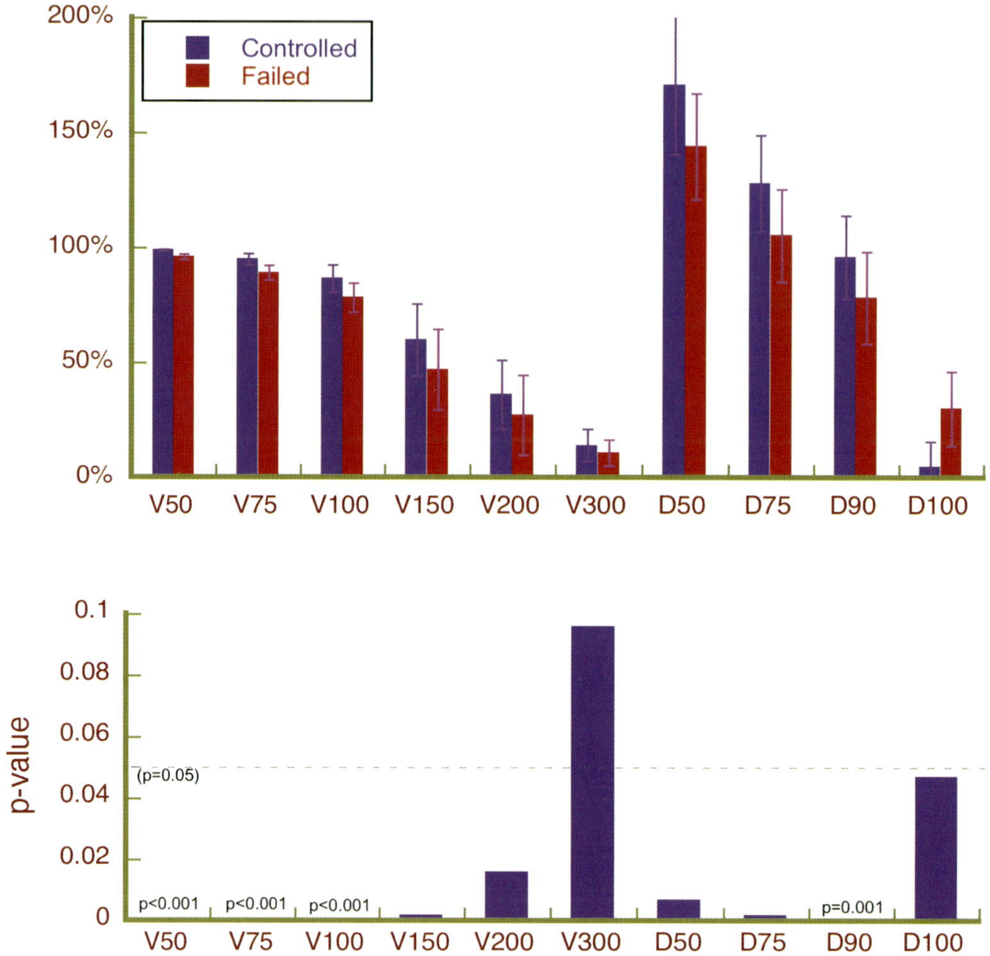

11-18. Vxx and Dxx values for patients with or without biochemical control after Pd-103 brachytherapy. The take home point here is that the dosimetric values tend to be lower in patients who are not cured.(HERSTEIN 07)

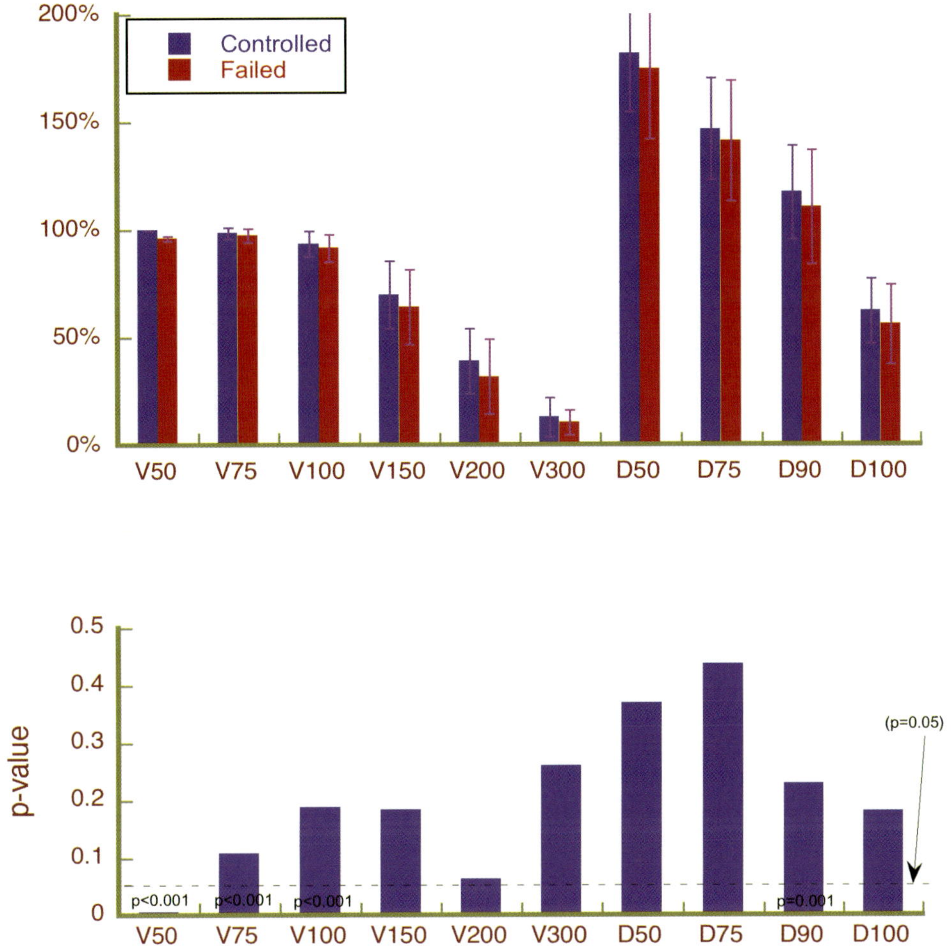

Figure 11-19. Vxx and Dxx values for patients with or without biochemical control after I-125 brachytherapy. As with Pd-103 in Figure 11-18, the dosimetric values tend to be lower in patients who are not cured.(HERSTEIN 07)

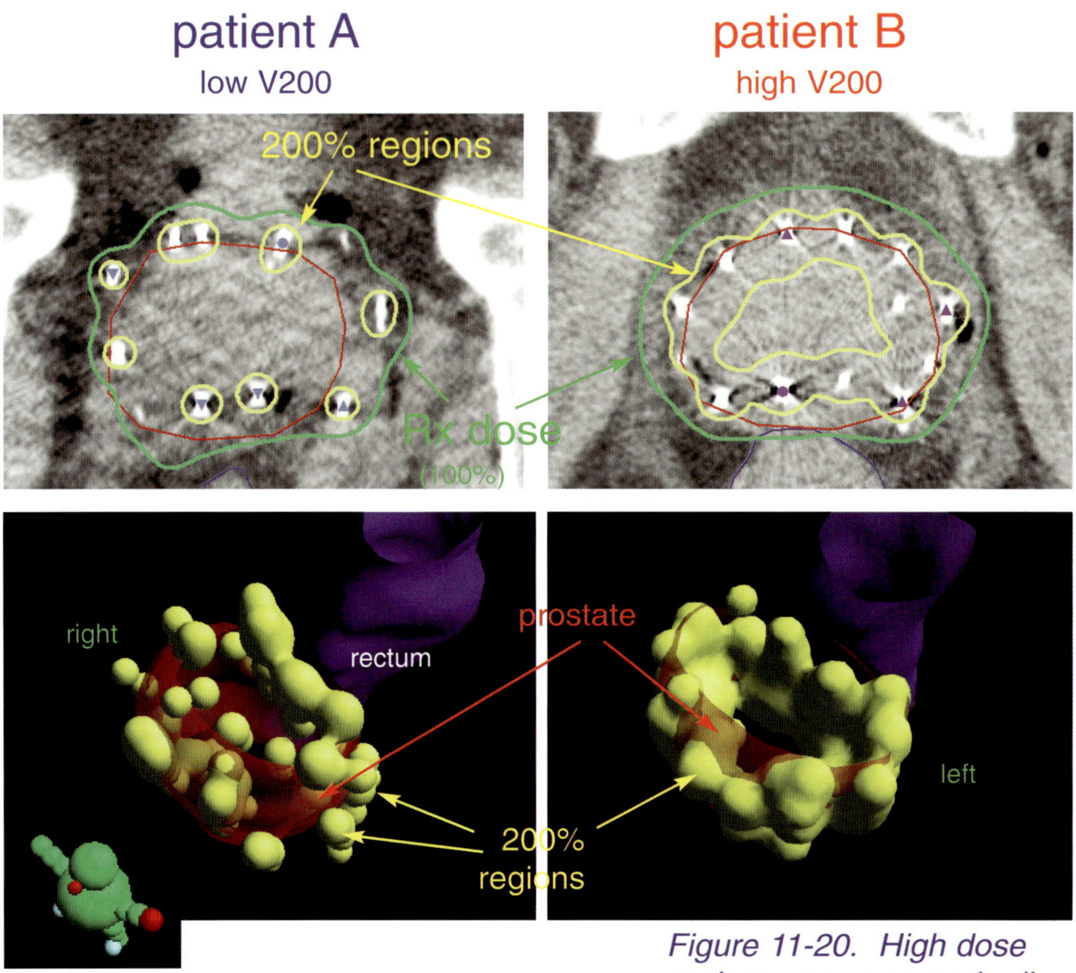

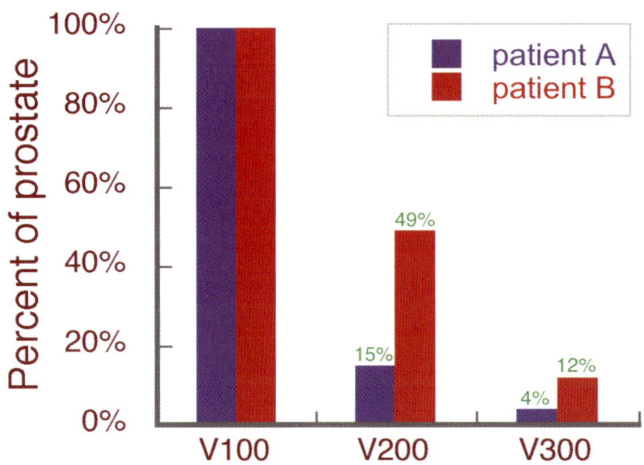

Figure 11-20. High dose regions can vary markedly betwen implants with similar V100s. These two patients each have a 100 of 100%, but have markedly different V200s and V300s. There appears to be little clinical relevance to high dose region variability, as long as the prostate is covered by the prescription dose, and the rectal and urethral doses are not excessive.(JONES, WALLNER 05)

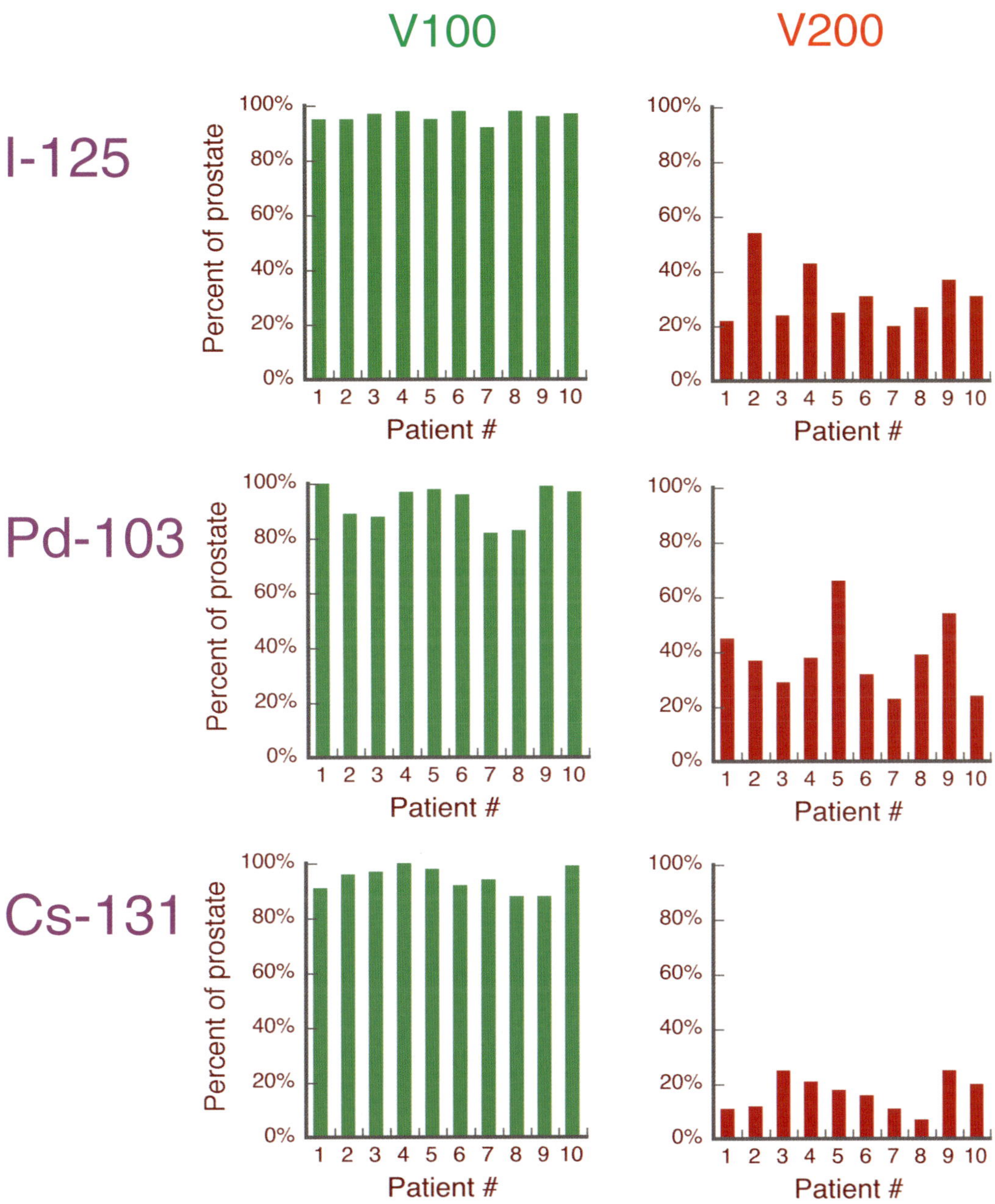

Figure 11-21. V100 and V200 for ten unselected I-125, Pd-103 or Cs-131 patients at the Puget Sound VA. High dose regions tend to be highest for Pd-103 and lowest for Cs-131.

obvious of which is fuzziness of the prostatic margins. A second major shortcoming is that the prostate size *changes* in the peri-implant period.

Defining the prostate

The prostatic margins are not sharply delineated on CT scan, and there is substantial subjectivity defining them. It is especially difficult to delineate the prostatic apex, as it blends with the pelvic floor musculature. Also, the lateral margins can be difficult to distinguish from the puborectalis muscles (see chapter 4). Inclusion of the puborectalis or levator ani musculature in the target volume or overly generous drawing of the prostatic apex leads to falsely large prostate volumes and falsely low V100s. The vagaries of prostatic margin interpretation can lead to substantial inter-observer variability in the post-implant dosimetric calculations.(CROOK, HAN, LEE)

Because of the potential for substantial inter-observer variability in the way CT images are interpreted, there is interest in switching to MR-based post-implant imaging, a move that is likely to become more practical in the future. But for now, CT-based dosimetry is the basis for most of what we know about implant analysis, and is considered the standard of care. Despite its image interpretation problems, it is important to point out that CT-based dosimetric studies have been fairly consistent between experienced implant groups, and that CT-based dosimetry does correlate with tumor control rates.

Prostate swelling

Getting implanted is tough on a prostate. Think about it—enemas beforehand, catheterization, a DRE or two, and 50 to 100 needle jabs. Throw in a post-implant cystoscopy and you've got a pretty battered gland—it shouldn't be surprising that it's swollen by the time you're done.

Numerous investigators have shown that the prostate volume increases by approximately 20% to 50% during the implant procedure, with substantial variability among patients (**Figures 11-22 and 11-23**). In some series, implant-related swelling primarily affected the antero-posterior prostatic dimension (**Figure 11-24**).(BADIOZAMANI, MERRICK 99) And the size increase is not just a TRUS or CT artifact—it's evident when comparing pre- and post-implant CT or MR.(WILLINS 98, WATERMAN 98).

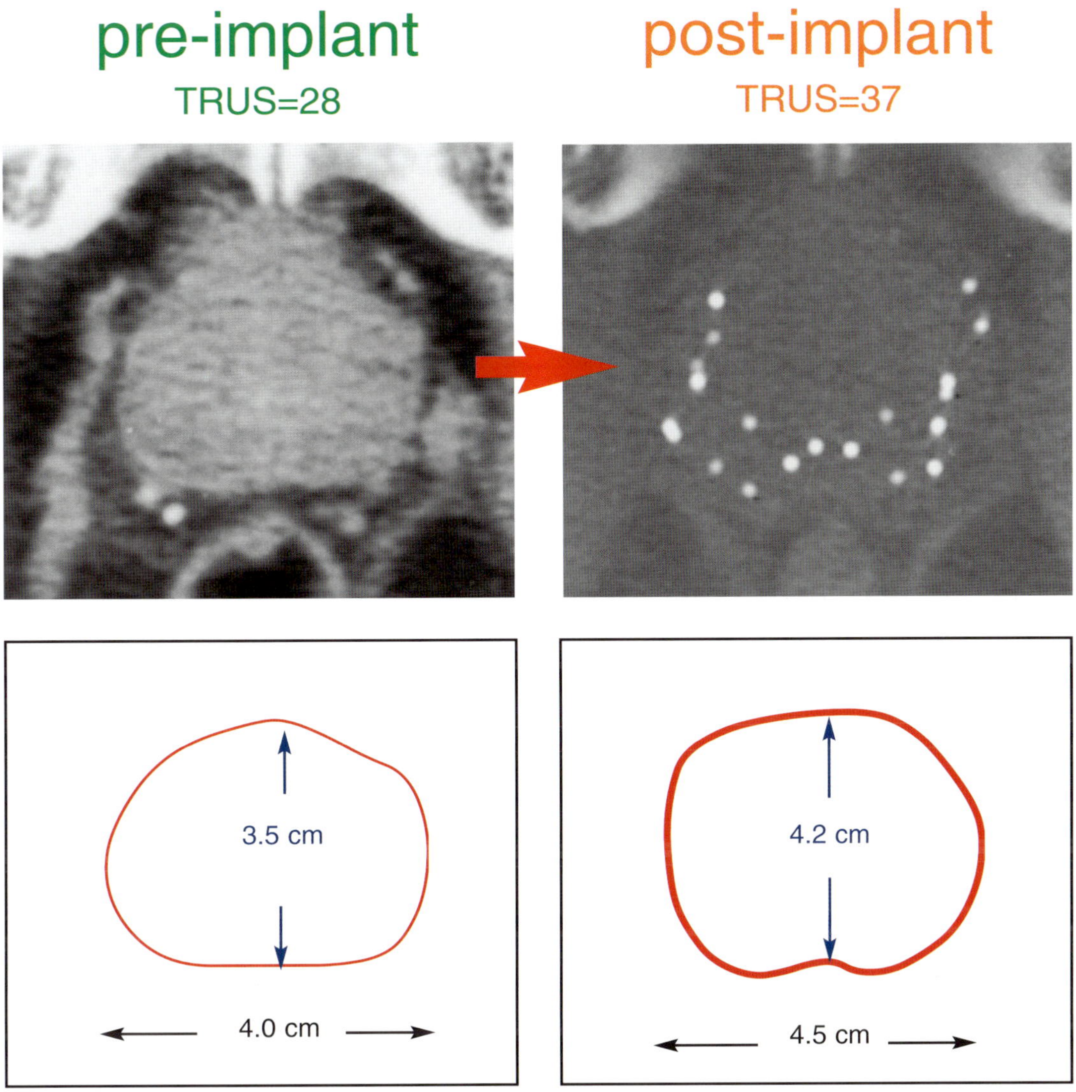

Figure 11-22. Typical pre-implant and post-implant CT (day 0) showing greatest increase in the anterior-posterior dimension.

The problem that implant-related swelling causes from a dosimetric perspective is that it increases the prostate volume on which post-implant evaluation is based. A bigger prostate volume makes target coverage inferior to what would be determined if it was based on the smaller, pre-implant prostate size. But the effect of implant-related swelling is not as great as the volume change would suggest. Willins showed that the target cover-

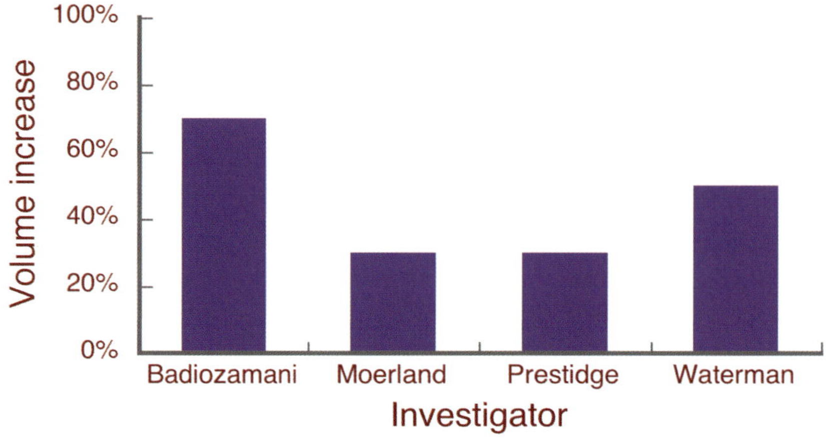

Figure 11-23. The degree of post-implant prostate swelling has been fairly consistent between reported series. Differences beetween series are likely due to differences in the way investigators interpret their images.(BADIOZAMANI, MOERLAND, PRESTIDGE, WATERMAN 98)

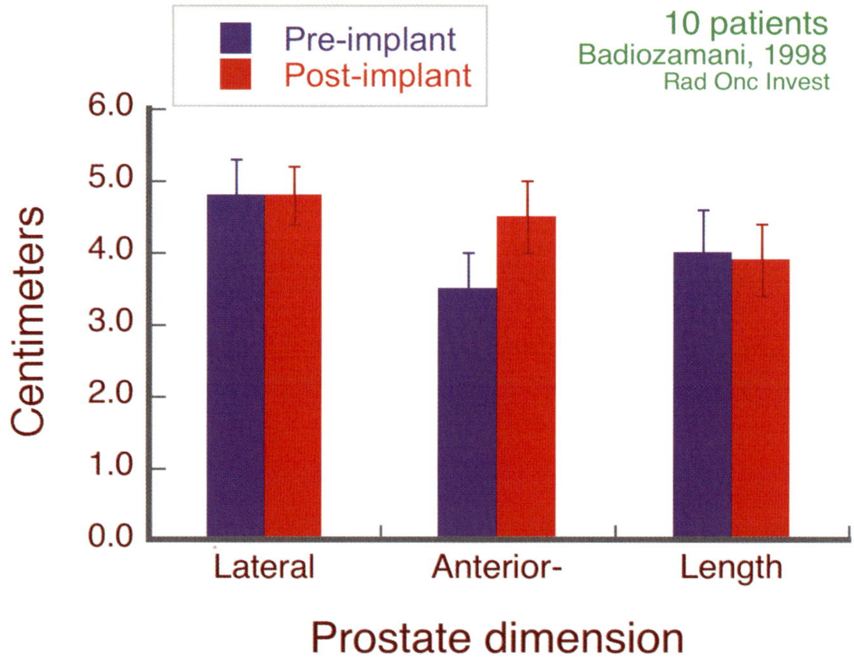

Figure 11-24. Prostatic dimensions before and after the implant procedure.

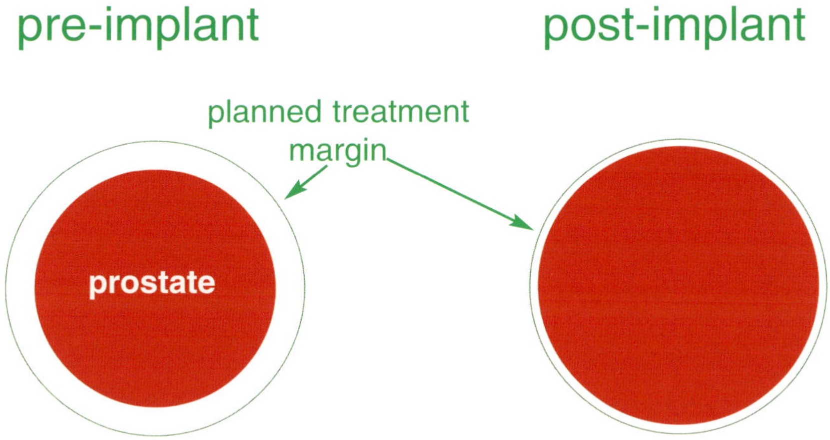

Figure 11-25. Why the post-implant prostate coverage is less affected than predicted by the degree of implant-related swelling. Generous treatment margins allow for swelling, such that most of the larger post-implant prostate volume is still within the prescription isodose volume.(MERRICK 98 AND 00)

Very important point

Pay attention here! Generous treatment margins protect against underdosage due to prostate swelling.

age fell an average of only 5%, despite an average prostate volume increase of 25%, the reason being that the addition of treatment margins in the pre-plan allows for a large degree of swelling, with most of the volume increase still inside of the prescription isodose volume (**Figure 11-25**).(WILLINS 98, WATERMAN 98, MERRICK) Merrick has championed the use of large treatment margins as a protective against edema-related underdosage.(MERRICK 98, MERRICK 00, BUTLER 00, REED 05) Waterman and colleagues showed that the magnitude of the volume increase is not related to the number of needles used, the radioisotope used, or the number of seeds.(WATERMAN 98)

Variability in the degree of implant-related swelling among patients is an impediment to establishing uniform guidelines for dosimetric evaluation in the setting of a changing target volume, especially in extreme cases.

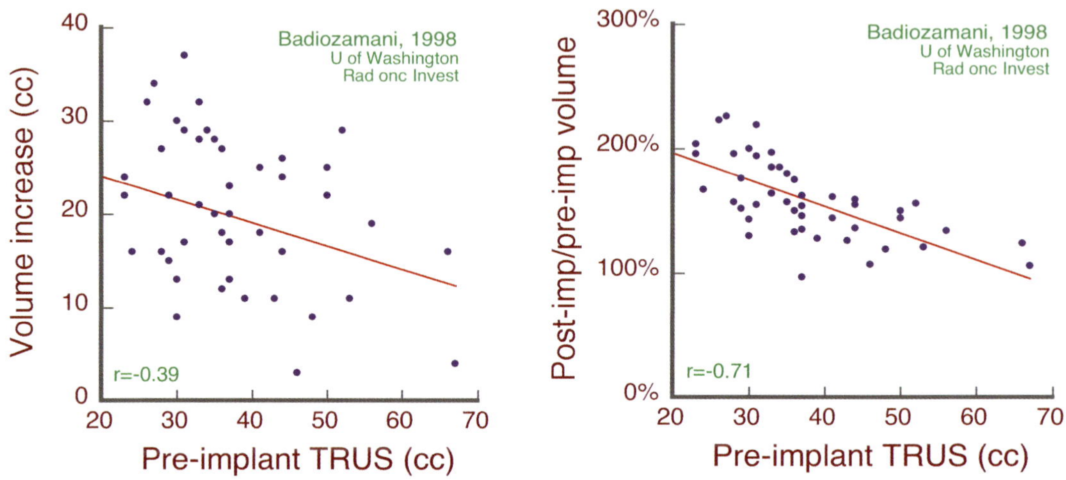

Figure 11-26. Absolute (left) and proportional (right) prostate volume increase as a function of pre-implant TRUS volume.

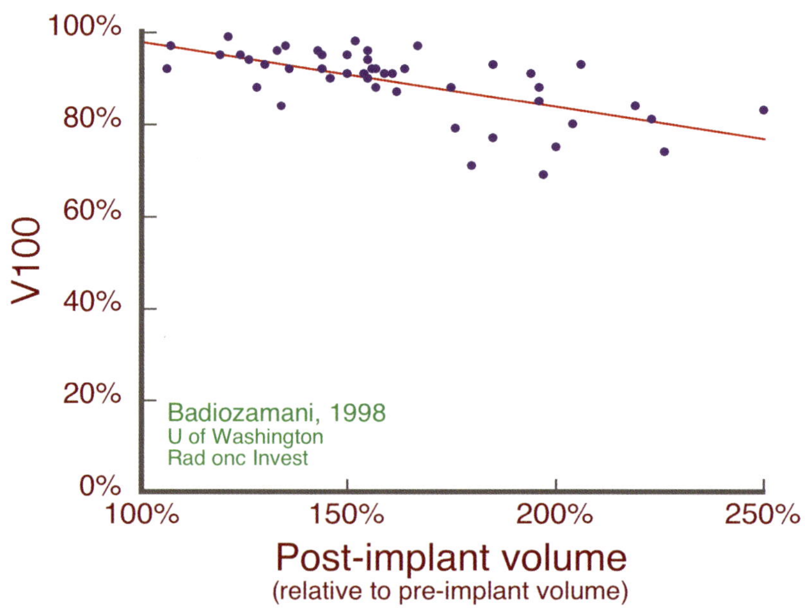

Figure 11-27. Fraction of post-implant prostate volume covered by prescription dose (V100) in relation to the degree of implant-related swelling.

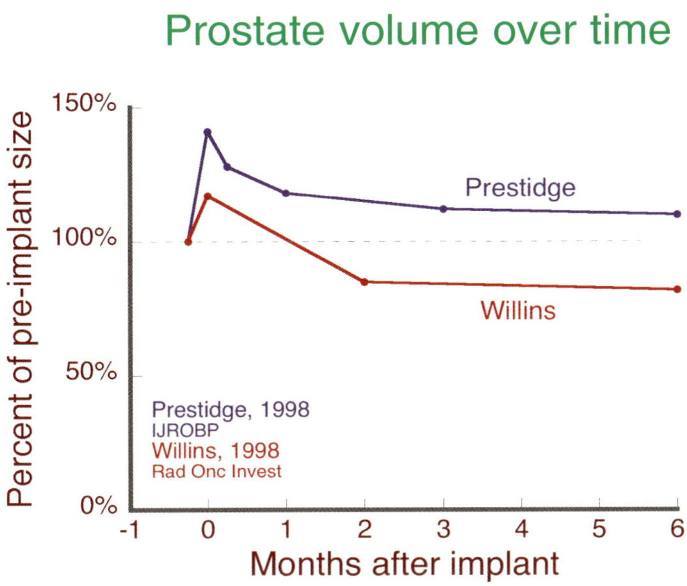

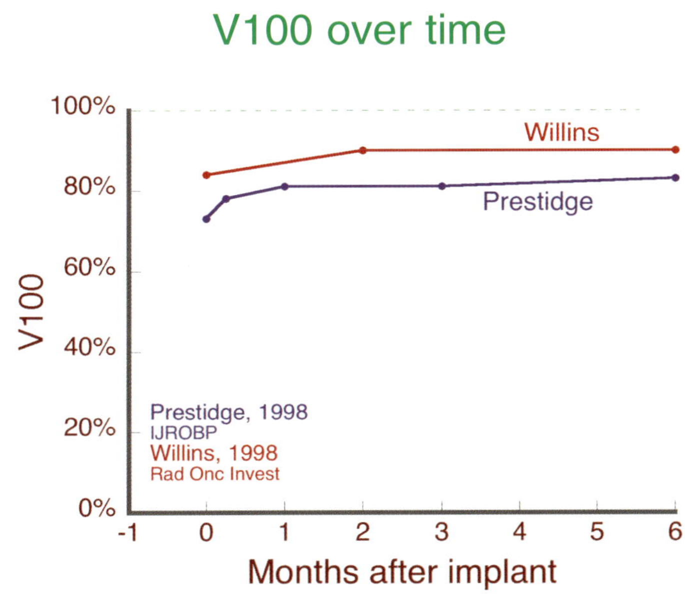

Figure 11-28. Time course of implant-related prostate swelling, and the corresponding V100s reported by two independent investigative teams.

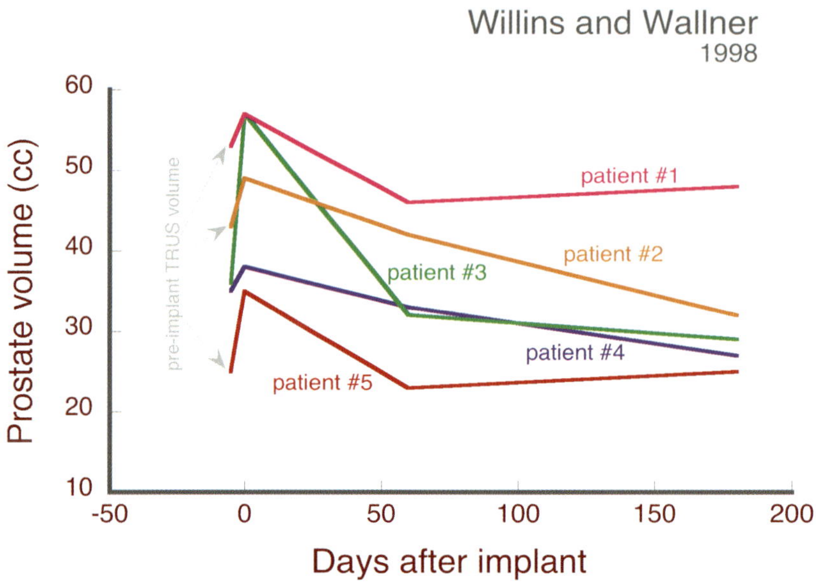

Figure 11-29. The degree of swelling and its resolution vary substantially among patients, making a uniform policy regarding its consideration in post-implant dosimetry difficult, at best.

With the intention of more effectively customizing treatment planning to the individual patient, Badiozamani and colleagues compared patients' degree of implant-related volume changes with multiple clinical parameters, including pre-implant volume, hormonal ablation, and pre-implant external beam radiation in 50 patients treated at the University of Washington. Their hope was to determine which patients required a larger planning treatment margin (TM) to ensure adequate post-implant prostate coverage. Overall, the post-implant prostate volume increased by an average factor of 1.7 (±0.34) compared to the pre-implant volume. The absolute volume change was similar in patients with small versus large pre-implant prostate volume, but the proportional change was less in patients with a larger prostate volume (**Figure 11-26**). As expected, the degree of post-implant target coverage was less in patients with greater volume increase (**Figure 11-26**). Because patients with a small pre-implant prostate had proportionately greater volume increase, their post-implant target coverage was generally less (**Figure 11-27**).

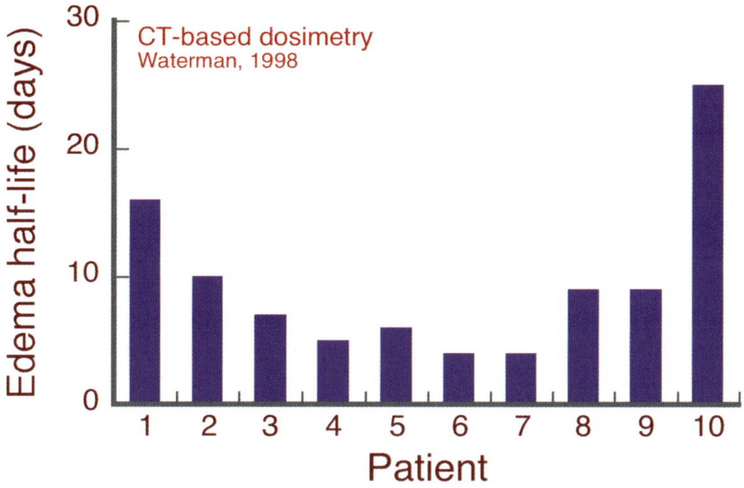

Figure 11-30. The time course of edema resolution is highly variable from one patient to the next, making the application of a standard correction factor in evaluating prostatic coverage impractical in the clinical setting.

While Badiozamani identified some trends regarding the degree of swelling in relation to pre-implant parameters, the most striking finding was the substantial scatter in the data for all parameters. This marked variabilty between patients precludes any predictive rule that might be applied to predict swelling from one patient to the next.

One way to account for the degree of swelling is to base the post-implant dosimetry on the pre-implant volume, somehow registered with the post-implant seed locations. Doing so may be the most realistic way to assess how well the pre-plan was executed, but it's a dubious policy in regards to optimizing cancer eradication. Most of the dose will be delivered while the prostate is still larger than the pre-treatment volume. Pretending that the prostate is smaller than it is during that time may make the physician feel better, but would not help eradicate cancer if the implant does not cover the prostate sufficiently.

Swelling resolution
The confounding effect of implant-related prostate swelling is exacerbated by the variable resolution of swelling in the post-implant period. In order to

characterize the post-implant prostate volume changes, investigators have analyzed serial scans.(WILLINS 98, WATERMAN 98) In general, the prostate volume returns to its pre-implant size by two months, and prostate coverage increases by about 5% to 10% (**Figure 11-28**).

Delaying the post-implant scan

Another way to circumvent the added uncertainty of implant-related prostatic swelling is to wait one or two months to obtain post-implant dosimetry films, allowing time for much of the implant-related swelling to resolve. This is another unwise idea. The problem with waiting to get the evaluation scan is that if target coverage is determined at that time to be inadequate, adding seeds so long after the initial procedure would be suboptimal. It is in the patient's best interest to identify an inadequate implant as early as possible, and correct it sooner rather than later. For teams that are new to brachytherapy, immediate scanning and same-day dosimetric assessment should also help compress the learning curve, revealing mistakes soon after the fact to make it easier to figure out ways to correct them. As accurate intra-operative evaluation becomes more available, we believe that more and more brachytherapists will move toward day 0 dosimetry.(ORIO,REED, GONG)

Mathemetical correction for swelling

Investigators have devised elegant formulas to account for the degree of swelling resolution over time when calculating prostate coverage.(CHEN) Unfortunately, such correction factors are clinically useless, because implant-related volume changes are so inconsistent from one patient to the next (**Figures 11-29 and 11-30**).

PLANNED WITH TRUS, EVALUATED BY CT?

Perhaps the biggest conceptual problem with CT-based dosimetry is that it is not based on TRUS, the usual treatment planning imaging modality. One could argue that whatever modality is used to plan an implant should also be used to assess it. The most obvious potential problem with using different imaging modalities is the tendency to derive larger prostate volumes from CT scan, compared to TRUS. In fact, the accuracy of TRUS versus CT is still a contentious topic, and the importance of crossing imaging modalities is uncertain. However, this problem should be minimized if CTs are not overread to include the levator ani muscles with the prostatic volume (see chapter 4).

ASSESSING DOSE TO THE TUMOR ITSELF

Current practice is to assess the dose to the entire prostate, considering it to be uniformly at risk of cancerous involvement. More detailed dosimetric evaluation of dose to the cancerous areas specifically will likely be possible and desirable in the future. Unfortunately, while assessing the dose to the tumor itself is conceptually appealing, current imaging techniques do not allow accurate delineation of cancer within the prostate.(SCHEIDLER) Even if this were possible, it would likely be best to continue to evaluate the dose to the entire prostate, to maximize the likelihood of eradicating microscopic synchronous cancers.

WHAT TO DO WITH AN INADEQUATE IMPLANT

Uh-oh. Regardless of one's level of experience, there will be cases in which the degree of target coverage appears insufficient (**Figure 11-31**). Although there are no clearly established criteria for adequate target coverage, there will be cases in which an implant is grossly suboptimal by customary standards. While you might quibble about the significance of a V100 of 83% versus 80%, most reasonable people would get concerned with a value below 80%. If the V100 is below that, you've got a problem that you need to address (**Table 11-3**).

The first thing to do when an implant seems inadequate is to review the site of the positive pre-treatment biopsies. If the involved portion of the prostate is covered well by the prescription dose, and the biopsies were negative elsewhere, tumor control *might* not be compromised by underdosage of the apparently uninvolved regions. Of course, this assumes that those portions of the prostate with negative biopsy tissue truly are free of cancer, a certain leap of faith.

If the prescription dose coverage is suboptimal, and you are having trouble deciding on the adequacy of an implant, it may help to run the coverage at slightly lower dose levels—try the 80% isodose lines. It is likely that the full current prescription doses are not needed to eradicate cancer and that coverage of the cancerous regions by the 80% isodose line is adequate. But again, this is an admittedly big assumption. Another option for borderline inadequate implants is to repeat the evaluation CT one month later, to see how the coverage looks. But remember, the V100 typically improves by only about 5% to 10% (see Figure 11-28). So if you have really bad coverage, a delayed CT scan is unlikely to resolve the issue.

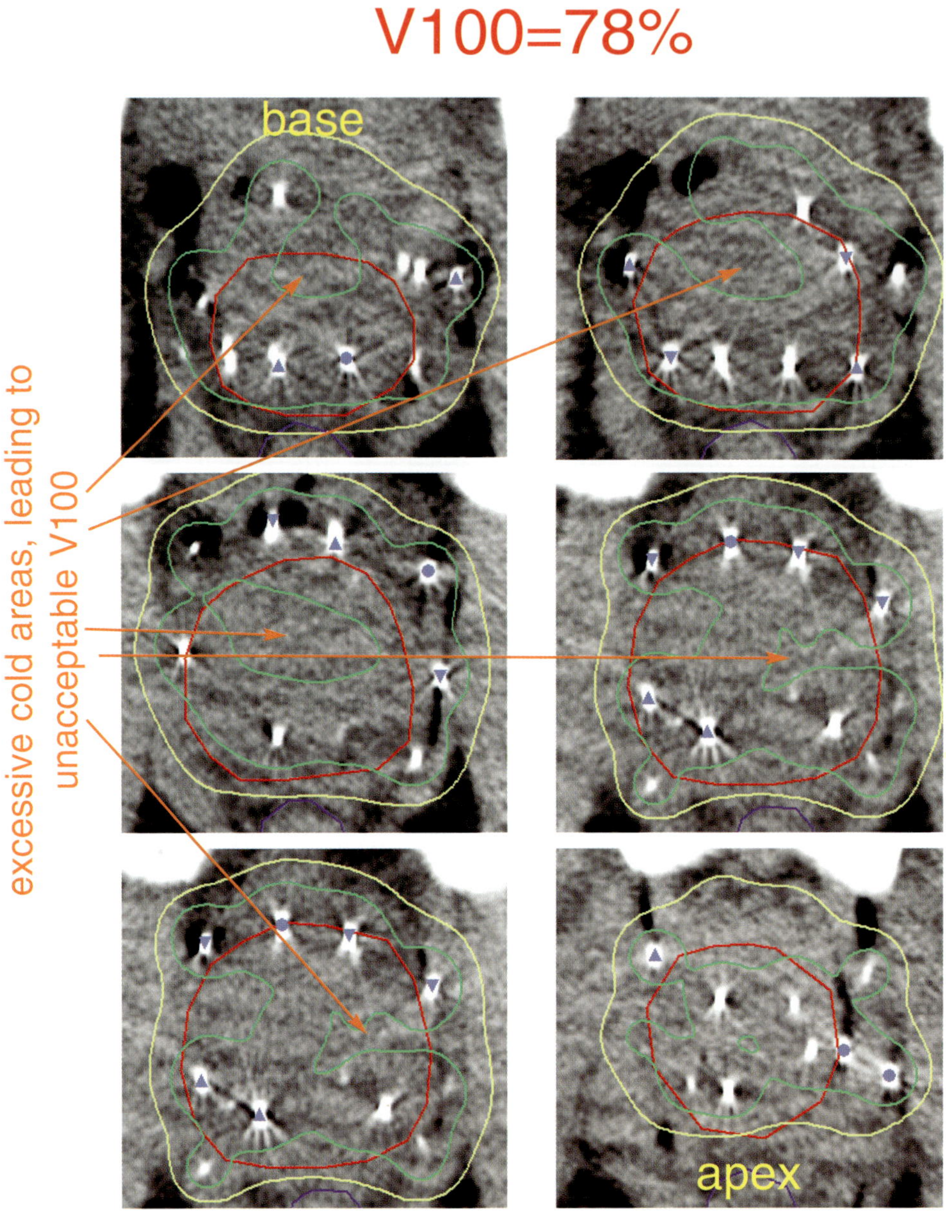

Figure 11.31. This is a great example of a bad implant. The V100 of 78% is too low. Cold spots are everywhere—anterior, posterior, lateral and central. You'd have do something about this one!

Table 11-3. Some considerations in assessing a low V100.

- Look at the degree of swelling
  - -if more than normal, would be more accepting of slightly inferior coverage
  - -consider rescanning at one month postimplant, to let swelling resolve
- Look at where the cold spots are
  - -if anterior, less significant in terms of cancer eradication
- Look at site(s) of positive biopsies
  - -if positive where the implant is cold, greater impetus to supplement the implant

There are a number of corrective options in cases where prostatic coverage is deemed deficient, but ignoring the problem is not one of them. The first thing we do is discuss the situation with the patient. Although it is painful to admit an inadequate job, there's no realistic way around it. Of course patients would also like to ignore the issue and call it a day, but we really do not think that is a good idea either. We're dealing with cancer here. If you miss the chance for cure, and your patient goes on to develop metastatic disease because you ignored a technical problem that could have been fixed...well, you can finish this story yourself.

There are two reasonable choices to fix an inadequate implant—either add some external beam radiation, or go back and add seeds (**Table 11-4**). Adding supplemental external beam radiation is a murky proposition, which should be approached with caution. It's one thing to add supplemental external radiation to a prostate that has been treated with a relatively homogeneous implant. But it's another thing to add it to a prostate that has received a full therapeutic dose to some areas, and far less to others. Bringing the therapeutic dose to acceptable levels in the most under-dosed regions may mean over-treating other regions, and possibly risking complications. Using even the most sophisticated treatment planning technique to supplement just a portion of the gland is probably not realistic.

Probably the best way to correct an inadequate implant is to return to the operating room to add more seeds to the under-dosed region. To do so,

Table 11-4. Ways to correct a low V100.

- Add seeds
  - -medically most sensical
- Supplemental external beam radiation

use the post-implant CT to determine the dose to be delivered by the seeds already implanted. Then, on the post-plan, add seeds to cold areas, until most are eliminated and the V100 is up close to 100%. But keep in mind that rectal or urethral doses should be respected. Make a note of the number of seeds needed and where they should go. Hang a copy of the unretouched post-plan in the implant suite to refer back to at the time of touch-up. Implementing a touch-up is facilitated by the presence of seeds already implanted, which can act as a guide under fluoroscopy.(KEYES) Other than the embarrassment of telling a patient that his implant needs a touch-up, the final product is typically pretty good (**Figures 11-32 and 11-33**).

DOSIMETRY OF NORMAL TISSUES

Everything we've covered so far in this chapter relates to *prostate* coverage. The other role of post-implant dosimetry is to monitor normal tissue doses in order to minimize the likelihood of complications, while maintaining the high cure rates that are achievable with brachytherapy. The normal tissues at risk are primarily the urethra and rectum.

Urethral doses

Urethral doses have typically been calculated by leaving a urinary catheter in place to identify the urethra on post-implant CT scan images (**Figure 11-34**). A reasonable alternative to leaving the catheter in place is to arbitrarily use the central prostatic point on each CT slice as the urethral dose calculation point. Waterman showed that approximating the urethral point this way comes within 5% to 10% of the catheter-based point in the higher dose ranges, where the clinical effect is most relevant.(WATERMAN 00) The notable exceptions would be the occasional patient with a markedly asymmetric urethra. The close correlation between actual and arbitrary urethral dose calculations diminishes at the bladder neck, where the urethra tends to lie more anteriorly. Interestingly, the uncatheterized urethra often shows up faintly on CT, and can be traced fairly well in many patients (**Figure 11-**

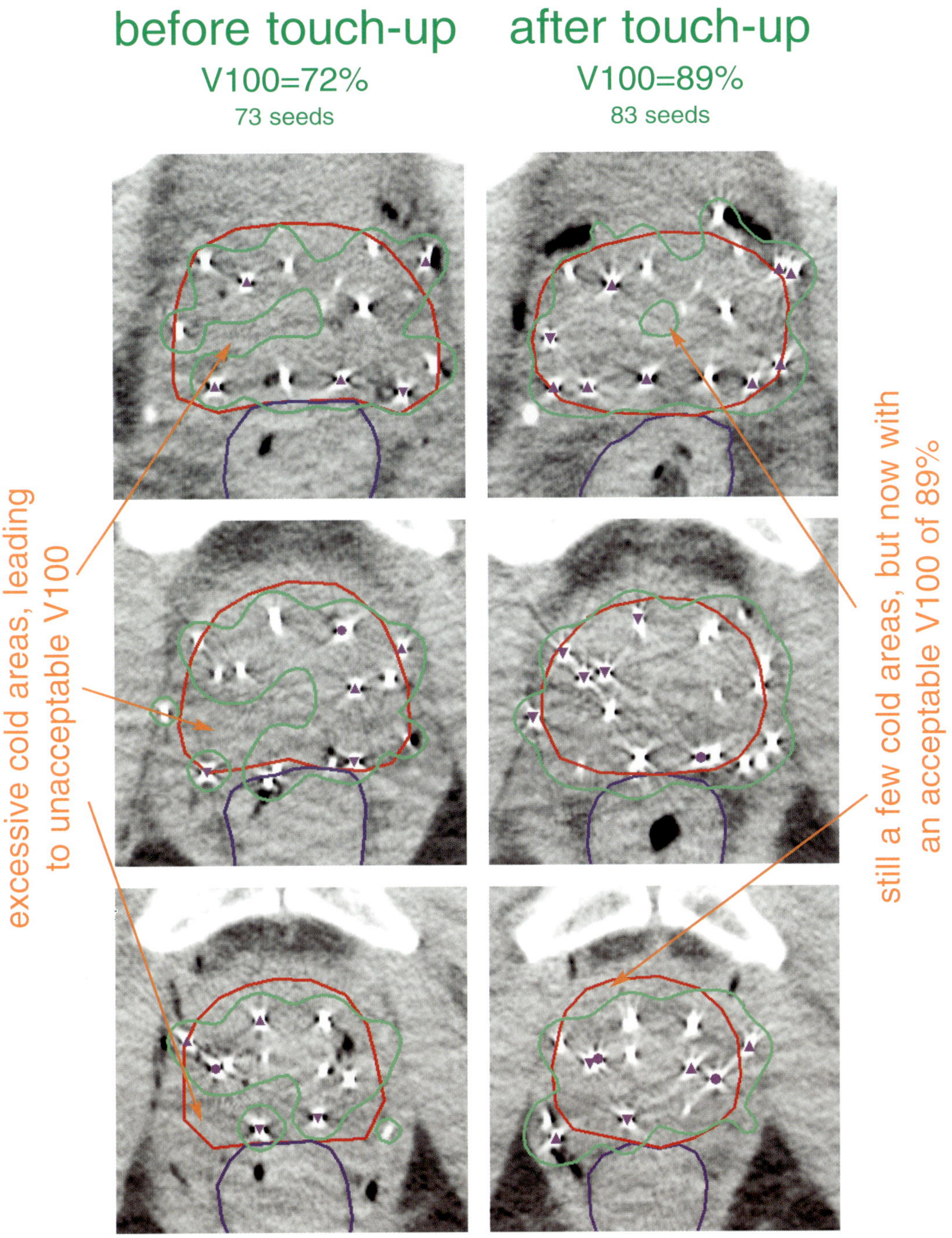

Figure 11-32. Touching up an inadequate implant. This patient had a day 0 post-implant V100 of 72%. He came back and had 10 additional seeds placed, raising the V100 to 89%.

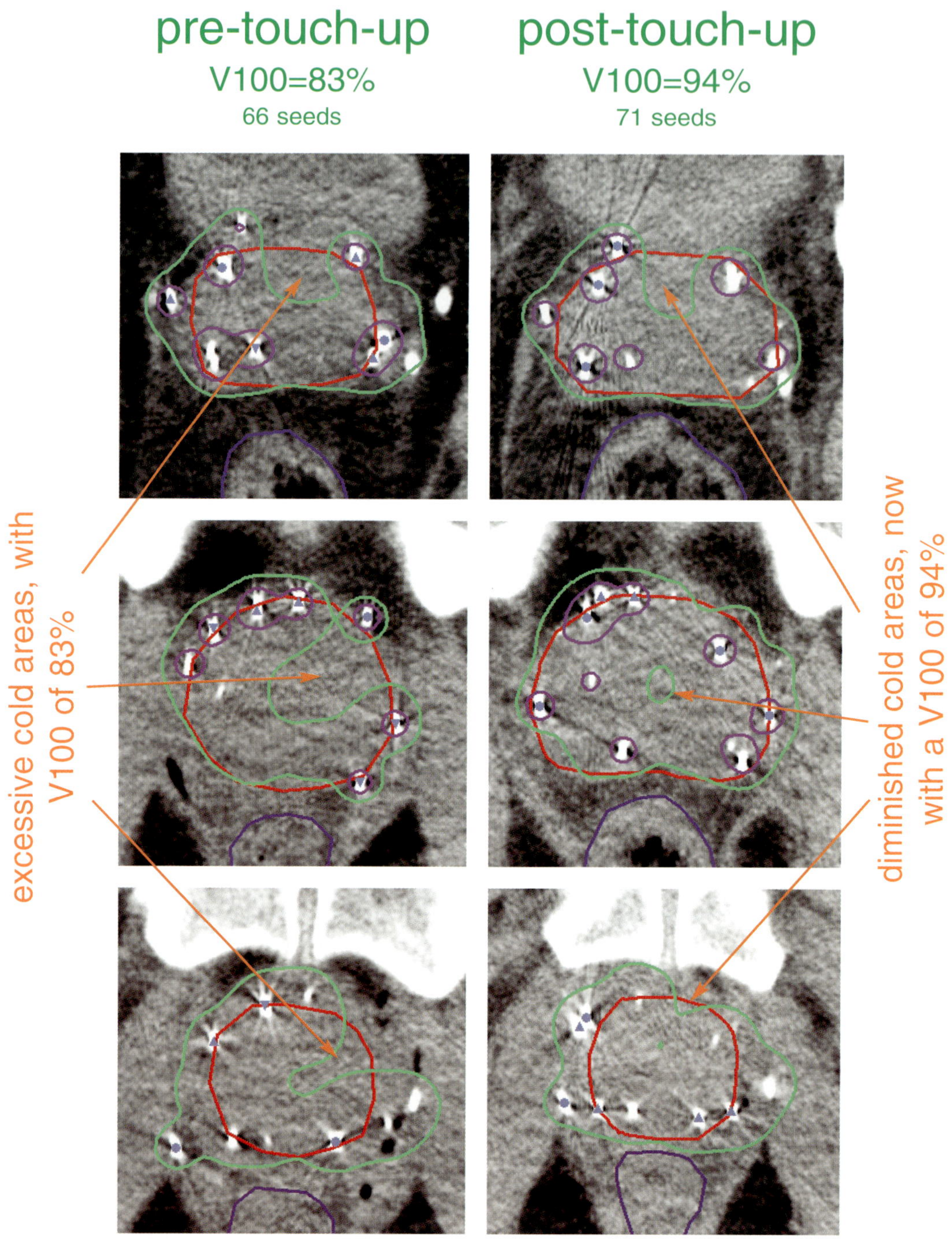

Figure 11-33. Touching up an inadequate implant. This patient had a post-implant V100 of 83%. Although above what we consider 80% acceptable, we brought him back for five additional seeds, raising the V100 to 93%.

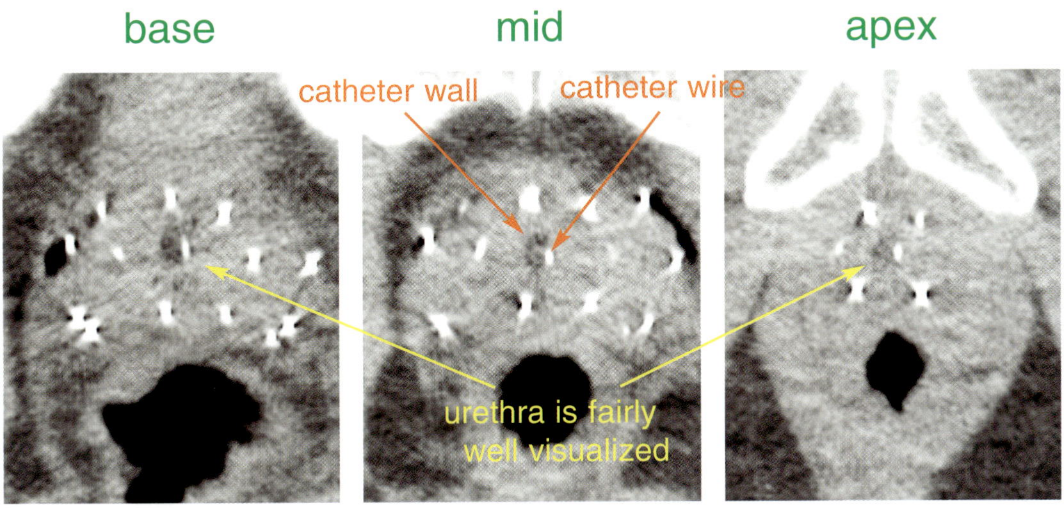

Figure 11-34. Examples of good urethral visibility, with a catheter in place.

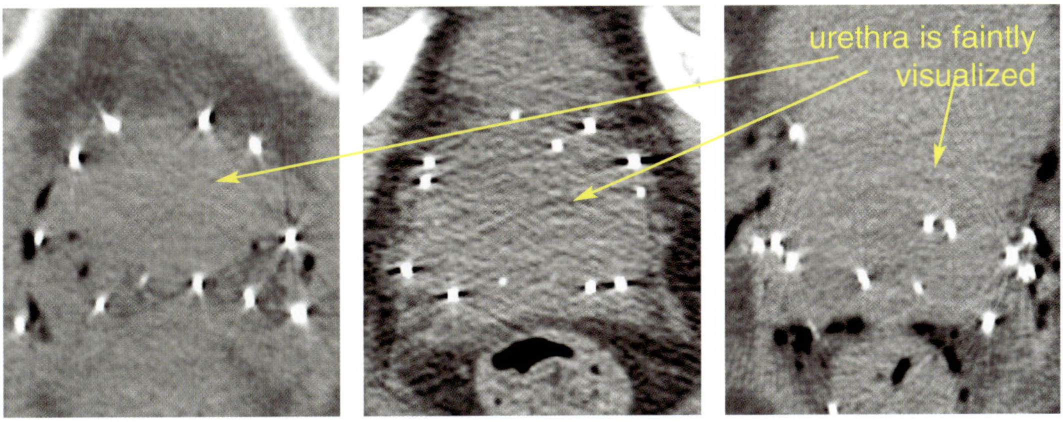

Figure 11-35. Examples of faint urethral visibility, without a catheter in place. Oftentimes, the urethra can be traced from one image to another, even without a catheter in place.

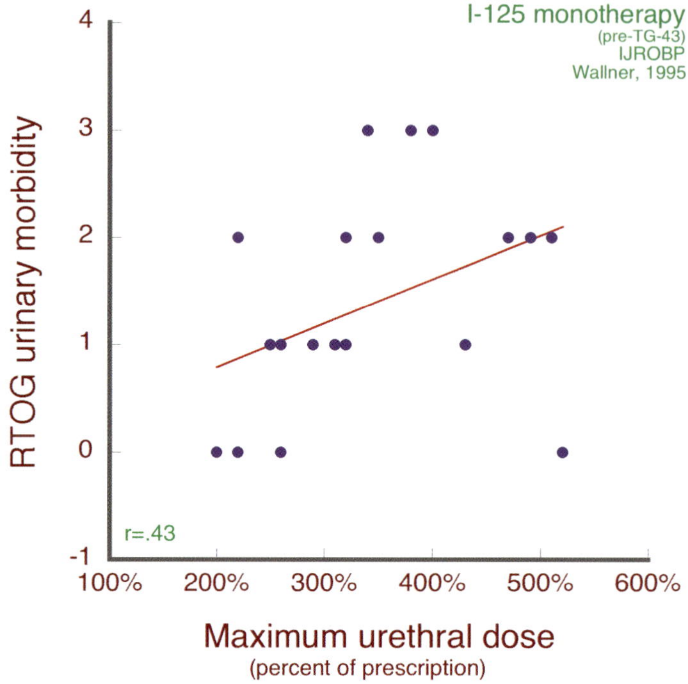

Figure 11-36. Maximum urethral dose versus RTOG post-implant urinary morbidity.

35).

In patients treated in the earlier days of transperineal implants, urinary morbidity correlated fairly well with the maximal central urethral dose. Patients with a maximum I-125 urethral dose below 250% of the prescription dose were less likely to develop substantial urinary morbidity (**Figure 11-36**). More sophisticated calculations, including the length of urethra that received greater than 400 Gy, were no better for predicting morbidity than the simple parameter of maximum dose. The maximum desirable urethral dose for Pd-103 or Cs-131 should presumably also be less than 250%. With a peripheral loading pattern, the central urethral dose can routinely be kept below 2.5 times the prescription dose (**Figures 11-37 through 11-39**).

Since the significance of excessive urethral doses was first reported in the mid-1990s, peripheral loading patterns have become standard. Accordingly, excessive urethral doses, like those seen in the early experience of Blasko and colleagues and Wallner and colleagues, are uncom-

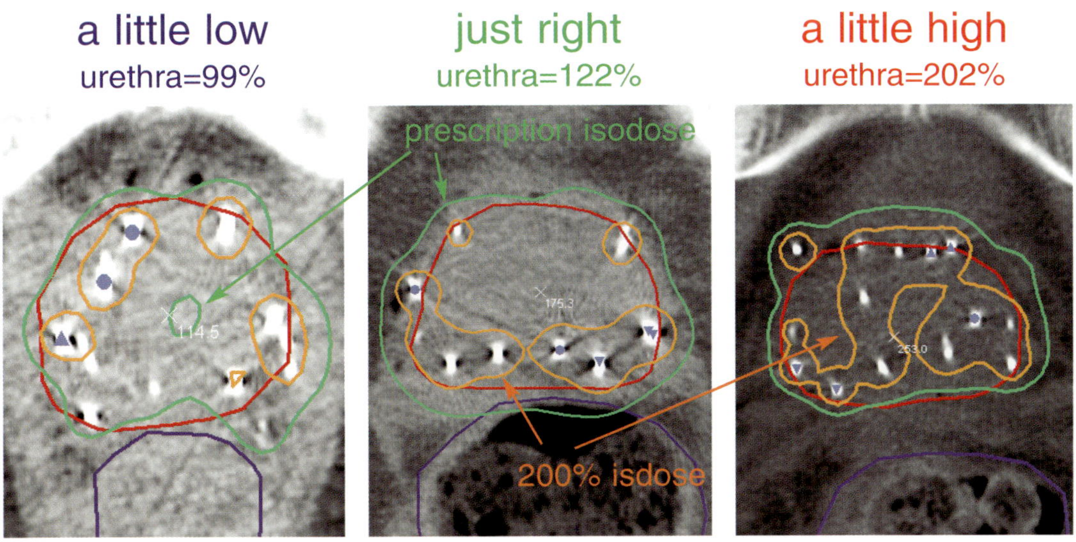

Figure 11-37. Examples of an acceptable range of central prostatic doses. The central dose for the patient on the left is slightly below prescription, something that one risks as you cut the dose too close in an effort to avoid urethral overdose. Note that the 200% isodose goes through the center of the prostate for the patient on the right.

mon. In fact, with peripheral loading patterns, no relationship between urethral doses and morbidity has been described, probably because the range in urethral doses is too limited.(MERRICK 99, ALLEN) Within a narrower dose range, differences in urethral morbidity are more likely related to individual physical or biologic factors than to radiation dose. Accordingly, urethral doses are currently not routinely calculated by most implant teams.

The desirable maximal urethral dose when brachytherapy is combined with beam radiation has also not been well documented. Extrapolating from the early report of Wallner and colleagues, and in the absence of data to the contrary, keeping it below 2.5 times the brachytherapy prescription dose seems prudent and practical.

RECTAL DOSES
Rectal complications are the most worrisome implant-related morbidities. They can cause major lifestyle problems for patients and can require major corrective surgery. The good news is that serious rectal complications are

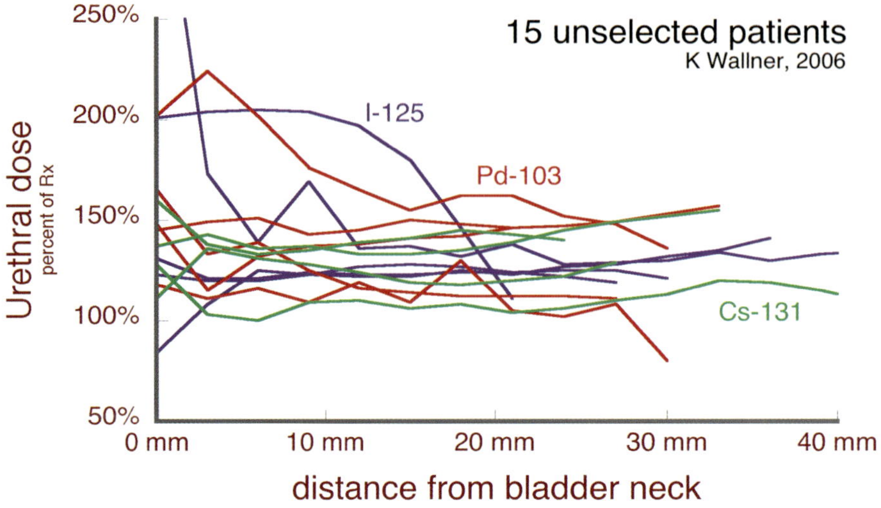

Figure 11-38. Typical I-125, Pd-103 or Cs-131 urethral doses with modified peripheral loading pattern, implanted by K Wallner in 2006.

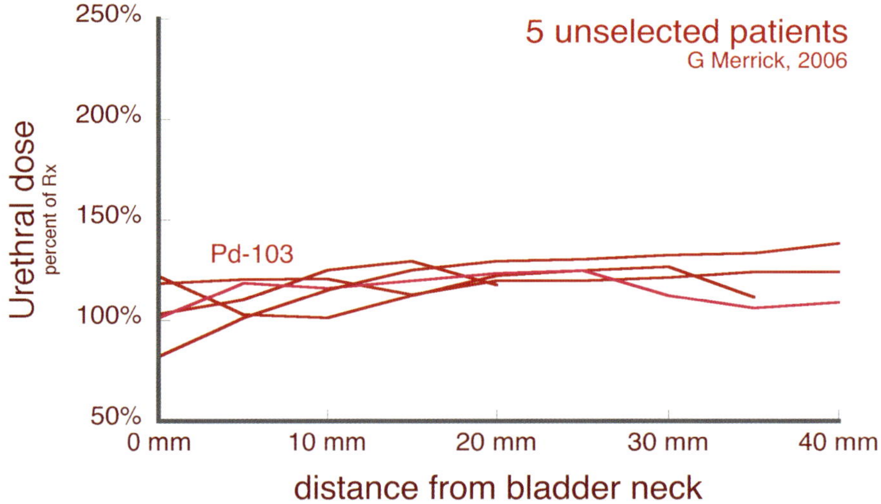

Figure 11-39. Typical Pd-103 urethral doses with modified peripheral loading pattern, implanted by G Merrick in 2006.

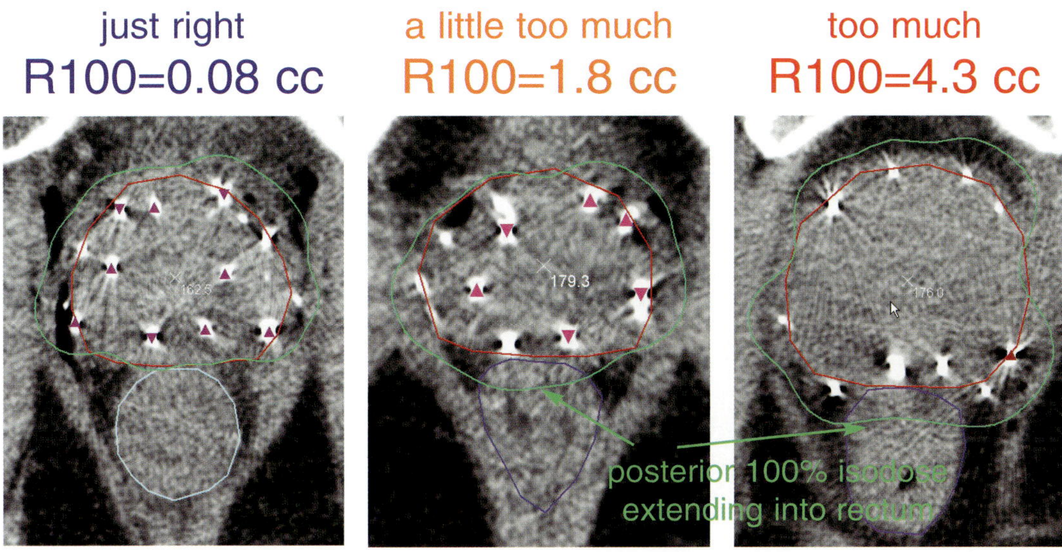

Figure 11-40. Examples of widely diffrerent R100s. The R100 for the patient on the left is 0.08 cc, a good thing as long as the posterior prostate is still covered. The R100 of 4.3 cc in the patient on the right is too high. If you are getting R100s of more than 1.0 cc on a regular basis, you need to stop and reconsider your technique.

uncommon. The bad news is that because they are uncommon, limited data exist regarding rectal tolerance doses. In some cases, the cause of a rectal complication is obvious—for example, when several seeds are placed in the rectal wall (see **Figure 11-8**). But most of the time, it's not so obvious why a particular patient develops a problem. To date, dosimetry has given only a partial answer.

Transverse isodose overlays show the potential for variability in rectal wall doses (**Figure 11-40**). A couple of mm difference in the how far the prescription isodose extends into the rectum makes a big differenece in the volume of rectum receiving a high radiation dose. Keep in mind that rectal doses may be artifactually increased by rectal filling (**Figure 11-41**).(MERRICK 00)

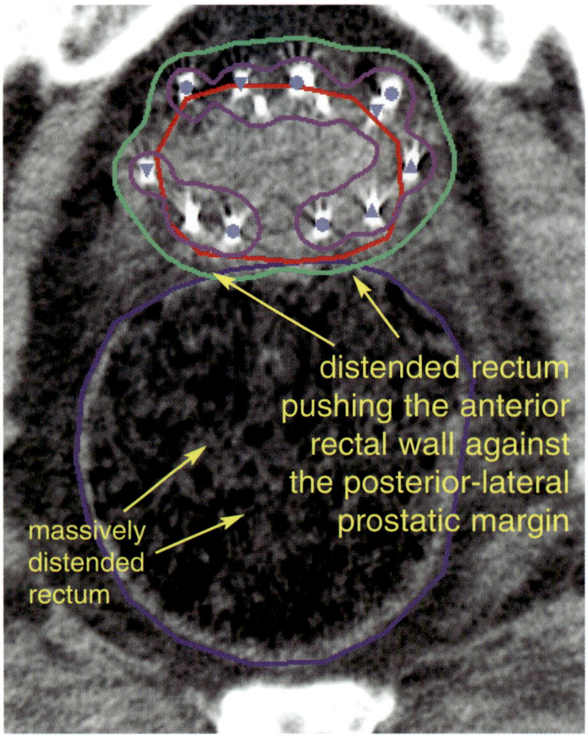

Figure 11-41. Rectal distension will push the anterior rectal wall against the prostate, falsely elevating the R100.

There are a variety of ways to quantify rectal doses. Mueller drew only the outer rectal wall, and considered the rectum as a solid structure. She used the dosimetric acronym *R100*, defined as the volume of rectum that receives the prescription dose or higher. Snyder made the process more complicated by drawing the inner and outer wall, and calculating the dose to the wall it itself.(SNYDER) The problem with trying to identify the inner wall is that it will change depending on the degree of rectal filling. In fact, Han and colleagues showed that rectal surface and volume doses are closely correlated and that all are predictive of implant-related proctitis (**Figure 11-43**).(HAN) So keep it simple. All of the examples shown in this book were calculated for an R100 identified only with the outer rectal wall identified, and the rectum considered as a solid structure.

Several investigators have correlated rectal wall doses with complications. There has been pretty good agreement that proctitis is unusual with an R100 of less than 1.0 cc (**Figure 11-44**).(SNYDER, WATERMAN, MUELLER)

While there is some statistical correlation between rectal doses and morbidity, any relationship seems loose, at best. Rectal complications are only

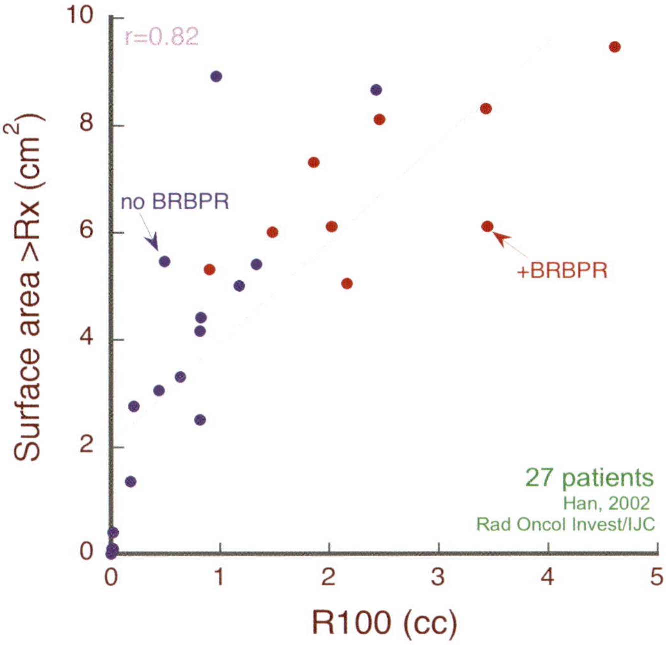

Figure 11-43. Scatter plots of rectal surface area versus rectal volume receiving greater than the prescription dose (R100). These parameters are closely related. So use what's simplest to quantify—the R100.

partially explained by higher doses—some patients who developed ulcerations did not appear to have excessive rectal wall doses, and most patients with higher doses did not suffer complications. Although rectal

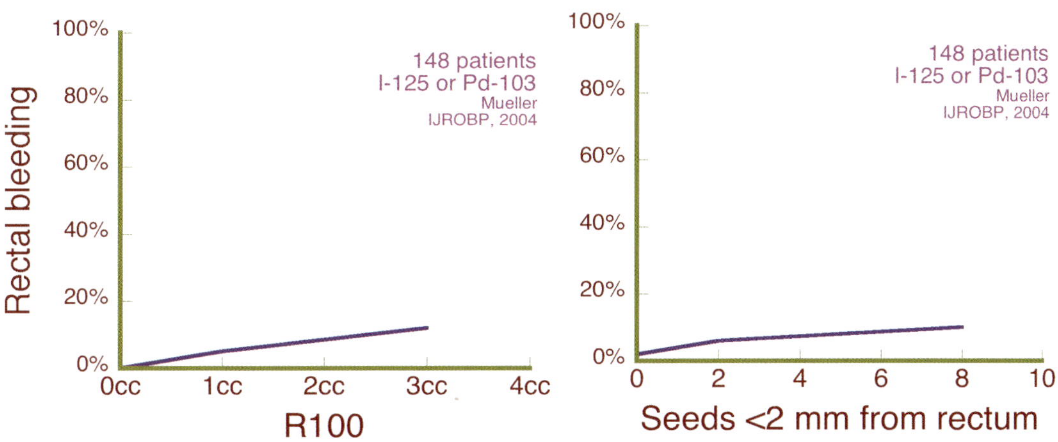

Figure 11-44. Incidence of rectal bleeding versus the volumes of rectum treated to prescription dose or higher (left) or the number of seeds 0–2 mm from the rectal wall (right).

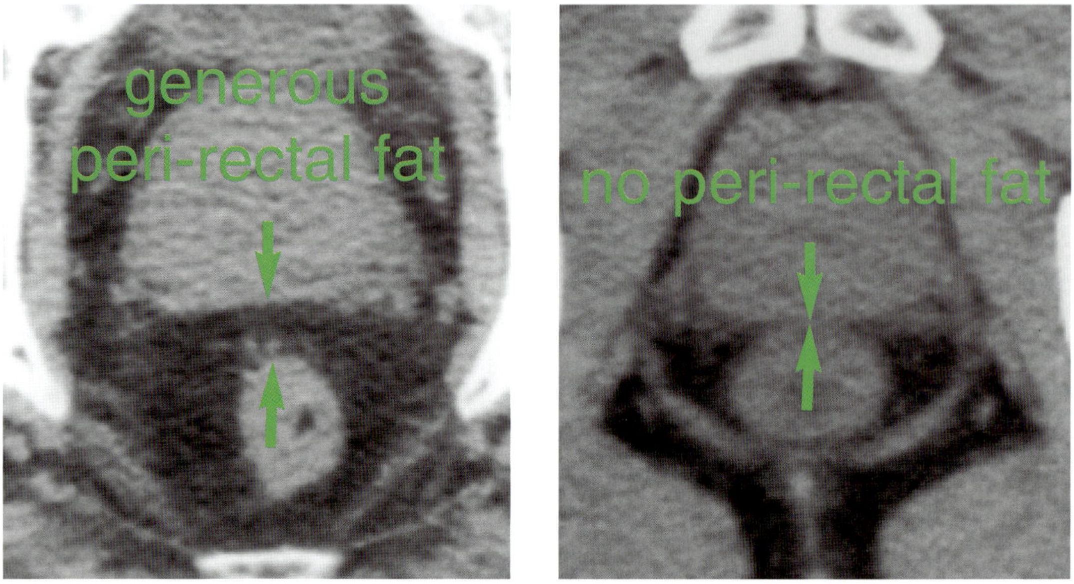

Figure 11-45. Patients with lesser degrees of perirectal fat are more likely to receive excessive rectal doses. Han and colleagues showed that patients like those on the right were more prone to develop post-implant proctitis. (HAN)

dose contributes to the likelihood of complications, it appears that some patients are predisposed to complications, perhaps by diabetes, smoking, genetic factors, or aberrant rectal wall blood supply. Han and colleagues showed that some patients may be predisposed to higher rectal doses due to a limited amount of perirectal fat, placing their rectum in closer proximity to the prostate (**Figure 11-45**). But remember, the prostatic apex always abuts the distal rectum, even in obese patients (see Chapter 21). High dose regions within the prostate do not appear to increase the risk of proctitis, provided that the rectal wall dose is not high.(HOWARD, TRAN)

Changes in rectal doses over the first few weeks may be a contributing factor to proctitis. The R100 typically increases by almost 1.0 cc from day 0 to day 30, as the prostate shrinks (**Figures 11-46 and 11-47**). Variability in this degree of R100 increase might partially explain why some patients develop proctitis while others don't despite similar R100s at one point in time.(REED 05, TAUSSKY)

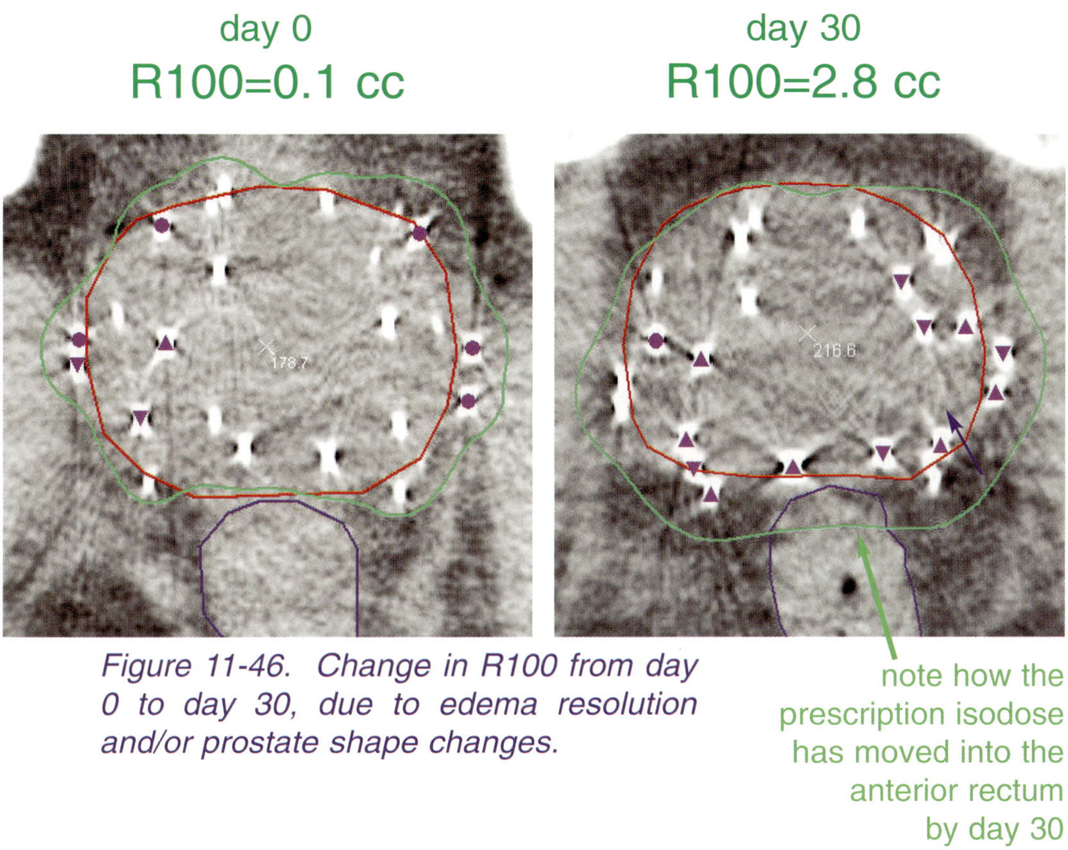

Figure 11-46. Change in R100 from day 0 to day 30, due to edema resolution and/or prostate shape changes.

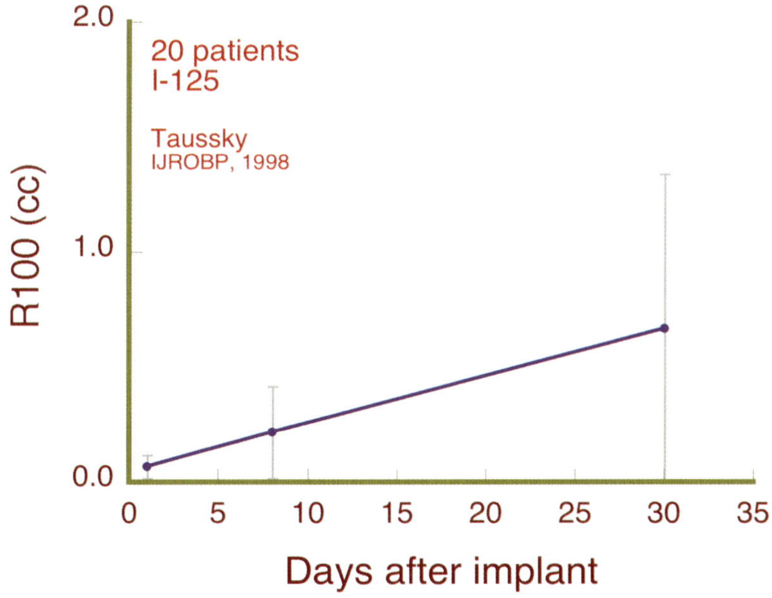

Figure 11-47. Changes in R100 over time.

DOSIMETRY POLICIES IN YOUR PRACTICE

It is a blessing that dosimetric calculations can help maximize cure rates and minimize complications. Prostate brachytherapy probably lends itself to meaningful quality assurance more than most of radiation therapy, for which actual dose delivery is typically not accurately quantified. And the price of prostate brachytherapy quality assurance is still small compared to the overall costs of care.

Adequate prostate coverage should be verified in every patient, as part of a meaningful quality assurance program. In the early part of your brachytherapy experience, it would be prudent to do extensive dosimetric analysis including urethral and rectal doses, to be sure that your implants meet generally acceptable guidelines in regards to the risk of complications. Once you're confident that urethral and rectal doses are being kept within acceptable limits while still achieving adequate prostate coverage, some streamlining could be considered. In contrast to target coverage, routine calculation of urethral doses in every patient is probably not necessary. Detailed dosimetric studies correlating dosimetry with urinary complications were valuable in helping to establish dosimetry guidelines. In current practice, however, serious urinary complications are very low, and it seems reasonable to limit routine dosimetric analysis. We limit our urethral dose calculations to patients enrolled in research trials, or the occasional patient who develops a serious complication, in which case doses are calculated at the time the complication is discovered—typically long after the implant procedure. On the other hand, it's probably still a good idea to routinely monitor rectal doses.

REFERENCES

1. Allen Z, Merrick G, Butler E, et al. Detailed urethral dosimetry in the evaluation of prostate brachytherapy-related urinary morbidity. Int J Rad Oncol Biol Phys 2005; 62:981-987.

2. Amdur RJ, Gladstone D, Leopold KA, Harris RD. Prostate seed implant quality assessment using MR and CT image fusion. Int J Radiat Oncol Biolo Phys 1999; 43:67-72.

3. Anderson LL. A "natural" volume-dose histogram for brachytherapy. Med Phys 1986; 13:898-903.

4. Badiozamani K, Wallner K, Sutlief S, Ellis W, Blasko J, Russell K. Anticipating prostatic volume changes due to prostate brachytherapy. Radiat Oncol Invest 1999; 7:360-364.

5. Chen Z, Yue N, Wang X, Roberts KB, Peschel R, Nath R. Dosimetric effects of edema in permanent prostate seed implants: A rigorous solution. Int J Rad Oncol Biol Phys 2000; 47:1405-1419.
6. Crook J, Milosevic M, Catton P, et al. Interobserver variation in postimplant computed tomography contouring affects quality assessment of prostate brachytherapy. Brachytherapy 2002; 1:66-73.
7. DeLaney TF, Shipley WU, O'Leary MP, Biggs PJ, Prout GR. Preoperative irradiation and 125-Iodine implantation for patients with localized carcinoma of the prostate. Int J Radiat Oncol Biol Phys 1986; 12:1779-1785.
8. Dubois FD, Prestidge BR, Hotchkiss LA, Bice WS, Prete JJ. Source localization following permanent transperineal prostate intersititial brachytherapy using magnetic resonance imaging. Int J Radiat Oncol Biol Phys 1997; 39:1037-1041.
9. Fuks Z, Leibel SA, Wallner KE, et al. The effect of local control on metastatic dissemination in carcinoma of the prostate: Long term results in patients treated with 125-I implantation. Int J Radiat Oncol Biol Phys 1991; 21:337-347.
10. Gong L, Cho P, Han B, et al. Registration of prostate brachytherapy seeds with prostate anatomy for postimplant dosimetry. Int J Rad Oncol Biol Phys 2002; 54:1322-1330.
11. Han B, Wallner K. Dosimetric and radiographic correlates to prostate brachytherapy-related rectal complications. International Journal of Cancer 2002; 96:372-378.
12. Han B, Wallner K, Merrick G, Badiozamani K, Butler W. The effect of inter-observer differences in post-implant prostate CT image interpretation on dosimetric parameters. Med Phys 2003; 30:1096-1104.
13. Han B, Wallner K, Merrick G, Butler W, Sutlief S, Sylvester J. Prostate brachytherapy seed identification on post-implant TRUS images. Med Phys 2003; 30:898-900.
14. Herstein A, Wallner K, Merrick G, et al. There is a wide range of predictive dosimetric factors for I-125 and Pd-103 prostate brachytherapy . Am J Clin Onc 2007; in press.
15. Howard A, Wallner K, Han B, Schneider B, al e. Clinical course and dosimetry of rectal fistulas after prostate brachytherapy. JBI 2001; 17:37-42.
16. Jones S, Wallner K, Merrick G, Cavanagh W, Butler W. Clinical correlates of high brachytherapy dose regions within the prostate. Int J Rad Oncol Biol Phys 2002; 53:328-333.

17. Keyes M, Pickles T, Agranovich A, Kwan W, Morris WJ. 125-I reimplantation in patients with poor innitial dosimetry after prostate brachytherapy. Int J Rad Oncol Biol Phys 2004; 60:40-50.
18. Kollmeier M, Stock RG, Stone NN. Biochemical outcomes after prostate brachytherapy with 5-year minimal follow-up: Importance of patient selection and implant quality. Int J Rad Oncol Biol Phys 2003; 57:645-653.
19. Lee WR, deGuzman AF, McMullen K, McCullough DL. Dosimetry and cancer congrol after low-dose-rate prostate brachytherapy. Int J Rad Oncol Biol Phys 2005; 61:52-59.
20. Lee WR, Roach M, Michalski J, Moran B, Beyer D. Interobserver variability in quantifiers of prostate implant adequacy. Int J Rad Oncol Biol Phys 2002; 54:457-461.
21. Ling CC, Roy J, Sahoo N, Wallner K, Anderson L. Quantifying the effect of dose inhomogeneity in brachytherapy: Application to permanent prostatic implant with 125-I seeds. Int J Rad Oncol Biol Phys 1994; 28:971-978.
22. Merrick G, Butler W, Dorsey A. The effect of constipation on rectal dosimetry following prostate brachytherapy. Med Dosim 2000; 25:237-241.
23. Merrick GS, Butler WM. Modified uniform seed loading for prostate brachytherapy: rationale, design, and evaluation. Techniques in Urology 2000; 6:78-84.
24. Merrick GS, Butler WM, Dorsey AT, Lief JH. Potential role of various dosimetric quality indicators in prostate brachytherapy. Int J Rad Oncol Biol Phys 1999; 44:717-724.
25. Merrick GS, Butler WM, Dorsey AT, Lief JH. The dependence of prostate postimplant dosimetric quality on CT volume determination. Int J Rad Oncol Biol Phys 1999; 44:1111-1117.
26. Merrick GS, Butler WM, Dorsey AT, Walbert HL. Influence of timing on the dosimetric analysis of transperineal ultrasound-guided, prostatic conformal brachytherapy. Radiat Oncol Invest 1998; 6:182-190.
27. Moerland MA, Wijrdeman HK, Beersma R, Bakker CJG. Evaluation of permanent I-125 prostate implants using radiography and magnetic resonance imaging. Int J Radiat Oncol Biol Phys 1997; 37:927-933.
28. Mueller A, Wallner K, Merrick G, Cavanagh W, Butler W. Peri-rectal seeds as a risk factor for prostate brachytherapy-related rectal bleeding. Int J Rad Oncol Biol Phys 2004; 59:1047-1052.
29. Orio P, Wallner K, Merrick G, et al. Dosimetric parameters as predictive factors for biochemical control in patients with higher risk prostate

cancer treated with Pd-103 and supplemental beam radiation. Int J Rad Oncol Biol Phys 2007; 67:342-346.
30. Papagikos M, deGuzman AF, Rossi P, CMcCullough D, Clark P, Lee WR. Dosimetric quantifiers for low-dose-rate prostate brachytherapy: Is V100 superior to D90? Brachytherapy 2005; 4:252-258.
31. Potters L, Cao Y, Calugaru E, Torre T, Fearn P, Wang X. A comprehensive review of CT-based dosimetry parameters and biochemical control in patients treated with permanent prostate brachytherapy. Int J Rad Oncol Biol Phys 2001; 50:605-614.
32. Prestidge BR, Bice WS, Kiefer EJ, Prete JJ. Timing of computed tomography-based postimplant assessment following permanent transperineal prostate brachytherapy. Int J Radiat Oncol Biolo Phys 1998; 40:1111-1115.
33. Reddy EK, Krishnan L, Mebust WK, Weigel JW. External beam radiation vs Iodine-125 implantation in localized prostatic cancer. Endocurie/Hyper Oncol 1991; 7:179-183.
34. Reed D, Wallner K, Ford E, et al. Effect of post-implant edema on prostate brachytherapy treatment margins. Int J Rad Oncol Biol Phys 2005; 63:1469-1473.
35. Reed D, Wallner K, Narayanan S, Sutlief S, Ford E, Cho P. Intraoperative fluoroscopic dose assessment in prostate brachytherapy patients. Int J Rad Oncol Biol Phys 2005; 63:301-307.
36. Roy JN, Wallner KE, Chiu-Tsao S, Anderson LL, Ling CC. CT-based optimized planning for transperineal prostate implant with customized template. Int J Radiat Oncol Biol Phys 1991; 21:483-489.
37. Roy JN, Wallner KE, Harrington PJ, Ling CC, Anderson LL. A CT-based evaluation method for permanent implants: Application to prostate. Int J Radiat Oncol Biol Phys 1993; 26:163-169.
38. Scheidler J, Hricak H, Vigneron DB, et al. Prostate cancer: Localization with three-dimensional proton MR spectroscopy imaging*clinicopathologic study. Radiol 1999; 213:473-480.
39. Snyder KM, Stock RG, Hong SM, Lo YC, Stone NN. Defining the risk of developing grade 2 proctitis following 125-I prostate brachytherapy using a rectal dose-volume histogram analysis. Int J Rad Oncol Biol Phys 2001; 50:335-341.
40. Stock RG, Stone NN, Dahlal M, Lo YC. What is the optimal dose for 125-I prostate implant? A dose-response analysis of biochemical control, posttreatment prostate biopsies, and long-term symptoms. Brachytherapy 2002; 1:83-89.

41. Stock RG, Stone NN, Kao J, Ianuzzi C, Unger P. The effect of disease and treatment-related factors on biopsy results after prostate brachytherapy. Cancer 2000; 89:1829-1834.

42. Taussky D, Yeung I, Williams T, et al. Rectal-wall dose dependence on postplan timing after permanent-seed prostate brachytherapy. Int J Rad Oncol Biol Phys 2006; 65:358-363.

43. Tran A, Wallner K, Merrick G, Seeberger J, Armstrong J, Mueller A. Rectal fistulas following prostate brachytherapy. Int J Rad Oncol Biol Phys 2005; 63:150-154.

44. Vicini FA, Kestin LL, Martinez AA. The importance of adequate follow-up in defining treatment success after external beam irradiation for prostate cancer. Int J Rad Oncol Biol Phys 1999; 45:553-561.

45. Waehre H, Amellem O, Stenwig AE, et al. Deoxyribonucleic acid cytometry and histological findings before and after 125-Iodine implantation of primary prostate cancer. J Urol 1992; 148:838-842.

46. Wallner K, Merrick G, Sutlief S, True L, Butler E. High-dose regions versus likelihood of cure after prostate brachytherapy. Int J Rad Oncol Biol Phys 2005; 62:170-174.

47. Wallner K, Merrick G, True L, Sutlief S, Cavanagh W, Butler W. I-125 versus Pd-103 for low risk prostate cancer: Preliminary biochemical outcomes from a prospective randomized mulitcenter trial. Int J Rad Oncol Biol Phys 2003; 57:1297-1303.

48. Wallner KE, Roy J, Harrison L. Dosimetry guidelines to minimize urethral and rectal morbidity following transperineal I-125 prostate brachytherapy. Int J Radiat Oncol Biol Phys 1995; 32:465-471.

49. Waterman FM, Dicker AP. Determination of the urethral dose in prostate brachytherapy when the urethra cannot be visualized in the postimplant CT scan. Med Phys 2000; 27:448-451.

50. Waterman FM, Dicker AP. Impact of postimplant edema on V100 and D90 in prostate brachytherapy: can implant quality be predicted on day 0? Int J Rad Oncol Biol Phys 2002; 53:610-621.

51. Waterman FM, Dicker AP. Probability of late rectal morbidity in I-125 prostate brachytherapy. Int J Rad Oncol Biol Phys 2003; 55:342-353.

52. Willins J, Wallner K. CT-based dosimetry for transperineal I-125 prostate brachytherapy. Int J Rad Oncol Biol Phys 1997; 39:347-353.

53. Willins J, Wallner KE. Time-dependent changes in CT-based dosimetry of I-125 prostate brachytherapy. Radiat Oncol Invest 1998; 6:157-160.

54. WM B, Merrick G, Dorsey A, Lief JH. Isotope choice and the effect of edema on prostate brachytherapy dosimetry. Med Phys 2000; 27:1067-1075.

12

Post-operative care

One of the major advantages of brachytherapy is that peri-operative care is relatively simple. Serious complications or hospital readmissions after brachytherapy are very infrequent.(HAN) However, patients typically experience marked urinary and rectal symptoms and need ready access to medical advice, even if only by phone.

There is a wide range of acceptable ways to manage patients post-operatively, with little data to support one approach over another. The pages ahead mostly summarize our own experience and biases.

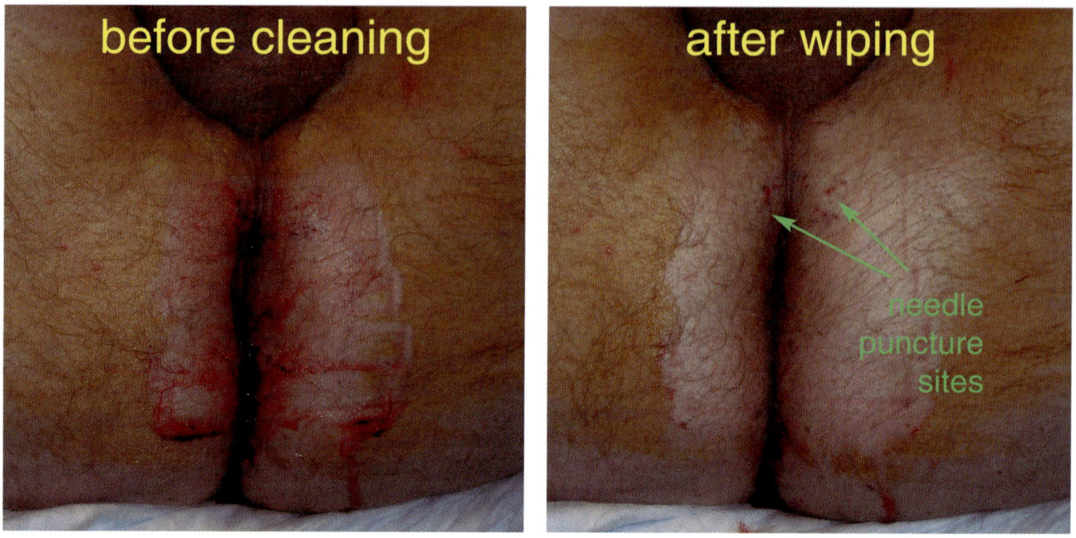

Figure 12-1. Perineal skin immediately after procedure. Application of a dressing is impractical. Infections are almost unheard of.

SKIN CARE

After withdrawing the last needle, the perineum should be cleaned with a damp cloth (**Figure 12-1**). Any additional skin care is of questionable value. Povidine-iodine solutions or other cleansing agents are better saved for the OR staff than the patient. The benefit of post-implant perineal icepacks is questionable. Application of a perineal dressing is impractical. Patients are instructed to shower with soap after returning home, several hours after the implant. Implant-related perineal infection is almost unheard of.

CATHETER REMOVAL

A urinary catheter is commonly used for the implant procedure. There is no known relation between catheter removal time and the risk of post-implant urinary retention. Blasko, Merrick and Wallner advocate catheter removal upon completion of the procedure. M. Dattoli prefers to keep it in overnight, a policy that prevent re-catheterization in some patients who would otherwise need it.

Patient who have not urinated within six hours of catheter removal will likely need to to be re-catheterized. Re-catheterization should be individualized, depending on the patient's level of discomfort.

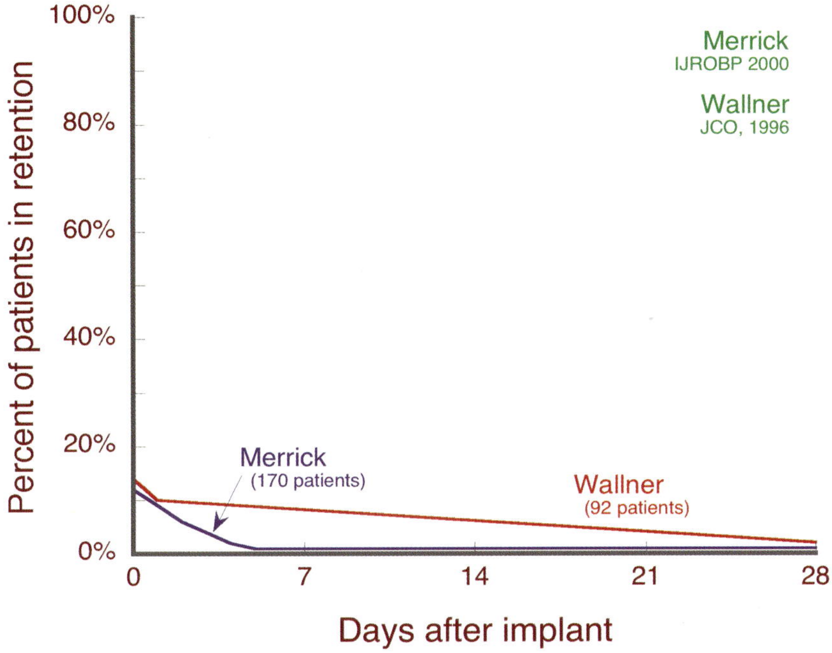

Figure 12-2. Resolution of retention after I-125 or Pd-103 implantation. Most patient were managed with intermittent catheterization or an indwelling catheter with intermittent voiding trials. In patients who develop retention, we prefer to proceed right away to intermittent self-catheterization, rather than use an indwelling catheter.(WALLNER 96, MERRICK 00)

GOING HOME

Patients are typically sent home after recovery from anesthesia. They are usually asked to stay within a one-hour drive of the hospital for the first day afterwards, unless arrangements can be made to be seen in a local emergency room if an acute problem develops. If a patient lives more than an hour away, it is probably best that they stay in a hotel close to the hospital.

URINARY RETENTION

Urinary retention is the most common acute implant-related complication and is almost impossible to predict for a given patient (see chapter 12). Fortunately, it typically resolves rapidly (**Figure 12-2**). Prophylactic alpha

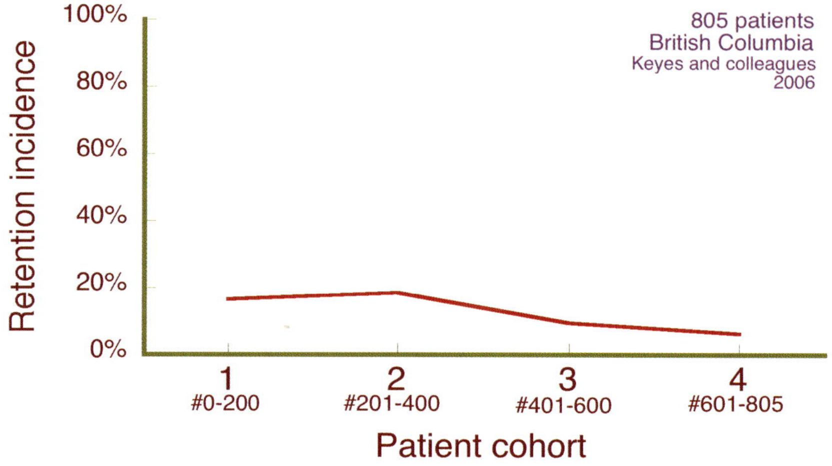

Figure 12-3. Incidence of acute urinary retention with increasing experience.(KEYES)

blockers do not appear to decrease the need for short-term catheterization.(MERRICK, ELSHAIKH)

Post-implant retention usually resolves spontaneously within twenty-four hours. Patients who still cannot urinate by the second post-implant day will need longer catheterization. How you manage prolonged retention in these less fortunate patients can make a big difference in their post-implant experience. A better option than reinserting an indwelling catheter is to instruct patients in self-catheterization—those patients willing to give it a try generally prefer it over an indwelling catheter. Intermittent catheterization avoids the irritation of the constant presence of a catheter, and allows a more normal lifestyle. It also allows patients to urinate spontaneously as they improve, rather than waiting for a voiding trial. Considering that most patients do well with intermittent self-catheterization, a suprapubic catheter should be reserved only for those who cannot or will not self-catheterize and can't tolerate an indwelling catheter.

Nearly all cases of post-implant retention resolve spontaneously within a few days of implantation. Surgical intervention, including transurethral resection or incision of the prostate (TURP or TUIP) or a suprapubic catheter, should be avoided in favor of longer term intermittent self-

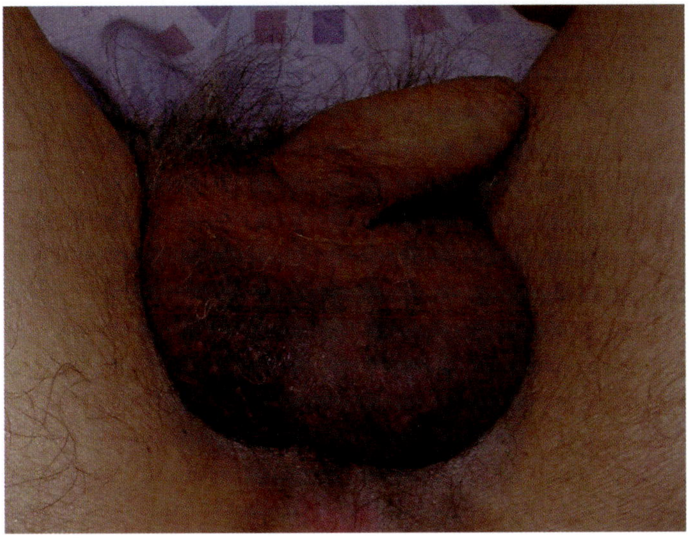

Figure 12-4. Scrotal bruising 10 days after an implant procedure.

catheterization or indwelling Foley catheter (see chapter 15).(HU, LANDIS, MERRICK 04)

In the authors' experience, the likelihood of retention has diminished substantially over the past ten years, a finding borne out by other groups (**Figure 12-3**).(KEYES) The explanation for the decrease is unclear, and is likely multi-factorial. Post-implant retention is a rarity after brachytherapy under local anesthesia (K Wallner, unpublished data).

HEMATURIA

Most patients have a minor degree of post-implant gross hematuria, lasting for one to 14 days. Occasional patients will pass clots for a longer time. The amount of bleeding is usually minimal, but patients occasionally pass larger amounts, possibly from a urethral tear or minor bladder injury. When that happens, a Foley catheter can be placed and irrigated until clear. Hemodynamically significant post-implant bleeding is rare. Catheter placement usually tamponades and stops the bleeding immediately. We typically leave the catheter in for three days. Diagnostic cystoscopy or surgical intervention is usually unnecessary.

DYSURIA IN THE FIRST POST-OPERATIVE WEEK

Patients typically experience substantial dysuria in the immediate post-operative period, presumably due to needle-related trauma. This initial dysuria subsides substantially within 24 hours. Taking nonsteroidal anti-inflammatory drugs (NSAID) for several hours after implantation can help with acute discomfort. Bleeding problems, even with immediate use of NSAIDs, are rare. Narcotics generally do not help to alleviate the acute dysuria. Prophylactic alpha-1 blockers are routinely prescribed by some brachytherapists, and may prevent dysuria.(MERRICK)

Patients are instructed not to drink extra fluids during the first few hours following implantation, because it can exacerbate their already troublesome urinary problems. They should start drinking extra fluids the morning *after* the implant, and continue doing so for three days, possibly decreasing the likelihood of a urinary infection.

SCROTAL BRUISING
Patients commonly develop scrotal and perineal bruising several days after the procedure. (**Figure 12-4**). It resolves spontaneously, but it should be mentioned beforehand because its unexpected appearance can be disconcerting.

INFECTION
Peri-operative urinary infections are unusual, regardless of whether antibiotics are used (see chapter 7).(WALLNER 96, DICKER) Late infections occur occasionally, and should be treated appropriately. Epididymitis occurs in approximately 1% of patients, at variable times after implantation.(HOFFELT)

PAIN
Post-operative pain (apart from dysuria) is usually limited to minor perineal discomfort. More significant post-operative pain is unusual. Narcotic analgesics should not be routinely prescribed. Patients who experience pain requiring narcotics should be carefully assessed for an unusual circumstance.

URINARY BLEEDING
Microscopic hematuria is commonly noted in routine urinalyses, but has not been rigoruosly characterized. It is important to recognize brachytherapy as a possible cause so as to avoid unwarranted work-ups. Clinically apparent gross hematuria occurs months to years following implantation in approximately 10% of patients.(BARKER) It is nearly always self-limited, but may persist for weeks or months, usually intermittently. Cystoscopic exam usually reveals a pale prostatic urethra, typically with scattered telangiectasias, which are presumably the source of bleeding. Cauterization, lasering or resection are rarely needed, and could make the situation worse.

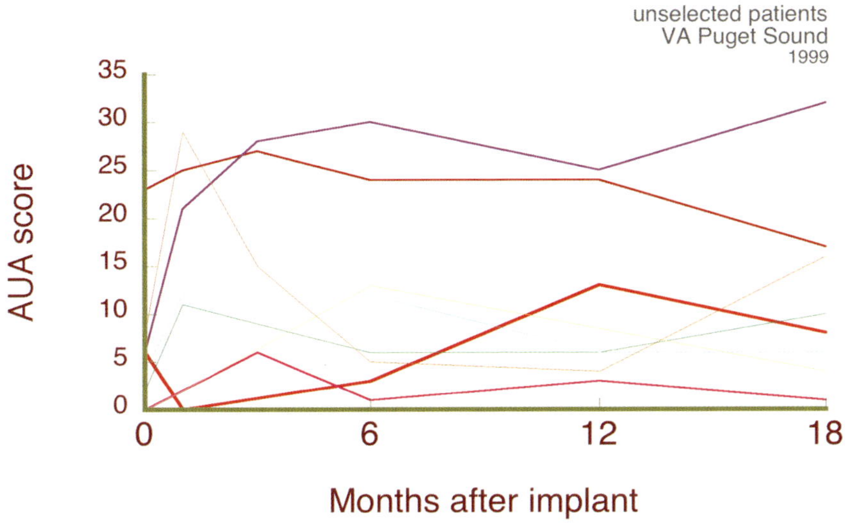

Figure 12-5. Post-implant AUA scores in different patients. Patients vary tremendously in how quickly their symptoms resolve—be flexible in regard to alpha-blocker use. Many patients don't need them at all, while others need higher doses for extended periods of time.

Late bleeding can be distressing for patients, and is the cause for frantic calls to the physician. Because it occurs late, it's relationship to brachytherapy is often not recognized initially. A work-up to rule out other causes may be justified.

If and when to pursue a work-up for other causes of post-implant hematuria is a source of consternation. We generally do not vestigate microscopic hematuria, assuming it to be related to early or late radiation prostatitis. Even in the absence of brachytherapy, the need to investigate microscopic hematuria is a subject of debate.(RODGERS)

We generally do no pursue an aggressive work-up for gross hematuria, unless it persists for longer than three months. If so, preliminary testing with IVP, CT and urinary cytology seems reasonable, although the accuracy of all three tests is open to some question.(RODGERS) If we are con-

Dysuria

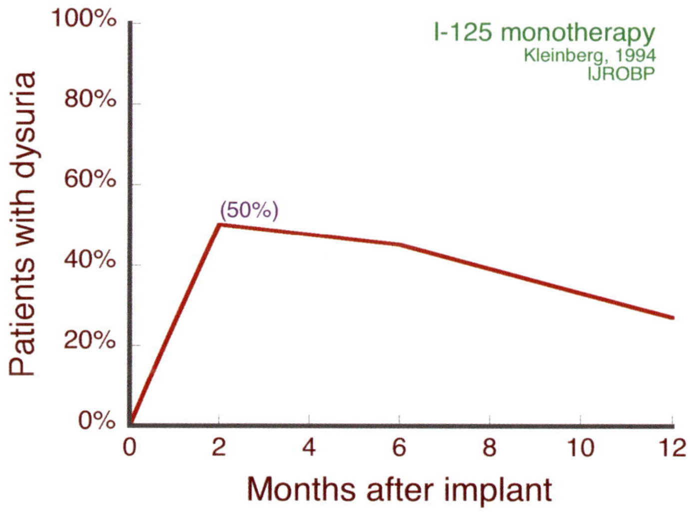

Figure 12-6. Average dysuria and AUA scores in the post-implant period.
(KLEINBERG, GELBLUM)

AUA scores

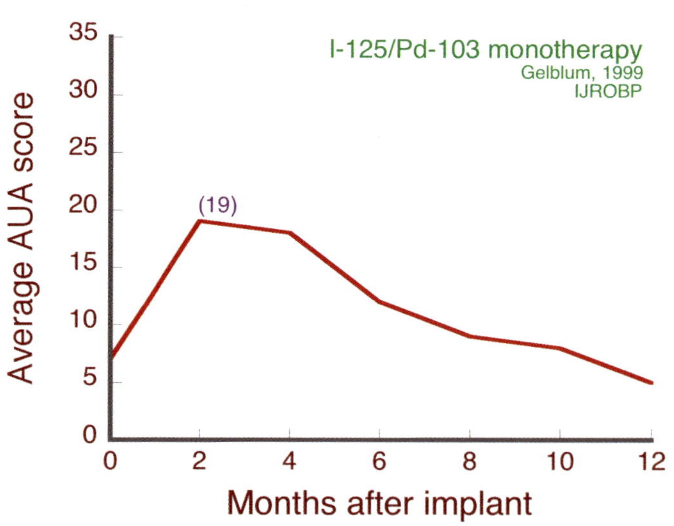

Table 12-1. Alpha blockers.

Generic	Brand	Tablet strength	Approximate Cost/tablet
doxazosin	Cardura™	1, 2, 4, 8 mg	$1.10
tamsulosin	Flomax™	0.4 mg	$1.40
terazosin	Hytrin™	1, 2, 5, 10 mg	$1.10
allfuzosin	Uroxatral	10 mg	$1.40

cerned about excessive implant-related hematuria or wish to rule out other causes, cystoscopic evaluation may be needed.(KHADRA)

URINARY SYMPTOMS AFTER THE FIRST WEEK

Nearly all patients develop symptoms of radiation prostatitis, including dysuria, daytime frequency, nocturia, and urgency (**Figures 12-5 and 12-6**). Radiation-related symptoms generally start one to two weeks following implantation, and are due to *urethral* inflammation, not to *cystitis*. At least half of patients report dysuria, typically with a severity of 3–4 on a 0–10 scale.(MERRICK)

If no medications are routinely prescribed, about half of patients do not have severe enough urinary symptoms to request medication.(WALLNER 96) The other half are symptomatic enough to prefer treatment. Selective alpha-1 adrenergic blockers are by far the most effective treatment for radiation prostatitis (**Table 12-1**). Terazocin (Hytrin™), doxazosin (Cardura™), or tamsulosin (Flomax™) are remarkably effective in relieving radiation-related obstructive symptoms, usually within an hour or two of ingestion.(CRAWFORD)

It was surprising to us that the only randomized trial testing the use of alpha blockers in the post-implant setting showed only modest benefit.(ELSHAIKH) The relatively small benefit of alpha-blockers after brachytherapy reported by Elshaikh and colleagues is far less than reported in retrospective studies, and should be clarified in another prospective, randomized trial.

Table 12-2. Varous remedies that are worth a try for patients with difficult-to-control dysuria.

<u>Alpha blockers</u>

doxazosin (Cardura)
tamsulosin (Flomax)
terazosin (Hytrin)
allfuzosin (Uroxatral)
dibenzyline

<u>phenozopyridine concoctions</u>

Azo-standard	Uricalm
Baridium	Urodine
Eridium	Urogesic
Geridium	Viridium
Pyridium	

<u>Anti-spasmodics (anticholinergics)</u>

Ditropan	Enablex
Detrol	Oxytrol
Vesicare	Sanctura

<u>NSAIDs</u>

ibuprofen
celebrex
meloxicam (Mobic)

<u>Misc</u>

pentoson polysulfate/Elmiron (for interstitial cystitis)
Prosed (for just about everything!)
K citrate/Urocit-K (alkinizing agent)
pentoxyphyline/Trental

Four alpha blockers are currently FDA-approved for relief of urinary obstructive symptoms. The older agents—doxazosin and terazosin—are most frequently associated with bothersome vasodilation, including dizziness and orthostatic hypotension.(DJAVAN) Newer, more selective alpha blockers include tamsulosin (Flomax™) and alfuzosin (Uroxatral™). Both agents are similarly effective against urinary obstructive symptoms as older agents, and are less likely to cause orthostatic hypotension.(ref) Another advantage of the newer, more selective blockers is that they do not need to be titrated upward with initial use. In patients who have trouble with all standard alpha-blockers, a trial of an older blocker, dibenzyline, might be considered (M Dattoli).

The usual starting dose for terazocin or doxazosin is 1 or 2 mg at night, and 0.4 mg for tamsulosin. There is a risk of hypotension, especially when first starting alpha blockers. Hypotensive episodes are probably more likely in older, thin patients, but patients should be warned about this when first starting the medication.

Some patients do well taking the drugs once daily. Although all four drugs are said to have twenty-four-hour action, patients often do better if they take two or more daily doses. In general, the total daily dose of prazosin or terazosin should be kept below 10 mg; above that, patients commonly experience fatigue. The authors have prescribed up to six Flomax™ (2.4 mg total) daily with few side effects.

Although the newer alpha-blockers appear to have similar efficacy, there is increasing appreciation of their particular side effects. It is now widely appreciated that tamsulosin causes retrograde ejaculation in 5-10% of patients, an effect that may lead to drug discontinuation.(ref) Alfuzosin appears have less adverse sexual effects, and may actually improve sexual function in patients with coexisting BPH.(NICKEL)

In addition to alpha blockers, anticholinergics are often helpful with radiation-related urinary symptoms.(RUGGIERi) Despite the classic teaching that anticholinergics (**Table 12-2**) are useful only for spasm, it is difficult to predict from clinical history whether anticholinergics will help brachytherapy patients. Combining or substituting alpha blockers and anticholinergics is best done on a trial basis for patients who get insufficient relief from an alpha-blocker alone.

Recalcitrant symptoms

While most patients tolerate post-implant radiation prostatitis with little or minor medical intervention, a minority will be substantially bothered despite maximal institution of the usual medications. For these "problem patients" there is a dizzying array of potential remedies, some more drastic than oth-

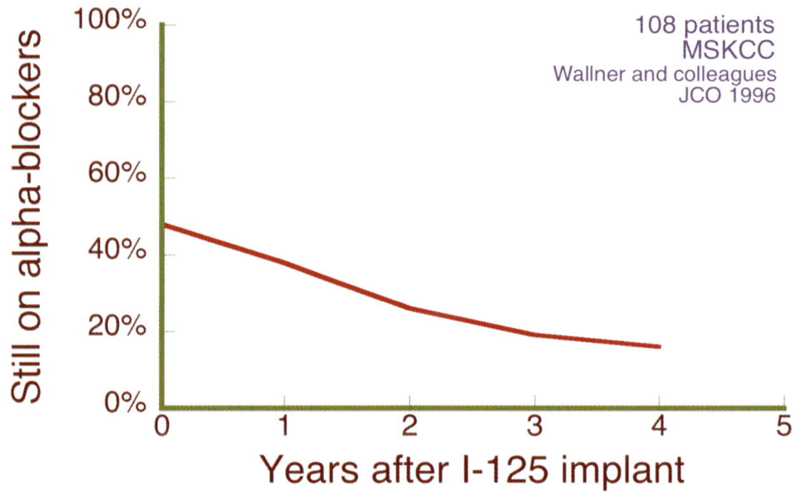

Figure 12-7. Percentage of patient still using alpha-blockers after I-125 implantation.(WALLNER 96)

ers (**Table 12-2**). We have been amazed at the hit or miss response to these various remedies. But we have also been impressed that one or more will occasionally be miraculously effective for a given patient. We can't always make sense of what works, but they're worth a try. Narcotics are not a good idea; they seldom work well for radiation prostatitis and they carry the potential for psychological dependence.

Think long-term

Radiation prostatitis typically begins to remit within several months of implantation, and at some point most patients stop their alpha-blockers (**Figures 12-7**). Patients can try decreasing their medication for one or two days. If symptoms of radiation prostatitis persist, alpha-blockers can be restarted and stopped again in a month or two. There is much variability among patients in their time to resolution of radiation-related symptoms and in their response to medication, so that patients and physicians should be flexible regarding the way that mediations are taken. To keep things in perspective regarding the 20% of patients still using alpha-blockers at one year, keep in mind that many men in the prostate cancer age range are on alpha-blockers even without having had an implant.

It is fairly common for patients to have an exacerbation of their prostatitis symptoms 6 to 12 months after implantation, about the same time they frequently experience a temporary rise ("spike") in their PSA (see chapter 13). The mechanism for these temporary symptom exacerbations is unknown, but temporary reinstitution of alpha-blockers may be called for. While late urinary infections are distinctly uncommon, urine cultures should be done as clinically indicated.

PHYSICAL ACTIVITY

Patients are instructed to avoid strenuous physical activity for one to two days following implantation. After that, all restrictions are lifted. This policy seems prudent in the post-anesthesia setting, with some possibility of bleeding. Having said that, however, many patients have ignored our advice to limit their activity and we have rarely seen any problem related to vigorous activity in the peri-operative period.

Physical activity generally alleviates urinary obstructive symptoms, the mechanism of which is unclear.(ORSINI) Regular exercise should be encouraged as part of the treatment for post-implant obstructive urinary symptoms (and for other good reasons as well). Some patients experience discomfort with perineal pressure, and avoid activities like bicycling. The authors are unaware, however, of any adverse effects from perineal pressure.

DIETARY CHANGES

Despite innumerable recommendations in physicians' recommendations to patients, there is no documented benefit to dietary changes in the post-implant period. Avoidance of caffeine and alcohol might help.

SEXUAL ACTIVITY

There is no published information regarding ill effects from sexual activity in the post-implant period. Surprisingly, some patients engage in sex the night of the implant, and we're unaware of any problems with that apart from some discomfort with ejaculation (see chapter 16).

Theoretically, one or more seeds could be passed with the ejaculate, although this is apparently very rare. It may be prudent to recommend condom use for four months after I-125 and one month after Pd-103.

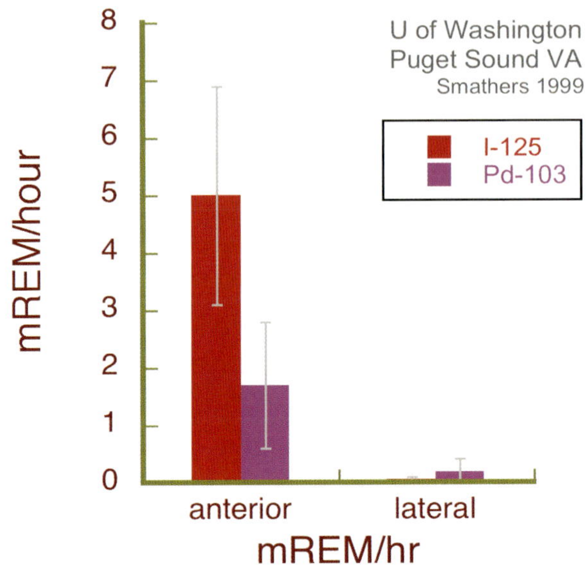

Figure 12-8. Exposure rates at the anterior and lateral skin surfaces with I-125 versus Pd-103.(SMATHERS)

RECTAL BLEEDING

Patients may have some bright red blood per rectum in the immediate post-operative period, presumably due to inadvertent piercing of the rectal mucosa or to procedure-related hemorrhoidal exacerbation. Bleeding due to radiation itself is very unlikely in the first six post-implant months (see chapter 15).

RADIATION PROTECTION

Implants generate little radiation detectable at the skin surface. The dose rate at the skin surface immediately following a full dose I-125 implant is approximately 2–10 mR/hour. The typical exposure at skin surface with full dose Pd-103 implant is 1–5 mR/hour. There is no data regarding the risk to humans from such low exposure rates. Extrapolating from much higher dose rates, regulations have been advanced limiting the total annual dose to 100 mREM for the general public. Accordingly, the *safe* total exposure time at the anterior skin surface would be approximately 20 hours for I-125 and 50 hours for Pd-103 (**Figures 12-8 & 12-9**). Of course, the "safe" exposure times would increase with each radionuclide half-life that passes.

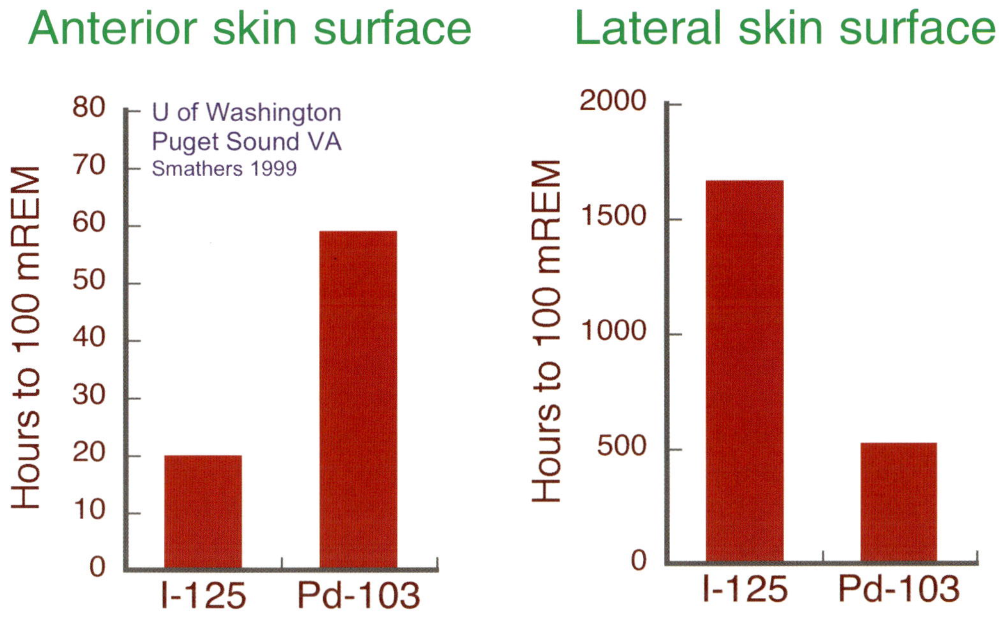

Figure 12-9. Approximate exposure times at anterior and lateral skin surfaces needed to reach NRC annual limits for the general public (100 mrem).(SMATHERS)

Lead underwear (*Radiation Guard*)

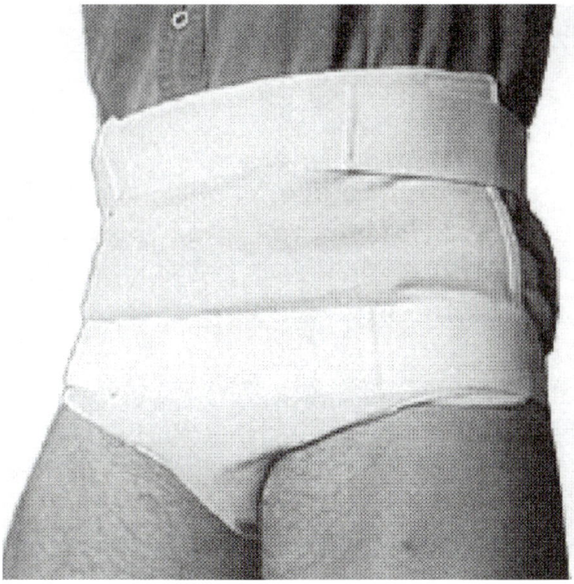

Figure 12-10. Lead-lined shield, worn over underwear, will stop more than 95% of I-125 emissions and 99% of Pd-103 emissions (Atlantic Nuclear, Canton, MA, 800-878-9118).

Exposure to others can be decreased with increased distance from the patient. The exposure at one meter from the pelvic skin surface is virtually undetectable with a conventional clinical ionization chamber. Exposure to others can be almost eliminated by wearing a lead apron fabricated from lead-lined sheeting or purchased from a radiology supply company (**Figure 12-10**).

PSA DETERMINATIONS

The proper timetable for post-implant PSA determinations is still unclear. Until recently, it was common to get the first follow-up PSA one month after the procedure. However, PSA values taken before two years will not be used to make a clinical decision, because readings commonly rise between one and two years, and then fall again (see chapter 13). Even when PSA rises occur, a follow-up biopsy would not be recommended until two years, because of the high rate of false positives before that time (see chapter 13). A reasonable compromise between patients' desire for information about their course and the fact that early PSAs usually don't mean much is to get PSAs every six months for the first two years, and annually thereafter. If the PSA is greater than 1.0 ng/ml at the two-year mark and is not falling, a repeat prostate biopsy should be considered, providing the patient is a potential candidate for salvage therapy.

Patients with markedly elevated pre-treatment PSA or elevated prostatic acid phosphatase should probably be monitored at six-month intervals from the day of implantation, because they are at higher risk of having metastatic disease. A rapidly rising PSA would be an indication to obtain a bone scan to look for possible bone metastases, which may warrant early hormonal ablation.

IT'S USUALLY EASY

In general, there is minimal need for physician intervention in the post-operative period. Problems that do occur typically can be managed over the telephone. Low-tech interventions such as listening, providing explanations and reassurance, and the liberal use of alpha-blockers are generally all that is needed. Surgical intervention is rarely required. Tincture of time is the best remedy for nearly all implant-related problems. It's important, however, that patients have easy access to a physician or nurse clinician for advice in coping with post-implant symptoms. **Second and third opinions should be sought before proceeding with any surgical intervention for seemingly intractable implant-related problems.**

REFERENCES

1. Barker J, Wallner K, Merrick G. Gross hematuria after prostate brachytherapy. Urol 2003; 61:408-411.
2. Crawford E, Kavanagh B. The role of alpha-blockers in the management of lower urinary tract symptoms in prostate cancer patients treated with radiotherapy. Am J Clin Onc 2006; 29:517-523.
3. Dicker AP, Figura AT, Waterman FM, al e. Is there a role for antibiotic prophylaxis in transperineal interstitial permanent prostate brachytherapy? Techniques in Urology 2000; 6:104-108.
4. Djavan B, Chapple C, Milani S, Marberger M. State of the art on the efficacy and tolerability of alpha1-adrenoceptor antagonists in patients with lower urinary tract symptoms suggestive of benign prostatic hyperplasia. Urology 2004; 64:1081-1088.
5. Elshaikh M, Ulchaker J, Reddy C, et al. Prophylactic tamsulosin (Flomax) in patients undergoing prostate I-125 brachytherapy for prostate carcinoma: Final report of a double-blind placebo-controlled randomized study. Int J Rad Oncol Biol Phys 2005; 62:164-169.
6. Gelblum DY, Potters L, Ashley R, Waldbaum R, Wang X, Leibel S. Urinary morbidity following ultrasound-guided transperineal prostate seed implantation. Int J Rad Oncol Biol Phys 1999; 45:59-67.
7. Han BH, Demel KC, Wallner KE, Young L. Patient reported short-term complications after prostate brachytherapy. J Urol 2001; (in press).
8. Hoffelt S, Wallner K, Merrick G. Epididymitis after prostate brachytherapy. Urol 2004; 63:293-296.
9. Hu K, Wallner KE. Urinary incontinence in patients who have a TURP/TUIP following prostate brachytherapy. Int J Radiat Oncol Biol Phys 1998; 40:783-786.
10. Keyes M, Schellenberg D, Moravan V, et al. Decline in urinary retention incidence in 805 patients after prostate brachytherapy: The effect of learning curve? Int J Rad Oncol Biol Phys 2006; 64:825-834.
11. Khadra MH, Pickard RS, Charlton M, Powell PH, Neal DE. A prospective analysis of 1,930 patients with hematuria to evaluate current diagnostic practice. J Urol 2000; 163:524-527.
12. Kleinberg L, Wallner K, Roy J, et al. Treatment-related symptoms during the first year following transperineal I-125 prostate implantation. Int J Radiat Oncol Biol Phys 1994; 28:985.
13. Landis D, Wallner K, Locke J, et al. Late urinary morbidity after prostate brachytherapy. Brachytherapy 2002; 1:21-26.

14. Merrick G, Butler W, Wallner K, Galbreath R. Effect of transurethral resection on urinary quality of life after permanent prostate brachytherapy. Int J Rad Oncol Biol Phys 2004; 58:81-88.

15. Merrick GS, Butler WM, Dorsey AT, al e. Influence of prophylactic dexamethasone on edema following prostate brachytherapy. Techniques in Urology 2000; 6:117-122.

16. Merrick GS, Butler WM, Lief JH, Dorsey AT. Temporal resolution of urinary morbidity following prostate brachytherapy. Int J Radiat Oncol Biolo Phys 2000; 47:121-128.

17. Merrick GS, Butler WM, Wallner KE, Lief JH, Galbreath RW. Prophylactive versus therapeutic alpha blockers following permanent prostate brachytherapy. Urol 2002; 60:650-655.

18. Nickel JC, Elhilali M, Emberton M, Vallancien G. The beneficial effect of alfuzosin 10 mg once daily iin "real-life" practice on lower urinary tract symptoms)LUTS), quality of life and sexual dysfunction in men with LUTS and painful ejaculation. European Urology 1006; 97:1242-1246.

19. Orsini N, RashidKhani B, Andersson S, Karlberg L, Johansson J, Wolk A. Long-term physical activity and lower urinary tract symptoms in men. J Urology 2006; 176:2546-2550.

20. Rodgers M, Hempel S, Aho T, Kelly, JD, Kleijnen J, Westwood M. Diagnostic tests used in the investigation of adult haematuria: A systematic review. BJU International 2006; 98:1154-1160.

21. Smathers S, Wallner KE, Lai K, et al. Radiation safety parameters following prostate brachytherapy. Int J Radiat Oncol Biol Phys 1999; 45:397-399.

22. Wallner KE, Roy J, Harrison L. Low risk of perioperative infection without prophylactic antibiotics for transperineal prostate brachytherapy. Int J Radiat Oncol Biol Phys 1996; 36:681-683.

23. Wallner KE, Roy J, Harrison L. Tumor control and morbidity following transperineal I-125 implantation for Stage T1/T2 prostatic carcinoma. J Clin Oncol 1996; 14:449-453.

13

Supplemental beam radiation

Supplemental external beam radiation has long been added to brachytherapy in the definitive therapy of cervical, endometrial, and tongue cancers, the rationale being that brachytherapy eradicates large central tumor masses while beam radiation eradicates microscopic disease outside of the implant volume. Similarly, supplemental beam radiation has long been combined with Ir-192 prostate brachytherapy, with substantial success.(MARTINEZ) So when TRUS-based transperineal I-125 and Pd-103 brachytherapy emerged in the late 1980s, the concept of combining brachytherapy with external beam radiation was similarly adopted for

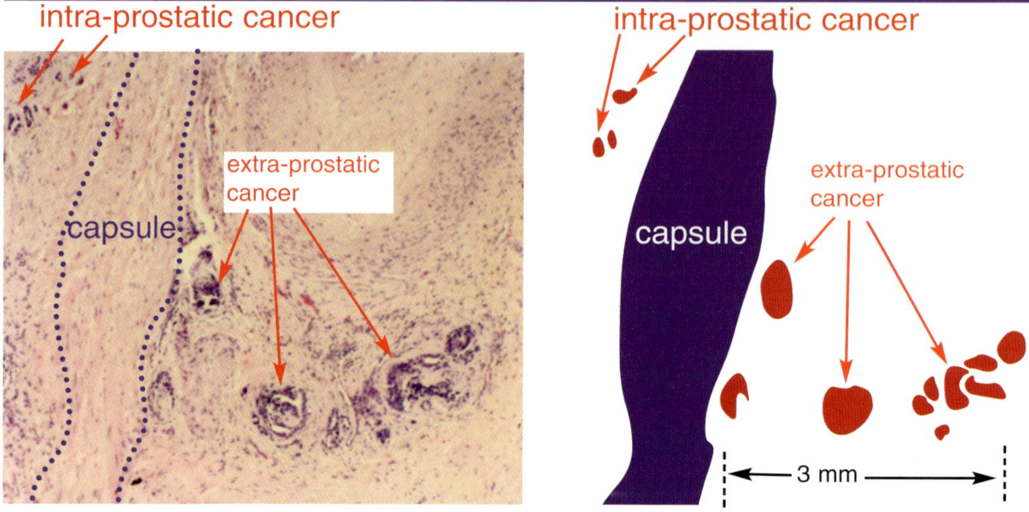

Figure 13-1. Advanced ECE—in this prostatectomy specimen, cancer has penetrated the capsule, extending approximately 3 mm outside of capsular margin. The cancer is still within the margin of resection (not visible here). This degree of ECE probably would be included within the cancercidal isodose of an implant (see Figure 11-10) (courtesy of L. True).

many patients. The external beam fields typically used are just large enough to cover the prostate with a 2–4 cm margin (see chapter 6).

For a while, there was general agreement as to which patients should receive supplemental external radiation—those with a pre-treatment PSA above 10 or a Gleason score above 6. While the tumor control rates with this policy have been favorable, several areas of clinical investigation have cast a lot of doubt on the need for supplemental beam radiation. First, results with implant alone, even in patients with higher PSA and Gleason scores, have been remarkably good in experienced hands.(BLASKO 00, MERRICK 01) Second, detailed pathology studies have revealed that the radial extent of extra-prostatic cancer extension, even in patients with higher PSA and Gleason scores, is surprisingly limited.(DAVIS, SOHAYDA, TEH) Although almost universally accepted in the early days of TRUS-based implants, it turns out that the role of supplemental external radiation is one of the most questionable aspects of prostate brachytherapy.

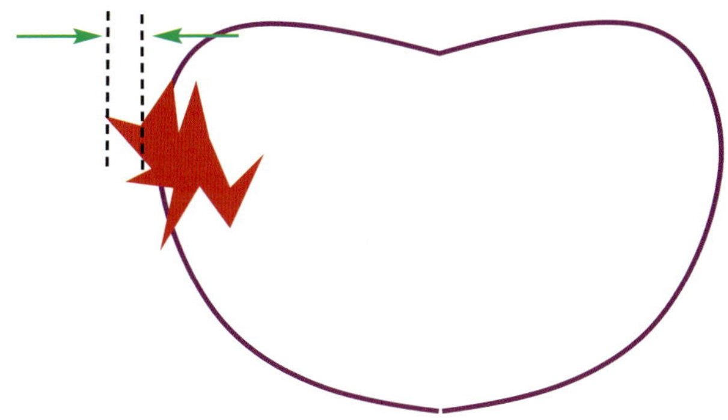

Figure 13-2. As cancer breaches the prostatic capsule, it extends radially. The potential for radial extension is the rationale for seeking greater peripheral coverage with supplemental external beam radiation.

RATIONALE FOR BEAM RADIATION
There are four rationales for using supplemental external beam radiation:

1. *enhance coverage of peri-prostatic tissue*
2. *escalate dose to intra-prostatic tumor*
3. *make up for a technically inadequate implant*
4. *sterilize pelvic lymph nodes*

Each of these rationales seem logically compelling. But with more clinical data, the validity of each has come into question.

Extra-capsular cancer
The primary rationale for supplemental beam radiation is to increase the coverage of the peri-prostatic region, helping to sterilize extra-capsular cancer extension (ECE) (**Figure 13-1**). The prostatic capsule is a collection of fibrous layers of variable thickness, without a distinct margin. Cancers commonly achieve varying degrees of ECE by the time of diagnosis (**Figure 13-2**).(SAKR, SATTAR) Patients with early ECE are still curable, providing the extra-capsular tumor can be eradicated. The most compelling evidence for their curability is that cure with radical prostatectomy is still possible in the setting of ECE, assuming that the surgical margins are

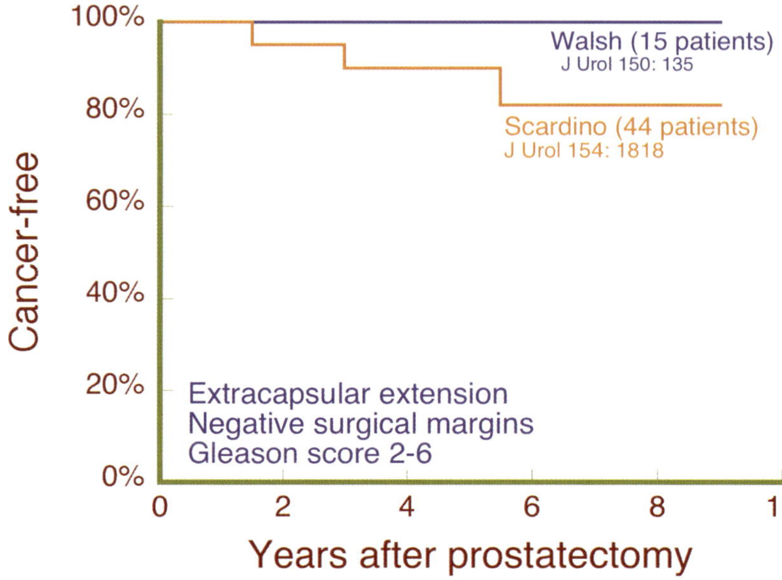

Figure 13-3. Disease-free survival for T1/T2 prostatectomy patients with limited ECE and negative margins. Such patients are still highly curable surgically, despite the presence of ECE.(OHORI, EPSTEIN)

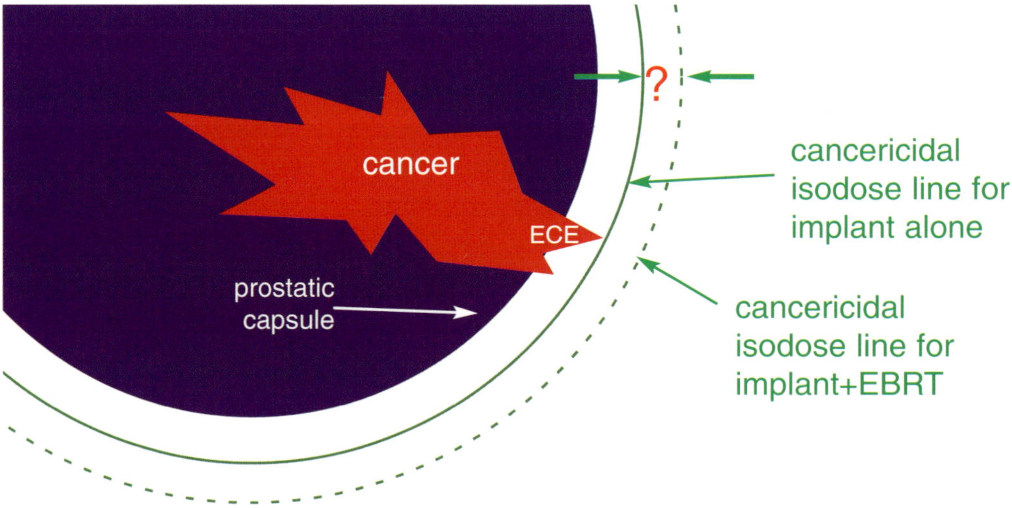

Figure 13-4. A major theoretical issue regarding supplemental beam radiation is whether it is needed to assure that the cancercidal isodose encompasses any and all ECE.

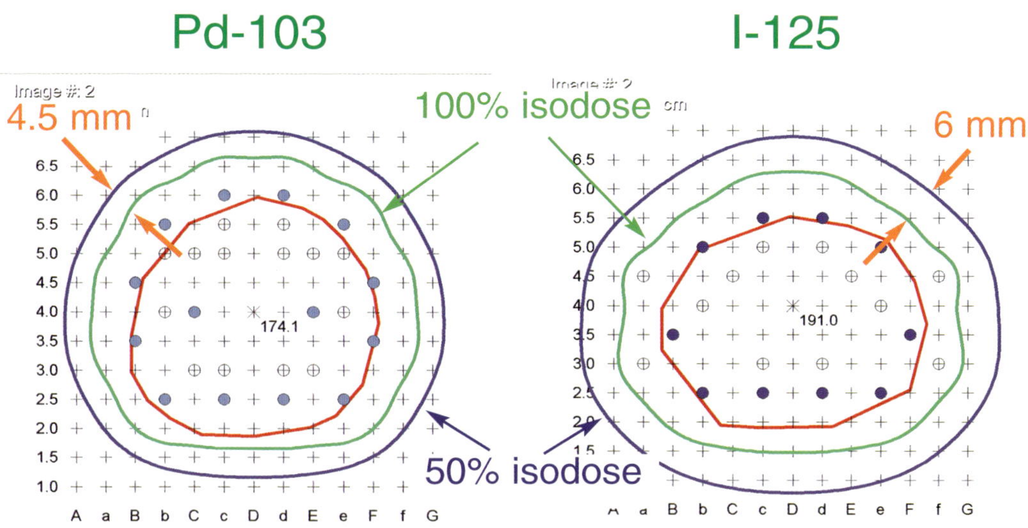

Figure 13-5. It's not known exactly how much extra therapeutic margin supplemental beam radiation provides, but a perusal of two typical monotherapy plans gives an estimate. Assuming that 45 Gy beam radiation brings the 50% brachytherapy isodose up to a cancericidal level, then beam radiation would increase the treatment margin by about 4–6 mm.

clear of cancer (**Figure 13-3**). And considering the high cure rates with radiation, the same must hold true—patients with capsular penetration are still curable if the cancercidal radiation dose encompasses all EPE. Unfortunately, the precise cancercidal margin with implant alone or combined with supplemental beam radiation is unclear, partly because no one knows precisely what the cancericidal dose is (**Figure 13-4**)! Assuming the cancericidal effect of 45 Gy given with external beam radiation is approximately that of a half-dose implant, supplemental beam radiation should increase the therapeutic margin by approximately 4-6 mm by moving the effective dose at the 50% implant dose line to the 100% line.(**Figures 13-5**).

Guidelines for adding supplemental beam radiation were initially extrapolated from surgical pathology studies, whereby the likelihood of ECE was correlated with pre-treatment PSA and Gleason score (**Figures 13-6 and 13-7**). Although the likelihood of EPCE is a continuum with increasing PSA or Gleason score, the generally accepted cutoff for adding beam radiation

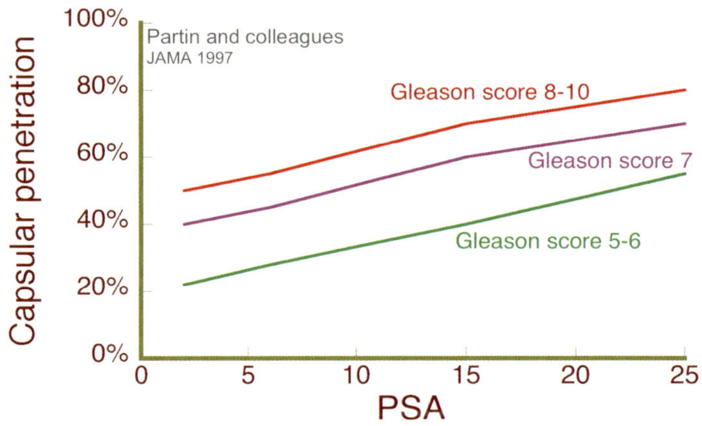

Figure 13-6. Likelihood of ECE in patients with Stage T1c-T2a tumors, versus Gleason score and PSA, based on data from JHU. (PARTIN)

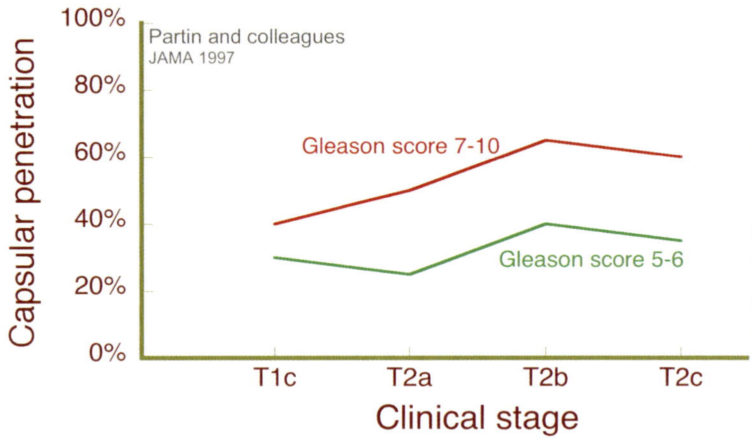

Figure 13-7. In comparison to PSA and Gleason score, the effect of clinical stage on the likelihood of ECE is minor, due to subjective nature of the exam and because palpable abnormalities are likely to be unrelated to cancer.(PARTIN)

Very important point

Why the Partin Tables are unduly frightening

The *Partin Tables* have been misinterpreted by both physicians and patients to mean that patients with EPE are not curable. In fact, a large percentage of patients with EPE are still curable, surgically or with brachytherapy, provided that the EPE is still encompassed within the surgical margins, or within the cancercidal dose range. This should be stressed to patients, who otherwise believe that their high likelihood of EPE is synonymous with a high likelihood of treatment failure.

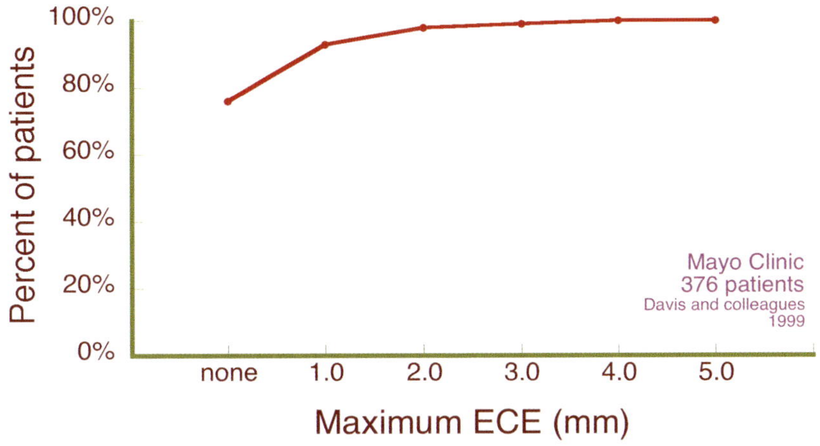

Figure 13-8. Nearly all cases of ECE are limited to within 3 mm of the prostatic capsule.(DAVIS)

has been a PSA of 10 ng/ml or a Gleason score of 7. Stage has been a less-used criterion, due to the subjectivity of the digital rectal exam and the fact that most patients are now diagnosed with non-palpable disease (**Figure 13-7**).

Most pathology studies of ECE address only its *incidence*, not its radial distance from the prostatic capsule. The *Partin Tables*, for instance, have been misinterpreted by doctors and patients alike to equate ECE with incurability.(PARTIN) More recent studies of the *radial* extent of ECE have rekindled the debate regarding its clinical significance and the rationale for supplemental beam radiation.(TEH, DAVIS, SOHAYDA)

Using prostatectomy specimens, Dr. Brian Davis from the Mayo Clinic and Dr. Chris Sohayda from Cleveland Clinic correlated radial ECE with pretreatment PSA and Gleason score (**Figures 13-8 and 13-9**). In what came as a real surprise to most oncologists, ECE was limited to within 3 mm of the prostatic edge in most of their patients. Accordingly, a radiation treatment margin (TM) of 3 mm should suffice. Since brachytherapy alone can consistently achieve a TM of 3 mm or more, the rationale for adding beam radiation to achieve a wider treatment margin was re-opened to debate (**Figure 13-10**).(MERRICK 02)

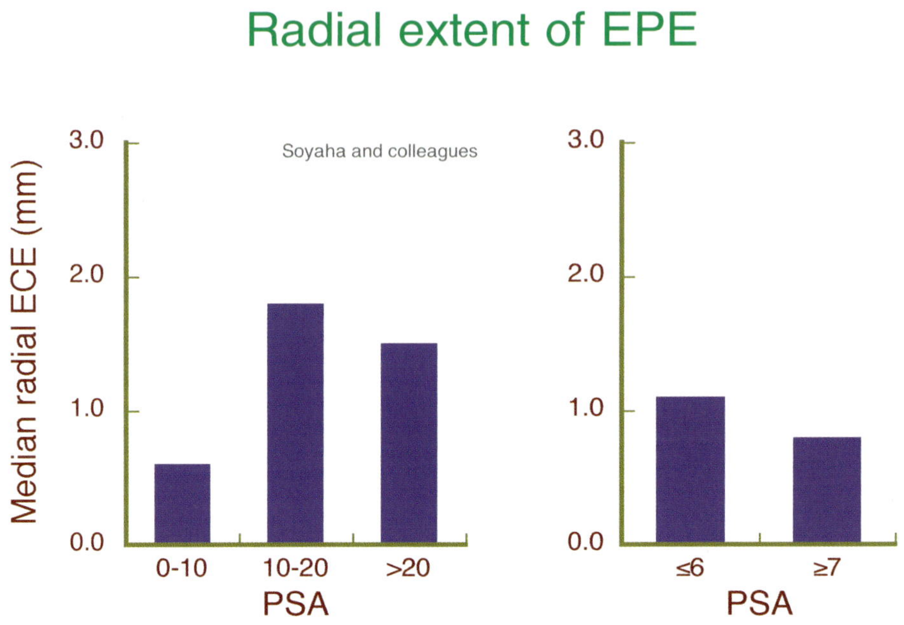

Figure 13-9. The magnitude of EPE, measured perpendicular to the prostatic capsule, versus pretreatment PSA or Gleason score.(SOHAYDA)

While clinically important, the EPE work by Davis and colleagues comes with two caveats. First, some patients had positive surgical margins, and must have had greater radial cancer extension than reported. Secondly, hemosiderin and eosin staining used by Davis might underestimate radial extension as evaluated by PCR staining.(THEODORESCU)

Dose escalation

The second rationale for adding beam radiation to an implant is to increase the intra-prostatic radiation dose. Quantifying the biologic dose of monotherapy versus combined treatment is not readily doable. Simple addition of implant and beam doses is not radiobiologically legitimate. Orton and colleagues estimated dose translations between modalities, but such estimates are plagued by ignorance of in vivo radiobiologic parameters used.(ORTON) Simpler estimates, expressed as percent of full monotherapy doses, suggest that the biological effect of combined modality is higher than standard brachytherapy or beam doses alone (**Figure 13-11**). But is a higher dose than that achieved with an implant alone needed?

Average treatment margins achieved

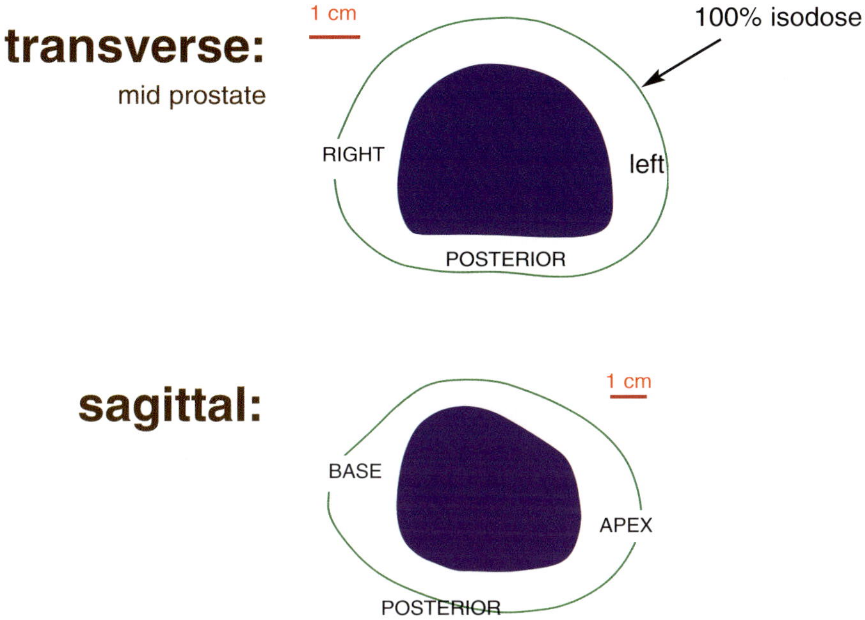

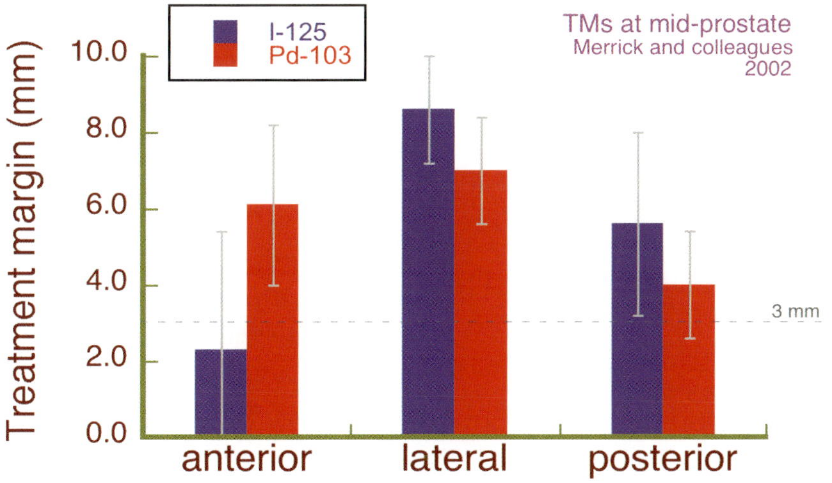

Figure 13-10. Average treatment margins achieved in an unselected series of 26 patients randomized to I-125 versus Pd-103. The TMs, measured on post-implant day 0 CT, exceeded the minimum 3 mm desirable in 87% of points overall MERRICK *03)*

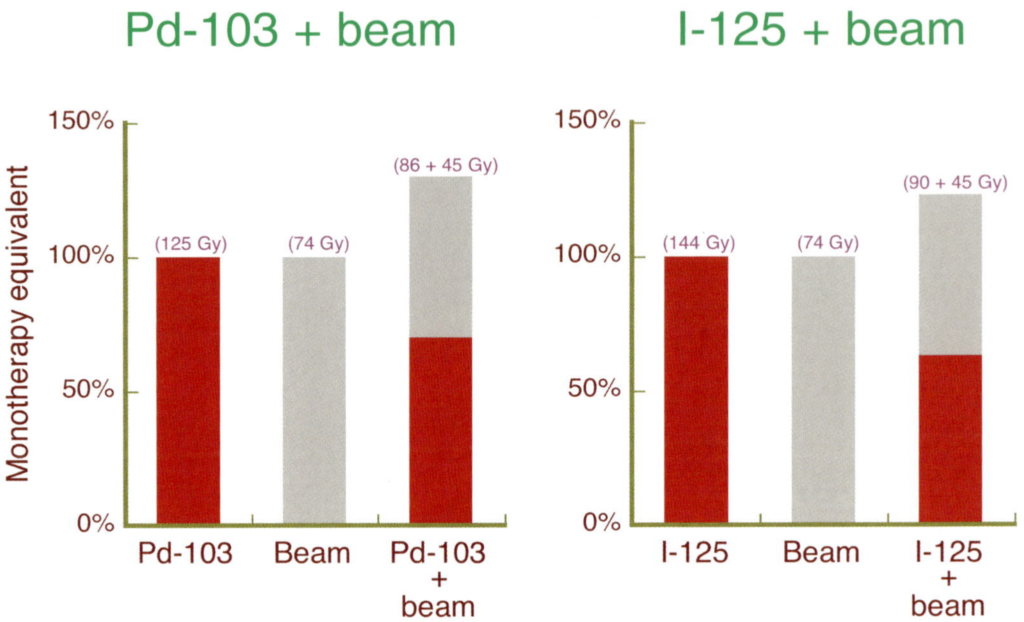

Figure 13-11. Approximation of biologically effective doses of brachytherapy therapy alone versus brachytherapy combined with supplemental external beam radiation, based on simple proportions of monotherapy doses.

Based on the high rates of negative post-implant biopsies that have been consistently reported, it does not appear that intra-prostatic dose escalation is needed—the real problem is the possibility of metastatic disease, not intra-prostatic tumor eradication.(PRESTIDGE, SHARKEY)

Very important point

Why brachytherapy may be more effective than surgery

The potential for capsular penetration extending beyond the surgical margins is part of the theoretical appeal of brachytherapy. Patients with capsular penetration extending beyond the likely surgical margin, may have a higher likelihood of cure with the wider therapeutic margin achieved with brachytherapy (**Figure 13-4**).

Inadequate implants

No matter how skilled you are, you will occasionally do an implant that does not cover the prostate as generously as you would like. Adding supplemental beam radiation should increase the peri-prostatic coverage by several mil-

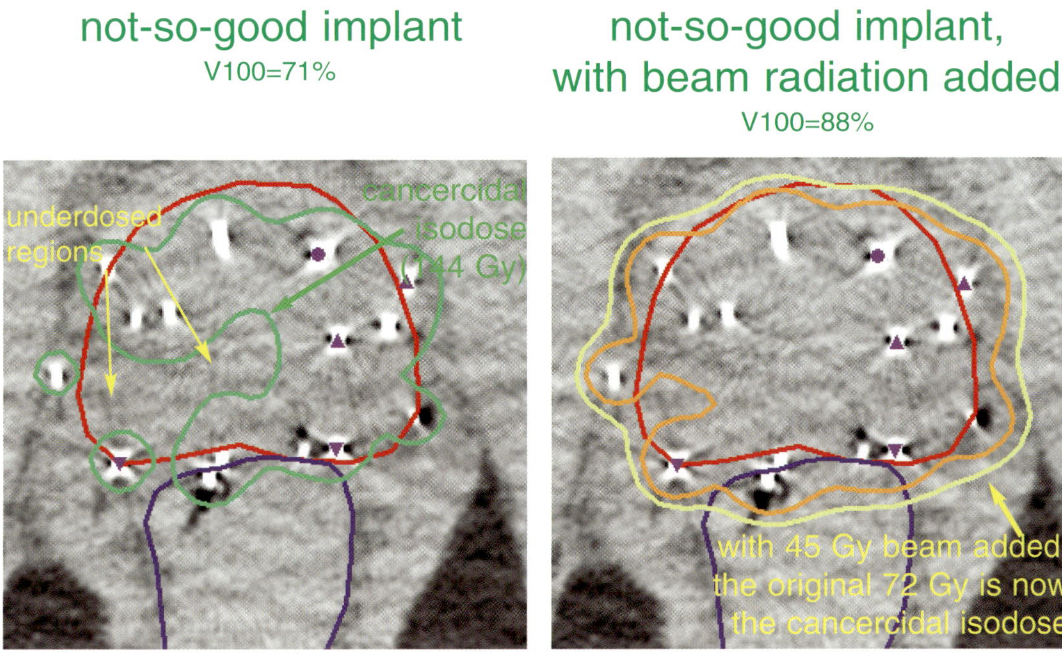

Figure 13-12. By increasing the therapeutic margin, supplemental external beam radiation improves prostatic coverage of an inadequate implant. In this case, only 71% of the post-implant prostate volume was covered by the 144 Gy monotherapy prescription dose (left). If 45 Gy supplemental beam radiation is added to this inadequate implant, and assuming that the original 72 Gy implant isodose line now represents the cancercidal 144 Gy isodose, approximately 3 mm would be added to the treatment margin (right). Theoretically, the V100 would increase from 71% to 88%.

limeters, decreasing the clinical impact of a technically inadequate implant (**Figure 13-12**).

There is meager clinical evidence that adding supplemental beam can make up for a technically inferior implant. In a retrospective analysis, Potters reported no benefit to supplemental beam radiation, regardless of whether D90 was considered in multivariate analysis.(POTTERS 03)

For a novice brachytherapist who's not yet up to speed with technique, use of beam radiation is more appealing than to someone who's already highly

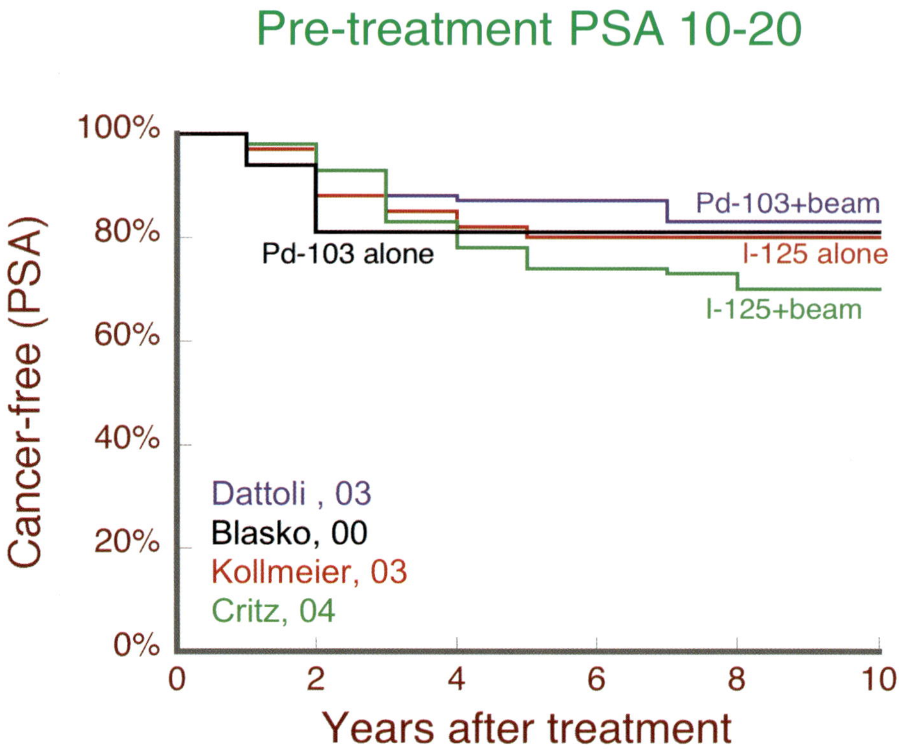

Figure 13-13. Biochemical tumor control for patients with pre-treatment PSA of 10 to 20 ng/ml, treated with brachytherapy, with or without supplemental beam radiation.(KOLMEIER, BLASKO 00, CRITZ 04, DATTOLI 03) The most striking finding, apart from the fact that all of the curves level off at relatively high levels, is that they are all so similar. Although the biochemical endpoints differ between studies, with longer follow-up the definition of biochemical failure makes little difference.(LU, KESTIN)

skilled. Brachytherapists who consistently achieve generous treatment margins are unlikely to need the extra margin afforded by supplemental beam radiation.(CHOI, MERRICK 03, ORIO)

Treating pelvic lymph nodes
A fourth rationale for combining brachytherapy with external beam radiation is to treat pelvic lymph nodes, a highly contentious subject in itself. Retrospective studies have almost uniformly shown that nearly all patients

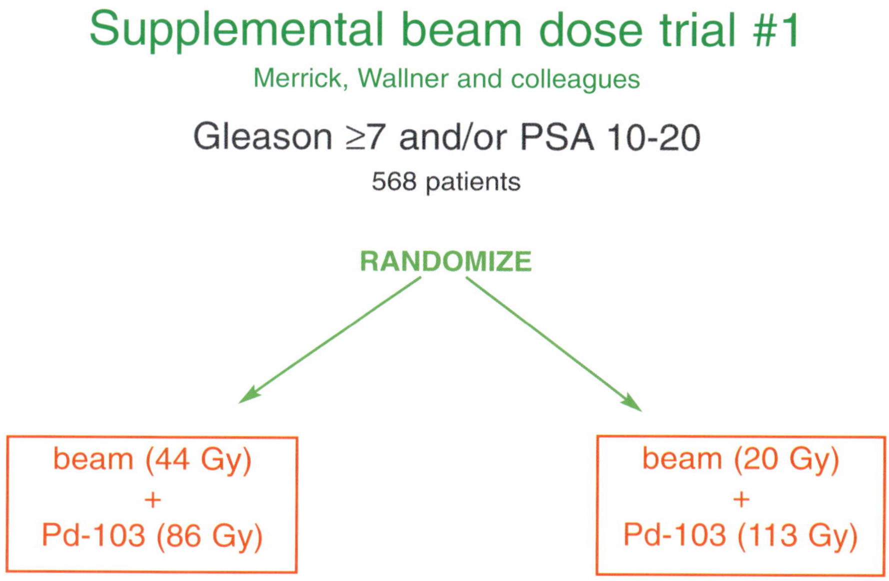

Figure 13-14. Design of completed trial to compare moderate- versus low-dose supplemental external beam radiation (568 patients randomized).

with known lymph node involvement ultimately develop metastatic cancer, regardless of therapy.(LEIBEL) And large, prospective randomized trials have failed to show a clinically meaningful benefit of lymph node treatment.(PILIPECH, ROACH, ASBELL) One randomized trial did show a small benefit of adding whole pelvic radiation with hormonal therapy to prostate radiation. However, the increase in disease-free survival was small, and there was no cancer-specific survival benefit.(ROACH) It is not unreasonable to add pelvic radiation in patients at high risk for nodal involvement, but supporting data is skimpy, at best.

Clinical results

The use of supplemental beam radiation remains a subject of intense theoretical debate. In the meantime, emerging clinical data are also casting increasing doubt on its use routine use. Longer-term series with monotherapy or with supplemental beam radiation, show similar 5-year freedom from failure rates, casting doubt on the beam's contribution to cancer eradication (**Figure 13-13**).(BLASKO 00)

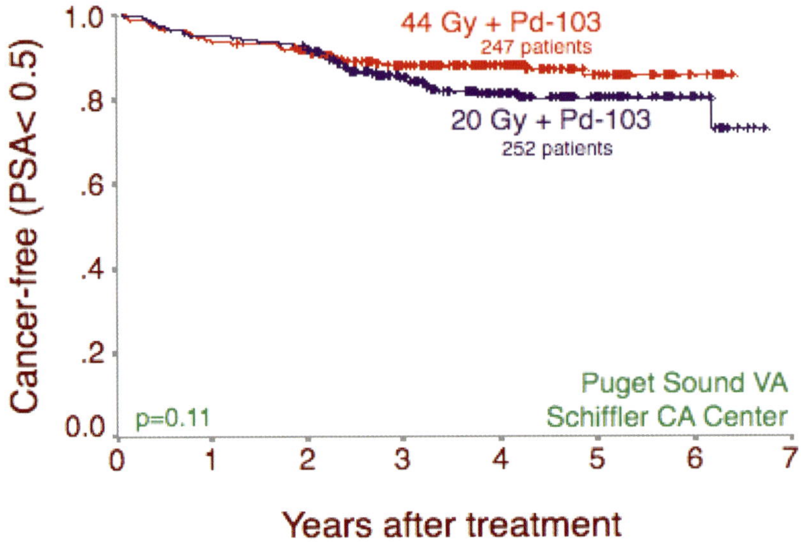

Figure 13-15. Biochemical cancer control rates for 499 intermediate risk patients randomized to 20 Gy versus 44 Gy supplemental beam radiation. There is a non-signficant trend to higher biochemical control in patients who recieved 44 Gy beam.

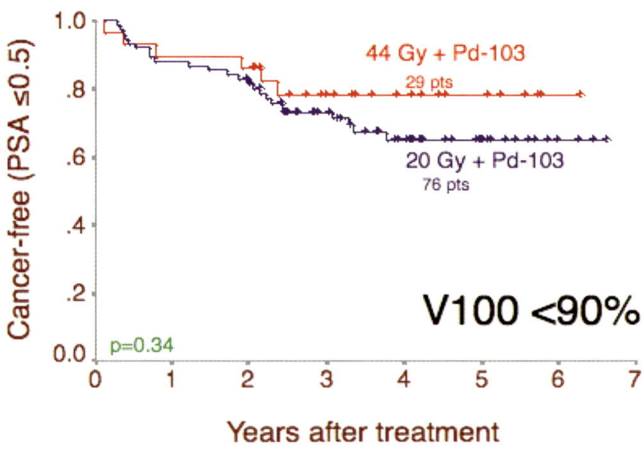

Figure 13-16. Biochemical cancer control rates for patients with V100s above or below 90%. The trend to better biochemical control in patients who recieved 44 Gy appears to be limited to patients with cooler implants.

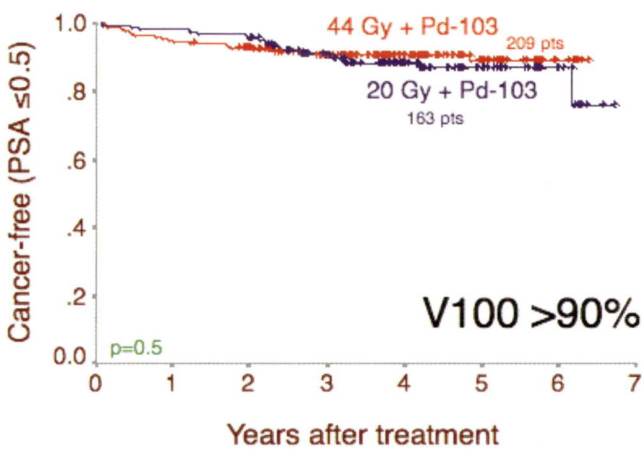

Supplemental beam dose trial #2

Merrick, Wallner and colleagues

Gleason ≥7 and/or PSA 10-20

420 patients

RANDOMIZE

beam (20 Gy)
+
Pd-103 (113 Gy)

Pd-103 (125 Gy)

Figure 13-17. Design of ongoing trial to compare 20 Gy versus no supplemental external beam radiation (220 patients randomized as of May 2007).

RTOG Supplemental beam

Prestidge and colleagues

Gleason ≥7 and/or PSA 10-20

1520 patients

RANDOMIZE

beam (44 Gy)
+
implant

implant alone

Figure 13-18. Design of RTOG trial designed to compare brachytherapy with or without supplemental external beam radiation. Implants could be performed with either I-125 or Pd-103.

In a more rigorous attempt to decipher the need for supplemental beam radiation, Merrick, Wallner and colleagues are conducting a series of large, prospective randomized studies sequentially decreasing the dose of supplemental beam. Their rationale for gradually decreasing the dose was akin to that underlying the Wilms' tumor studies performed in the 1980s, in which the doses of beam radiation were gradually decreased through a series of randomized trials.(THOMAS)

In the first trial, 568 patients were randomized to 44 Gy versus 20 Gy supplemental beam, with the implant doses adjusted accordingly (**Figure 13-14**). Preliminary analyses show a slight decrement in cancer control with less beam radiation (**Figures 13-15 and 13-16**).(WALLNER) However, the trend to lower biochemical control in 20 Gy patients appeared to be limited to those with cooler implants. While waiting for the 20 Gy versus 44 Gy results to mature, the same investigators are randomizing an additional 600 implant patients between 20 Gy supplemental beam and *no* supplemental beam (**Figure 13-17**). Preliminary outcomes should be available by 2010.

In a more direct test of the need for supplemental beam radiation, investigators with RTOG opened a trial in 2005 to randomize intermediate risk patients to an implant alone or combined with 45 Gy beam radiation (**Figure 13-18**). Accrual has been slow, and it is unclear whether the trial will be completed.

DIAGNOSTIC IMAGING

Rightly or wrongly, the general consensus has been to use PSA and grade as the principle criteria by which to determine use supplemental external beam radiation, even though such criteria are plagued by their imprecision in predicting radial ECE. Diagnostic imaging is a potentially more precise way to determine the need for supplemental external radiation, with the rationale being that ECE identified on imaging would be an indication for the wider treatment margins afforded by beam radiation. Unfortunately, CT and TRUS are remarkably unreliable ways to diagnose ECE, with investigators unanimously concluding that the sensitivity and accuracy are insufficient to evaluate ECE or seminal vesicle invasion.(ENGELER, PLATT, RIFKIN)

MR scanning is much more likely to provide useful information about the presence and extent of ECE, allegedly capable of detecting 3 mm of ECE (**Figure 13-19**).(SCHIEBLER) Because patients with ECE of less than 3 mm

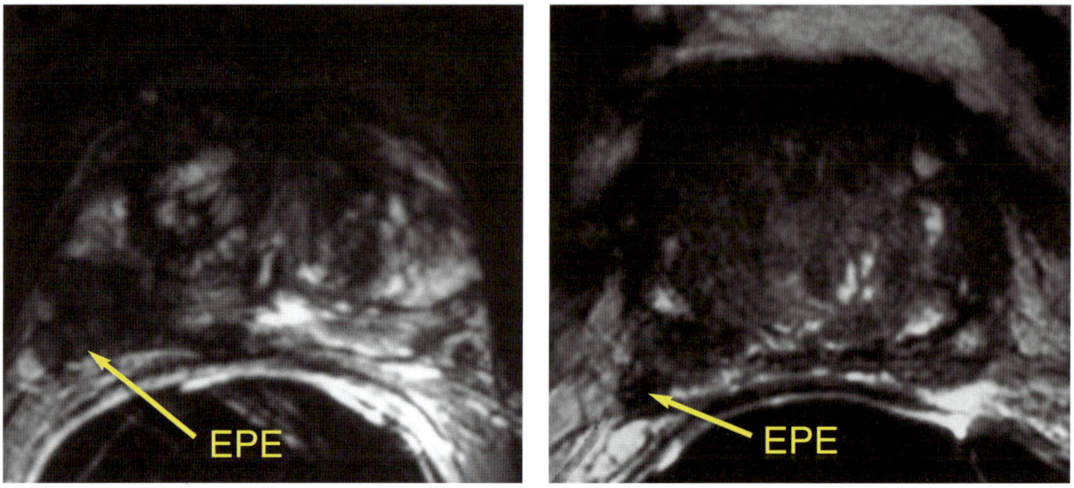

Figure 13-19. Examples of extra-prostatic cancer extension (arrows) on transverse MR (courtesy of Dr. Daniel Clarke).

should be highly curable with the cancercidal dose margin of an implant alone, it seems logical that if MR does not reveal ECE, monotherapy would be appropriate. Conversely, those patients with MR-detected EPE presumably have greater than 3 mm radial extent and might benefit from supplemental radiation (or larger implant treatment margins that deliver full doses to all ECE disease). Following this strategy, Clarke and colleagues reported high cure rates with beam radiation plus seeds for MR-based T3 disease. Their treatment strategy includes extra-prostatic implantation of all MR-detected ECE.(CLARKE)

D'Amico and coworkers have made considerable efforts to define which patients are most likely to benefit from MR staging.(D'AMICO) The problem with routine MR scanning in low-risk patients is that only a small percent of them will have their treatment altered by the test findings. The incidence of ECE on pathology specimens is only 20% to 30%, and of those, only approximately 10% will be detected by MR (**Figures 13-19 & 13-20**). MR has higher sensitivity for ECE in patients with high-grade cancer or high PSA, presumably because their ECE is greater and hence more readily detected.

Color Doppler ultrasound might also be a valuable tool to detect substantial ECE, and to direct such sites for more generous seeding or supple-

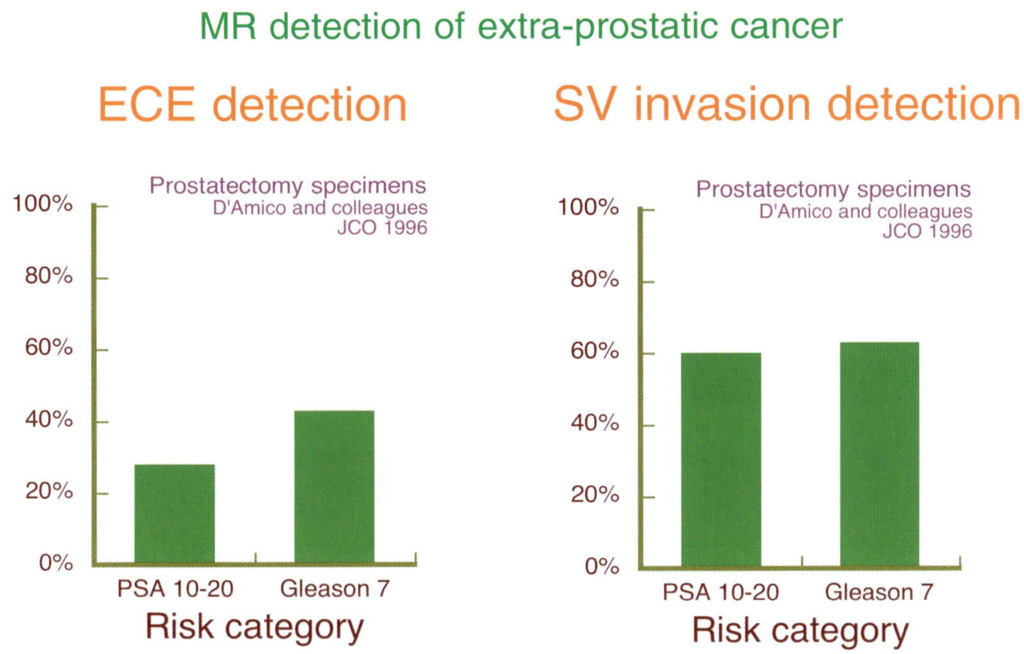

Figure 13-20. Sensitivity of MR in detecting EPE, based on pretreatment PSA or Gleason score. With a low PSA or Gleason score, there is little likelihood of detecting EPE. Although sensitivity is greater at higher PSA, those patients should be assumed to have substantial ECE even if not detected radiographically. So it's unclear that MR really adds to their management.(D'AMICO)
sensitivity =true-positive/(true-positive+false negative)

mental beam radiation. The use of Doppler-assisted biopsy for cancer detection has met with mixed results.(KRAVCHICK) However, M Dattolli uses Doppler TRUS extensively to detect and treat peripheral areas suspicious for cancer (**Figure 13-21**).

The ability to evaluate the presence and extent of ECE would go a long way to making more rational use of supplemental external beam radiation. Unfortunately, all imaging modalities are of limited or unproven value for diagnosis of ECE, and especially in evaluating its radial extent. The principle limitation with MR studies to date is that they may not distinguish between minimal ECE, which should be highly curable with implant alone,

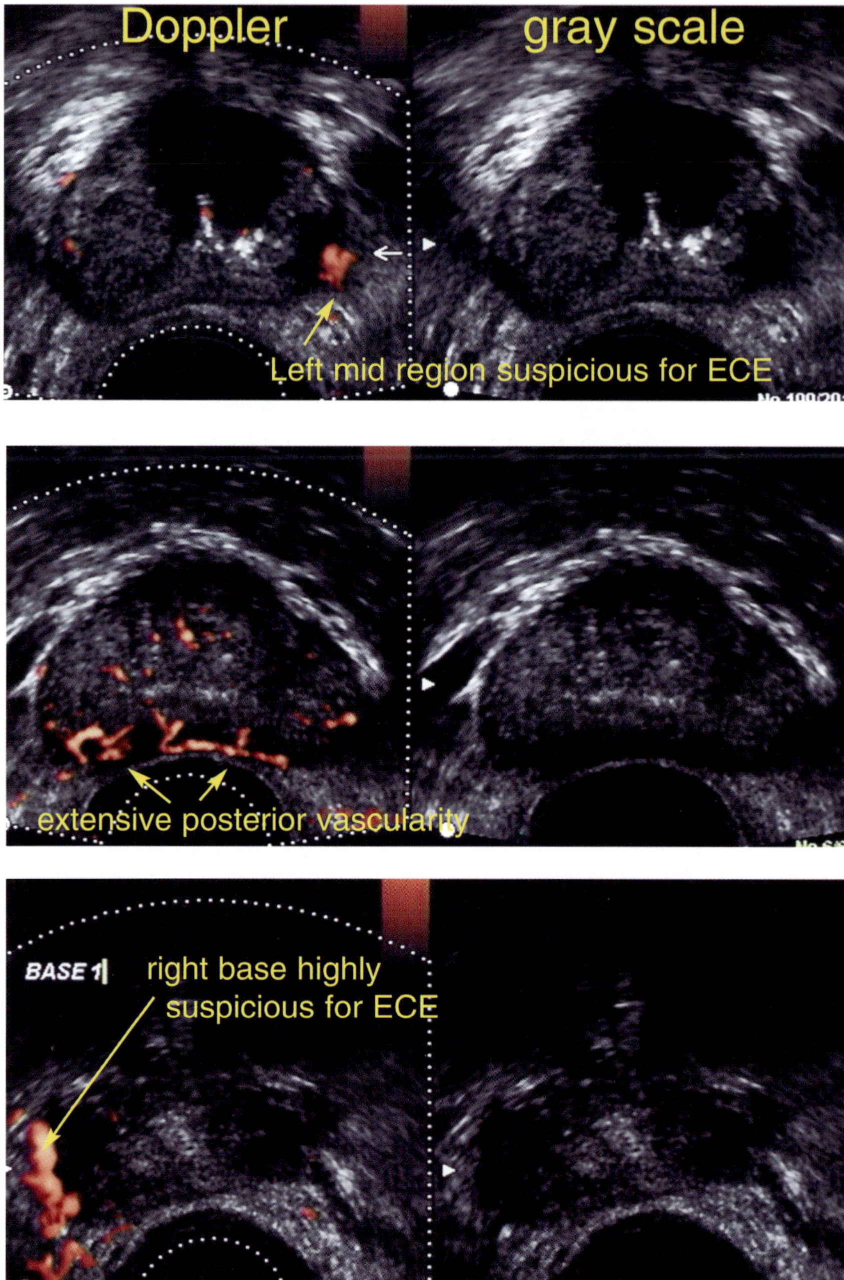

Figure 13-21. Power mode Doppler-identified peripheral regions that appear highly suspicious for ECE.

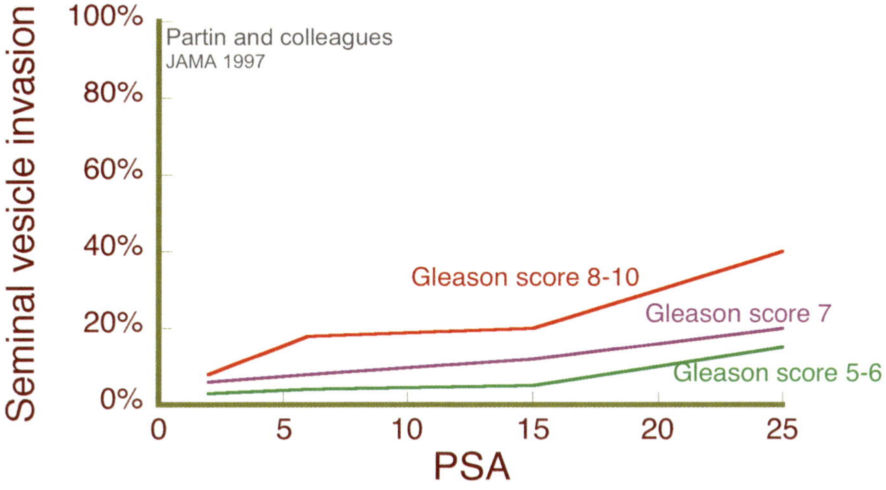

Figure 13-22. Likelihood of seminal vesicle invasion in patients with Stage T1c-T2a tumors in relation to Gleason score and PSA.(PARTIN)

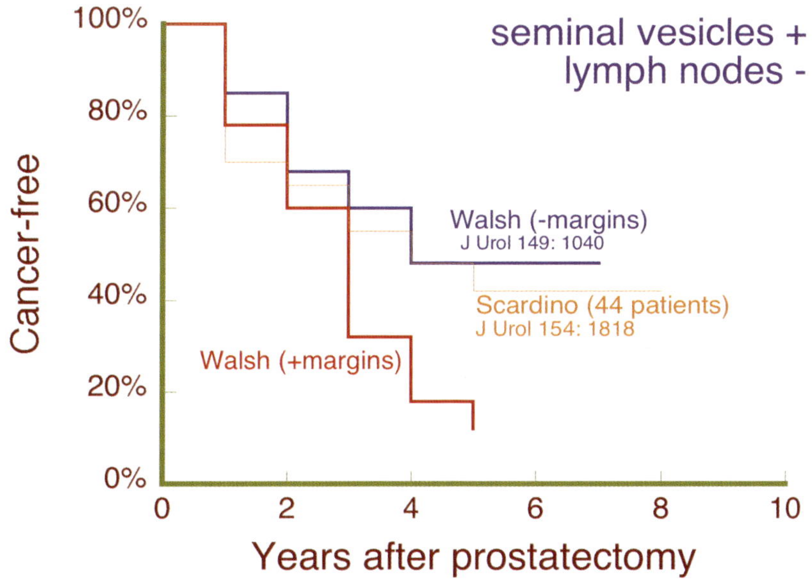

Figure 13-23. Freedom from failure for patients with seminal vesicle involvement. It appears that a small proportion of patients may be cured, if the lymph nodes and surgical margins are negative.

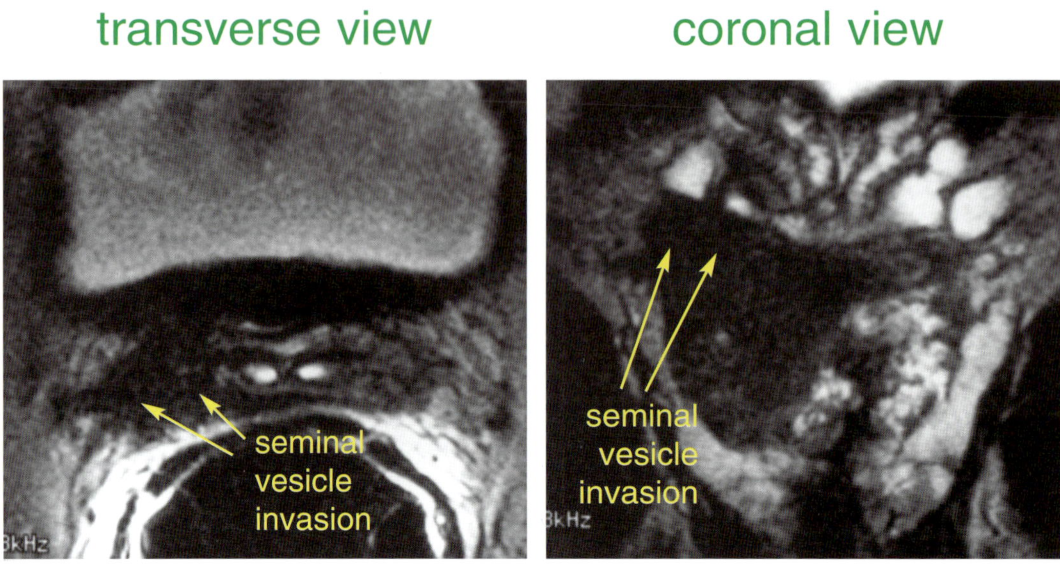

Figure 13-24. MR showing right-sided seminal vesicle invasion on transverse and coronal view (courtesy of Dr. Daniel Clarke).

versus more substantial ECE, which may call for supplemental external radiation to enhance the cancercidal treatment margin. Proper studies to address these issues would require correlating radial EPE measurements on prostatectomy specimens with pre-surgical MR findings.

Seminal vesicles

The likelihood of invasion of the peri-vesicle tissue or the muscular wall of the seminal vesicles is related to PSA and Gleason score, and is associated with a high likelihood of post-prostatectomy recurrence (**Figures 13-22 and 13-23**). (EPSTEIN 93) Judging from prostatectomy series, *some* patients with early seminal vesicle involvement are still surgically curable. Presumably, a few are also curable with radiation.

The seminal vesicles are irregular structures that change their shape and position as the bladder expands and contracts. They cannot be treated adequately with brachytherapy alone, due to rapid dose fall-off outside of the prostate.(STOCK) Seeds cannot be reliably placed in the distal portions of the seminal vesicles because the vesicles move when pushed by a needle tip, and seeds tend to migrate after being ejected in their vicinity.

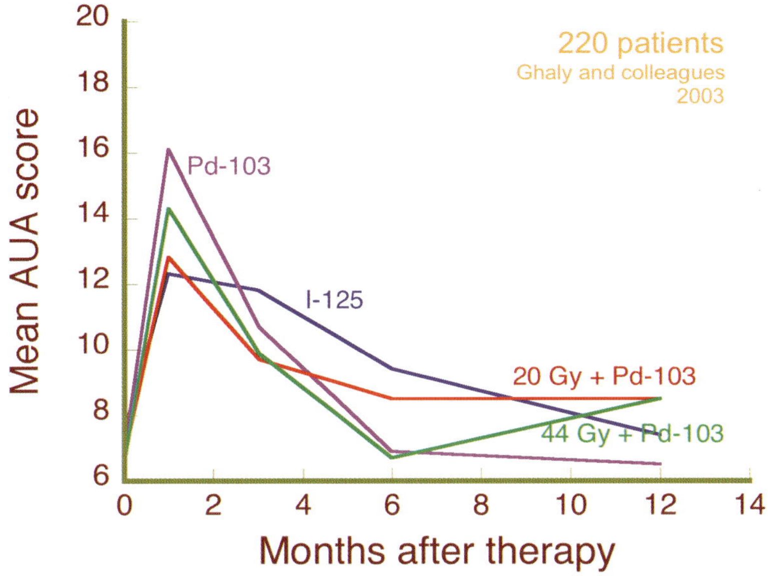

Figure 13-25. Urinary morbidiity in patients with or without supplemental beam.

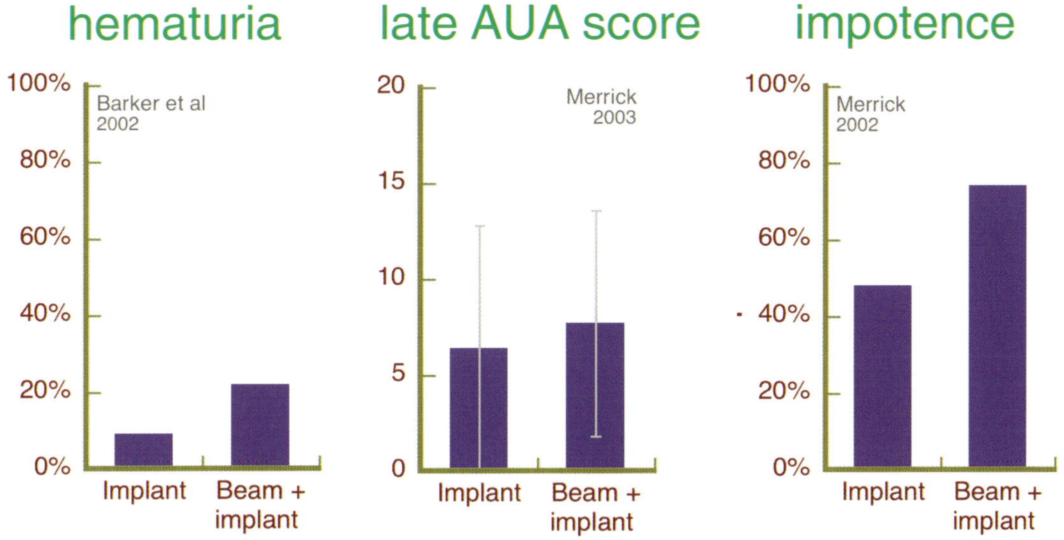

Figure 13-26. Various morbidities appear to be increased by the addition of supplemental beam radiation.

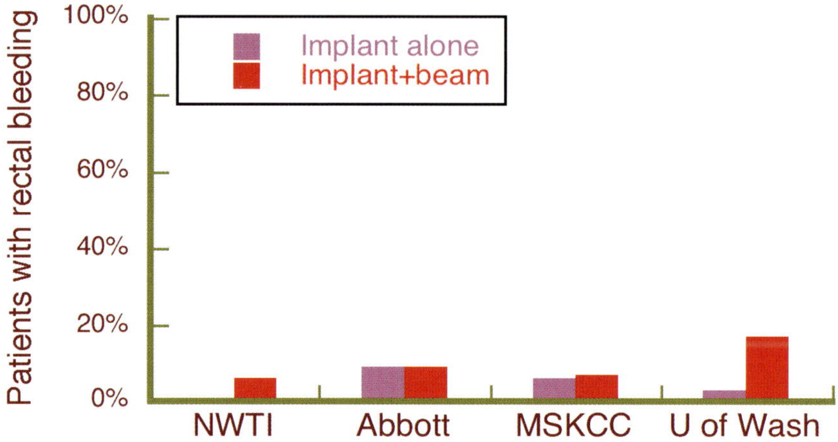

Figure 13-27. Incidence of implant-related rectal bleeding after brachytherapy, with or without supplemental external beam radiation.(BLASKO, KAYE, GELBLUM, HAN)

Perhaps the best use of pre-implant diagnostic imaging is to rule out seminal vesicle invasion, a task for which MR is fairly accurate (**Figure 13-24**).(D'AMICO) But even so, questions remain as to MR's relevance in relation to therapy. Early seminal vesicle invasion, still compatible with cure, is frequently limited to within a few mm of the prostatic capsule, potentially well covered by implant alone.(DAVIS, MICHIGAN) More extensive seminal vesicle invasion, beyond the high-dose region of an implant, may well be synonymous with distant disease, so that adding external beam radiation would have no impact on a patient's ultimate prognosis. As in the case of ECE, the accuracy of MR needs to be correlated with the *degree* of vesicle invasion before a stronger argument can be made for its routine use as a pre-brachytherapy staging modality.

MORBIDITY OF SUPPLEMENTAL BEAM

While there is substantial doubt about the value of supplemental beam radiation in the setting of good quality brachytherapy, there is no doubt that it adds to morbidity. Early urinary morbidity may be *less* with combined therapy (**Figure 13-25**). However, a myriad of longer-term morbidities, including hematuria, obstructive symptoms and impotence have been shown to increase with the addition of beam radiation (**Figure 13-26**). Early and late proctitis are also probably increased(**Figure 13-27**).(BITTNER)

Table 13-1. Traditional criteria for adding supplemental beam radiation.

Generally accepted:	PSA >10 Gleason ≥7 clinical T2c/T3
Less accepted:	extensive tumor in biopsy (>10 mm) bilateral positive biopsies perineural invasion ECE by MR

One must weigh the added morbidity and cost of supplemental beam radiation against its questionable clinical benefit.

CURRENT PRACTICE

The role of supplemental beam radiation is likely to be debated for years to come. Fortunately, the necessity for adding supplemental beam radiation should be clarified through ongoing rigorous clinical studies. In the meantime, the generally accepted criteria for treatment with implant alone are PSA″10, Gleason score ″7 and clinical stage T1-T2b (**Table 13-1**). Patients with a PSA >10, Gleason ≥8 or T3 tumor on digital rectal exam have typically been given supplemental beam radiation. In borderline cases, extensive tumor in the biopsy sample or the presence of perineural invasion would favor the use of supplemental beam radiation, on the assumption that they are associated with increased radial extent of extraprostatic cancer extension.

REFERENCES

1. Asbell SO, Krall JM, Pilepich MV, Baerwald H. Elective pelvic irradiation in stage A2, B carcinoma of the prostate: Analysis of RTOG 77-06. Int J Radiat Oncol Biol Phys 1988; 15:1307-1316.

2. Barker J, Wallner K, Merrick G. Gross hematuria after prostate brachytherapy. Urol 2003; 61:408-411.

3. Bittner N, Wallner K, Merrick G, et al. Time gap between Pd-103 prostate brachytherapy and supplemental beam radiation versus morbidity and the likelihood of cure. submitted 2007.

4. Blasko JC, Grimm PD, Sylvester JE, Badiozamani KR, Hoak D, Cavanagh W. Palladium-103 brachytherapy for prostate carcinoma. Int J Rad Oncol Biol Phys 2000; 46:839-850.

5. Blasko JC, Ragde H, Grimm PD. Transperineal Ultrasound-Guided Implantation of the Prostate: Morbidity and Complications. Scand J Urol Nephrol Suppl 1991; 137:113-118.

6. Choi S, Wallner KE, Merrick G, Butler W. Treatment margins predict biochemical outcomes after prostate brachytherapy. Cancer Journal (Scientific American) 2004; 10:175-180.

7. Clarke DH, Banks SJ, Wiederhorn AR, et al. The role of endorectal coil MRI in patient selection and treatment planning for prostate seed implants. Int J Rad Oncol Biol Phys 2001; in press.

8. Critz F. Summary of simultaneous irradiation for prostate cancer. Urology 2004; 64:633-636.

9. D'Amico AV, Whittington R, Malkowicz SB, Schultz D. Critical analysis of the ability of the endorectal coil magnetic resonance imaging scan to predict pathologic stage, margin status, and postoperative prostate-specific antigen failure in patients with clinically organ-confined prostate cancer. J Clin Oncol 1996; 14:1770-1777.

10. Dattoli M, Wallner K, True L, Cash J, Sorace R. Long-term outcomes following EBRT + Pd-103 for higher risk prostatic carcinoma: influence of prostatic acid phosphatase. Cancer 2003; 97:979-983.

11. Davis BJ, Haddock MG, Wilson TM, al e. Treatment of extraprostatic cancer in clinically organ-confined prostate cancer by permanent intersititial brachytherapy: Is extraprostatic seed placement necessary? Techniques in Urology 2000; 6:70-77.

12. Engeler CE, Wasserman NF, Zhang G. Preoperative assessment of prostatic carcinoma by computerized tomography: Weakness and new perspectives. Urol 1992; 40:346-350.

13. Epstein JI, Carmichael M, Walsh PC. Adenocarcinoma of the prostate invading the seminal vesicle: definition and relation of tumor volume, grade and margins of resection to prognosis. J Urol 1993; 149:1040-1045.

14. Epstein JI, Carmichael MJ, Pizov G, Walsh PC. Influence of capsular penetration on progression following radical prostatectomy: A study of 196 cases with long-term followup. J Urol 1993; 150:135-141.

15. Gelblum DY, Potters L. Rectal complications associated with transperineal interstitial brachytherapy for prostate cancer. Int J Rad Oncol Biol Phys 2000; 48:119-124.

16. Ghaly M, Wallner K, Merrick G, et al. The effect of supplemental beam radiation on prostate brachytherapy-related morbidity: Morbidity outcomes from two prospective randomized multicenter trials. Int J Rad Oncol Biol Phys 2003; 55:1288-1293.

17. Han B, Wallner K. Dosimetric and radiographic correlates to prostate brachytherapy-related rectal complications. International Journal of Cancer 2002; 96:372-378.

18. Kaye KW, Olson DJ, Payne JT. Detailed preliminary analysis of 125 iodine implantation for localized prostate cancer using percutaneous approach. J Urol 1995; 153:1020-1025.

19. Kestin LL, Vicini FA, Ziaja EL, Stromberg JS, Frazier RC, Martinez AA. Defining biochemical cure for prostate carcinoma patients treated with external beam radiation therapy. Cancer 1999; 86:1557-1566.

20. Kollmeier M, Stock RG, Stone NN. Biochemical outcomes after prostate brachytherapy with 5-year minimal follow-up: Importance of patient selection and implant quality. Int J Rad Oncol Biol Phys 2003; 57:645-653.

21. Kravchick S, Cytron S, Peled R, London D, Sibi Y, Ben-dor D. Optimal combinations for detection of prostate cancer: Systematic sextant and laterally directed biopsies versus systematic sextan and color dopplar-targeted biopsies. Urology 2004; 63:301-305.

22. Leibel SA, Fuks Z, Zelefsky MJ, Whitmore W. The effects of local and regional treatment on the metastatic outcome in prostatic carcinoma with pelvic lymph node involvement. Int J Rad Oncol Biol Phys 1993; 28:7-16.

23. Lu J. Statistical aspects of evaluating treatment and prognostic factors for clinically localized prostate cancer. Seminars in Urol Oncol 2000; 18:83-92.

24. Martinez A, Gustafson G, Gonzales J, et al. Dose escalation using conformal high-dose-rate brachytherapy improves outcome in unfavorable prostate cancer. Int J Rad Oncol Biol Phys 2002; 53:316-327.

25. Merrick G, Bulter W, Wallner K, et al. The importance of radiation doses to the penile bulb vs. crura in the development of postbrachytherapy erectil dysfunction. Int J Rad Oncol Biol Phys 2002; 54:1055-1062.

26. Merrick G, Butler W, Wallner K, Galbreath R, Kurko BS, Cleavinger S. Long-term urinary quality of life following permanent prostate brachytherapy. Brachytherapy 2003; 2:147-157.

27. Merrick G, Wallner K, Butler W, et al. Brachytherapy in men aged ″54 years with clinically localized prostate cancer. BJU International 2006; 98:324-328.

28. Merrick GS, Butler WM, Wallner KE, Burden LR, Dougherty JE. Extracapsular dose distribution following permanent prostate brachytherapy. Am J Clin Onc 2003; 26:178-189.
29. Ohori M, Wheeler TM, Kattan MW, Goto Y. Prognostic significance of positive surgical margins in radical prostatectomy specimens. J Urol 1995; 154:1818-1824.
30. Orio P, Wallner K, Merrick G, et al. Dosimetric parameters as predictive factors for biochemical control in patients with higher risk prostate cancer treated with Pd-103 and supplemental beam radiation. Int J Rad Oncol Biol Phys 2007; 67:342-346.
31. Orton CG, Webber BM. Time-dose factor (TDF) analysis of dose rate effects in permanent implant dosimetry. Int J Radiat Oncol Biol Phys 1977; 2:55-60.
32. Partin AW, Kattan MW, Subong ENP, Walsh PC. Combination of prostate-specific antigen, clinical stage, and Gleason score to predict pathological stage of localized prostate cancer. JAMA 1997; 277:1445-1451.
33. Pilepich M, Krall J, Sause W, et al. Prognostic factors in carcinoma of the prostate: analysis of RTOG 75-06. Int J Rad Oncol Biol Phys 1987; 13:339-349.
34. Platt JF, Bree RL, Schwab RE. The accuracy of CT in the staging of carcinoma of the prostate. American Journal of Radiology 1987; 149:315-318.
35. Prestidge BR, Hoak DC, Grimm PD, Ragde H, Cavanagh W, Blasko JC. Posttreatment biopsy results following interstitial brachytherapy in early-stage prostate cancer. Int J Radiat Oncol Biol Phys 1997; 37:31-39.
36. Rifkin MD, Zerhouni EA, Gatsonis CA, Quint LE. Comparison of magnetic resonance imaging and ultrasonography in staging early prostate cancer. NEJM 1990; 323:621-626.
37. Roach M, DeSilvio M, Valicenti R, et al. Whole-pelvis, "mini-pelvis," or prostate-only external beam radiotherapy after neoadjuvant and concurrent hormonal therapy in patients treated in the Radiation Therapy Oncology Group 9413 trial. Int J Rad Oncol Biol Phys 2006; 66:647-653.
38. Sakr WA, Wheeler TM, Blute M, al e. Workgroup 2: Staging and reporting of prostate cancer*sampling of the radical prostatectomy specimen. Cancer 1996; 78:366-368.
39. Sattar AA, Noel J-C, Vanderhaeghen J-J, Schulman CC, Wespes E. Prostate capsule: Computerized morphometric analysis of its components. Urol 1995; 46:178-181.

40. Schiebler ML, Schnall M, Pollack HM, al e. Current role of MR imaging in the staging of of adenocarcinoma of the prostate. Radiol 1993; 189:339.
41. Sharkey J, Chovnick SD, Behar RJ, Perez R, al e. Minimally invasive treatment for localized adenocarcinoma of the prostate: Review of 1048 patients treated with ultrasound-guided palladium-103 brachytherapy. J Endourol 2000; 14:343-350.

42. Sohayda C, Kupelian PA, Levin JS, Klein EA. Extent of extracapsular extension in localized prostate cancer. Urol 2000; 55:382-386.
43. Stock RG, Lo Y, Gaildon M, Stone NN. Does prostate brachytherapy treat the seminal vesicles: A dose-volume histogram analysis of seminal vesicles in patients undergoing combined Pd-103 prostate implantation and external beam irradiation. Int J Rad Oncol Biol Phys 1999; 45:385-389.
44. Teh B, Bastasch M, Mai W, Butler E, Wheeler TM. Predictors of extracapsular extension and its radial distance in prostate cancer: Implications for prostate IMRT, brachytherapy, and surgery. Cancer J 2003; 9:454-460.
45. Theodorescu D, Frierson H, Sikes R. Molecular determination of surgical margins using fossa biopsies at radical prostatectomy. J Urology 1999; 161:1442-1448.
46. Thomas PRM, Tefft M, Compaan PJ, al e. Results of two radiation therapy randomizations in the third National Wilms' Tumor Study. Cancer 1991; 68:1703.
47. Wallner K, Merrick G, True L, et al. 20 Gy versus 44 Gy supplemental beam radiation with Pd-103 prostate brachytherapy:Early biochemical outcomes from a prospective randomized multi-center trial. Radiother and Oncol 2005; 75:307-310.

14

Hormonal therapy

It has long been known that removing androgen stimulation shrinks prostate cancer, primarily through enhanced apoptosis.(SHARIFI) Surgical castration, DES, LHRH agonists and anti-androgens have all been used extensively for clinical hormonal ablation (**Table 14-1**). The various methods of androgen ablation are similarly effective at decreasing prostate volume, but with varying side effects.

RATIONALE FOR ADJUVANT HORMONAL THERAPY

There are two rationales for combining androgen deprivation with brachytherapy—physical and biologic. Decreasing the prostate size

Table 14-1. Hormonal therapies.

Drug class	agents	site of action	mechanism
gonadotropin-releasing hormone (GnRH) agonists	leuprolide (Lupron) goserelin (Zolodex)	anterior pituitary	down regulation of GnRH receptors
androgen receptor antagonists	fluamide (Eulexin) bicalutamide (Casodex) nilutamide (Nilandron)	prostate glands	inhibits intracellular androgen binding
5 alpha-reductase inhibitors	finasteride (Proscar) duasteride (Avodart)	prostate glands	decreased conversion of testosterone to DHT

decreases the volume of rectum, bladder, and small bowel receiving beam radiation.(ZELEFSKY, FORMAN) The same should hold true for brachytherapy rectal wall doses, conceivably decreasing the risk of complications.(WATERMAN) Additional physical advantages to implanting a hormonally downsized prostate include easier access to the anterior prostate in patients for

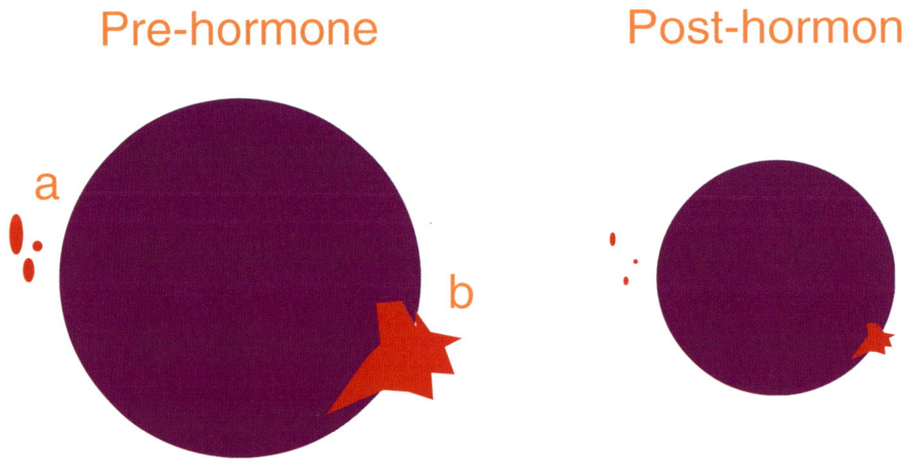

Figure 14-1. The physical effect of hormonal therapy on the degree of extraprostatic cancer extension (ECE) depends on which scenario, **a** *or* **b***, occurs in vivo. If cancer shrinks but remains at a given distance from the prostatic margin, hormonal therapy won't increase the likelihood of eradicating early EPE. However, if the radial extent of cancer decreases (scenario* **b***), adjuvant hormonal therapy could increase the likelihood of ECE eradication.*

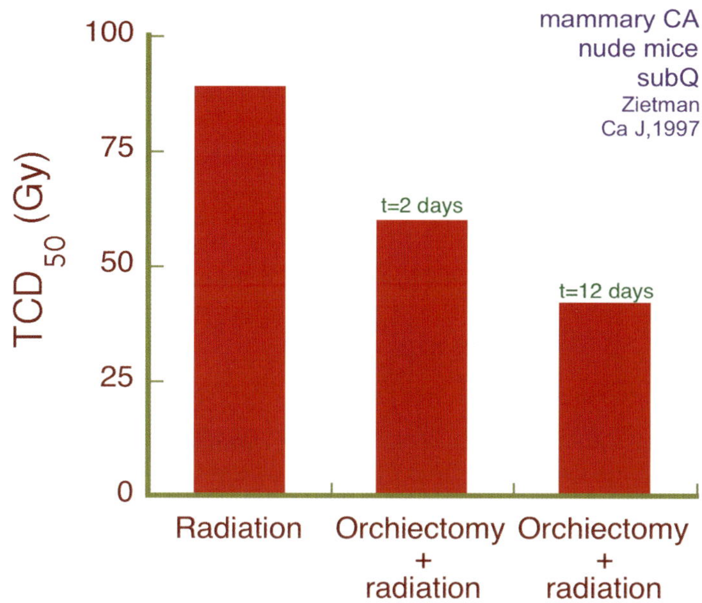

Figure 14-2. Radiation dose required to control 50 percent of androgen-dependent mammary tumors in mice. The hormonal sensitizing effect was greater if more time elapsed between orchiectomy and radiation, possibly due to continued tumor shrinkage with longer antiandrogen effect. (t = time between orchiectomy and radiation)(ZIETMAN)

whom pubic arch interference would otherwise be a problem, and a reduction in the number of seeds needed.

Perhaps the most clinically important potential advantage of hormonally down-sizing the prostate is the possibility that it could facilitate eradication of extracapsular cancer extension (ECE), if the shrinkage means that ECE retracts back toward the prostatic margin (**Figure 14-1**). However, there arae no studies regarding the effect of hormonal therapy on the magnitude of EPE.

In addition to the potential for physical advantages to hormonal downsizing, hormonal deprivation *may* enhance radiation sensitivity. Adjuvant therapy could favorably alter the oxygen milieu of prostate cancer.(RIPPLE) Zietman and colleagues showed that hormonal deprivation increases the

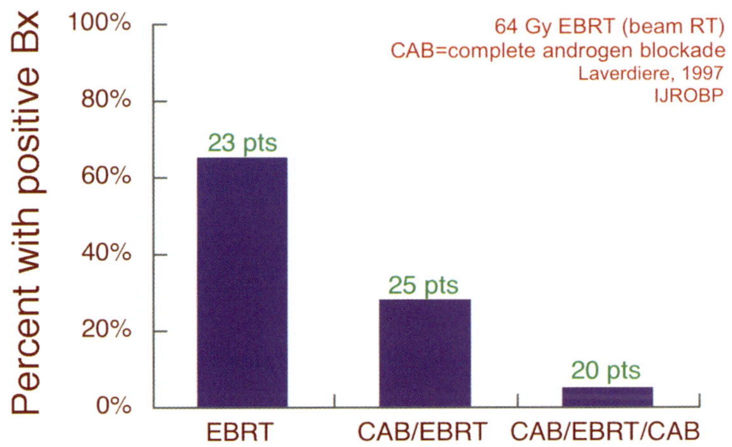

Figure 14-3. Positive biopsy rates after 64 Gy external beam radiation alone, beam radiation preceded by three months androgen blockade, or beam preceded (three months) and followed (six months) by androgen blockade.(LAVERDIERE)

radiation sensitivity of androgen-dependent mammary tumors, carried in nude mice.(ZIETMAN) The radiation sensitivity enhancement was most marked if hormonal deprivation was complete more than 48 hours prior to radiation, possibly due to greater volume reduction (**Figure 14-2**). While Zietman and colleagues are to be congratulated for bringing some scientific rigor to the exploration of the biologic effect of hormonal manipulation, the clinical relevance of their experiments in a subcutaneous, transplantable mouse mammary tumor to human prostate cancer is uncertain.

Laverdiere and colleagues reported that androgen blockade decreases the likelihood of a positive biopsy after conventional dose external beam radiation.(LAVERDIERE) The effect was most marked if androgen blockade was continued for six months after completion of external radiation (**Figure 14-3**). The findings seem compelling but might be another example of temporary cancer suppression, without a real change in the cure rate. Longer biochemical follow-up should clarify this issue. The general applicability of Laverdiere's work is hampered by the small patient numbers and incomplete follow-up biopsies.

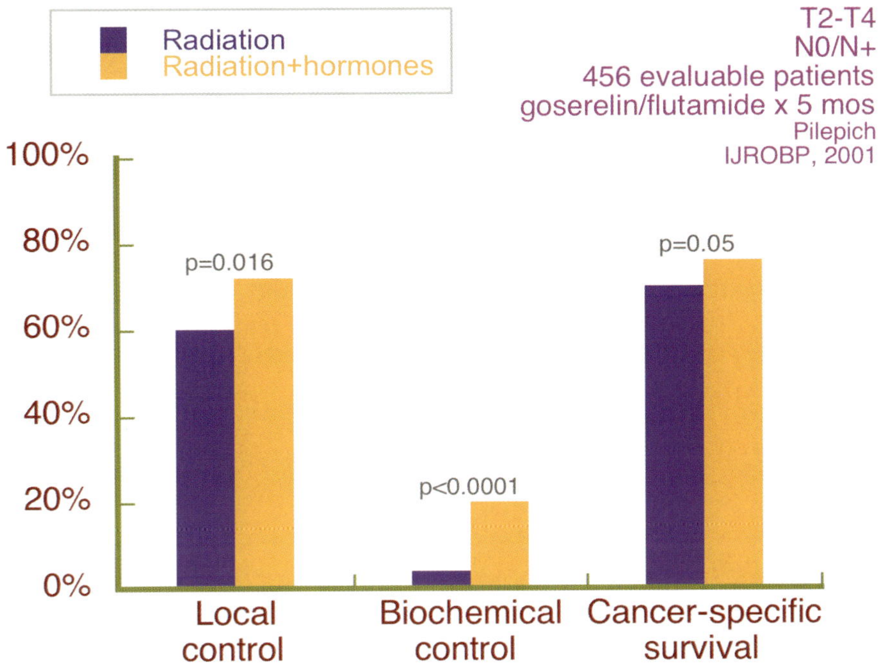

Figure 14-4. Typical of adjuvant hormonal therapy, patients with locally advanced tumors treated with 65-70 Gy ±hormone showed progressively smaller improvements in local, biochemical and disease-specific survival, respectively.

Two large randomized RTOG clinical trials of hormonal ablation combined with radiation have shown a benefit in terms of suppressing overt metastases, but no difference in survival (**Figure 14-4**).(PILEPICH 97 & 95) The most likely explanation is that androgen ablation suppresses the clinical, biochemical, and pathologic evidence of cancer after beam radiation, but does not enhance tumor eradication. This explanation would be consistent with multiple negative surgical trials demonstrating a lower positive margin incidence but no change in cancer-free survival with pre-surgical hormonal ablation.(KLOTZ)

To date, three studies has shown a survival benefit with adjuvant hormonal therapy and external beam radiation.(BOLLA, D'AMICO, PILEPICH) In the EORTC trial, patients with clinical stage T3-T4 (any histology) or high grade T2 tumors had a statistically significant improvement in five year

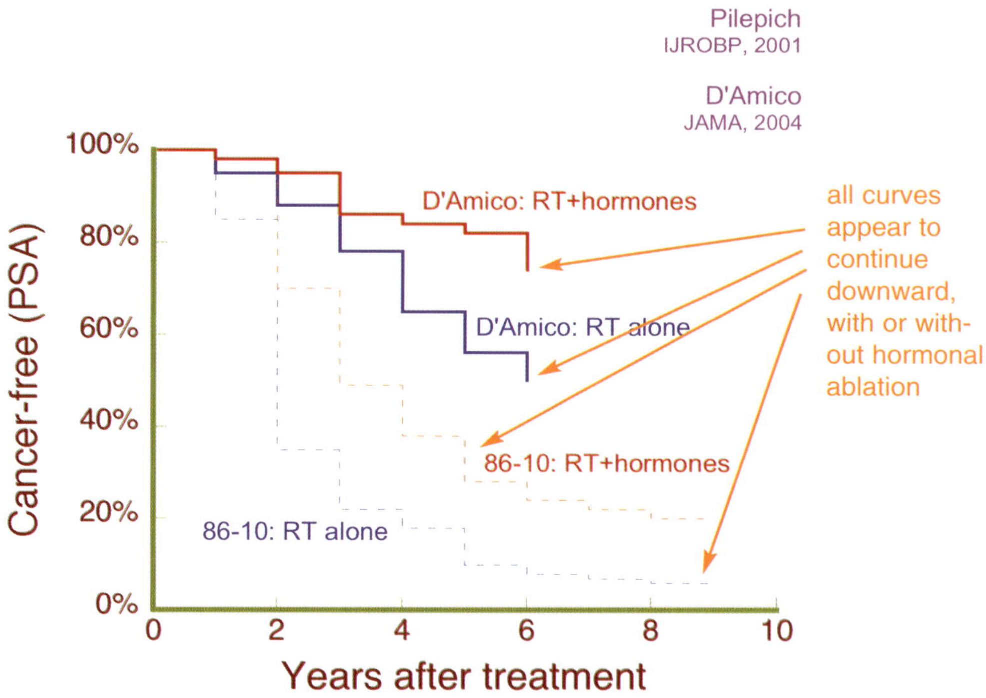

Figure 14-5. Although clinically evident tumor recurrence is delayed with hormonal deprivation, there is no apparent plateau on the disease-free survival curves, raising the question of whether or not hormonal therapy actually increases the likelihood of cure.

overall and disease-free survival. These EORTC findings have been criticized partly because more than 25 percent of the adjuvant patients were still receiving hormonal therapy at the time of the analysis.

D'Amico and colleagues randomized 206 patients to 70 Gy EBRT with or without six months of androgen ablation. They showed a reduction in death from prostate cancer at five years following treatment. While statistically significant, the number of events was very small—six prostate cancer related deaths in the control arm versus none in the androgen ablation arm. Additionally, the 70 Gy beam radiation given was low, even by standards at the time the trial was conducted (1995-2001), so that its relevance to modern doses typically used for intermediate to high-risk patients is unclear.

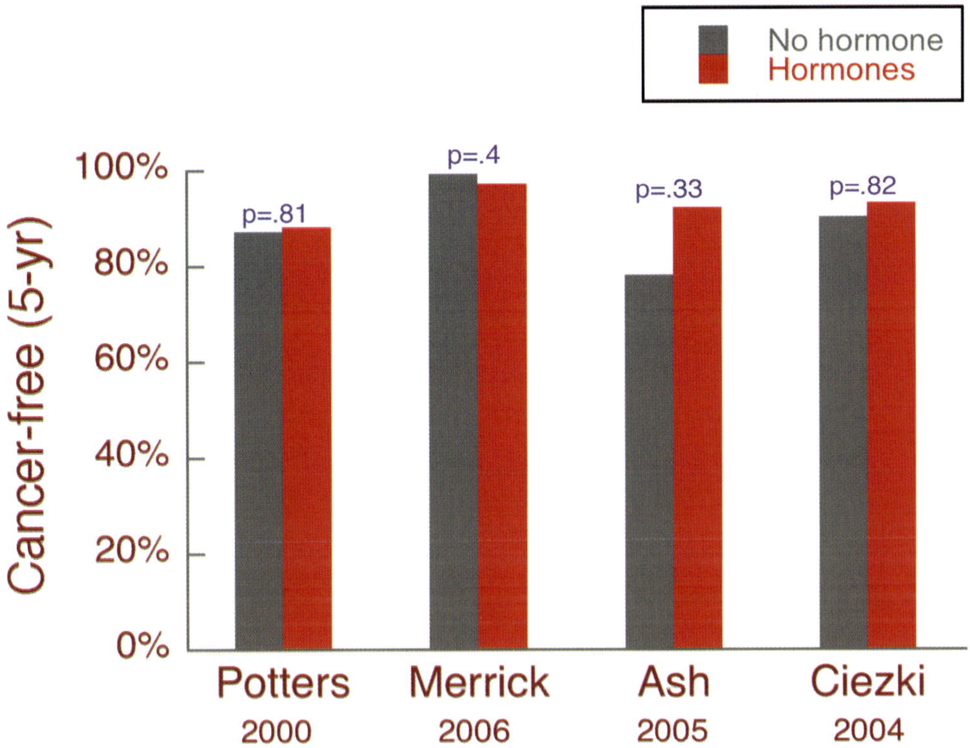

Figure 14-6. Retrospective studies of hormonal ablation in low risk brachytherapy patients.

Roach and colleagues randomized 1,292 eligible patients to four treatment arms, two of which included whole pelvic radiation and two of which included neoadjuvant or adjuvant hormonal therapy. The neoadjuvant hormonal therapy arm with whole pelvic had the lowest likelihood of death from prostate cancer, but the absolute differences were small. Nonetheless, the trial has renewed some clinicians' flagging enthusiasm for whole pelvic radiation and hormonal therapy in high risk patients.(ROACH)

Probably the biggest problem with most radiation + hormone trials has been the lack of a clear plateau and the survival curves (**Figure 14-5**). This lack of a plateau suggests that the ultimate cancer control rates will be very low within the patient groups treated with beam radiation, with or without hormonal ablation. Such low cancer eradication rates, even in major centers, has to make one question whether beam radiation, without

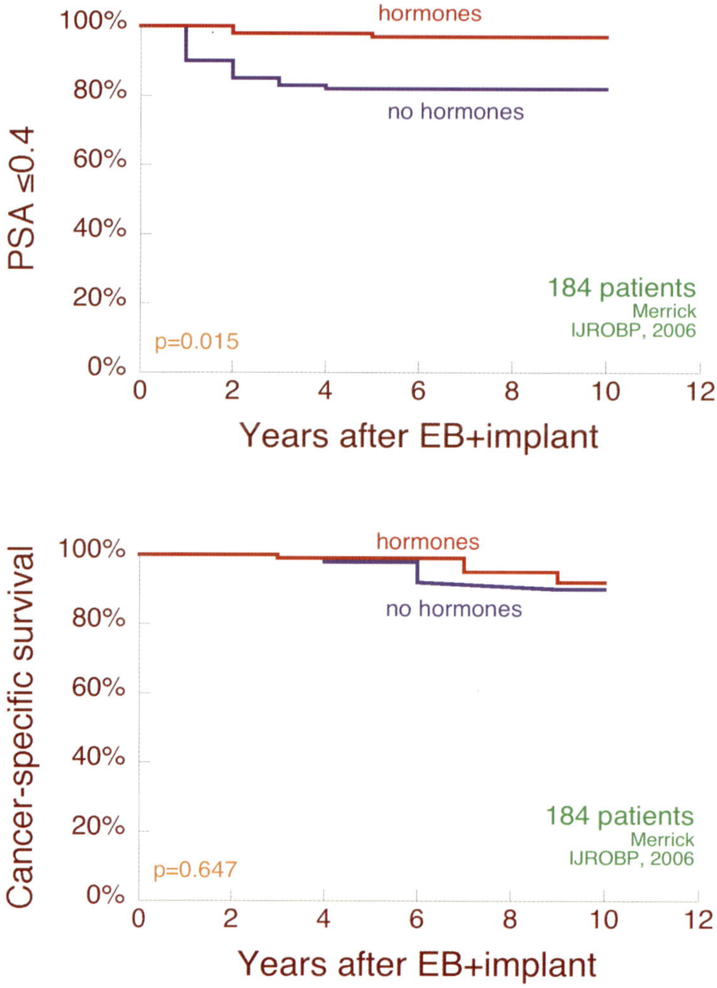

Figure 14-7. Biochemical versus cause-specific survival for high risk paitents.(Merrick 06).

brachytherapy, is such a good idea for patients with more locally advanced cancers.

CLINICAL STUDIES WITH BRACHYTHERAPY

There are no *in vitro*, *in vivo*, or controlled clinical studies regarding the effect of hormonal ablation on brachytherapy radiation sensitivity. Retrospective clinical studies have shown little benefit in low-risk patients (**Figure 14-6**).

Favorable results in uncontrolled studies of higher-risk brachytherapy patients receiving combined androgen blockade may be explained by bet-

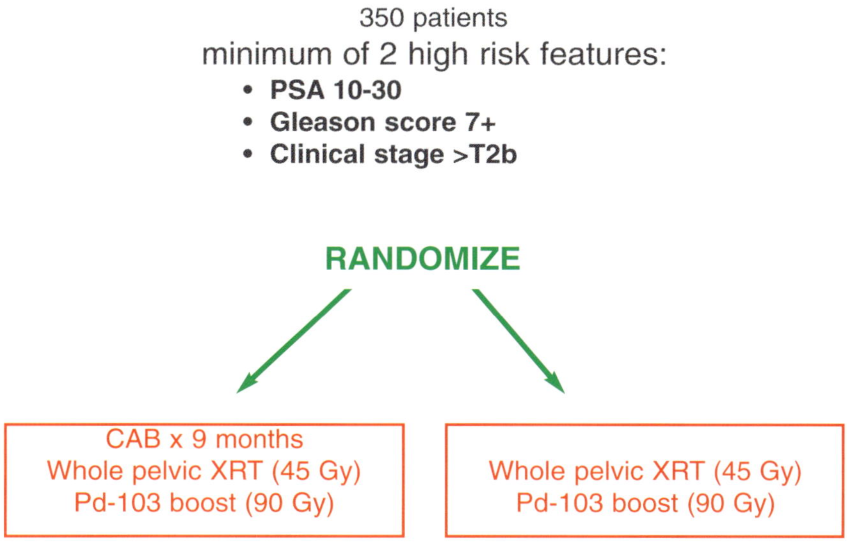

*Figure 14-8. Ongoing prospective randomized study of hormonal ablation with brachytherapy-based treatment.(*MERRICK*)*

ter local control with brachytherapy, rather than adjuvant hormonal therapy.(SYLVESTER, COPP) A retrospective, matched-pair analysis of implant patients by Potters and colleagues showed no difference in biochemical freedom from relapse in patients with or without androgen deprivation prior to brachytherapy, regardless of PSA or Gleason score.(POTTERS) The same was reported by Dattoli and colleagues for patients with locally advanced disease.(DATTOLI 03) Merrick and colleagues showed an hormone therapy-related improvement in freedom from biochemical failure only in high risk patients (**Figure 14-7**).(MERRICK 06)

Based largely on subgroup analysis of RTOG 85-31 and a prospective randomized trial using inadequate beam radiation, many otherwise rational oncologists are convinced that adjuvant hormonal therapy enhances cure in patients with higher risk disease.(D'AMICO 04, LAWTON 05) To test the use of hormonal therapy with adequate local radiation, Merrick and colleagues have begun accruing 350 high risk patients (PSA 10-30 ng/ml and Gleason score $\geq$7) to a randomized trial of 45 Gy whole pelvic radiation and a Pd boost, with or without six months of androgen ablation (**Figure 14-8**).

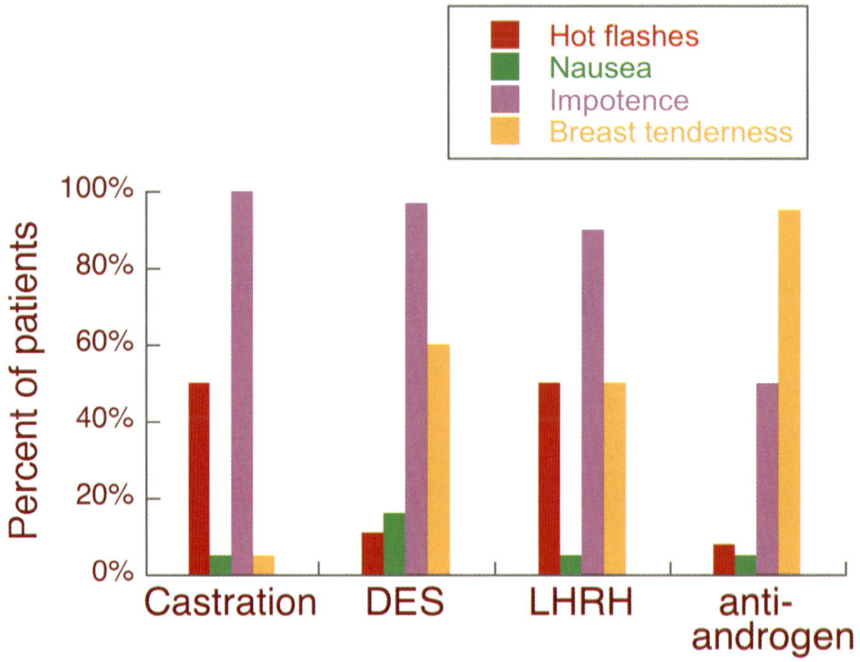

Figure 14-9. Side effects of the various hormone treatments are generally similar.(COX, SMITH, LEUPROLIDE STUDY GROUP)

MORBIDITY FROM HORMONAL THERAPY

While its affect on cancer eradication continues to be studied, it has become clearer that long-term hormonal therapy has the potential for substantial adverse effects. In addition to the long-appreciated side effects (**Figure 14-9**) a potential for fatigue, osteopenia, muscle weakness, anemia and cognitive impairment associated wtih prolonged androgen ablation are becoming better described (**Table 14-2**).(SHARIFI)

Additionally, it has been amply documented that the effects of LHRH use extend far beyond the nominal activity duration. Only about half of patients will return to pre-therapy androgen levels by 12 months after discontinuing therapy. Almost a third are still suppressed three years after stopping their medication (**Figure 14-10**). Better appreciation of the adverse effects and the true duration of hormonal therapy is spurring efforts to use it in less harmful ways. Two areas of clinical interest include limiting the duration of

Table 14-2. Adverse effects of androgen ablation. (Sharifi)

hot flashes
decreased bone denstify
impotence
anemia
increased BMI
increased cholesterol
glucose intolerance
mood changes, depression
decreased cognitive function

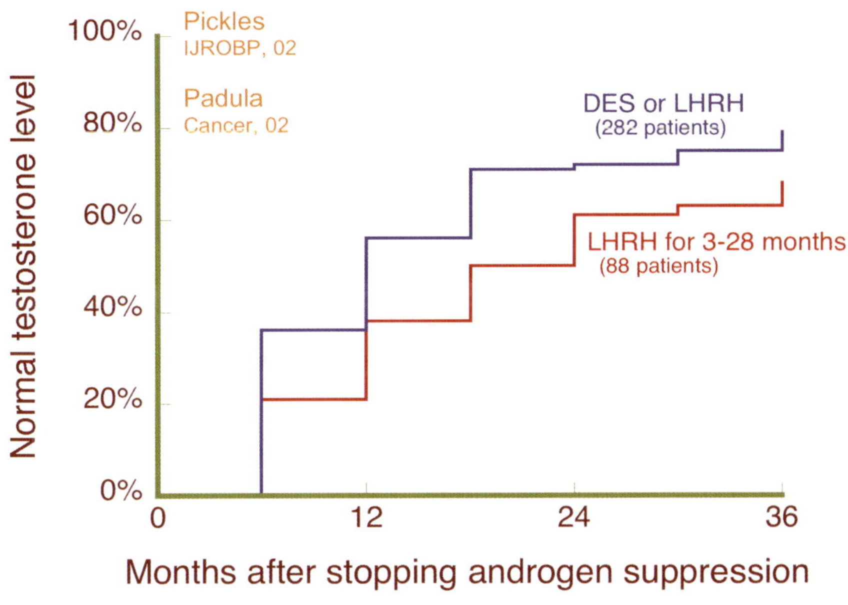

Figure 14-10. Prolonged time to normalization of testosterone in the majority of patients treated witth adjuvant DES or LHRH androgen suppression.

ablation, and substituting anti-androgens for LHRH agonists.(SHARIFI, MERRICK 06)

REFERENCES

1. Ash D, Al-Qaisieh B, Bottomley D, Carey B, Joseph J. The correlation between D90 and ooutcome for I-125 seed implant monotherapy for localized prostate cancer. Radiother and Oncol 2006; 79:185-189.
2. Bolla M, Collette L, Blank L. Long-term results with immediate androgen suppression and external irradiation in patients with locally advanced prostate cancer (an EORTC study): A phase III randomized trial. Lancet 2002; 360:103-106.
3. Ciezki J, Klein E, Angermeier K, et al. A retrospective comparisoin of androgen deprivation (AD) vs no AD among low-risk patients treated with brachytherapy, external beam radiotherpy, or radical prostatectomy. Int J Rad Oncol Biol Phys 2004; 60:1347-1350.
4. Copp H, Bissonette E, Theodorescu D. Tumor control outcomes of patients tretaed with trimodality therapy for locally advanced prostate cancer. Urology 2005; 65:1146-1151.
5. Cox R, Crawford E. Estrogens in the treatment of prostate cancer. J Urol 1995; 154:1991-1998.
6. D'Amico A, Manola J, Loffredo M, Renshaw A, DellaCroce A, Kantoff P. 6-month androgen suppression plus radiation therapy alone for patients with clincally localized prostate cancer: A randomized controlled trial. JAMA 2004; 292:821-827.
7. Forman JD, Kumar R, Haas G, Montie J. Neoadjuvant hormonal downsizing of localized carcinoma of the prostate: Effects on the volume of normal tissue irradiation. Ca Invest 1995; 13:8-15.
8. Group LS. Leuprolide versus diethylstibestrol for metastatic prostate cancer. N Eng J Med 1984; 311:1281-1286.
9. Klotz LH, Goldenberg SL, Jewett M, Barkin J, al e. CUOG randomized trial of neoadjuvant androgen ablation before radical prostatectomy: 36-month post-treatment PSA results. Urol 1999; 53:757-763.
10. Laverdiere J, Gomez JL, Cusan L, Suburu ER. Beneficial effect of combination hormonal therapy administered prior and following external beam radiation therapy in localized prostate cancer. Int J Rad Oncol Biol Phys 1997; 37:247-252.

11. Lawton C, Winter K, Grignon D, Pilepich M. Androgen suppression plus radiation versus radiation alone for patients with Stage D1/pathologic node-positive adenocrcinoma of the prostate: updated results based on

national prospective radnomized trial Radiation Therapy Oncology Group 85-31. J Clin Oncol 2005; 23:800-807.
12. Merrick G, Butler W, Wallner K, Galbreath R, Allen Z, Adamovich E. Androgen-deprivation therapy dies not impact cause-specific or overall survival after permanent prostate brachytherapy. Int J Rad Oncol Biol Phys 2006; 65:669-677.
13. Padula G, Zelefsky MJ, Venkaatraman ES, et al. Normalization of serum testosterone levels in patients treated with neoadjuvant hormonal therapy and three-dimensional conformal radiotherapy for prostate cancer. Int J Rad Oncol Biol Phys 2002; 52:439-443.
14. Pickles T, Agranovich A, Berthelet E, et al. Testosterone recovery following prlonged adjuvant androgen ablation for prostate carcinoma. Cancer 2000; 94:362-367.
15. Pilepich M, Winter K, John M, et al. Phase III Radiation Therapy Onolocy Group (RTOG) trial 86-10 of androgen deprivation adjuvant to defiinitive radiotherapy in locally advanced carcinoma of the prostate. Int J Rad Oncol Biol Phys 2001; 50:1243-1252.
16. Pilepich MV, Caplan R, Byhardt RW, Lawton CA. Phase III trial of androgen suppression using goserelin in unfavorable-prognosis carcinoma of the prostate treated with definitive radiotherapy: Report of Radiation Therapy Oncology Group Protocol 85-31. J Clin Oncol 1997; 15:1013-1021.
17. Pilepich MV, Sause WT, Shipley WU, Krall JM. Androgen deprivation with radiation therapy compared with radiation therapy alone for locally advanced prostatic carcinoma: A randomized comparative trial of the Radiation Therapy Oncology Group. Urol 1995; 45:616-623.
18. Potters L, Torre T, Ashley R, al e. Examining the role of neoadjuvant androgen deprivation in patients undergoing prostate brachytherapy. J Clin Oncol 2000; 18:1187-1192.
19. Ripple M, Henry W, Rago R, Wilding G. Prooxidant-antioxidant shift induced by androgen treatment of humna prostate carcinoma cells. J National Cancer Inst 1997; 89:40-48.
20. Roach M, DeSilvio M, Valicenti R, et al. Whole-pelvis, "mini-pelvis," or prostate-only external beam radiotherapy after neoadjuvant and concurrent hormonal therapy in patients treated in the Radiation Therapy Oncology Group 9413 trial. Int J Rad Oncol Biol Phys 2006; 66:647-653.
21. Sharifi N, Gulley J, Dahut W. Androgen deprivation therapy for prostate cancer. JAMA 2005; 294:238-244.

22. Smith M, Goode M, Zietman A, McGovern F, Lee H, Finkelstein J. Bicalutamide monotherapy versus leuporolide monotherapy for prostate cancer: Effects on bone mineral density and body composition. J Clin Oncol 2004; 22:2546-2553.

23. Sylvester J, Blasko JC, Grimm PD, al e. Neoadjuvant androgen ablation combined with external-beam radiation therapy and permanent interstitial brachytherapy boost in localized prostate cancer. Molecular Urology 2000; 3:231-236.

24. Zelefsky MJ, Leibel SA, Burman CM, Kutcher GJ. Neoadjuvant hormonal therapy improves the therapeutic ratio in patients with bulky prostatic cancer treated with three-dimensional conformal radiation therapy. Int J Radiat Oncol Biol Phys 1994; 29:755-761.

25. Zietman AL, Nakfoor BM, Prince EA, Gerweck LE. The effect of androgen deprivation and radiation therapy on an androgen-sensitive murine tumor: An in vitro and in vivo study. Ca J 1997; 3:31-36.

15

Who Can't Have One

> **Stupidity alert!**
> Published patient selection recommendations for brachytherapy include some great examples of baseless physician recommendations.(HAKENBERG)

There is no question that certain patients are not good candidates for brachytherapy. Particular pre-treatment conditions *may* predispose patients to implant-related problems. Unfortunately, we still lack a reliable set of criteria to determine beforehand who is going to develop trouble. Age, prostate size, and urinary obstructive symptoms are among myriad alleged selection criteria (**Table 15-1**). However, currently perceived criteria are generally based on physicians' assumptions rather than an objective look at the data. A lack of data has fueled the proliferation of opinions regarding contraindications to brachytherapy (**Figure 15-1**). This predisposition of physicians to make recommendations in the absence of data

Table 15-1. Alledged contraindications to brachytherapy.

- young age
- pubic arch interference
- risk of urinary retention
- high AUA score
- prostate volume
- prior prostatitis
- penile prosthesis
- median lobe hypertrophy
- adverse pathologic features on biopsy
- prostatic calculi
- obesity
- inflammatory bowel disease
- prior pelvic surgery
- prior radiation

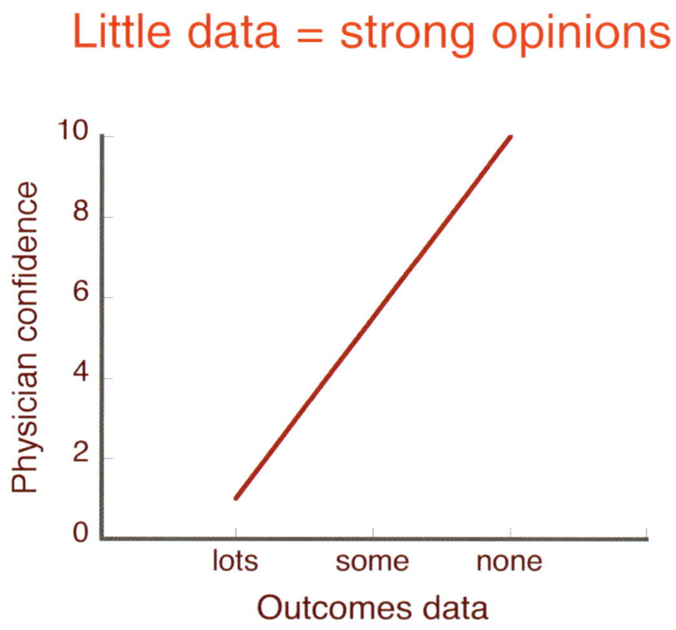

Figure 15-1. Lack of data has not impeded the proliferation of opinions regarding contraindications to prostate brachytherapy.

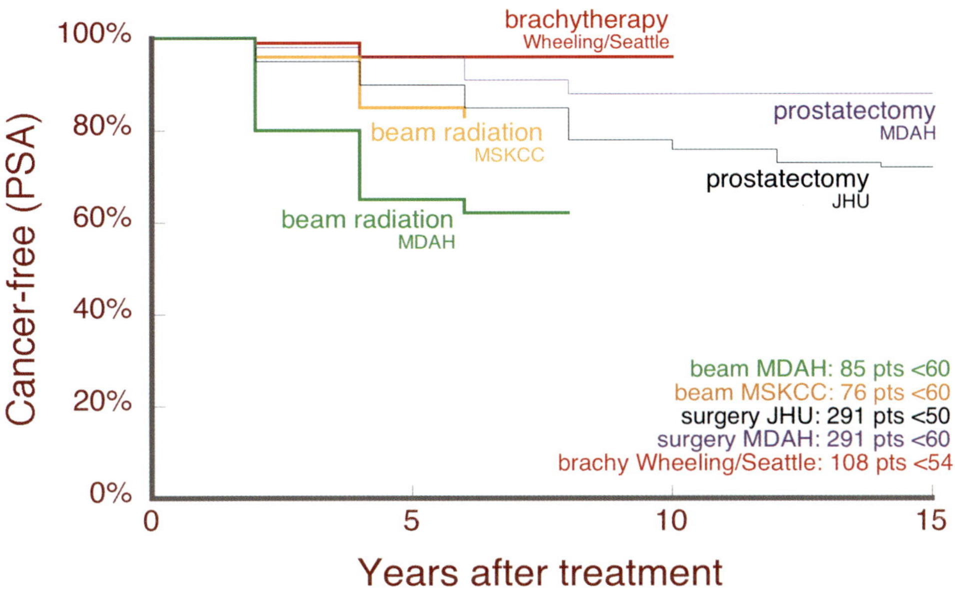

Figure 15-2. Likelihood of biochemical cancer control in younger patients treated with beam, brachy or prostatectomy at highly published centers. The patient mix in all series was primarily low risk, with a minority of higher-risk patients. The external beam series used ASTRO criteria for biochemical failure. The beam results would look even worse if absolute critiera were used, as was the case for the implant and prostatectomy series.(MERRICK, ROSSER 02, ZELEFSKY, KHAN, ROSSER 06)

can reach ridiculous extremes.(KOVACS, HAKENBERG) The next forty-some pages is a commonsensical review of the evidence (or lack thereof) regarding the validity of selection criteria.

AGE

There has been a reluctance among oncologists to recommend brachytherapy for younger patients, primarily due to the lack of long-term tumor control data. Overall, age itself has no consistent effect on the likelihood of cure following prostatectomy, brachytherapy or external beam radiation (**Figure 15-2**).(FREEDMAN, MERRICK 06, JOHNSTONE) D'Amico and colleagues have reported worse outcomes in elderly patients treated with external beam radiation for higher-risk cancer. Their results should be

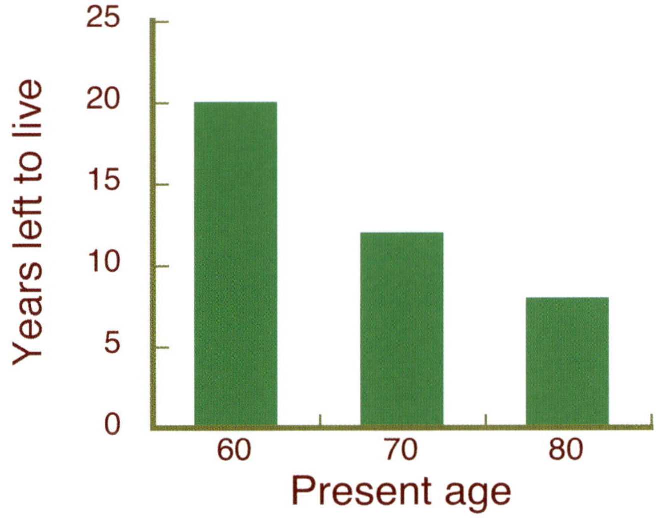

Figure 15-3. Approximate life expectancy for U.S. males versus present age.

interpreted cautiously, however, since their cancer control rates for all age groups were low compared to those achieved by most practitioners.(D'AMICO 02)

There has been some concern that younger patients, who are expected to live longer, may be at risk for secondary malignancies due to radiation exposure. To date, no excess incidence of radiation-related malignancies has been reported following retropubic implants from the 1970s, but longer follow-up data are needed to properly address this concern.(GUTMAN, MOON, LIAUW)

Another issue regarding brachytherapy and age is whether older patients will live long enough to benefit from eradication of prostate cancer. Because of its long natural history, patients with low-grade cancer or low PSA should have a life expectancy of ten years or more to justify treatment of their cancer. The *ten-year rule* is used because the likelihood of dying from low-grade, untreated prostate cancer is less than 10% at ten years, and probably even lower for patients with initial PSA less than 10 ng/ml.(ADOLFSSON) In reality, North American men in their 70s generally

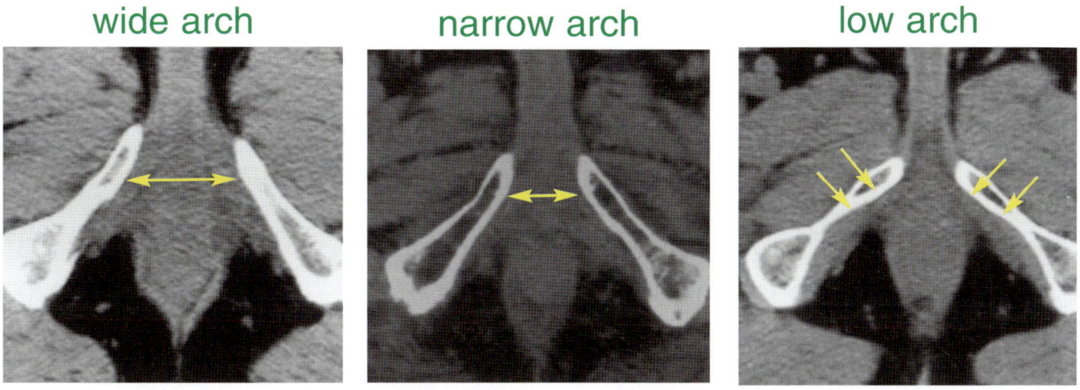

Figure 15-4. CT-based pubic arch visualization. The width of the arch is the distance between the medial aspects of the inferior pubic rami. Arch anatomy varies from narrow to wide. Some patients have a low-lying arch, whereby even if wide, it may interfere with placement of anterior needles.

have a life expectancy in excess of ten years, so that therapy for low-risk prostate cancer (PSA <10 ng/ml) is still reasonable (**Figure 15-3**). Patients with high-grade cancer or higher PSA at initial presentation are at risk of cancer death earlier and should be considered for treatment, even if their life expectancy is less than ten years. And before denying therapy to an elderly patient, keep in mind that we doctors are not all that adept at predicting longevity.(WILSON)

It is not clear whether older patients have any more or less difficulty with radiation prostatitis compared to younger men.

CLINICAL STAGE

Clinical stage has probably been one of the most misused parameters in the choice of treatment modality. It has been common misconception that brachytherapy should be limited to low stage patients—T1c and T2a. In fact, there is little correlation between clinical stage and pathological stage, except in the setting of obvious seminal vesicle invasion.(PHILIP)

PUBIC ARCH INTERFERENCE

Perhaps the most widely alleged contraindication to brachytherapy is pubic arch interference (PAI), whereby a relatively narrow pubic arch interferes with anterior needle insertion.(WALLNER 91, TINCHER) Pre-implant pelvic CT scans have been used to check for potential pubic arch interference, with

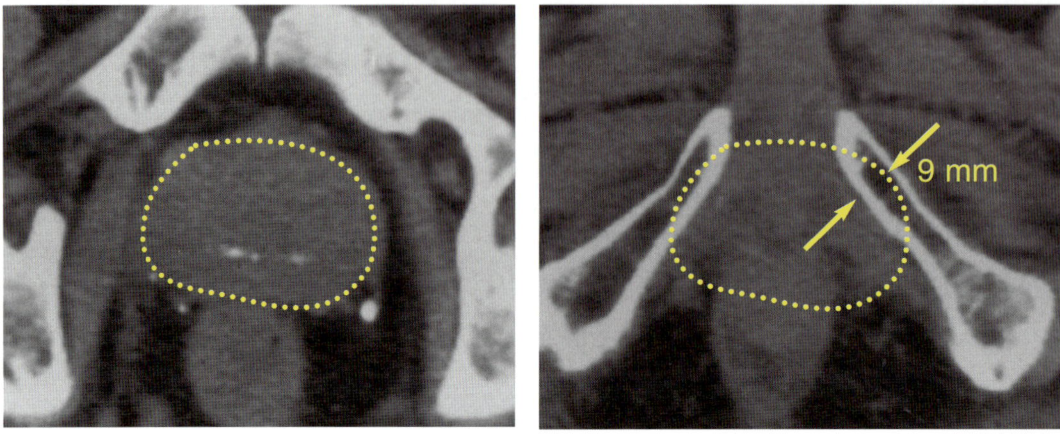

Figure 15-5. To assess the degree of pubic arch interference by CT, the largest prostate cross section is overlaid on the image with the narrowest-appearing pubic arch, using the CT scale as a registration point (not visible in figures here). This patient has 9 mm pubic arch interference.

the largest prostate cross section overlaid on the narrowest region of the arch (**Figure 15-4**). If there is substantial overlap of the pubic arch over the lateral or anterior prostate margins, it may be difficult to place needles in the shielded portion of the prostate using standard techniques. TRUS images can usually be substituted for CT-based arch assessment (**Figures 15-5 through 15-7**).(WALLNER 99)

In general, blockage of 25% of the prostate diameter, or blockage of more than 1 cm of prostate, has been considered excessive. Patients with this degree of interference have often been refused implantation, or given the option of pre-implant hormonal downsizing. But like nearly all alleged contraindications to prostate brachytherapy, there are limited data regarding the incidence and significance of PAI. Bellon and colleagues analyzed the pre-implant TRUS volumes and CT-based pubic arch studies of 97 unselected patients.(BELLON) As expected, there was considerable variability in pubic arch interference. Patients with larger prostate volumes generally had more pubic arch interference, but the degree of interference was only loosely related to the prostate volume (**Figure 15-8**). Even patients with very large prostate volumes are readily implantable, if they have a wide

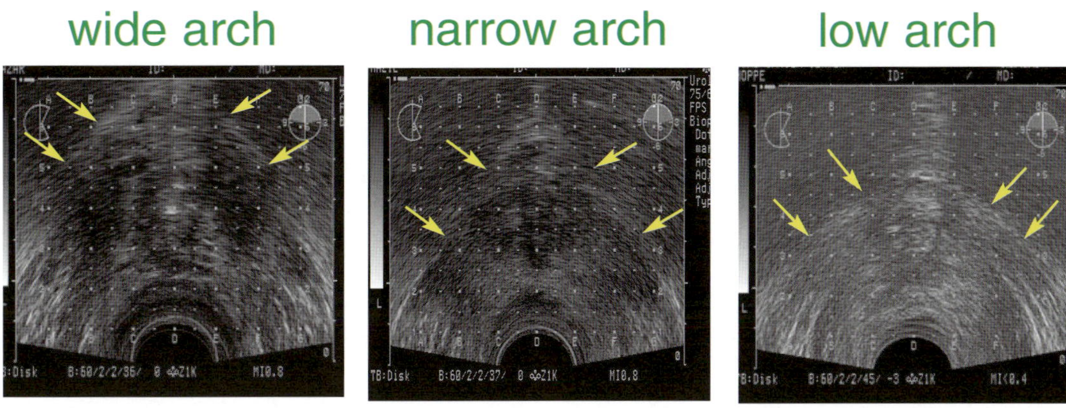

Figure 15-6. TRUS is usually adequate to assess the likelihood of pubic arch interference.

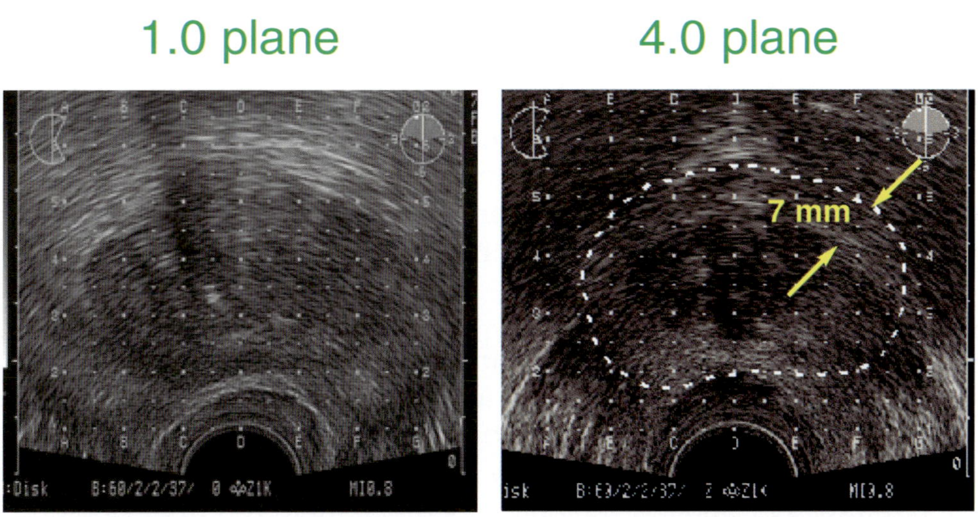

Figure 15-7. To assess the degree of pubic arch interference by TRUS, the largest prostate cross section (left) is overlaid on the image with the narrowest-appearing segment of pubic arch. This patient has 7 mm pubic arch interference.

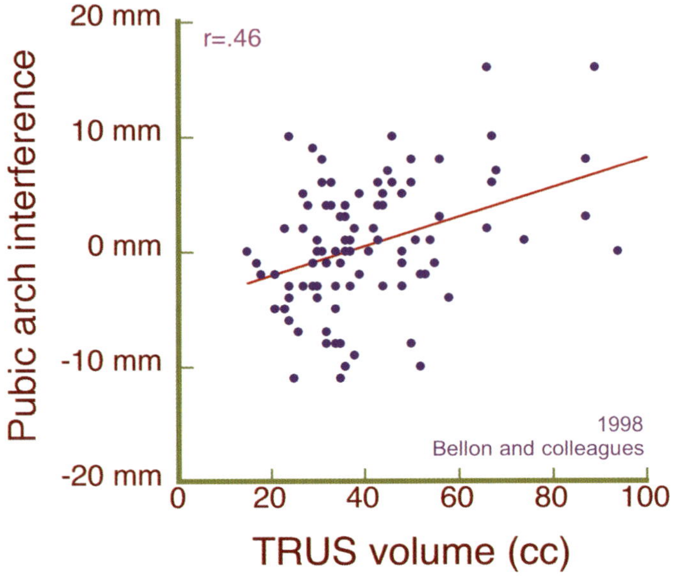

Figure 15-8. Prostate volume versus the degree of pubic arch interference.

pubic arch. Alternatively, some patients with very small prostate glands have substantial PAI, due to a very narrow pubic arch.

While the potential for pubic arch interference has received a lot of attention, its clinical significance is highly questionable. Several maneuvers, such as placing the patient in the extended lithotomy position or "steering" needles around the arch usually circumvents interference (see chapter 12). Using such strategies, nearly all patients can be implanted successfully by experienced clinicians, regardless of prostate size or the degree of PAI.

RISK OF URINARY RETENTION

Post-implant urinary retention is the most common acute morbidity of prostate brachytherapy, occurring in about 2% to 10% of patients (**Figure 15-9**). In most cases, retention lasts only a few days and is of no long-term consequence.(LANDIS, SHERERTZ) However, a small percentage of patients develop refractory retention, which might make them regret having chosen brachytherapy. Being able to identify those at high risk of refractory retention would be a big help in counseling prospective patients regarding their expected treatment-related complications. In fact, a dizzying array of criteria have been proposed as risk factors for urinary retention (**Table 15-2**).

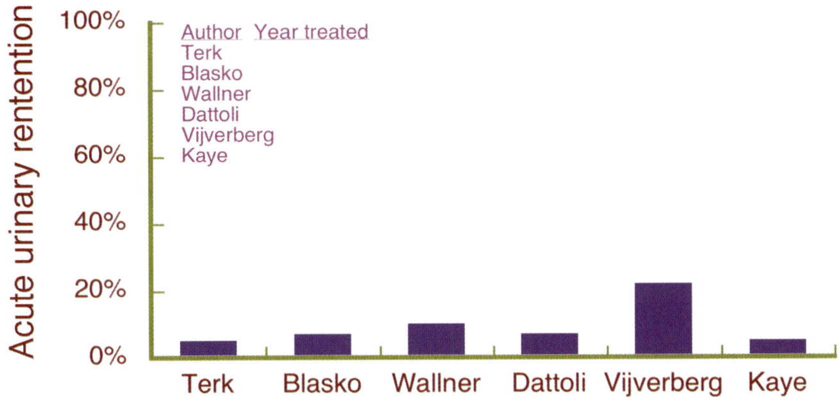

Figure 15-9. Likelihood of acute, post-implant urinary retention reported by various investigators.(TERK, BLASKO, WALLNER 96, DATTOLI, VIJVERBERG, KAYE)

Unfortunately, no single factor is associated with a risk of more than 20% to 30%.

Although patients with substantial pre-implant obstructive symptoms are at somewhat higher risk of developing post-implant urinary retention, the relationship between pre-implant obstructive symptoms and post-implant urinary obstruction is loose, at best. Terk, Stock, and Stone first showed that AUA scores are only a weak predictor of post-implant urinary obstruction (**Figure 15-10**). In a series of 62 patients followed prospectively at the University of Washington, there was little correlation between AUA score and acute urinary obstruction. While patients who developed retention tended to have higher pre-implant AUA scores, there was a remarkable

Table 15-2. Potential risk factors for post-implant urinary retention.

- high AUA score
- large prostate
- small prostate
- older age
- median lobe hypertrophy
- large postvoid residual
- low maximum flow rate

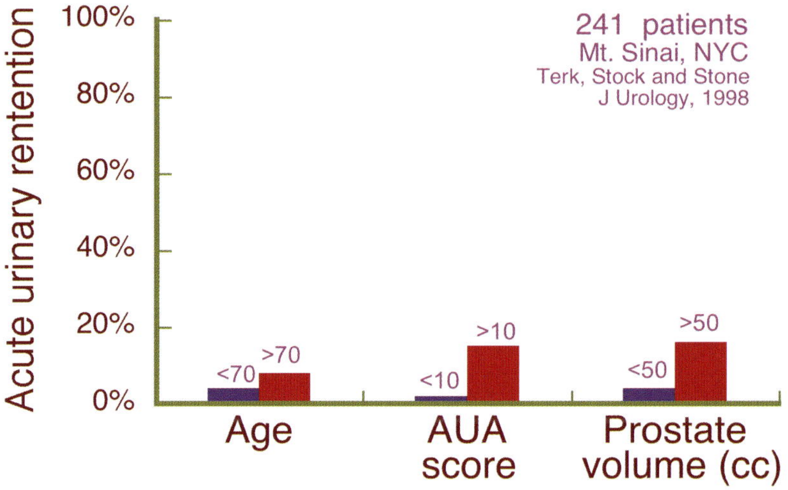

Figure 15-10. Likelihood of acute, post-implant urinary retention versus age, AUA scores, and prostate volume. In multivariate analysis, only AUA score was predictive of retention.

range of scores among those who did or did not develop retention (**Figure 15-11**).(LOCKE) Based on the loose statistical correlations of Terk and colleagues and the scatter in the University of Washington data, it is safe to say that AUA scores, in themselves, are not a *good* way to predict the likelihood of retention for an individual patient.

Prostate size has also long been assumed to be a good predictor of post-implant retention. In the Terk series, large prostate size was correlated with retention risk in univariate but not in multivariate analysis (**Figure 15-10**). Like the case for AUA scores, patients who developed retention tend to have larger pre-implant prostate volumes, but there's so much scatter in the data that prostate volume is *not* a useful parameter to predict an individual patient's risk of retention (**Figure 15-11**).(LOCKE) Most importantly, neither prostate size nor pre-implant IPSS scores were related to long-term urinary function.(GUTMAN)

Urodynamic studies including post-void residual urine volume or maximum flow rate appear to be weak predictors for post-implant retention (**Figure 15-12**). Pre-implant cystourethroscopy has been proposed as a way to

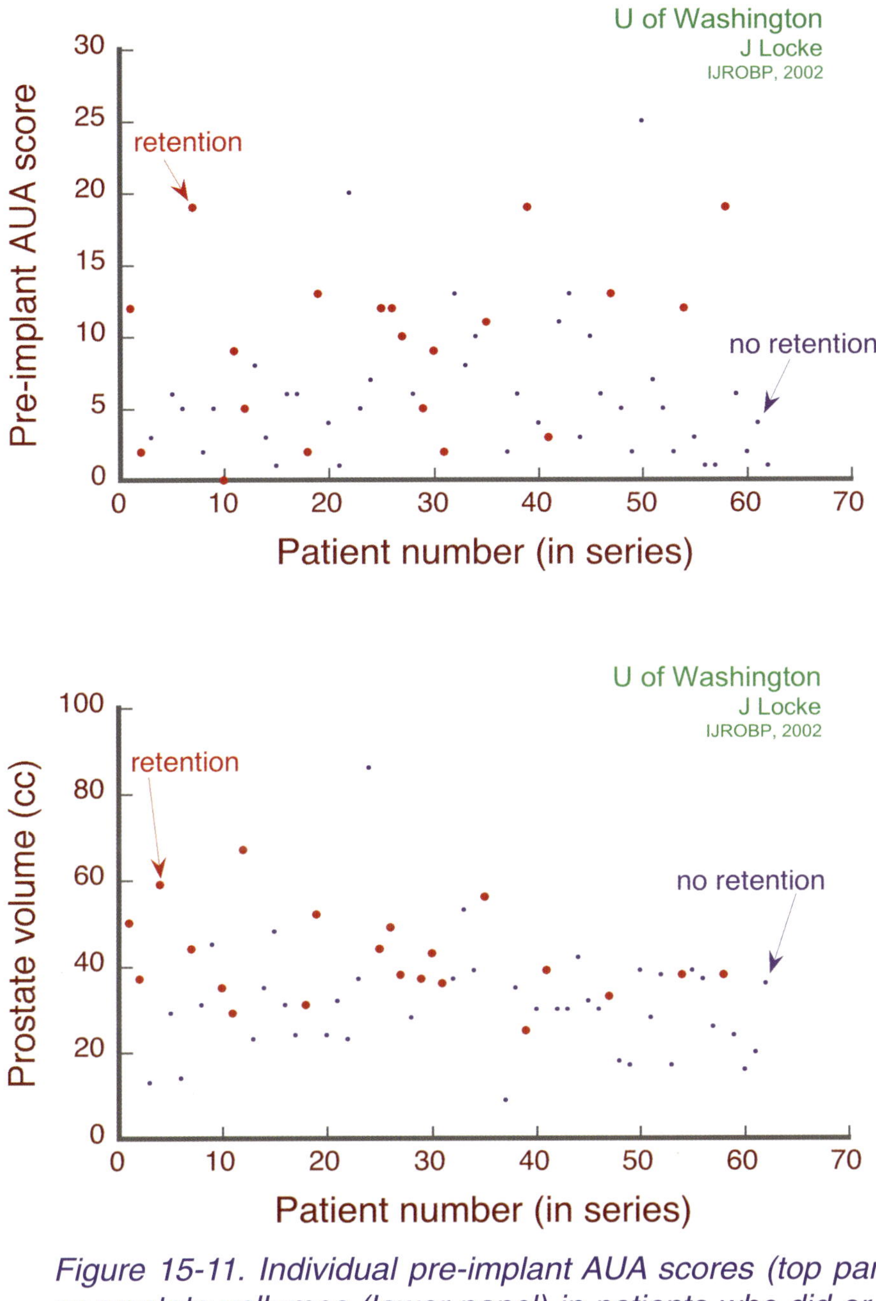

Figure 15-11. Individual pre-implant AUA scores (top panel) or prostate vollumes (lower panel) in patients who did or did not develop post-implant urinary retention at the University of Washington in 1998. The overall retention rate in this series was quite high. The point here is that it is not obvious, based on pre-implant AUA scores or prostate volumes, who is going to have a problem.

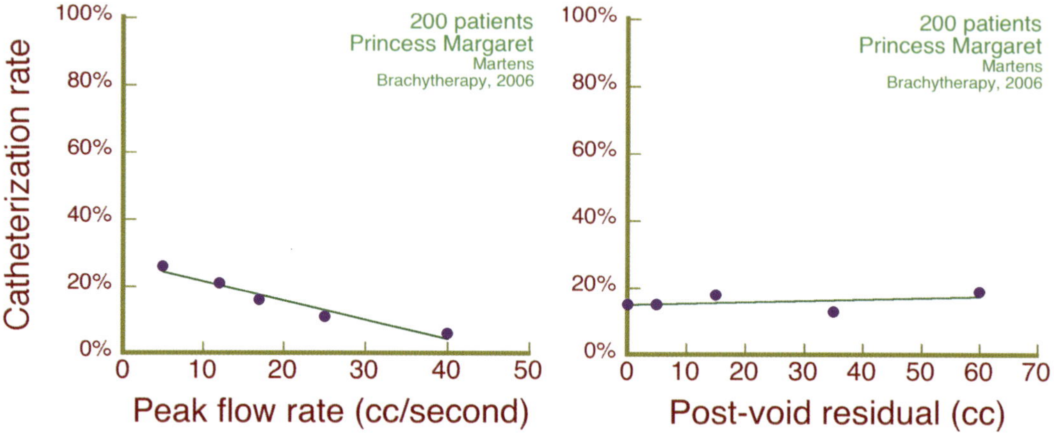

Figure 15-12. Post-implant urinary retention versus peak urinary flow rate (left) or post-void residual (right).

predict the risk of post-implant retention, with the assumption that mechanical obstruction predisposes patients to retention. Gray and colleagues, at the Puget Sound VA Hospital, prospectively performed pre- and post-implant cystourethroscopy on 15 implant patients. Their degree of pre-implant obstruction was rated using a 3-point scale, with the patients' pre-implant cystourethroscopic findings ranging from minimal to complete occlusion (**Figure 15-13**).(DIN) Nearly all patients had some increased physical obstruction following completion of the procedure, but there was little relationship between pre- or post-implant cystoscopic findings and post-implant retention (**Figure 15-14**). The investigators concluded that any correlation between cystourethroscopically identified obstruction and post-implant urinary retention that might be discerned in a larger patient sampling would likely be too weak to be used as a reliable predictor of post-implant retention in individual patients.

Transition zone

In addition to prostate volume, transition zone measurements have been used to predict patients' post-implant urinary morbidity (**Figure 15-15**). Thomas and colleagues claimed that the TZ volume was a good predictor of acute urinary retention, but their conclusions were based on a small

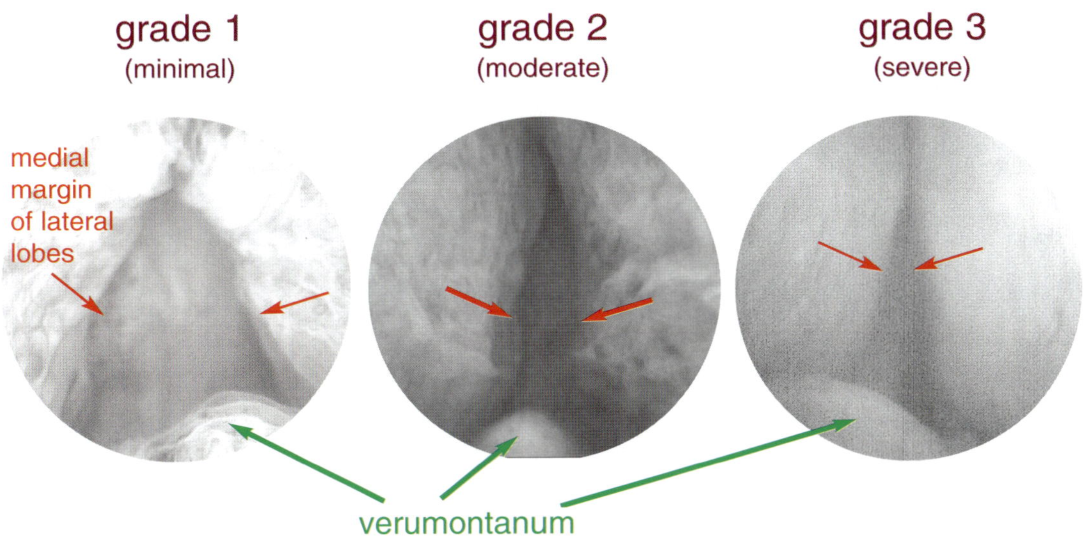

Figure 15-13. Cystourethroscopic view from verumontanum with minimal, moderate, and severe obstruction.

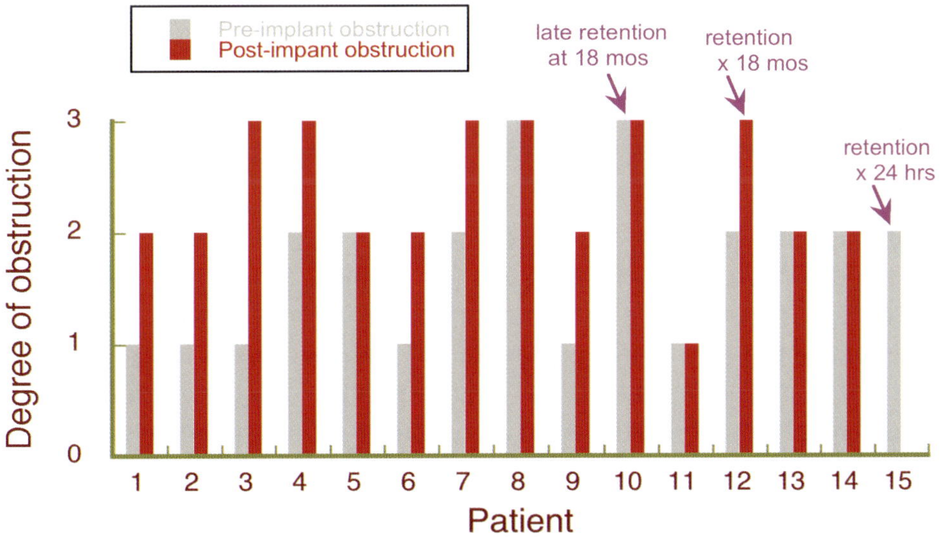

Figure 15-14. Pre- and post-implant cystoscopic urethral obstruction among 15 brachytherapy patients at the Puget Sound Health Care System, VA.(GRAY, YAP)

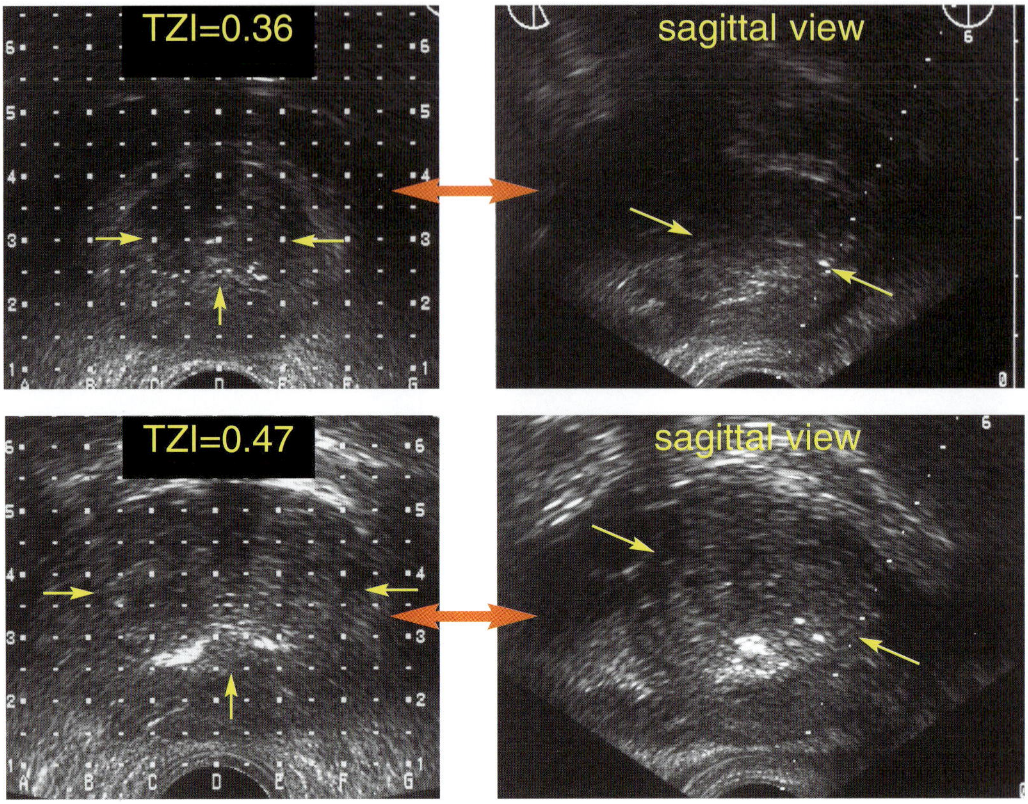

Figure 15-15. Examples of patients with small or large TZI . TZI is calculated by the ellipsoid formula(maximum prostate length, width and thickness on TRUS (width x height x length x pi/6).

number of patients (**Figure 15-16**).(THOMAS) Hinerman-Mulroy and colleagues, using a more robust database for analysis, found no relationship between transition zone index (transition zone volume/total prostate volume) and post-implant retention.(merrick 04, HINERMAN-MULROY) They did, however, show some correlation between the TZI and post-implant obstructive symptoms (**Figure 15-17**). A high TZI may be used to warn patients that they may experience more obstructive symptoms in the months following implantation.

While there is no dearth of conjecture regarding the risks for post-implant retention, the best that can be said with any certainty is that the overall risk of retention is low; if retention occurs it is typically short-lived; and acute

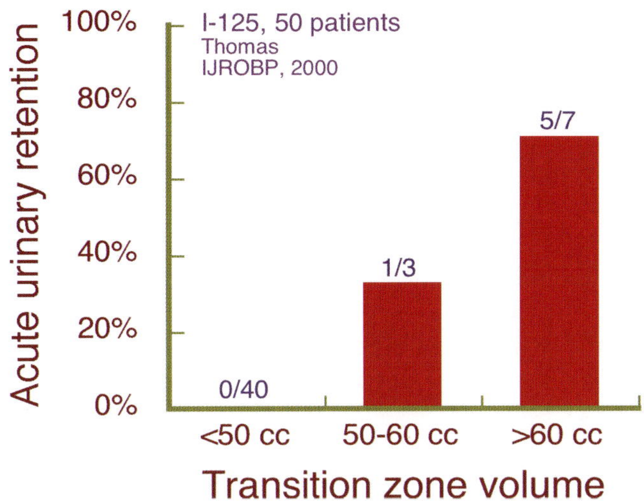

Figure 15-16. Transition zone volume versus likelihood of retention. While there is probably some relationship between TZ enlargment and post-implant morbditiy, this study was-based on a small number of patients.

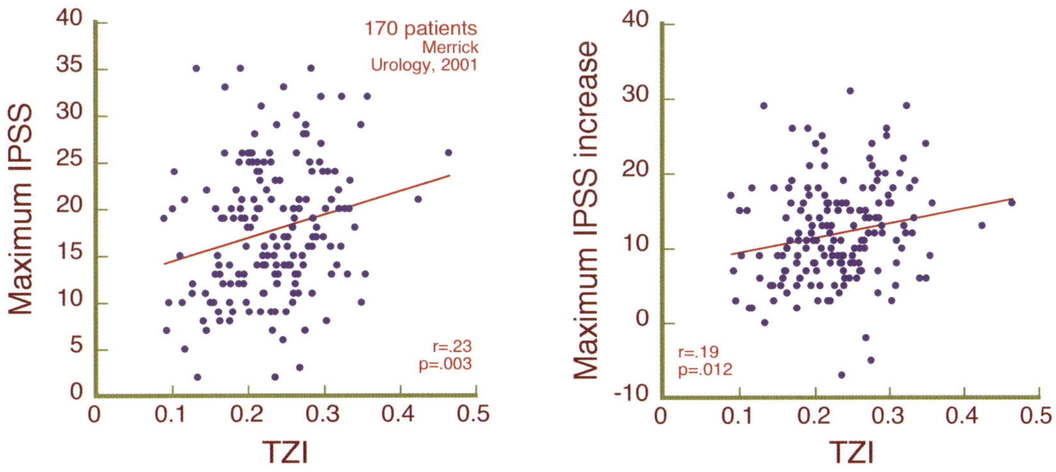

Figure 15-17. IPSS changes versus TZI.

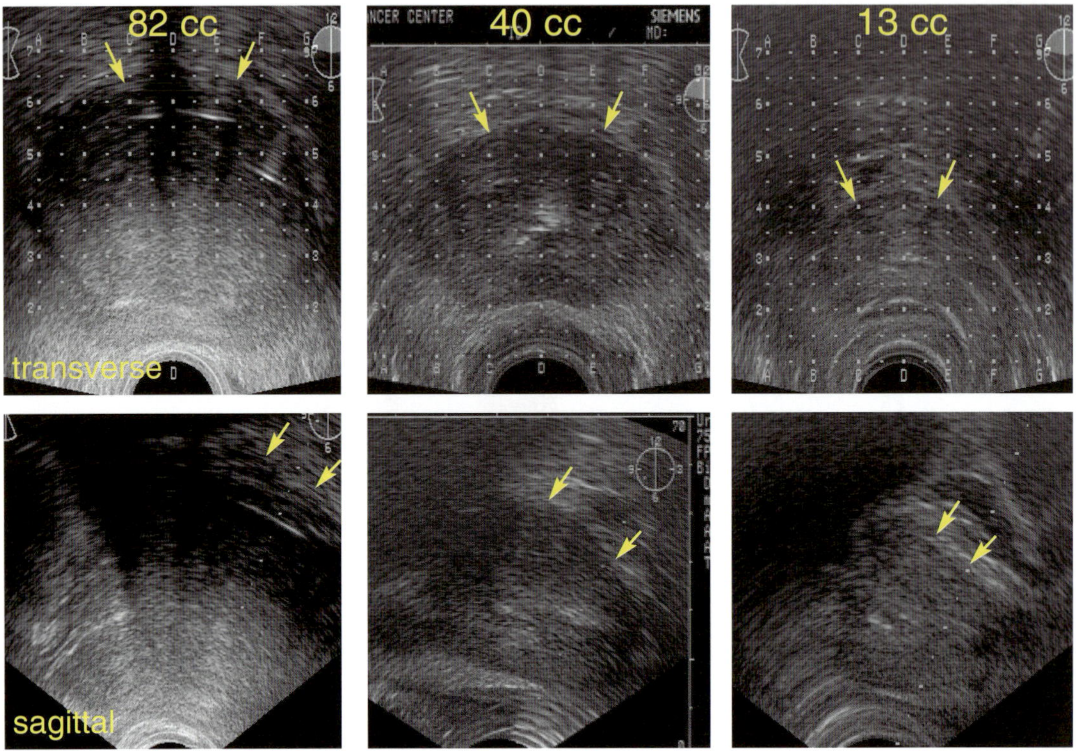

Figure 15-18. Transverse and sagittal TRUS images of 82 cc, 40 cc, and 13 cc prostate glands. Even at the tiny volume of 13 cc, there's plenty of room for seeds (arrows indicate anterior prostatic margin).

retention has little relationship to long-term urinary dysfunction.(LANDIS) Patients at high risk of retention are not reliably identifiable with known risk factors, despite numerous retrospective studies.(KEYES, CROOK) And the issue of identifying high risk patients seems less important over time, since the incidence of retention seems to decrease with experience.(KEYES)

EXTREME PROSTATE SIZE

Prostate size ranges widely, partly due to enlargement with advancing age (**Figure 15-18**). The extremes, both large and small, have long been considered by some to be contraindications to brachytherapy.

Big prostates

Large prostate size is widely believed to be a relative contraindication to brachytherapy, due to technical concerns and the perception that such

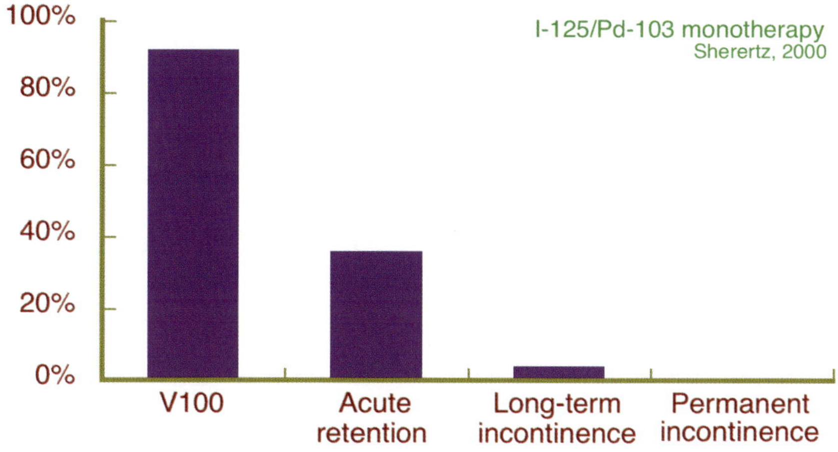

Figure 15-19. Long-term outcomes in 33 brachytherapy patients with prostate volumes greater than 50 cc.(WANG, SHERERTZ)

patients are at a higher risk of morbidity. Accordingly, patients with prostate volumes greater than 50–60 cc are commonly advised against brachytherapy or are placed on hormonal therapy prior to implant to shrink their gland. To help clarify the use of large prostate size as a contraindication to prostate brachytherapy, Wang and colleagues reviewed the dose volume histograms and post-implant course of 33 patients with a pre-implant prostate volume greater than 50 cc, which comprised 7% of the implants performed at the University of Washington. Despite typical implant-related volume increases of 2% to 50%, the V100 was at least 80% in all patients (**Figure 15-19**).

One concern in treating patients with large prostates is that the anterior/lateral portion of the prostate may not be adequately covered due to pubic arch interference of needle placement. In fact, five of the 33 patients' post-implant CT scans showed incomplete coverage of the anterior/lateral prostate margin. However, the dosimetric parameters were still well within the recommended range. Stock and colleagues also reported adequate prostate coverage for larger prostate glands.(STONE)

Twelve of the 33 patients from the University of Washington developed acute post-implant urinary retention, all developing within twenty-four hours of implantation. However, 85% of patients were catheter-free by one

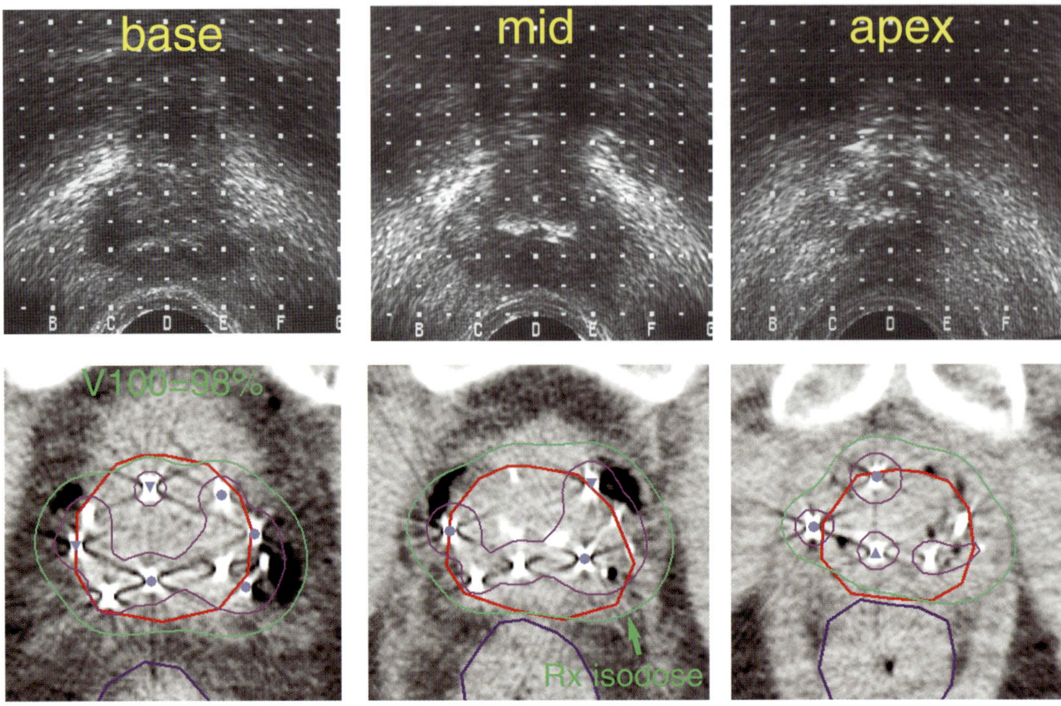

Figure 15-20. Pre-implant TRUS and post-implant CT of a 13 cc prostate. The post-implant volume (day 0) was 18 cc.

month and 96% were catheter-free by one year (**Figure 15-19**). Most patients eventually returned to more normal urinary function, even following prolonged intermittent self-catheterization.(SHERERTZ) The only disconcerting finding was that two of the 33 patients developed rectal fistulas. Oddly enough, detailed dosimetric analysis of these two cases showed relatively *low* rectal radiation doses.(HOWARD) One patient's fistula was likely related to a post-implant interstitial laser procedure. The second patient's fistula remains unexplained, but since his prostate was only 53 cc, volume per se was probably *not* related to his complication.

Although more data is needed, patients with larger prostate volume appear to have acceptable morbidity and satisfactory technical outcome, and the perception of large prostate volume being a contraindication to therapy is highly questionable.(KRUPSKI)

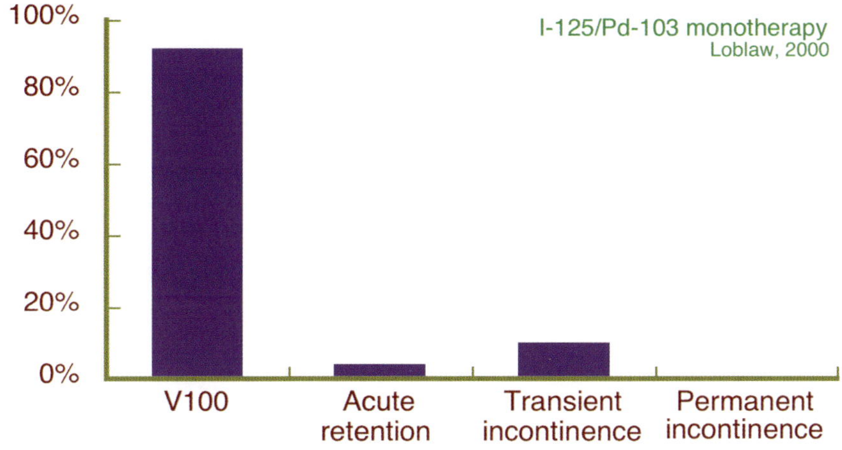

Figure 15-21. Short-term outcomes in 23 brachytherapy patients with prostate volumes less than 20 cc.

Cancer control rates with brachytherapy appear to be independent of prostate size.(MERRICK, LEHRER) In contrast, Kaminski and colleagues have reported worse biochemical outcomes in patients with large prostate glands treated with conformal beam radiation.(KAMINSKI)

Small prostates

Very small prostate volumes have been considered by some to be a contraindication to brachytherapy (**Figure 15-20**). Speculative rationales included the possibilities that small prostate glands lack sufficient tissue to hold enough seeds, that seeds inadvertently placed outside of the prostate would migrate, or that small prostate volumes might predispose patients to urinary complications.

To assess the impact of small prostate volume in brachytherapy patients, Loblaw and colleagues reviewed the clinical course of 30 consecutive, unselected patients with prostate gland volumes less than 20 cc, comprising 8% of patients treated at the University of Washington Medical Center.(LOBLAW) The median implant-related volume increase was 63%, somewhat higher than usual, but the median V100 was 92%. To calculate the incidence of seed migration, the number of seeds placed at the time of implant was compared with the number identified on post-implant Xrays (**Figure 15-21**). Patients lost an average of two seeds, consistent with prior reports not limited to patients with small prostate volumes.(WILLINS,

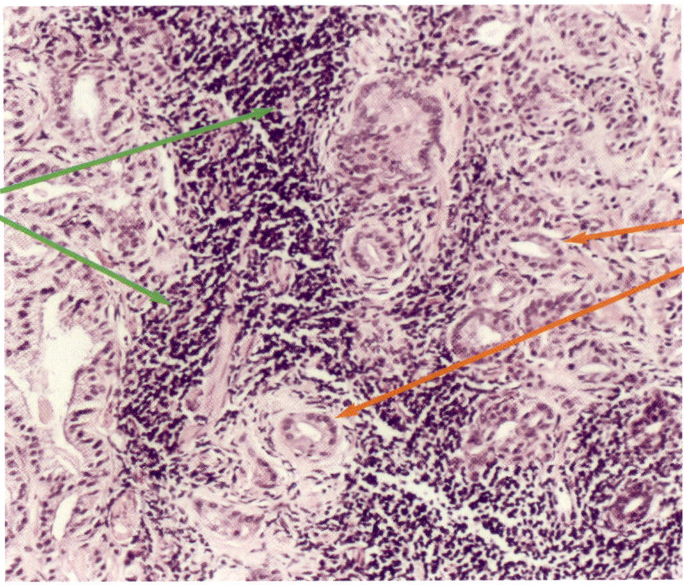

Figure 15-22. Diffuse, intense inflammatory infiltrate in pre-implant prostatic biopsy. Dense dark bands of infiltrating lymphocytes are seen between scattered cancerous glands.

SOMMENKAMP, MERRICK 00) Concerns regarding the possibility of excessive seed migration from small prostates were unfounded, despite the fact that a median of 31 seeds appeared to be outside of the prostatic margins, as identified on post-implant CT scan.

Of the 23 patients with longer follow-up information available, only one developed acute post-implant urinary retention, which resolved within two weeks of implantation. At last follow-up, patients' pre- and post-implant AUA scores were not substantially different, with the median AUA score rising from 7 to 8. Two patients reported mild, temporary post-implant urinary urge incontinence, lasting up to six months, but no patient had persistent incontinence (**Figure 15-21**). No serious rectal morbidity was encountered.

Patients with small prostate volumes appear to have acceptable morbidity and dose coverage, such that a small prostate volume should *not* be considered a contraindication to brachytherapy.

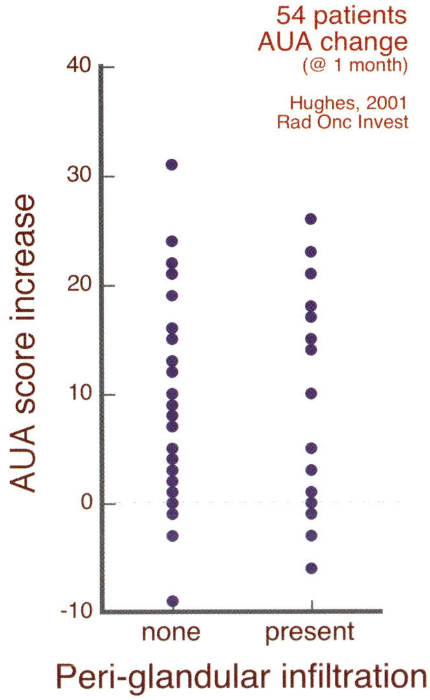

Figure 15-23. AUA score changes at one month following implant in patients with or without histologic evidence of prostatitis on pre-implant biopsy.

PROSTATITIS

Prostatitis is a poorly understood condition, often treated empirically with antibiotics. The diagnosis is usually based on clinical symptoms, unsubstantiated by biopsy or culture. A prior history of prostatitis has been considered by some to be a contraindication to brachytherapy. Aggarwal and colleagues summarized five brachytherapy patients with pre-implant clinical or pathologic evidence of prostatitis (**Figure 15-22**).(AGGARWAL) Two of the five patients developed post-implant urinary retention requiring short-term catheterization; both resolved spontaneously, and there was no other unusual morbidity in these patients.

In a more methodical study of the role of prostatitis as a contraindication to brachytherapy, Hughes and colleagues compared pre-implant clinical or pathological findings of prostatitis with patients' post-implant course.(HUGHES) No relation was seen between prostatitis and acute or chronic urinary morbidity (**Figure 15-23**).

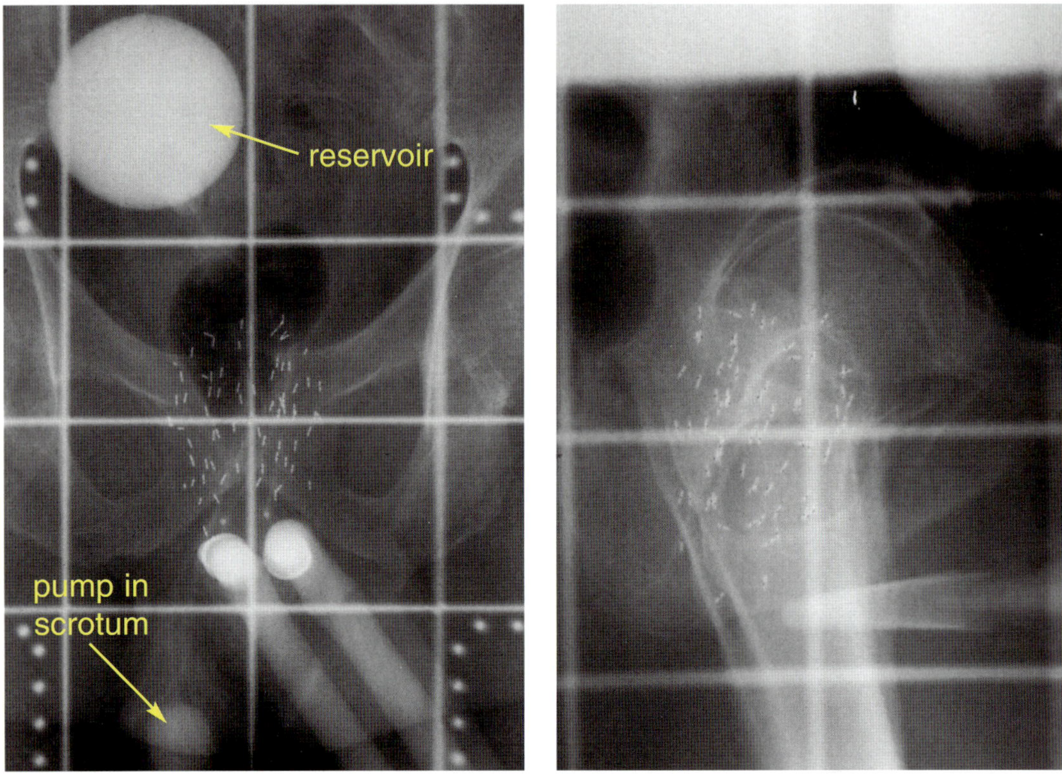

Figure 15-24. Post-implant plain films of a patient with an inflatable penile prosthesis.

Because radiation prostatitis and infectious prostatitis are both associated with frequent, painful urination and occasionally with acute urinary retention, it would seem logical that a prior history of infectious prostatitis would be a relative contraindication to prostate brachytherapy. However, available evidence fails to support a policy of withholding brachytherapy on the basis of clinical or histologic evidence of prostatitis. Even the benefit of prophylactic antibiotics in patients with pre-existing prostatitis remains unclear.(HUGHES)

PENILE PROSTHESIS

The presence of a penile prosthesis is a potential contraindication to brachytherapy, due to the possibility of peri-prosthetic infection or physical damage to the prosthesis. Li and colleagues reviewed five brachytherapy patients with a previously placed prosthesis, four of whom had semirigid,

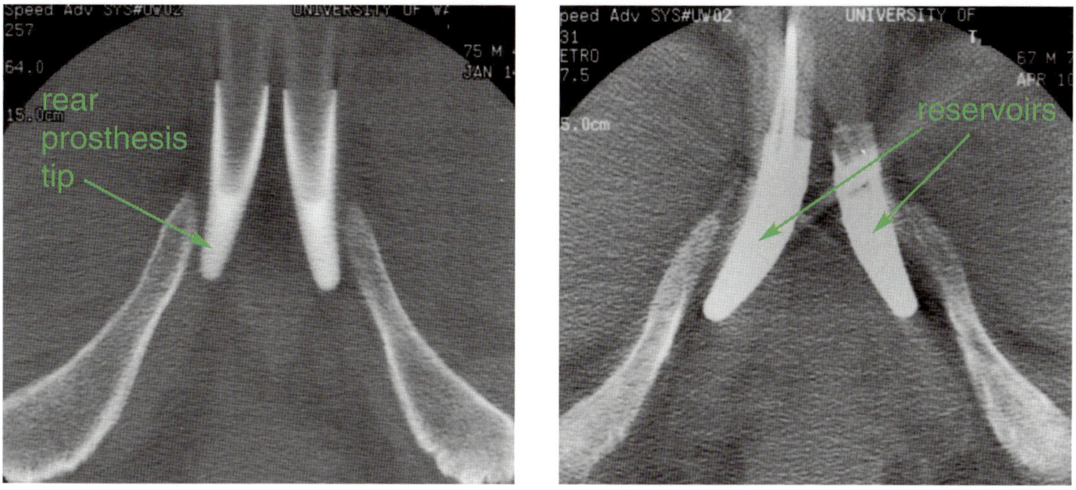

Figure 12-25. CT images showing penile prostheses near transperineal needle path.

malleable implants and one of whom had a three-piece inflatable prosthesis.(LI) Pretreatment computed tomography scans of the pelvis were reviewed to rule out significant pubic arch interference (**Figures 15-24 and 15-25**) and a broad spectrum intravenous antibiotic was administered. None of the four patients available for follow-up experienced prosthesis-related pain or infection in the first post-brachytherapy year. One patient, who had a three-piece implant 7 years prior to brachytherapy, reported a malfunction in his prosthesis 13 months after seed implantation. At the time of replacement, a connector tubing leak at the abdominal reservoir site was found, probably unrelated to the brachytherapy procedure. A fifth patient was lost to follow-up after the 24-hour postoperative period, but the implant procedure itself was uneventful. Based on this limited number of patients, it appears that concerns over prosthesis-related complications may be exaggerated. In fact, the prosthetic infection rate unrelated to brachytherapy has averaged only about 2%. And while late hematogenous seeding has been reported, nearly all prosthetic infections have been limited to the time of prosthesis placement.(CARSON, RADOMSKI, THOMALLA, DAVIS 92, SCHANNE, TIGUERT)

While brachytherapy appears to be safe in the setting of a penile prosthesis, several maneuvers may help prevent complications. First, preoperative, CT-based assessment of the pelvic anatomy can help evaluate the likelihood of pubic arch interference or striking the prosthesis. Additionally,

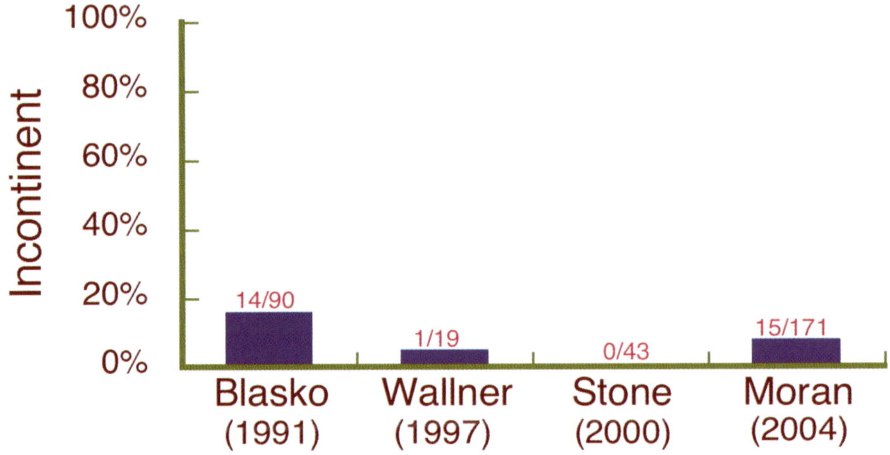

Figure 15-26. Incidence of post-implant urinary incontinence in patients with a prior TURP.

using the extended lithotomy position and taping the genitalia and scrotum anteriorly should help move the prosthesis anteriorly, away from the needle paths. Unfortunately, intra-operative TRUS is not of much help monitoring the position of the needles in relation to the prosthesis, because the prosthesis is not well visualized. Accordingly, patients should be warned that implant-related infectious or mechanical complications could arise.

TURP

There is continued controversy regarding brachytherapy in patients who have undergone transurethral resection of the prostate (TURP). In early reports from Blasko, Grimm, and Ragde, approximately 50% of such patients developed post-implant incontinence (see chapter 15). In more recent experience, however, the risk of incontinence in TURP patients has been low (**Figure 15-26**), probably because peripheral seed loading patterns avoid excessive urethral doses (see chapter 6).(WALLNER 97, STONE, MERRICK 03) Using the homogeneous loading patterns typical of the early practice of Blasko and colleagues, urethral doses can easily exceed three times the prescription dose. In contrast, urethral doses of 150% to 200% of the prescription are routinely attainable with a modified peripheral seed placement.(MERRICK 00) Avoiding excessive doses to the prostate apex

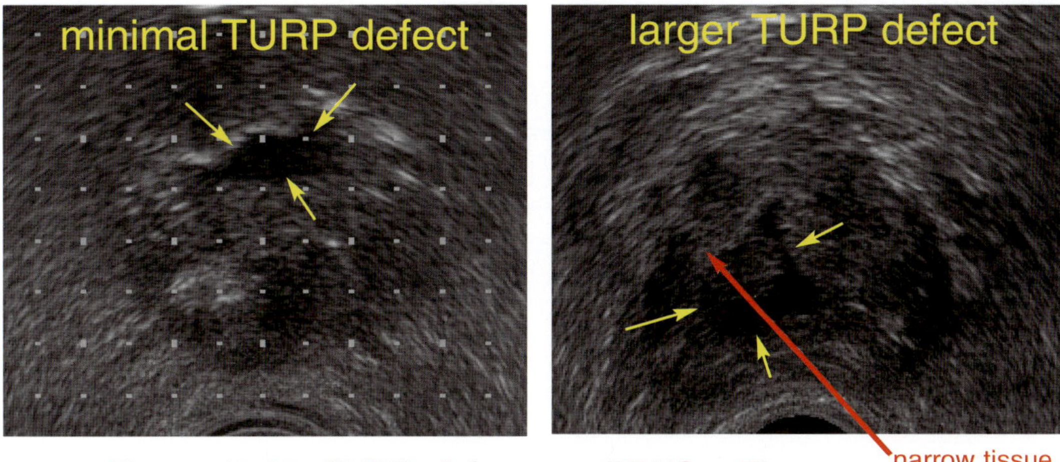

Figure 15-27. TURP defects on TRUS. The patient on the right has a larger defect, possibly placing him at higher risk of incontinence or seed loss.

and the external sphincter may be especially important in patients who have had a TURP.(MERRICK 03)

If brachytherapy is performed for a patient with prior TURP, there should probably be at least a 1.0 cm rim of tissue left around the TUR defect, to ensure sufficient tissue to hold the seeds. CT or TRUS are generally adequate to assess remaining tissue (**Figures 15-27 and 15-28**). A waiting interval of at least four weeks after TURP has been suggested, to allow adequate time for re-epitheliazation of the urethral lining, a recommendation based on experimental murine data.(SEYMORE) The risk of incontinence, if excessive urethral doses are avoided, is probably low. However, prospective brachytherapy patients with a prior TURP might be cautioned that they *may* be at higher risk of incontinence.

Perhaps more likely than the possibility of incontinence is the possibility of post-implant seed loss. Post TURP patients seem to have a higher chance of passing seeds in the post-implant period, and we routinely re-film them 1-3 days after their implant to check for loss. If re-scan shows substantial decrease in dose coverage, extra seeds are added.

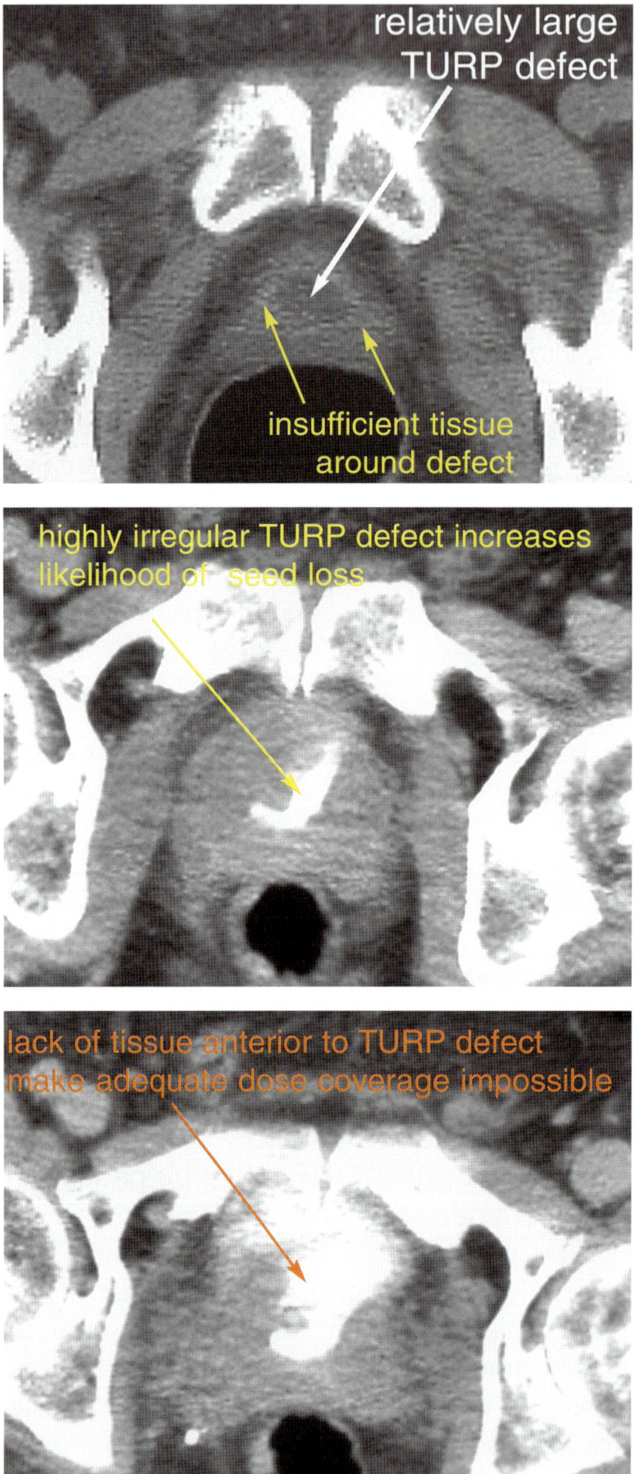

Figure 15-28. Examples of post-TURP patients we would not implant.

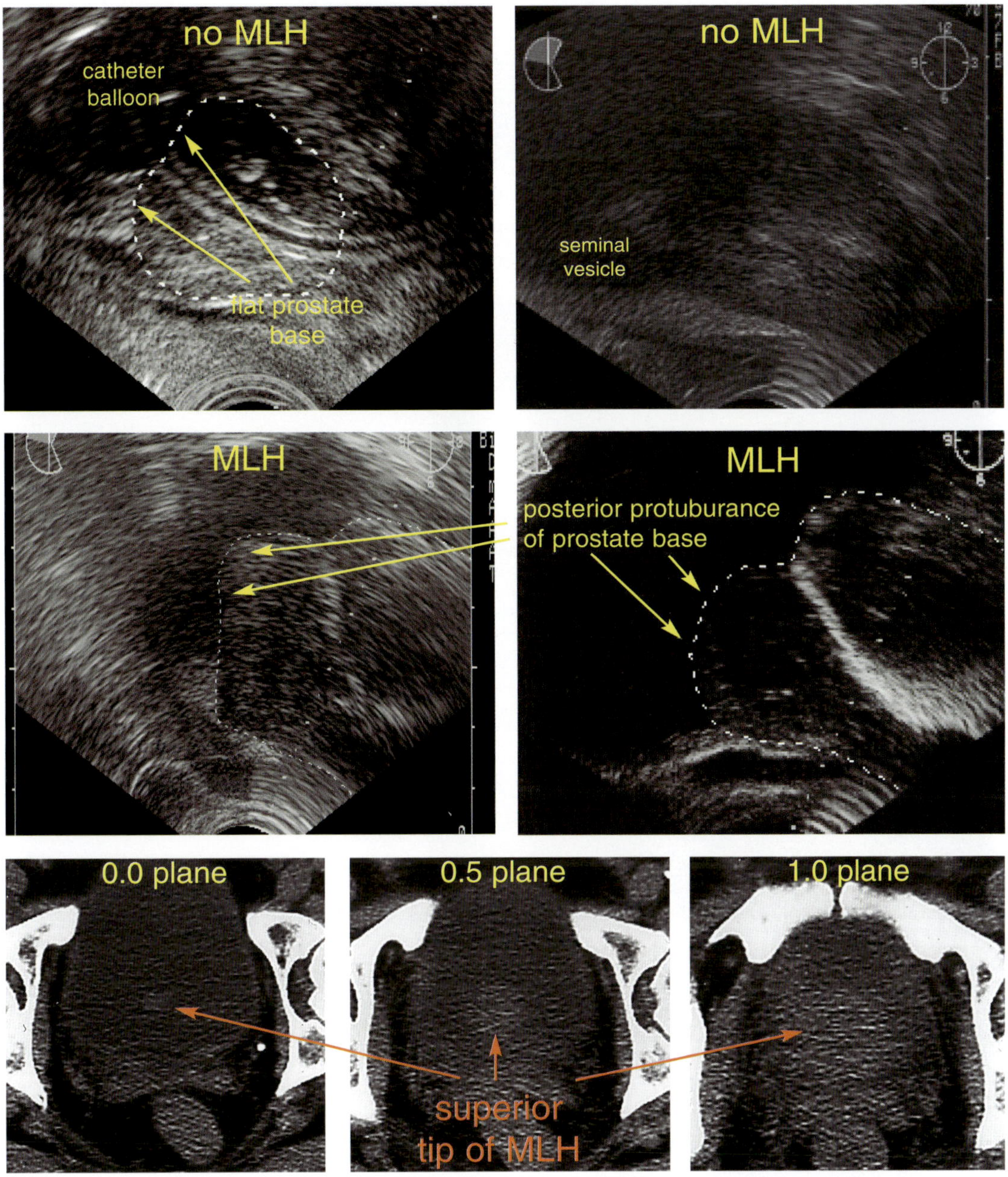

Figure 15-29. Top panels show normal prostatic contours, without median lobe hyperplasia (MLH). Middle panels show sagittal TRUS examples of median lobe hypertrophy. The lower panels show the intravesical component of prostatic hyperplasia on CT scan.

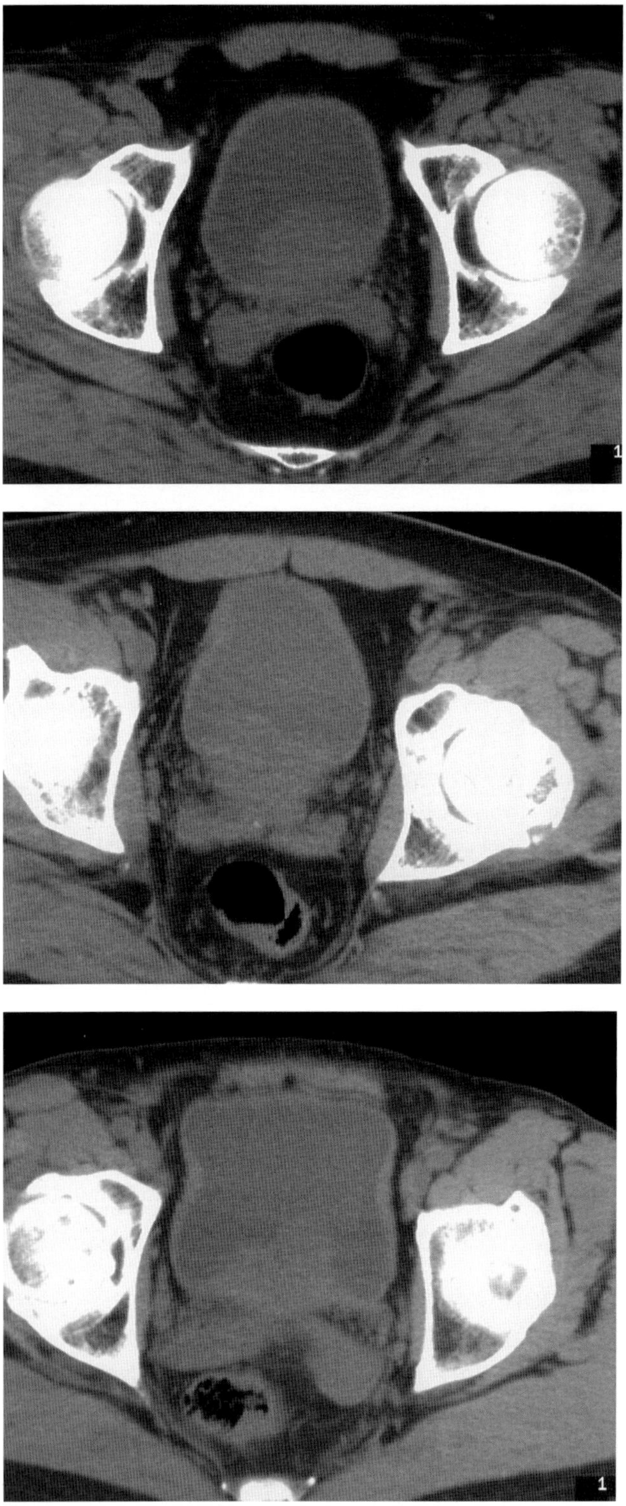

Figure 15-30. Examples of highly irregular MLH tissue growing into the bladder. We would be reluctant to implant these, due to concern about inadequate tissue coverage.

MEDIAN LOBE HYPERPLASIA

Median lobe hyperplasia (MLH) refers to protrusion of transitional zone tissue into the bladder (**Figure 15-29 and 15-30**).(DIN, WATSON, WALLNER 00) It has been suggested that MLH, or *intravesical prostatomegaly*, might be a contraindication to brachytherapy, either by increasing the risk of post-implant urinary morbidity or because of technical difficulties implanting the intravesical tissue. Wallner and colleagues reviewed the clinical course of eight brachytherapy patients with radiographic evidence of MLH.(WALLNER 00) There was no apparent association between the degree of MLH and pre-implant prostate volume or AUA score. Intra-operatively, MLH could be readily viewed by TRUS, and there was no particular difficulty placing seeds in the MLH tissue. Based on post-implant CT-based dosimetry, the base of the prostate, including the median lobe tissue, was completely covered by the prescription isodose in all cases. Two of the eight patients developed prolonged post-implant urinary retention and have been slow to improve. Longer-term follow-up is suggesting that such patients may also be slower to return to their baseline urinary function.(NGUYEN)

Despite some concern regarding brachytherapy in the setting of MLH, such patients don't appear to be at a substantially increased risk of post-implant urinary morbidity or inadequate target coverage. Considering that most MLH patients do well in the long term, there is little justification for prophylactic resection of hypertrophic tissue.

While MLH is not an insurmountable problem, it does pose a technical problem in that achieving full coverage is sometime tricky. We have turned down some patients with extensive MLH that seems likely to be difficult to adequately implant (Figure 15-30).

ADVERSE PATHOLOGIC FEATURES

High Gleason score, perineural invasion, and extensive tumor in the biopsy specimen have all been correlated with a higher likelihood of extra-prostatic cancer extension and of treatment failure, regardless of the modality used.(BASTAKY, GRANN, PARTIN, BOSTWICK, VILLERS) Although adverse pathologic features are associated with a higher likelihood of early extra-prostatic extension (ECE), such patients are apparently still highly curable. Brachytherapy, with or without supplemental external beam radiation, appears to be able to sterilize the ECE associated with adverse pathologic features (**Figure 15-31**), consistent with reports that nearly all cases of ECE are limited to within 3 mm of the prostatic capsule and readily covered

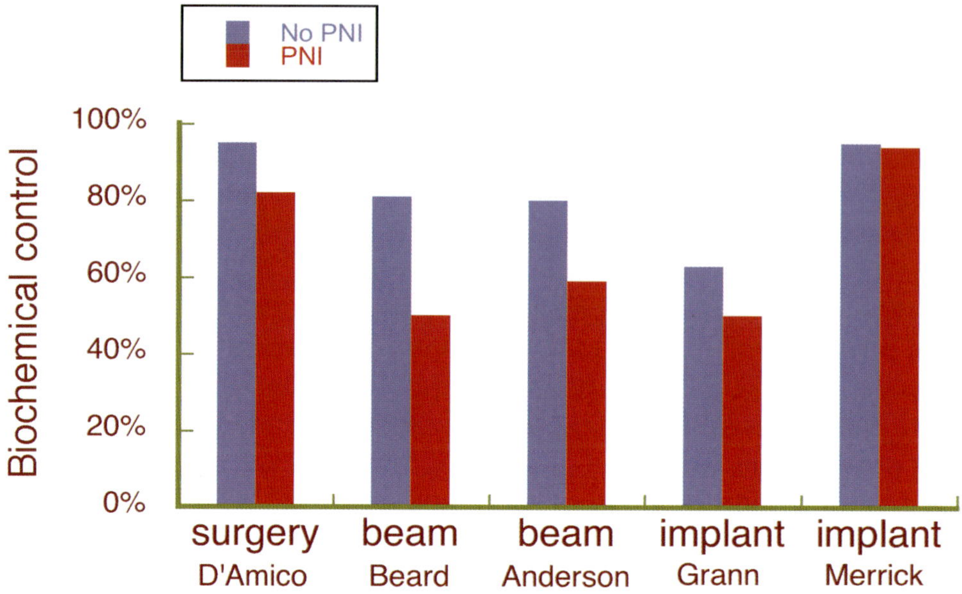

Figure 15-31. Freedom from biochemical recurrence for patients with or without perineural invasion from various series.

by an implant alone.(DAVIS 99) Unfortunately, no studies compare the presence of adverse pathologic features to the degree of radial ECE, the feature most relevant to brachytherapy. While there is no basis for using adverse pathologic features as a contraindication to brachytherapy, their presence has been used as an indication for adding supplemental external beam radiation (see chapter 11).

PROSTATIC ACID PHOSPHATASE

Like adverse pathologic features, patients with elevated prostatic acid phosphatase are at increased risk of cancer persistence after brachytherapy and after prostatectomy, so that PAP is not in itself a reason to choose one modality over the other.(refs) It might be used as an indication for adjuvant therapy.(TIERA, FANG)

LYMPH NODES

Patients with cancerous lymph nodes are at very high risk of treatment failure, and radiation of involved lymph nodes has not been found to increase the cancer control rates.(ASBELL) Patients with PSA <20 and Gleason ″7

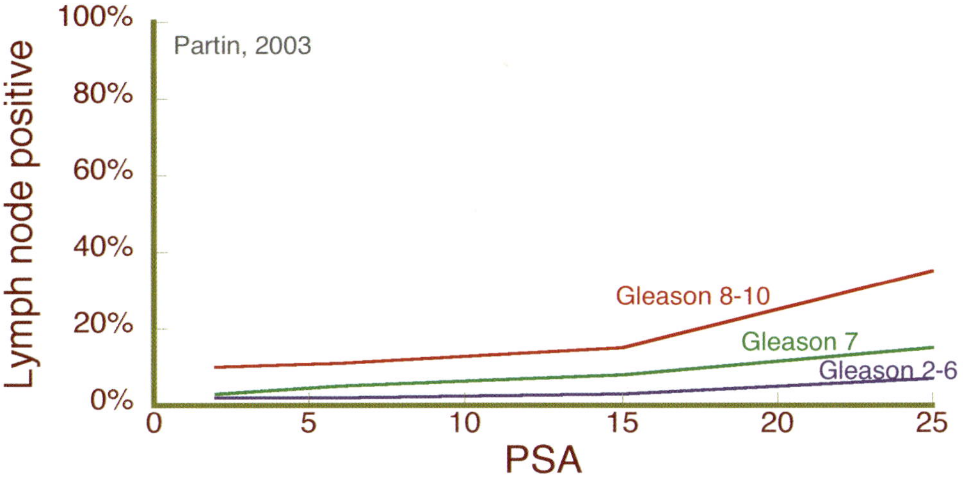

Figure 15-32. Likelihood of lymph node invasion in patients with stage T1c-T2a tumors, versus Gleason score and PSA.(PARTIN)

have a very low likelihood of lymph node involvement, and routine staging lymph node dissection is generally not warranted (**Figure 15-32**). In patients with a pretreatment PSA above 20 ng/ml, lymph node dissection should be considered, because the finding of positive lymph nodes is generally considered to be a contraindication to definitive local therapy. However, recent studies suggesting a benefit from radical prostatectomy in lymph node-positive patients may warrant a reappraisal of the role of brachytherapy in the setting of positive lymph nodes.(GHAVAMIAN, MESSING)

CALCIUM DEPOSITS

Prostatic calcium deposits (*calculi*) might be a (relative)contraindication to brachytherapy, if they interfere with needle insertion or if they induce dosimetric perturbation. In fact, needle penetration is not substantially impeded by calculi (**Figure 15-33**). The possibility of substantial dose attenuation due to absorption of low energy gamma radiation, however, remains to be elucidated.

OBESITY

Considering the high prevalence of obesity, surprisingly little has been reported regarding treatment of prostate cancer in obese patients. There is some evidence to suggest that obesity confers a better prognosis, per-

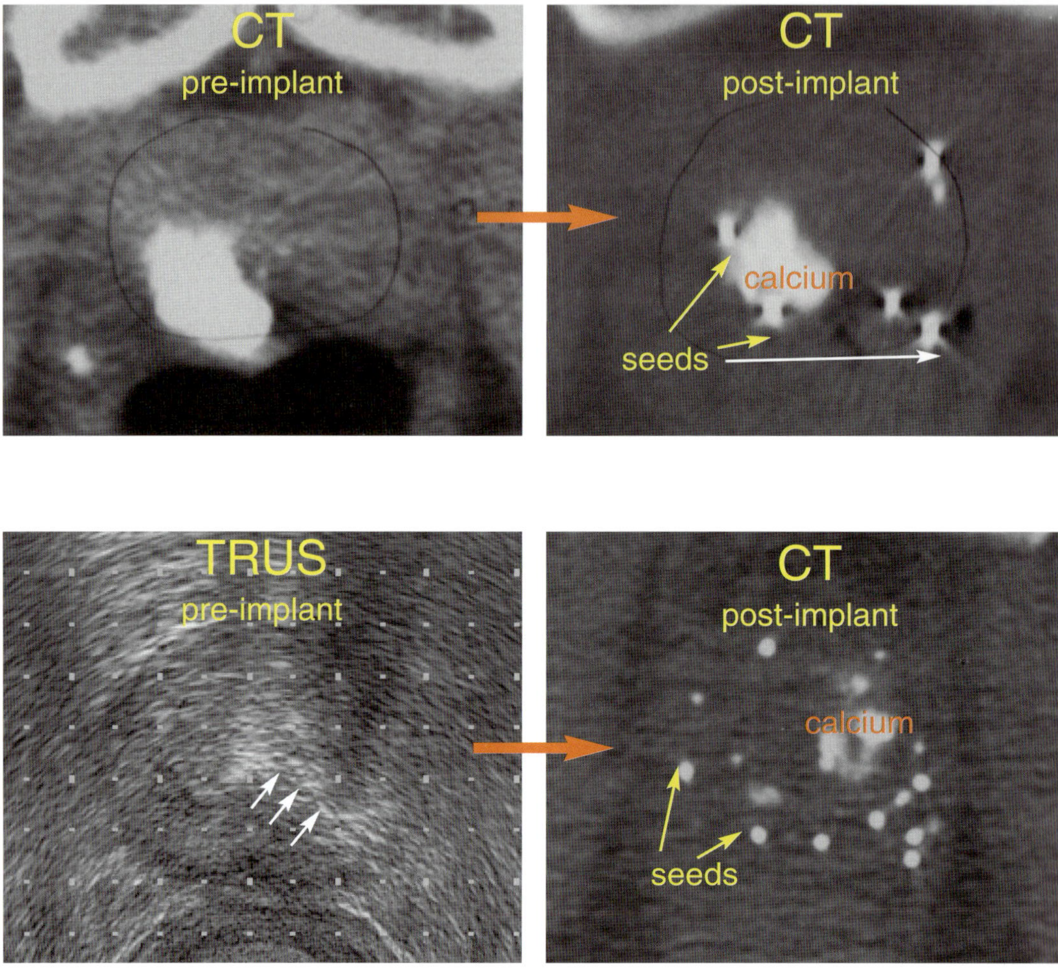

Figure 15-33. Calcium deposits. Top panels show pre- and post-implant CT images of a prostate with a large, dense deposit in the right side, that did not appear to interfere with seed placement. The lower panels show a large calculus on TRUS (arrows) that apparently did not interfere with seed placement, as seen on post-implant CT.

haps due to hormonal influences.(DANIELL) However, obesity can present technical difficulties, especially for prostatectomy and external beam radiation. Obese patients are more likely to develop postoperative complications, and are generally discouraged from surgery. They are more difficult to set up properly for external radiation, potentially increasing the risk of complications and decreasing the likelihood of cure using conformal radiation ports with small margins. In contrast, obesity poses a relatively minor problem for brachytherapy.(ROCKHILL) Operative setup can take longer, and there is less room to maneuver between the patient's legs, but this has not presented a huge problem (**Figures 15–34 and 15–35**). Standard 20 cm brachytherapy needles are almost always sufficient to reach the prostate, but 25 cm needles are commercially available. In experienced hands, clinical outcomes are unaffected by obesity.(MERRICK 02, MITSUYAMA)

INFLAMMATORY BOWEL DISEASE

The term *inflammatory bowel disease* (IBD) includes both ulcerative colitis and regional enteritis (Crohn's disease), which are chronic idiopathic inflammatory disorders of the gastrointestinal tract. While there is a widespread, scantily substantiated belief that IBD patients are at higher risk for radiation-related complications, there are only widely scattered mentions of bowel complications from external beam radiation in IBD patients with prostate cancer.(LEIBEL, WILLETT)

As an alternative to surgery, some IBD patients have been referred for brachytherapy, the rationale being that less rectal surface area would be irradiated (See Chapter 3). Grann and Wallner reported six patients treated with I-125, none of whom experienced unusual gastrointestinal morbidity.(GRANN) In a more recent brachytherapy series, Peters reported typical radiation reactions in 17 ulcerative colitis patients and seven Crohn's disease patients.(PETERS)

HOMOSEXUAL MEN

There is remarkably little data regarding treatment of prostate cancer in homosexual men.(BLANK, LEVINSON) The authors have treated several dozen gay men, but have not kept statistics regarding their outcomes. We believe, based on the literature and our personal experience, that sexual orientation is unrelated to outcomes.

TOBACCO

Smoking is bad. It's smelly, costly and increases the risk of heart disease, yellow teeth and bad breath. It also slightly increases the likelihood of biochemical failure and poorer urinary and rectal function.(MERRICK) It is unknown how the use of tobacco relates to outcomes after prostatectomy or beam radiation, but we suspect it is a risk factor for poorer results.

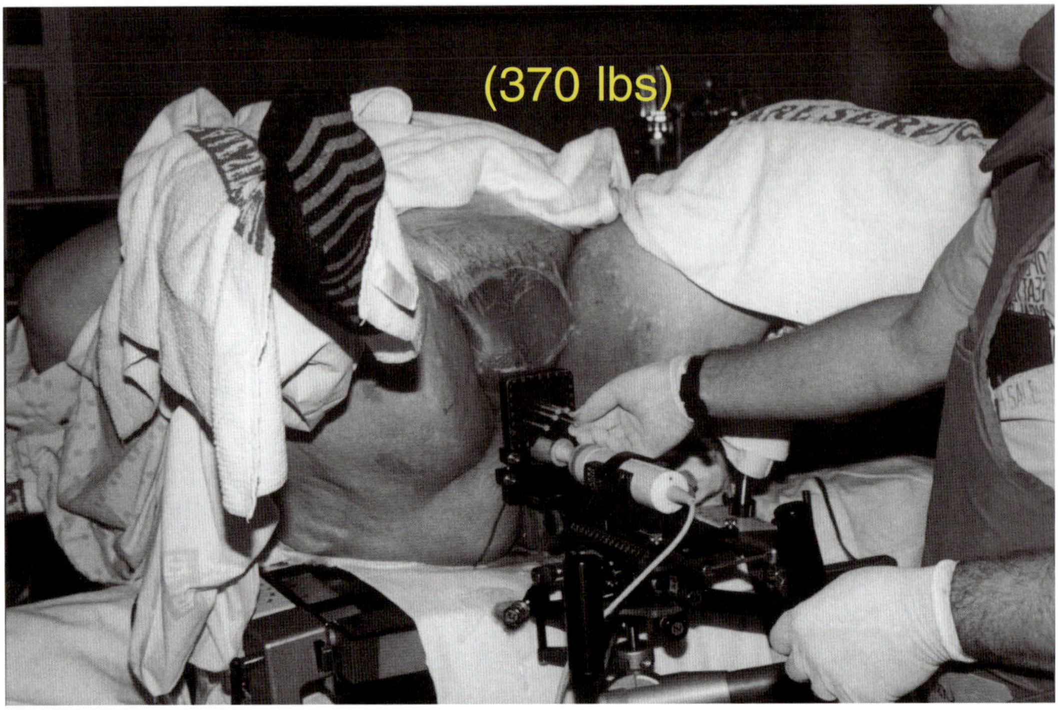

Figure 15-34. The implant procedure is not much different for massively obese patients. However, their fluoroscopic images are of poorer quality.

DIABETES MELLITUS

Diabetes does not appear to influence brachytherapy-related quality of life, except in that it increases the likelihood of development of impotence.(MERRICK)

RENAL TRANSPLANT RECIPIENTS

Treatment of prostate cancer in renal transplant recipients has received little attention. Prostatectomy outcomes appear to be unaffected in such patients.(HAFRON) There is a concern that external beam radiation might cause a hazard to the transplanted kidney, depending on its proximity to the prostate and the sophistication of the treatment planning available (**Figure 15-36**). Immunosuppression could place these patients at higher risk of cancer persistence. The authors have treated a handful of kidney transplant patients with brachytherapy, and are unaware of any adverse outcomes.

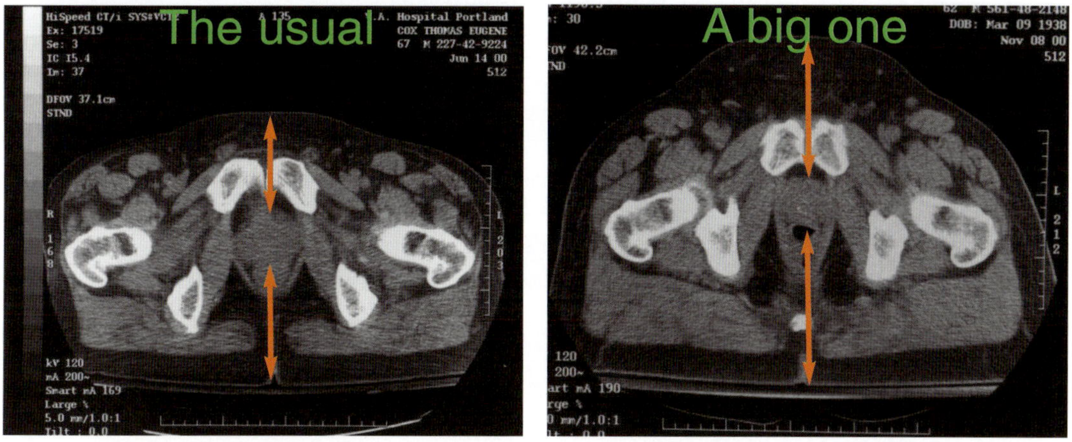

Figure 15-35. CTs of thin versus massively obese patients illustrating how much more tissue must be traversed to deliver external beam radiation, especially from the anterior and posterior directions.

PRIOR SURGERY

Prior pelvic surgery places patients at higher risk for external beam radiation-related bowel complications, presumably due to fixation of bowel within the abdomen or pelvis.(LANCIANO, WHELAN) Brachytherapy is probably less likely to cause bowel complications in patients with prior surgery, because it would entail less radiation to the bowel wall (see chapter 3), but no data are available.

PRIOR RADIATION

Patients with prior therapeutic pelvic radiation are presumably at higher risk for radiation-related complications. The most common scenarios are patients previously treated with intermediate-dose radiation for seminoma, or higher-dose radiation for colorectal carcinoma. If the dose to the rectal wall was greater than 40 Gy, brachytherapy would likely carry a moderate to high risk of significant complications, regardless of the time since the prior radiation. Prostatectomy may be preferable in these cases. However, because radiation may also increase the risk of surgery-related complications, such patients present unique and challenging situations, with no clearly "right" answer. The authors have treated a number of patients in this setting, with no recollection of subsequent serious complications, but few reports have appeared to specifically document the incidence of morbidity.(BATTERMANN) Re-irradiation in other sites has generally

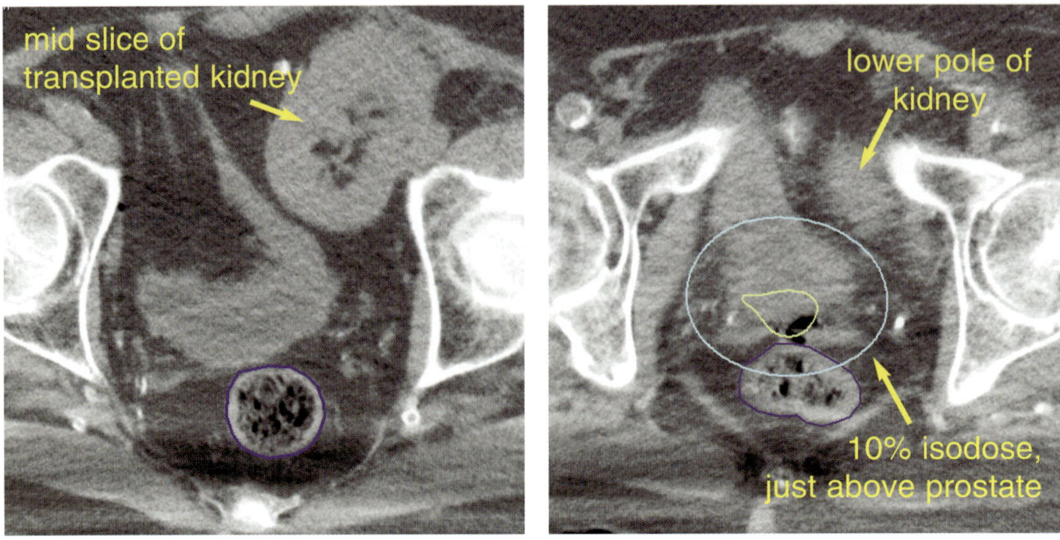

Figure 15-36. Renal transplant patient, showing minimal implant dose to his pelvic kidney.

been better tolerated than predicted radiobiologically, and it is likely reasonably safe in the setting of prostate cancer.(WONG, DE CREVOISIER) Our current policy is generally not to refuse brachytherapy to patients with prior pelvic radiation, but with an explanation and warning regarding the potential risk.

PRIOR PELVIC FRACTURES

Prior pelvic bone fracture may present a technical problem. One such patient was very difficult to implant, due to what seemed to be fibrosis at the inner margin of the pubic symphysis, making it difficult to traverse the arch (**Figure 15-37**).

REALLY BAD NUMBERS

Patients with a markedly elevated PSA or prostatic acid phosphatase have a very high likelihood of failing any treatment. Although their chance of cure is low, most brachytherapy series show some evidence of a plateau on the freedom-from-failure curve, such that there is likely a finite percentage of these patients who are curable (see chapter 14). Accordingly, if such patients otherwise have a life expectancy of more than five years,

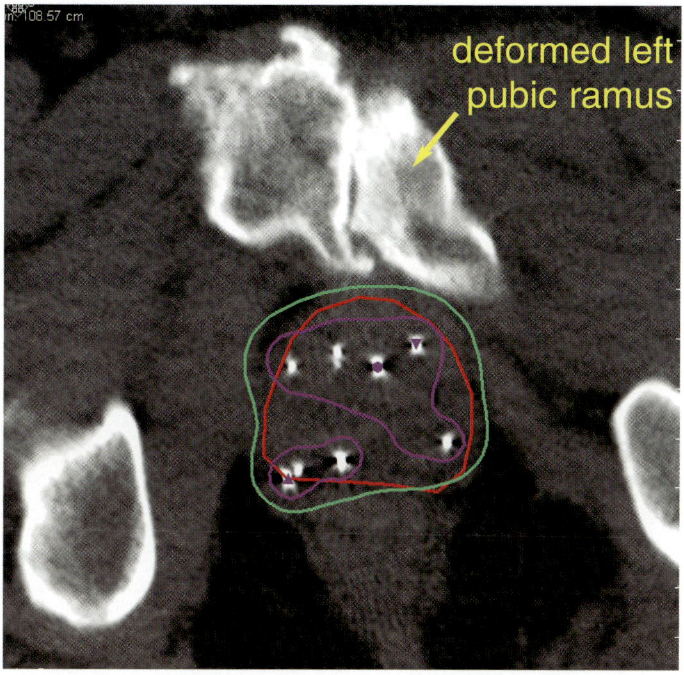

Figure 15-37. Patient with deformed pubic arch from prior pelvic fracture.

aggressive brachytherapy-based treatment is warranted once a reasonable effort to rule out distant metastases and lymph node metastases has been made. Newer imaging modalities and serum markers may help identify patients with micrometastases, who probably should not receive aggressive local therapy. (**Figure 15-38**).(DE LA PIEDRA, THURAIRAJA, MORRIS, KWEE)

RELATIVE VERSUS ABSOLUTE CONTRAINDICATIONS

While there is no shortage of opinions regarding the contraindications to brachytherapy, most are baseless. Reports to date have failed to establish any firm contraindication. That's not to say that all patients are great candidates for the procedure. Some factors, like prior urethral surgery, advanced age, obstructive symptoms, MLH, and pubic arch interference might be considered *relative* contra-indications, especially in the hands of

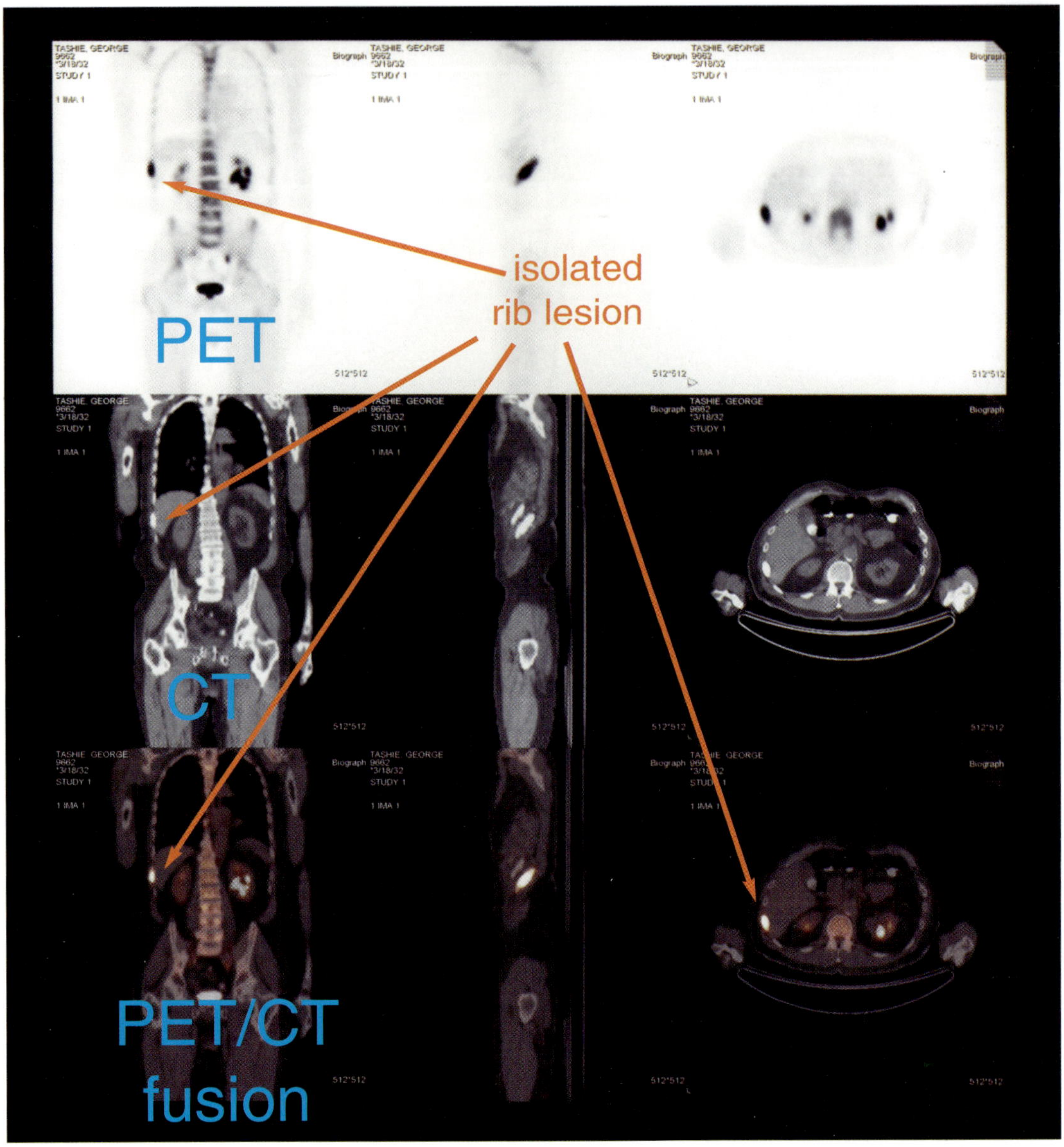

Figure 15-38. Example of remarkably clear PET/CT imaging of an isolated bone metastasis. Selective use of some combination of advanced imaging and serum markers might better identify patients who should not undergo brachytherapy for local disease.

novice brachytherapists. But even in situations where patients present with alleged contraindications, brachytherapy may still be their best choice, compared to the alternatives.

REFERENCES

1. Aggarwal S, Wallner KE, True LD, et al. Prostate brachtherapy in patients with prior evidence of prostatitis. Int J Radiat Oncol Biolo Phys 1999; 45:867-869.

2. Anderson P, Hanlon A, Patchefsky A, Al-Saleem T, Hanks G. Preineural invasion and Gleason 7-10 tumor predict increased failure in prostate cancer patients with pretreatment PSA <10 ng/ml treated with conformal external beam radiation therapy. Int J Rad Oncol Biol Phys 1998; 41:1087-1092.

3. Asbell SO, Krall JM, Pilepich MV, Baerwald H. Elective pelvic irradiation in stage A2, B carcinoma of the prostate: Analysis of RTOG 77-06. Int J Radiat Oncol Biol Phys 1988; 15:1307-1316.

4. Bastacky SI, Walsh PC, Epstein JI. Relationship between perineural tumor invasion on needle biopsy and radical prostatectomy capsular penetration in clinical stage B adenocarcinoma of the prostate. Am J Surg Path 1993; 17:336-341.

5. Battermann JJ. Feasibility of permanent implants for prostate cancer after previous radiotherapy in the true pelvis. Radiother Oncol 2000; 57:297-300.

6. Beard C, Chen M, Cote K, Loffredo M, Renshaw A, Hurwitz M. Perineural invasion is associated with increased relapse after external beam radiotherapy for men with low-risk prostate cancer and may be a maraker for occult, high-grade cancer. Int J Rad Oncol Biol Phys 2004; 58:19-24.

7. Bellon J, Wallner K, Ellis W, Cavanagh W, Blasko J. Use of pelvic CT scanning to evaluate pubic arch interference of transperineal prostate brachytherapy. Int J Radiat Oncol Biol Phys 1999; 43:579-581.

8. Blank T. Gay men and prostate cancer: Invisible diversity. J Clin Oncol 2005; 23:2593-2596.

9. Blasko JC, Ragde H, Grimm PD. Transperineal Ultrasound-Guided Implantation of the Prostate: Morbidity and Complications. Scand J Urol Nephrol Suppl 1991; 137:113-118.

10. Bostwick DG, Qian J, Bergstralh E, et al. Prediction of capsular perforation and seminal vesicle invasion in prostate cancer. J Urol 1996; 155:1361-1367.

11. Carson CC, Robertson CN. Late hematogenous infection of penile prosthesis. J Urol 1988; 139:50-52.
12. Crook J, Mclean M, Catton C, Yeung I, Tsihlias J, Pintilie M. Factors influencing risk of acute urinary retention after TRUS-fuided permanent prostate seed implantation. Int J Rad Oncol Biol Phys 2002; 52:453-460.
13. D'Amico A, Cote K, Loffredo M, Renshaw A, Chen M. Advanced age at diagnosis is an independent predictor of time to death from prostate carcinoma for patients undergoing external beam radiation threapy for clinically localized prostate carcinoma. Cancer 2003; 97:56-62.
14. D'Amico A, Wu Y, Chen M, Nash M, Renshaw A, Richie J. Perineural invasion as a predictor of biochemical outcome following radical prostatectomy for select men with clinically localized prostate cancer. J Urol 2001; 165:126-129.
15. Daniell HW. A better prognosis for obese men with prostate cancer. J Urol 1996; 155:220-225.
16. Davis BE, DeBrock BJ, Lierz MF, Weigel JW. Management of preexisting inflatable penile prosthesis during radical retropubic prostatectomy. J Urol 1992; 148:1198-1200.
17. Davis BJ, Pisansky TM, Wilson TM, et al. The radial distance of extraprostatic extension of prostate carcinoma: implications for prostate brachytherapy. Cancer 1999; 85:2630-2637.
18. De Crevoisier R, Bourhis J, Domenge C, Wibault P, al e. Full-dose reirradiation for unresectable head and neck carcinoma: experience at the Gustave-Roussey Institute in a series of 169 patients. J Clin Oncol 2001; 16:3556-3562.
19. de la Piedra C, Castro-Errecaorde N, Traba M, et al. Bone remodeling markers in the detection of bone metastases in prostate cancer. Clinica Chimica Acta 2003; 331:45-53.
20. Din K, Wildt M, Wijkstra H, Debruyne F, Rosette J. The correlation between urodynamic and cystoscopic findings in elderly men with voiding complaints. J Urol 1996; 155:1018-1022.
21. Fang C, Dattoli M, Wallner K, True L, Cash J, Sorace R. Prostatic Acid Phosphatase Predicts Cancer-Specific Survival in Patients with Intermediate to High Risk Prostate Cancer Treated with Palladium-103 Brachytherapy. 2007.
22. Freedman GM, Hanlon AL, Lee WR, Hanks GE. Young patients with prostate cancer have an outcome justifying their treatment with external beam radiation. Int J Radiat Oncol Biol Phys 1996; 35:243-250.

23. Ghavamian R, Bergstralh EJ, Blute ML, Slezak J, Zincke H. Radical retropubic prostatectomy plus orchiectomy versus orchietomy alone for pTxN+ prostate cancer: A matched comparison. Cancer 1999; 161:1223-1228.

24. Grann A, Gaudin PB, Raben A, Wallner KE. Pathologic features from prostate needle biopsy and prognosis after I-125 brachytherapy. Radiat Oncol Invest 1998; 6:170-174.

25. Grann A, Wallner K. Prostate brachytherapy in patients with inflammatory bowel disease. Int J Radiat Oncol Biol Phys 1998; 40:135-138.

26. Gray G, Wallner K, Roof J, Corman J. Cystourethroscopic findings before and after prostate brachytherapy. Techniques in Urology 2000; 6:109-111.

27. Gutman s, Merrick G, Butler W, et al. Severity categories of the International Prostate Symptom Score before, and urinary morbidity after, permanent prostate brachytherapy. BJU International 2005; 97:62-68.

28. Gutman S, Merrick G, Butler W, et al. Temporal relationship between prostate brachytherapy and the diagnosis of colorectal cancer. Int J Rad Oncol Biol Phys 2006; 66:48-55.

29. Hafron J, Fogarty J, Wiesen A, Melman A. Surgery for localized prostate cancer after renal transplantation. BJU International 2005; 95:319-322.

30. Hakenberg O, Wirth M, Hermann T, et al. Recommendations for the treatment of localized prostate cancer by permanent interstitial brachytherapy. Urol Int 2002; 70:15-20.

31. Howard A, Wallner K, Han B, Schneider B, al e. Clinical course and dosimetry of rectal fistulas after prostate brachytherapy. JBI 2001; 17:37-42.

32. Hughes S, Wallner K, Miller G, Miller S, True L. Pre-existing histologic evidence of prostatitis is unrelated to post-implant urinary morbidity. Radiat Oncol Invest 2001; 96 (supp):79-82.

33. Johnstone P, Riffenburgh R, Moul J, et al. Effect of age on biochemical disease-free outcome in patients with T1-T3 prostate cancer treated with definitive radiotherapy in an equal-access health care system: A radiation oncology report of the department of defense center for prostate research. Int J Rad Oncol Biol Phys 2003; 55:964-969.

34. Kaminski J, Hanlon A, Horwitz E, Pinover W, Mitra R, Hanks G. Relationship betwen prostate volume, prostate-specific antigen nadir, and biochemical control. Int J Rad Oncol Biol Phys 2002; 52:888-892.

35. Kaye KW, Olson DJ, Payne JT. Detailed preliminary analysis of 125 iodine implantation for localized prostate cancer using percutaneous approach. J Urol 1995; 153:1020-1025.
36. Keyes M, Schellenberg D, Moravan V, et al. Decline in urinary retention incidence in 805 patients after prostate brachytherapy: The effect of learning curve? Int J Rad Oncol Biol Phys 2006; 64:825-834.
37. Khan MA, Han M, Partin AW, Epstein J, Walsh P. Long-term cancer control of radical prostatectomy in men younger than 50 years of age: Update 2003. Urology 2003; 62:86-92.
38. Kovacs G, Potter R, Loch T, et al. GEC/ESTRO recommendations on temporary brachytherapy using stepping sources for localised prosate cancer. Radiother and Oncol 2005; 74:137-148.
39. Krupski T, Petroni GR, Bissonette EA, Theodorescu D. Quality-of-life comparison of radical prostatectomy and interstitial brachytherapy in the treatment of clinically localized prostate cancer. Urol 2000; 55:736-742.
40. Kwee S, Coel M, Lim J, Ko J. Prostate cancer localization with 18-Fluorine fluorocholine positron emission tomography. J Urology 2005; 173:252-255.
41. Lanciano RM, Martz K, Montana GS, Hanks GE. Influence of age, prior abdominal surgery, fraction size, and dose on complications after radiation therapy for squamous cell cancer of the uterine cervix. Cancer 1992; 69:2124-2130.
42. Landis D, Wallner K, Locke J, et al. Late urinary morbidity after prostate brachytherapy. Brachytherapy 2002; 1:21-26.
43. Lehrer S, Stone NN, Stock RG. Prostate cancer in a large prostate is associated with a decreased prostate specific antigen failure rate after brachytherapy. J Urol 2005; 173:79-81.
44. Leibel SA, Heimann R, Kutcher GJ. Three-dimensional conformal radiation therapy in locally advanced carcinoma of the prostate: preliminary results of a phase I dose-escalation study. Int J Radiat Oncol Biol Phys 1993; 26:55-65.
45. Levinson A, Nagler E, Lowe F. Approach to management of clinically localized prostate cancer in patients with humna immunodeficiency virus. Urology 2005; 65:91-94.
46. Li P, Wallner K, Ellis W, Blasko J, Corman JM. Prostate brachytherapy in patients with a penile prosthesis. Br J Urol 2001.
47. Liauw S, Sylvester J, Morris C, Blasko J, Grimm P. Second malignancies after prostate brachytherapy: Incidence of bladder and colorectal cancers in patients with 15 years of potential follow-up. Int J Rad Oncol Biol Phys 2006; 66:669-673.

48. Loblaw DA, Wallner K, Dibiase S, Russell K, Blasko J, Ellis W. Brachytherapy in patients with small prostate glands. Techniques in Urology 2000; 6:64-69.
49. Locke J, Ellis W, Wallner K, Cavanagh W, Blasko J. Risk factors for acute urinary retention requiring temporary intermittent catheterization after prostate brachytherapy: A prospective study. Int J Rad Oncol Biol Phys 2002; 52:712-719.
50. Martens C, Pond G, Webster D, Mclean M, Gillan C, Crook J. Relationship of the International Prostate Symptom score with urinary flwo studies, and catheterization rates following 125-I prostate brachytherapy. Brachytherapy 2006; 5:9-13.
51. Merrick G, Butler E, Wallner K, Galbreath R, Allen Z, Adamovich E. Prognostic significance of perineural invasion on biochemical progression-free survival after prostate brachytherapy. Urology 2005; 66:1048-1053.
52. Merrick G, Butler W, Galbreath R, Lief JH, Donzella J. Relationship between the transition zone index of the prostate gland and urinary morbidity after brachytherapy. Urology 2001; 57:524-529.
53. Merrick G, Butler w, Wallner K, et al. The impact of prostate volume and neoadvjuvant adrogen-deprivation therapy on urinary function following prostate brachytherapy. ca Journal Sci Am 2004; 10:181-189.
54. Merrick G, Butler W, Wallner K, Galbreath R, Allen Z, Adamovich E. Androgen-deprivation therapy dies not impact cause-specific or overall survival after permanent prostate brachytherapy. Int J Rad Oncol Biol Phys 2006; 65:669-677.
55. Merrick G, Butler W, Wallner K, et al. Permanent prostate brachytherapy-induced morbidity in patients with grade II and III obesity. Urol 2002; 60:104-108.
56. Merrick G, Wallner K, Butler W. Minimizing prostate brachytherapy-related morbidity. Urol 2003; 62:786-792.
57. Merrick G, Wallner K, Butler W, et al. Brachytherapy in men aged ″54 years with clinically localized prostate cancer. BJU International 2006; 98:324-328.
58. Merrick GS, Butler WM. Modified uniform seed loading for prostate brachytherapy: rationale, design, and evaluation. Techniques in Urology 2000; 6:78-84.
59. Messing EM, Manola J, Sarosdy M, Wilding G, Crawford ED, Trump D. Immediate hormonal therapy compared with observation after radical prostatectomy and pelvic lymphadenectomy in men with node-positive prostate cancer. NEJM 1999; 341:1781-1788.

60. Mitsuyama H, Wallner K, Merrick G. Treatment of prostate cancer in obese patients. Oncol 2006; 20:1191-1197.
61. Moon K, Stukenborg G, Keim J, Theodorescu D. Cancer incidence after localized therapy for prostate cancer. Cancer 2006; 107:991-998.
62. Moran B, Stutz M, Gurel M. Prostate brachytherapy can be performed in selected patients after transurethral resection of the prostate. Int J Rad Oncol Biol Phys 2004; 59:392-396.
63. Morris M, Akhurst T, Osman I, et al. Fluorinated deoxyglucose positron emission tomography imaging in progressive metastatic prostate cancer. Urology 2002; 59:913-918.
64. Nguyen J, Wallner K, Han B, Ellis W, Sutlief S. Increased long-term urinary morbidity in brachytherapy patients with median lobe hyperplasia. Brachytherapy 2002; 1:42-47.
65. Partin AW, Yoo J, Carter HB, et al. The use of prostate specific antigen, clinical stage and Gleason score to predict pathological stage in men with localized prostate cancer. J Urol 1993; 150:110-114.
66. Peters C, Cesaaretti J, Stone NN, Stock RG. Low-dose rate prostate brachytherapy is well tolerated in patients with a history of inflammatory bowel disease. Int J Rad Oncol Biol Phys 2006; 66:424-429.
67. Philip J, Roy S, Ballal M, Foster C, Javle P. Is a digital rectal examination necessary in the diagnosis and clinical staging of early prostate cancer? BJU International 2005; 95:969-971.
68. Radomski SB, Herschorn S. Risk factors associated with penile prosthesis infection. J Urol 1992; 147:383-385.
69. Rockhill J, Wallner K, Hoffman C, Hummel S, Arthurs S. Prostate brachytherapy in massively obese patients. Brachytherapy 2002; 1:54-60.
70. Rosser C, Kamat A, Wang X, et al. Biochemical disease-free survival in men younger than 60 years with prostate cancer treated with radical prostatectomy. Urology 2006; 67:769-773.
71. Schanne FJ, Carpiniello V, Chaiken D. Radical prostatectomy in patients with indwelling inflatable penile prosthesis. Urol 1998; 52:715-716.
72. Seymore CH, El-Mahdi AM, Schellhammer PF. The effect of prior transurethral resection of the prostate on post radiation urethral strictures and bladder neck contractures. Int J Radiat Oncol Biol Phys 1986; 12:1597-1600.
73. Sherertz T, Wallner K, Wang H, Sutlief S, Russell K. Long-term urinary function after transperineal brachytherapy for patients with large prostate glands (submitted) 2002.

74. Stone NN, Ratnow ER, Stock RG. Prior transurethral resection does not increase morbidity following real-time ultrasound-guided prostate seed implantation. Techniques in Urology 2000; 6:123-127.
75. Stone NN, Stock RG. Prostate brachtherapy in patients with prostate volumes ≥50 cm3: dosimetric analysis of implant quality. Int J Rad Oncol Biol Phys 2000; 46:1199-1204.
76. Taira A, Merrick G, Wallner K, Dattoli M. Reviving the acid phosphatase test for prostate cancer. Oncology 2007.
77. Terk MD, Stock RG, Stone NN. Identification of patients at increased risk for prolonged urinary retention following radioactive seed implantation of the prostate. J Urol 1998; 160:1379-1382.
78. Thomalla JV, Thompson ST, Rowland RG, Mulcahy JJ. Infectious complications of penile prosthetic implants. J Urol 1987; 138:65-67.
79. Thomas MD, Cormack R, Tempany CM, al e. Indentifying the predictors of acute urinary retention following magnetic-resonance-guided prostate brachytherapy. Int J Rad Oncol Biol Phys 2000; 47:905-908.
80. Thurairaja R, Iles R, Jefferson J, Persad R. Serum amino-terminal propeptide of Type 1 procollagen (P!NP) in prostate cancer: A potential predictor of bone metastases and prognosticator for disease progression and survival. Urologia Internationalis 2005; 76:67-71.
81. Tiguert R, Hurley PM, Gheiler EL, et al. Treatment outcome after radical prostatectomy is not adversely affected by a pre-existing penile prosthesis. Urol 1998; 52:1030-1033.
82. Tincher SA, Kim RY, Ezekiel MP, al e. Effects of pelvic rotation and needle angle on pubic arch interference during transperineal prostate implants. Int J Rad Oncol Biol Phys 2000; 47:361-363.
83. Vijverberg PLM, Kurth KH, Blank LECM, Dadhoiwala NF, de Reijke THM, Koedooder K. Treatment of localized prostatic carcinoma using the transrectal ultrasound guided transperineal implantation technique. European Urology 1992; 21:35-41.
84. Villers A, McNeal JE, Redwine EA, Freiha FS. The role of perineural space invasion in the local spread of prostatic adenocarcinoma. J Urol 1989; 142:763-768.
85. Wallner K, Ellis W, Russell K, Cavanagh W, Blasko J. Use of TRUS to predict pubic arch interference of prostate brachytherapy. Int J Rad Oncol Biol Phys 1999; 43:583-585.
86. Wallner K, Lee H, Wasserman S, Dattoli M. Low risk of urinary incontinence following prostate brachytherapy in patients with a prior TURP. Int J Radiat Oncol Biol Phys 1997; 37:565-569.

87. Wallner KE, Chiu-Tsao S, Roy J, et al. An Improved Method for Transperineal Prostate Implants. J Urol 1991; 146:90-95.
88. Wallner KE, Roy J, Harrison L. Tumor control and morbidity following transperineal I-125 implantation for Stage T1/T2 prostatic carcinoma. J Clin Oncol 1996; 14:449-453.
89. Wallner KE, Smathers S, Sutlief S, Corman J, Ellis W. Prostate brachytherapy in patients with median lobe hyperplasia. International Journal of Cancer 2000; 90:152-156.
90. Wang H, Wallner K, Sutlief S, Blasko J, Russell K, Ellis W. Transperineal brachytherapy in patients with large prostate glands. International Journal of Cancer 2000; 90:199-205.
91. Watson LR. Ultrasound anatomy for prostate brachytherapy. Seminars in Urol Oncol 1997; 13:391-398.
92. Whelan TJ, Dembo AJ, Bush RS, et al. Complications of whole abdominal and pelvic radiotherapy following chemotherapy for advanced ovarian cancer. Int J Rad Oncol Biol Phys 1992; 22:853-858.
93. Willett CG, Ooi C, Zietman AL, et al. Acute and late toxicity of patients with inflammatory bowel disease undergoing irradiation for abdominal and pelvic neoplasms. Int J Radiat Oncol Biol Phys 2000; 46:995-998.
94. Wilson J, Clarke M, Ewings P, Graham J, Macdonagh R. The assessment of patient life-expectancy: how accurate are urologists and oncologists? BJU International 2004; 95:794-798.
95. Wong W, Buskirk S, Schild S, Prussak K, Davis B. Combined prostate brachytherapy and short-term androgen deprivation therapy as salvage therapy for locally recurrent prostate cancer after external beam irradiation. J Urology 2006; 176:2020-2024.
96. Yap J, Wallner K, Gray G. Cystourethroscopic findings and long-term urinary function after prostate brachytherapy. JBI 2000; 16:257-262.
97. Zelefsky MJ, Marion C, Fuks Z, Leibel SA. Improved biochemical disease-free survival of men younger than 60 years with prostate cancer treated with high dose conformal external beam radiotherapy. J Urology 2003; 170:1828-1832.

16

Post-implant cancer assessment

Evaluating treatment efficacy for early-stage prostate cancer is hampered by the cancer's long natural history and by imprecise methods of assessing tumor control. Ideally, *survival* should be the endpoint by which efficacy is judged. However, survival analysis requires long follow-up, because most men with early stage disease aren't at risk for cancer-related death until ten years or more have passed.(ADOLFSSON) So in the shorter term, we've come to rely on digital rectal exam, repeat biopsies, and PSA to assess the effect of treatment. Unfortunately, all three measures are fraught with interpretive pitfalls, partly due to peculiarities in the post-brachytherapy setting. As brachytherapy becomes more widely practiced, it is important that physicians be aware of potential interpretive pitfalls. Failing to do so places patients at risk for errors, ranging from needless worry to unnecessary salvage therapy.(REED) In fact, it is important that physicians *and* patients be made aware of the potential interpretive pitfalls, because so many patients track their own PSA closely and may become overly alarmed at certain PSA changes.

DIGITAL RECTAL EXAM

Until PSA was introduced, the digital rectal exam (DRE) was the most commonly used method to evaluate treatment results, with local control assessment based on regression of palpable tumor. Reliance on palpability is complicated by the subjectivity of the DRE and the fact that most tumors diagnosed in the PSA era are not palpable even prior to therapy (Stage T1c). Even for palpable tumors, the correlation between tumor regression on rectal exam and local or distant recurrence is tenuous. Perez and colleagues showed that patients with Stage C disease did poorly, despite a high degree of tumor regression by DRE.(PEREZ)

PSA has rendered routine follow-up DRE nearly obsolete. In the absence of a rising PSA, repeat prostatic biopsies rarely show residual cancers, and a DRE is presumably even less likely to detect disease persistence.(ZELEFSKY) Similarly, after prostatectomy, a palpable tumor recurrence in the absence of a rising PSA is virtually unknown.(OBEK, POUND)

PROSTATE SPECIFIC ANTIGEN

PSA is a much more sensitive and objective measure of residual cancer than DRE. It has dramatically decreased the interval preceeding detection of cancer persistence. Following external beam radiation or brachytherapy, patients' PSAs typically decline markedly, reflecting local tumor regression. The rate of decline is highly variable and has not, in itself, been consistently correlated with prognosis (**Figure 16-1**).(RITTER, KAVADI) In the post-brachytherapy setting, any relation between the rate of decline and prognosis is made especially murky by the occurrence of temporary PSA rises (see below). For the majority of patients, it is pretty obvious in the first two to three years, whether or not their cancer has been eradicated. However, a substantial minority of patients exhibit a fluctuating or delayed pattern of PSA change, such that their cancer status is open to question (**Figure 16-2**).

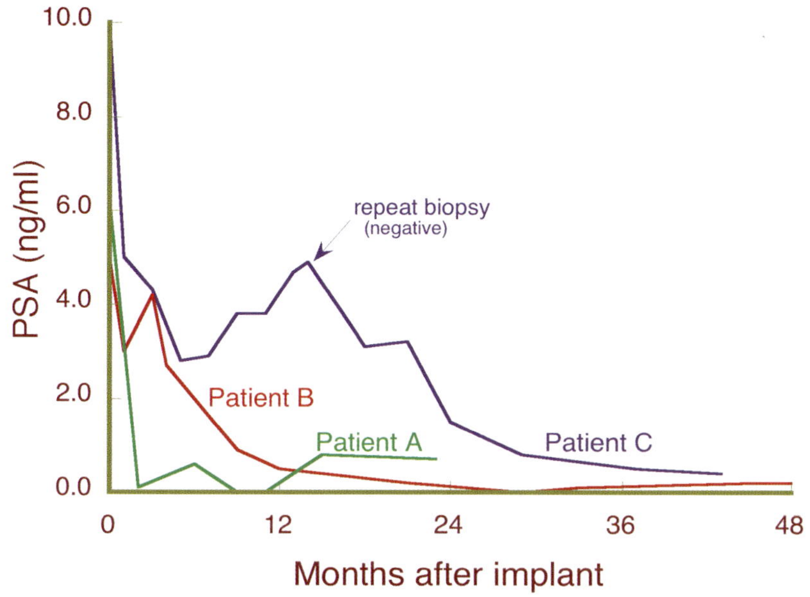

Figure 16-1. Various typical post-implant PSA changes. There is striking variability in the rate of PSA decline. Patients A and B dropped below 1.0 ng/ml at one and nine months, respectively. Patient C took three years to reach nadir. He was biopsied at two years because of postimplant PSA rise near the one-year mark (negative), and eventually fell below 0.5 ng/ml.

Although the rate of PSA decline is of uncertain significance, nearly all investigators have found that the *nadir* PSA correlates well with the likelihood of cure. The relationship between PSA nadir levels and disease-free status is a continuum down to low levels (**Figure 16-3**). However, there is no single nadir PSA value that guarantees against late biochemical failure. Additionally, because of the great variability in the rate and consistency of PSA declines after brachytherapy, the optimal time to allow for nadiring to occur is unknown—some patients nadir at six months, while others take six years.

The simplest and most sensible way to classify patients' disease status is to use an absolute PSA criteria (**Figure 16-4**). While an absolute criteria of 1.0 ng/ml was most popular during the 1990s, there is an increasing tendency to use 0.5, 0.4 or even 0.2 ng/ml as the cutoff for disease eradica-

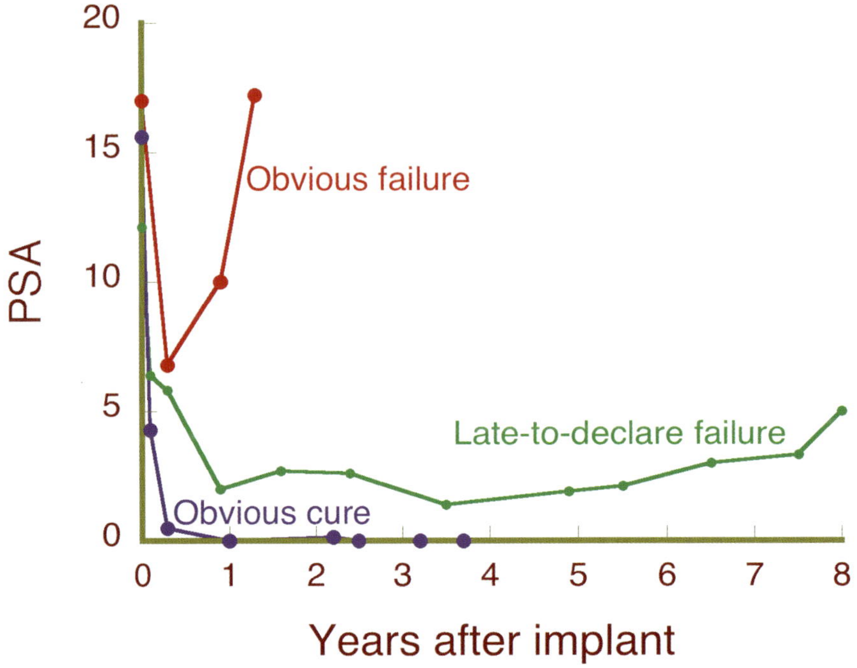

Figure 16-2. For most patients, it's pretty obvious in the first two or three years whether or not their cancers have been eradicated.

tion.(CRITZ 00. MERRICK, WALLNER, DATTOLI 07) Keep in mind, though, that no matter how low the nadir value, an individual patient is not guaranteed a cure. And while low post-treatment PSA values are associated with a low *likelihood* of cancer recurrence, even some patients with undetectable post-implant PSA will ultimately develop late biochemical failure.

Early, mainstream investigators were quick to adopt an absolute PSA value as the critera for biochemical failure.(HANKS 1996) However, when it became obvious how poor the control rates were with external beam radiation, a fix was rapidly devised. As an alternative to using nadir or absolute values to assess post-treatment cancer status, a 1997 ASTRO consensus panel advocated the use of a rising PSA as an indicator of persistent cancer.(ASTRO) Specifically, three consecutive rises, back-dated to midway between the nadir and the first rise, was recommended. The conceptual appeal of using a *rising* value as the criteria for cancer recurrence is that some PSA nadirs, while not below 1.0 ng/ml, may remain stable for several

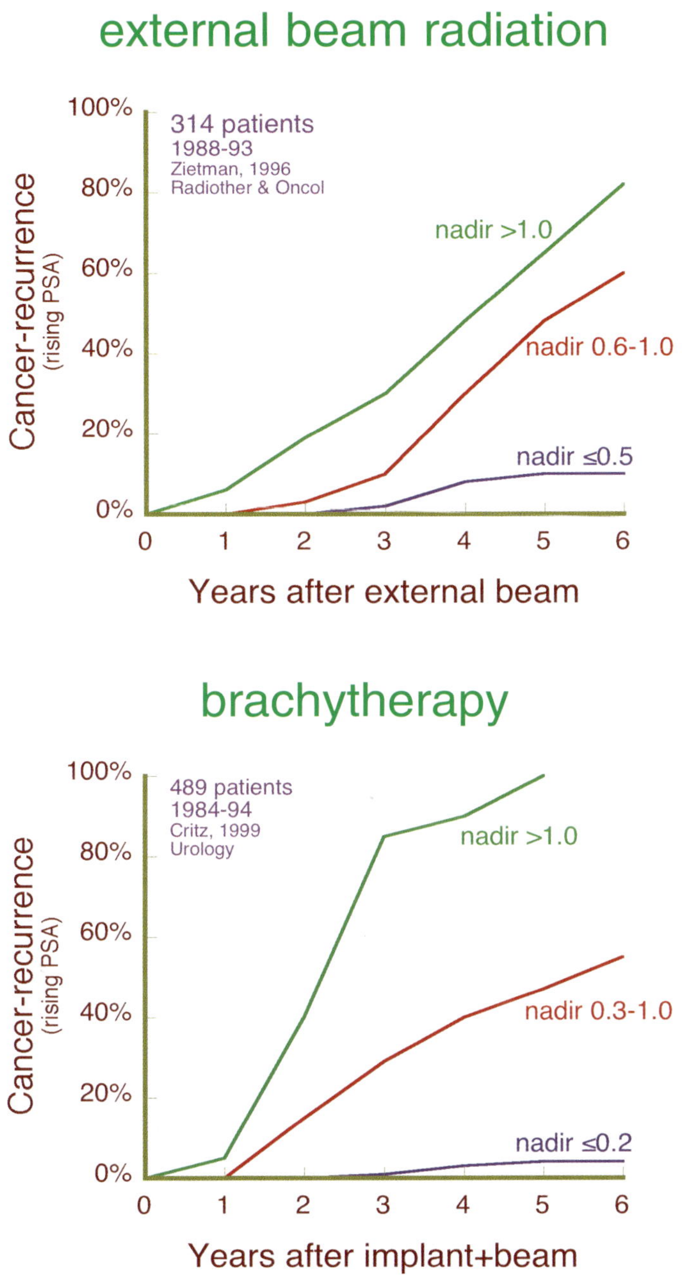

Figure 16-3. These were two of the ealiest studies to demonstrate the likelihood of subsequent biochemical failure as a function of post-treatment PSA. It has been known for many years that nearly all patients with a post-radiation nadir PSA ≥1.0 ng/ml will ultimately fail biochemically. The vast majoirty of patients with a nadir <0.5 ng/ml will remain in biochemical control.(ZIETMAN, CRITZ)

years or more. More recently, a "nadir+2" definition has been proposed, requiring a rise to 2 ng/ml above nadir, not back-dated. Nadir + 2 may be less subject to PSA bounce and post-hormonal PSA surge.(KUBAN 06)

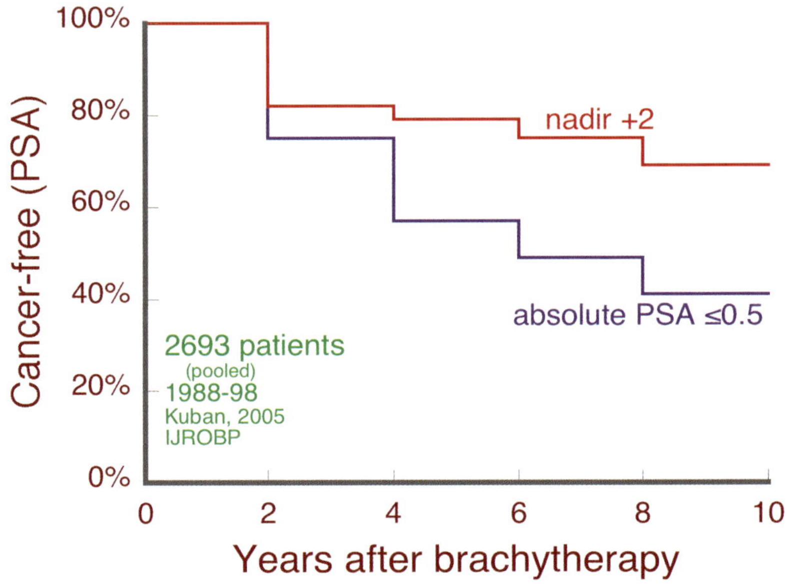

Figure 16-4. PSA-based cancer-free rates using biochemical control criteria of nadir+2 versus an absolute PSA <0.5. Using lax critieria like ASTRO or nadir+2 makes the control rate look better.

In practice, the ASTRO consensus criteria or more recent modifications make the disease-free curve look better in the first five to ten years, because many patients who would be scored failures based on a high nadir PSA will, in fact, require several years to show a persistent PSA rise. In other words, the ASTRO criteria delayed the bad news, making treatment appear more effective than it is (**Figure 16-5**). Debate over the preferability of the ASTRO criteria versus use of nadir values to score patients' cancer status has continued for almost 10 years.(KUBAN 06) With longer follow-up, however, the criteria used becomes less important because almost all cancer recurrences eventually declare themselves by a rising PSA, regardless of the nadir value.(VICINI, HANLON)

Whatever criteria are used to define biochemical failure, there will always be some ambiguous cases, probably the most common of which is the patient whose last PSA is slightly higher than previous values, but still below an arbitrary nadir criteria for tumor control. Ambiguous cases usu-

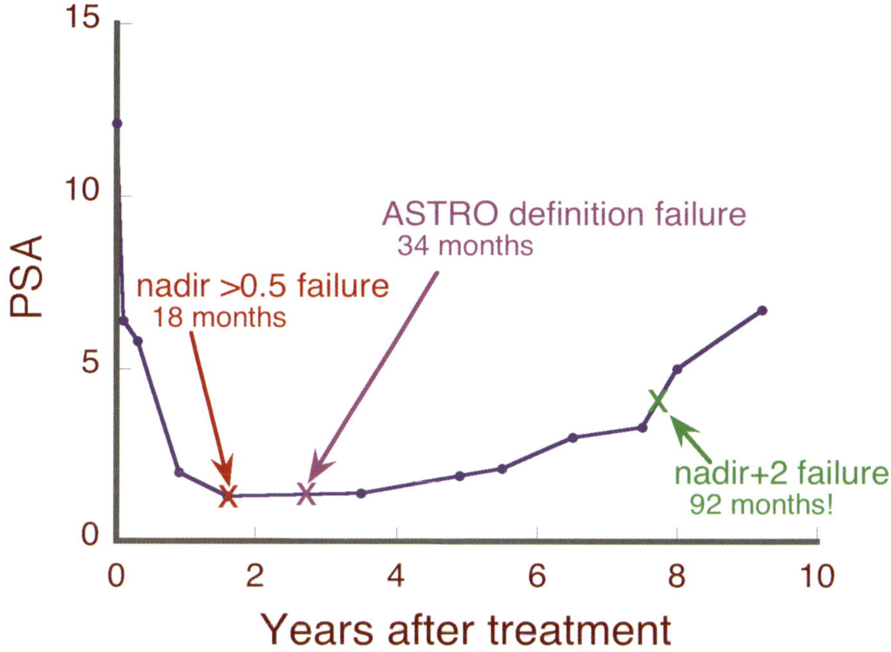

Figure 16-5. The major difference between using an absolute nadir value versus a rising PSA as a marker of disease status is that patients are scored as having failed much sooner when using a nadir parameter. A high nadir value is almost certainly indicative of residual cancer, but it may take several years for residual cancer to begin to grow and to cause the PSA to rise. Researchers who use a modifed ASTRO definition can carry such patients on the books as being "controlled", knowing that nearly all of them will ultimately fail.

ally account for only a small fraction of the total and they should not have a substantial statistical effect on reported cancer-free rates. Additionally, with longer follow-up, these ambiguous cases become less frequent.

TEMPORARY PSA RISES

While the prognostic importance of nadir values applies to both external beam radiation and brachytherapy, there are some peculiar aspects of post-treatment PSAs that seem specific to brachytherapy. *Temporary PSA rises*, also referred to as *PSA bumps, bounces* or *spikes,* occur commonly between 12 and 36 months after implantation (**Figures 16-6, 16-7 and 16-**

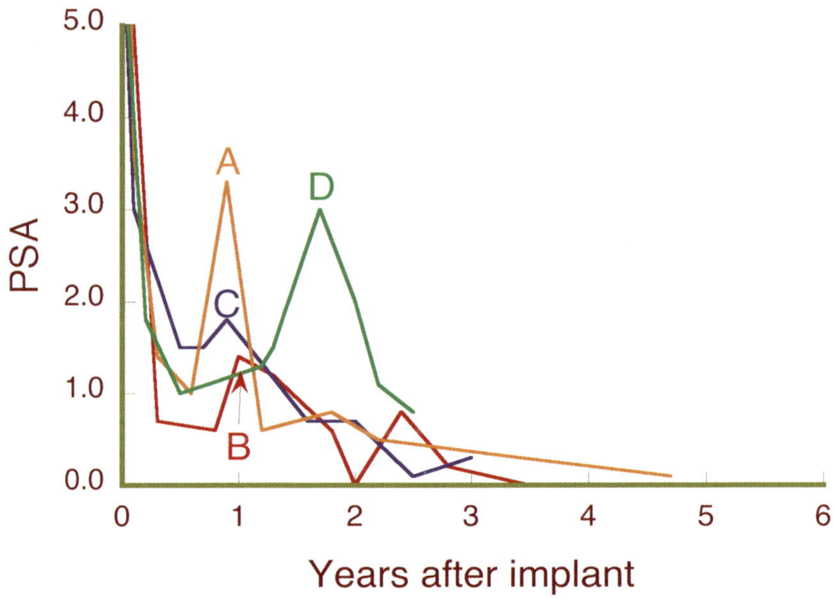

Figure 16-6. Typical examples of temporary PSA rises following brachytherapy. Note double rises in patients A and B.

8). The occurrence of PSA spikes was first reported in the first edition of Prostate Brachytherapy made Complicated (1997). The next published report came in 2000.(CRITZ)

The magnitude of most temporary rises is less than 2.0 ng/ml, but rises as high as 16 ng/ml have been reported (**Figure 16-7**).(CRITZ 00, CAVANAGH) The incidence of temporary rises depends partly on how often PSAs are taken, and what magnitude of increase is considered a *rise*. If PSAs are taken at the typical 4 to 6 months intervals and *any* increase is considered, then about one-third of patients will experience a spike or bump.(**Figures 16-9**). Approximately one-fourth of patients who spike will have two or more spikes.(MERRICK)

The likelihood of a temporary rise is independent of pre-treatment PSA, Gleason score, or use of supplemental external beam radiation (**Figure 16-10**). In multi-variate analysis of 218 hormone-naive brachytherapy patients, Merrick and colleagues reported that age, V150 and clinical stage were predictors of a spike. However, the absolute differences between

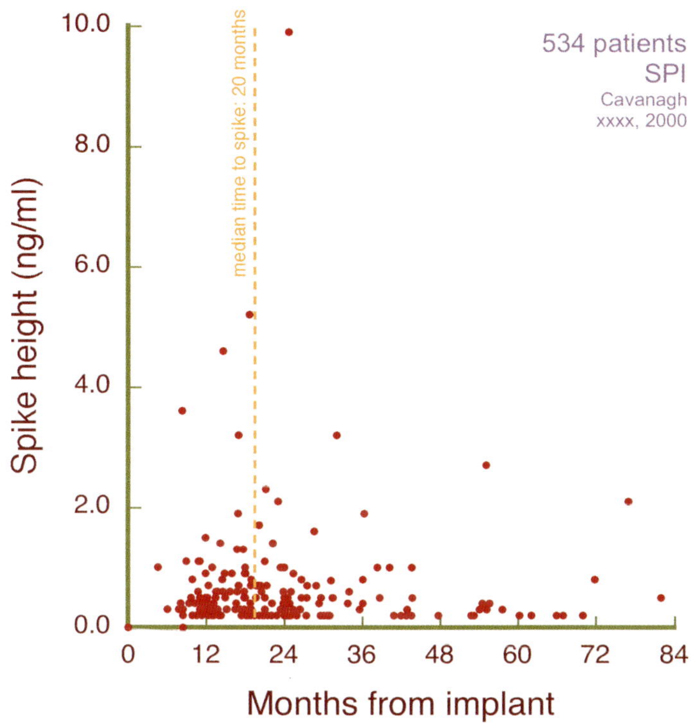

Figure 16-7. Magnitude of PSA spike peak versus time after brachytherapy. (CAVANAGH)

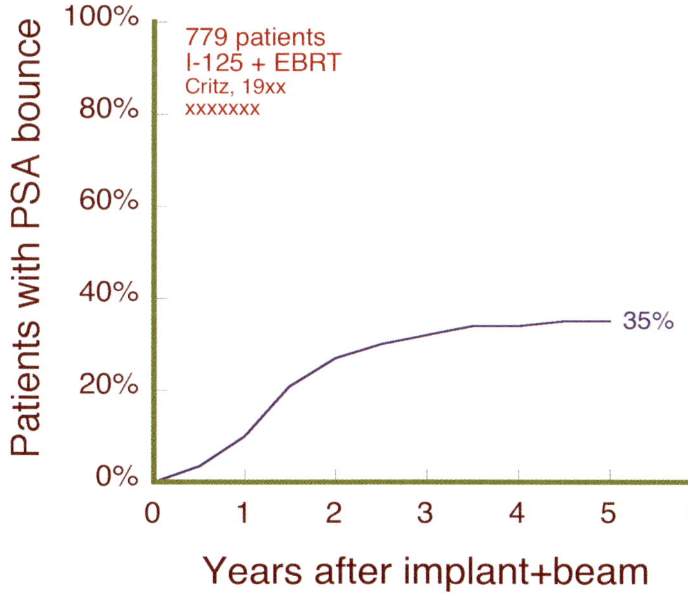

Figure 16-8. The incidence of a temporary PSA rise is greatest between one and two years postimplant.(CRITZ 00)

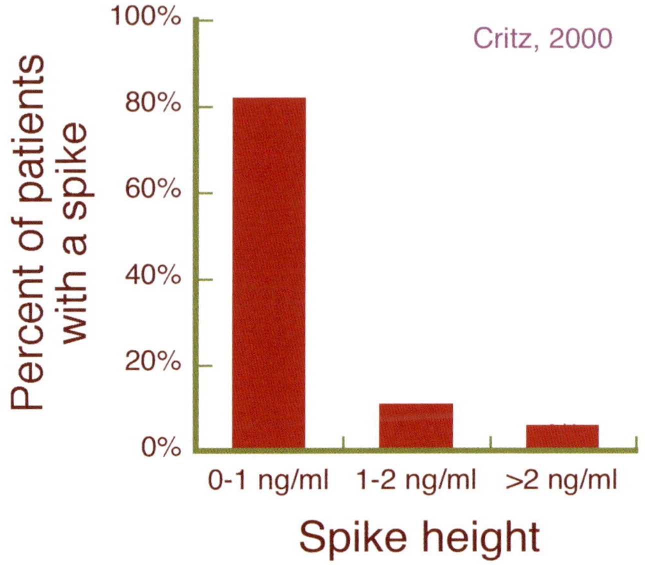

Figure 16-9. Of patients who experience a temporary PSA rise, 82% had an increase of 1.0 ng/ml or less, and only 6% had an increase of greater than 2.0 ng/ml.(CRITZ 00)

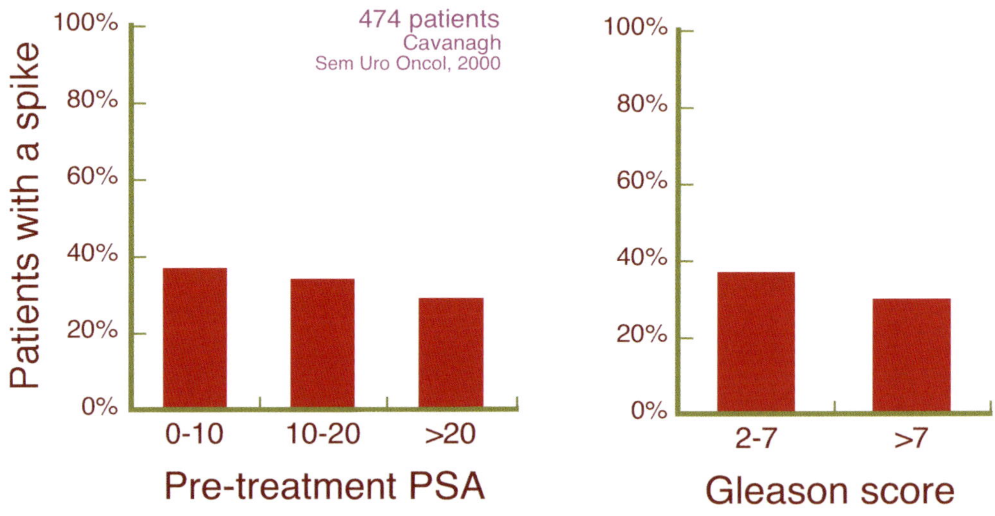

Figure 16-10. The likelihood of a patient demonstrating a temporary PSA rise is independent of pretreatment PSA or Gleason score.(CAVANAGH)

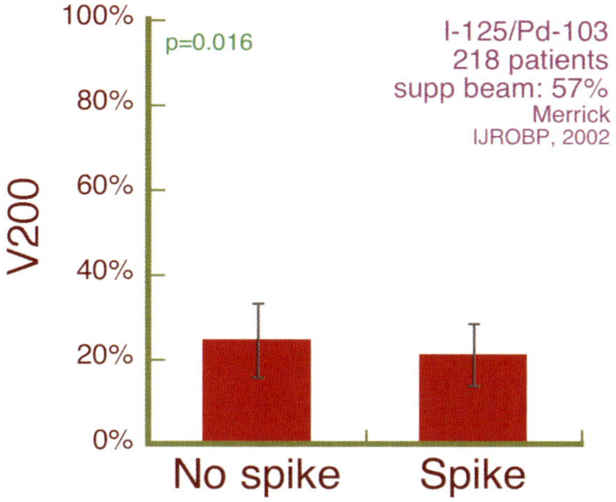

Figure 16-11. Likelihood of PSA spike versus V200.(MERRICK)

parameters and the occurrence of a spike were small, so that the clinical utility of these parameters is probably not sufficient to help decipher a spike from an early biochemical failure (**Figure 16-11**).(MERRICK) Das and colleagues reported an association between spike height and precipitating factors such as ejaculation, proctitis, instrumentation.(DAS) Such precipitating factors, however, are fairly common occurrences in the post-implant period, and any relationship, in a given patient, could easily be fortuitous. As a rule, any PSA increase less than 10 ng/ml in the first two post-implant years is very likely to turn out to be a spike, but the only way to know is to wait a few months and repeat the test at least twice.

While they make for a lot of patient and physician anxiety, the long-term prognosis for PSA spike patients appears similar to patients without a spike.(CAVANAGH, CRITZ 00) Temporary post-treatment rises seem to correspond to late recurrence of radiation-related urinary symptoms.(CESARETTI) Spikes also occur in approximately 25% of external beam radiation patients.(HORWITZ)

While there is currently no clear explanation for the occurrence of spikes, it's important to be aware of them because of the tendency of physicians and patients to panic with any PSA rise. To minimize the degree of panic, it's a good idea to warn patients in advance of the possibility of temporary

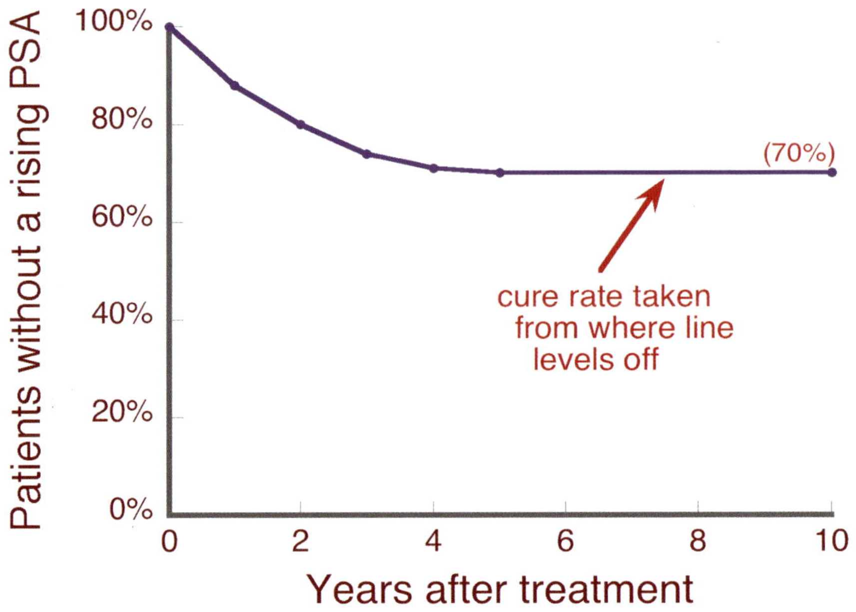

Figure 16-12. Cure rates are determined by where the freedom-from-cancer curve plateaus. If there is no plateau, no estimate of a cure rate can be made.

PSA rises. Multiple investigators agree that there is no negative significance to a PSA spike after beam radiation or brachytherapy.(PATEL, ROSSER, AKYOL, MERRICK 02)

An appreciation of the frequent occurrence of temporary PSA rises is especially crucial in patients for whom a salvage prostatectomy would be considered. To the uninitiated, it seems commonsensical that a rising PSA in the first three post-implant years would be an indication for salvage prostatectomy. Not so fast. Any consideration of a salvage procedure during that time should be approached with great reluctance. In fact, for patients with a pre-treatment PSA less than 20 ng/ml, a post-treatment PSA rise is far more likely to be temporary as opposed to a true indication of cancer persistence. The clinical dilemma of a rising PSA in the first three post-implant years is made doubly confusing when a post-implant biopsy in the same period is positive, because biopsies also may take two years or more to revert to negative (see below).(PRESTIDGE, SMATHERS, REED) The common occurrence of temporary PSA rises is further impetus to insist that investi-

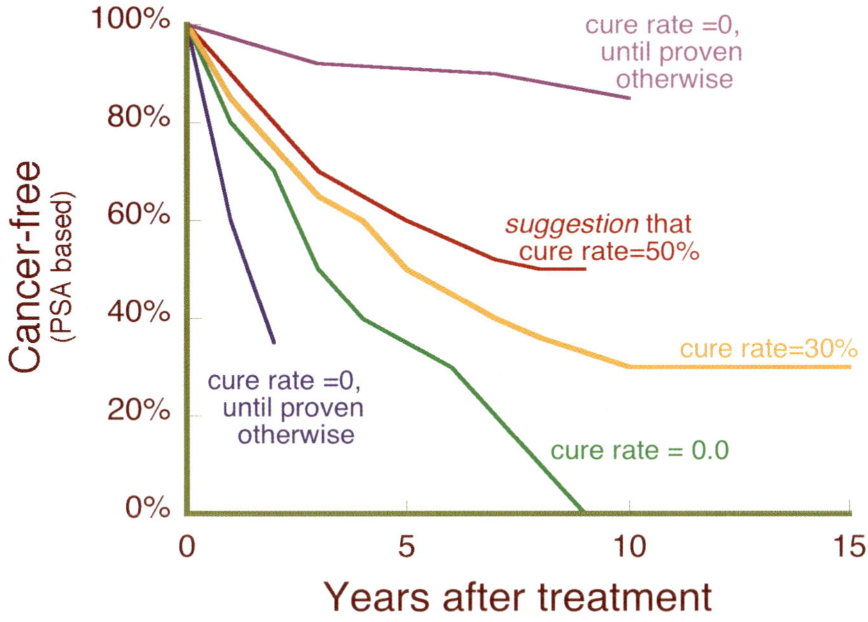

Figure 16-13. We repeat: cure rates are determined by where the freedom-from-cancer curve plateaus. If there is no plateau, no estimate of a cure rate can be made. This a very important point, because treatment outcomes are often published showing curves like the purlple one at the top, with a statement that the cure rate at 10 years is 85%, even though the trajectory is clearly still downward.

gators use longer follow-up times before reporting PSA-based cancer control rates after brachytherapy.(SHIPLEY)

CURE RATES

When tracking groups of patients at risk of cancer recurrence, there is no universally accepted definition of *cure*. With nearly all types of cancer, there is an initial rapid failure rate, followed by a leveling off of the curves, as the percent of the remaining patients with persistent cancer falls. Ideally, the cure rate (proportion of patients who will remain free of cancer) should be assessed at the time after which no more failures will occur (**Figure 16-12**). However, with prostate cancer there is probably no time, with any treatment modality, after which *no* more failures will occur—there

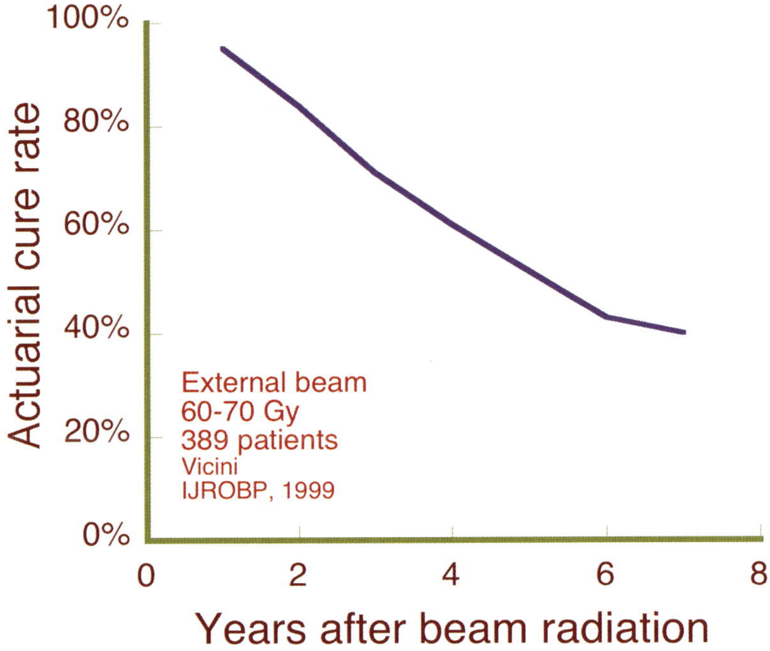

Figure 16-14. Due to the time required for post-treatment PSAs to start rising in patients with residual cancer, calculated cure rates are typically lower with longer follow-up.(VICINI)

is usually a small but persistent late failure rate. Some late failures could be due to second malignancies within the prostate, but differentiating late recurrences from second primaries is not currently practical. From a practical standpoint, that point on the survival curve at which the failure rate decelerates to near zero is generally taken as the *cure rate*. It would more appropriately be referred to as the *apparent* or *approximate* cure rate.

While actuarial statistics are generally a more realistic statistical method than straight percentages, they can still favorably bias the data, especially with short follow-up times. Patients with short follow-up may make the initial portion of the curve look more favorable, simply because there has not been sufficient time for many of the treated patients to manifest clinical or biochemical failure, especially if the ASTRO requirement for three successive rises is used (**Figure 16-14**).(VICINI) Favorable statistical bias with

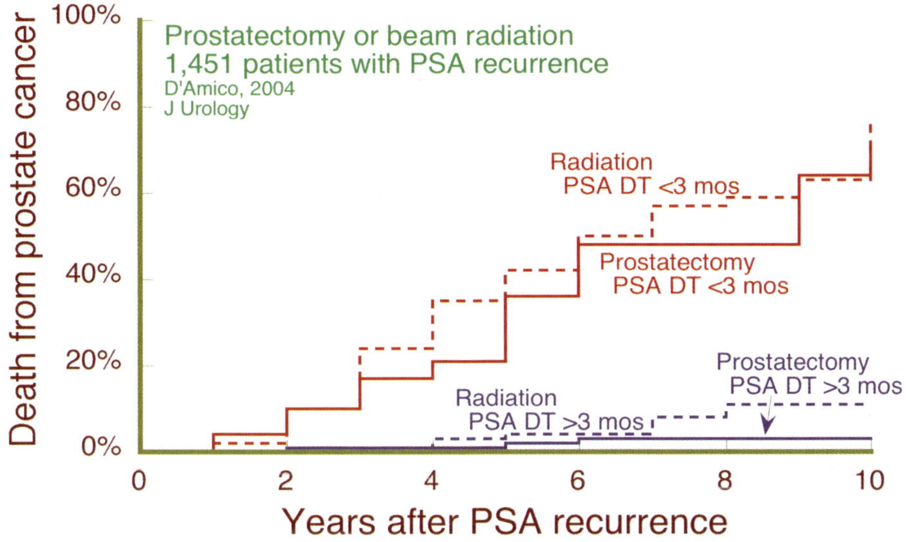

Figure 16-15. PSA doubling times versus incidence of distant mets over time.

short follow-up has rightly lead some investigators to call for exclusion of patients with less than 2.5 years follow-up.(SHIPLEY)

LOCAL VERSUS DISTANT FAILURE

A rising PSA is a general marker of disease progression—it does not in itself distinguish between local and distant failure. However, the rate of PSA rise helps distinguish between local and distant failures. After external beam radiation, patients with rapidly rising PSA (doubling time less than 12 months) are more likely to have distant metastases.(LEE, RITTER, SARTOR, POLLACK) However, the rate of rise is not a very specific criteria for local versus distant failure, because there is a large amount of overlap between the groups. To date, there are limited data specific to brachytherapy regarding the rate of PSA rise and the site of failure.

DOUBLING TIMES

There is strong evidence that PSA doubling times predict the time to overt metastatic disease and death from prostate cancer. To date, the relationship between PSA velocity and overt clinical recurrence has been shown most elegantly for beam radiation and prostatectomy. The relationship between doubling times and cancer-specific mortality has been remarkably

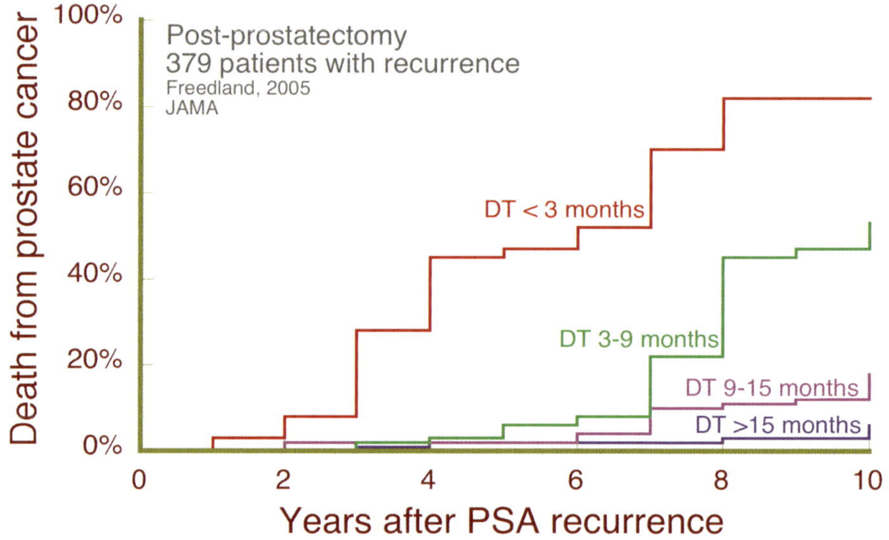

Figure 16-16. PSA doubling times and prostate-specific death following biochemical recurrence after prostatectomy.(FREEDLAND)

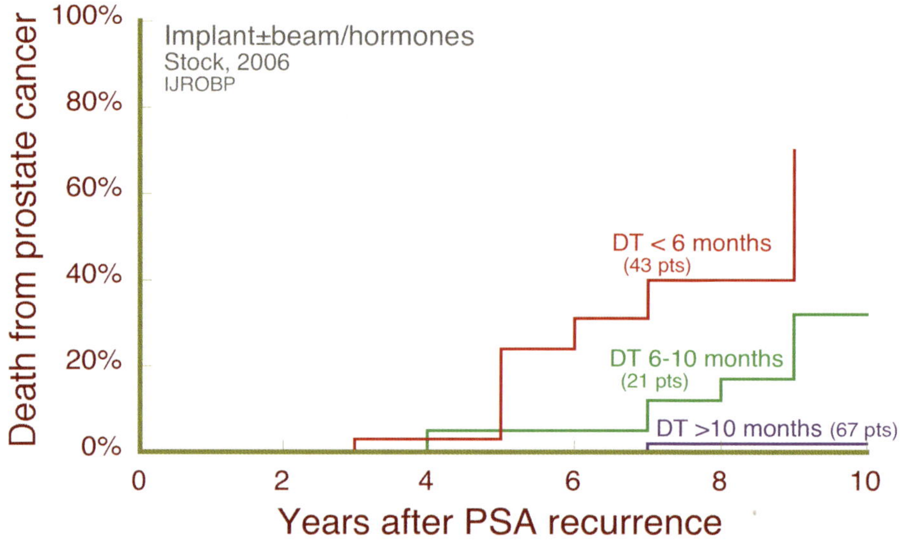

Figure 16-17. PSA doubling times and prostate-specific death following biochemical recurrence after brachytherapy. (STOCK)

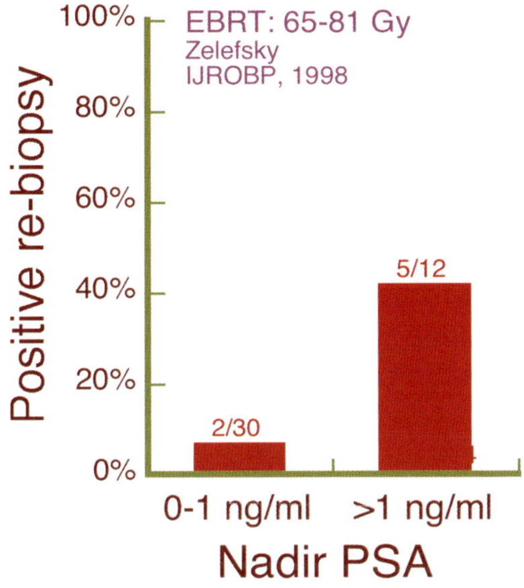

Figure 16-18. Likelihood of a positive re-biopsy after external beam radiation in patients with a non-rising nadir PSA below or above 1.0 ng/ml.(ZELEFSKY)

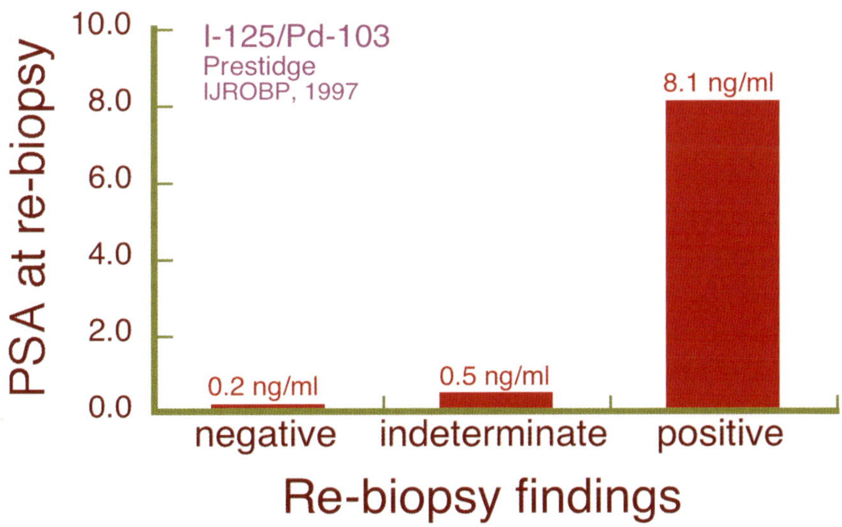

Figure 16-19. PSA at time of repeat biopsy correlated biopsy results.(PRESTIDGE)

consistent between the two modalities (**Figures 16-15 through 17**). However, the picture is bound to be fuzzier with brachytherapy due to PSA spikes that can occur as long as four years after treatment, so that interpreting an individual patient's PSA pattern can be difficult in the first few post-implant years.(STOCK 03)

POST-TREATMENT BIOPSIES

Post-treatment biopsy has been used sporadically to assess intra-prostatic tumor eradication. Compared to digital rectal exam, post-treatment prostatic biopsies always show a higher incidence of residual tumor. And in nearly all reported series, patients with histologically viable tumor have a greater likelihood of developing local recurrence and distant metastases.(KUBAN, SCARDINO) Some authors have argued that histologically viable tumor is irrelevant, but this is wishful thinking. The only series that failed to show worse outcomes in patients with positive follow-up biopsies was that by Cox and Kline.(COX) Their results were clouded, however, by the fact that some patients received hormonal ablation and that the biopsies were done under digital rather than TRUS guidance.

Post-implant biopsies are conceptually appealing, but their routine use is limited by ambiguity in interpretation of biopsy samples and the fact that biopsies are almost always negative in patients with a low PSA at the time of biopsy (**Figures 16-18 & 16-19**).(PRESTIDGE, ZELEFSKY 98) Immunostains have not been of much use so far, but they have the potential to help distinguish between a true biochemical failure versus a temporary PSA rise.(CROOK, BRAWER)

The majority of biopsies are clearly negative or positive. However, a small percentage show residual cancer with radiation effect, and have been termed *indeterminate* (**Figure 16-20**). With time, most indeterminate samples become negative, suggesting that substantial radiation effect is indicative of tumorcidal damage, which simply needs more time to become histologically evident (**Figure 16-21**). (PRESTIDGE) Positive or indeterminate biopsies are especially vexing in the doubly confusing situation of a temporary PSA rise in the first three post-implant years (**Figures 16-22, 16-23**).(SMATHERS, REED) Unfortunately, there's no way at present to be sure whether one is dealing with a true cancer recurrence or two transient phenomena. Color Doppler-directed biopsies might help decipher between cancer involution and cancer persistence (**Figure 16-24**). Take a minute to study **Figure 16-25** and then **Figure 16-26** to get a feel for how tough it can

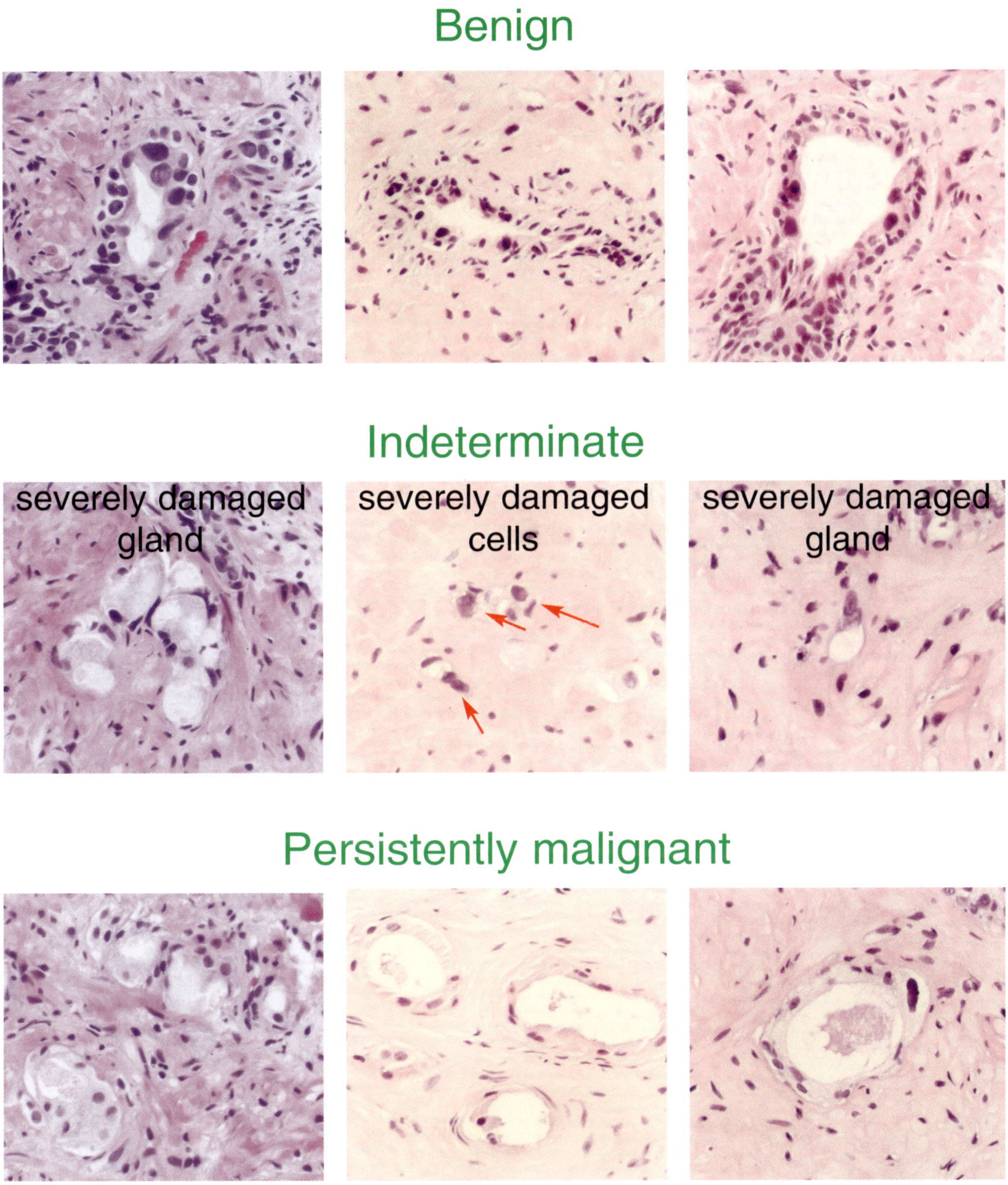

Figure 16-20. Findings on post-implant prostate biopsy range from irradiated noncancerous glands (top panels), to highly radiation-damaged glands of uncertain biologic potential for growth (middle panels), to what appear to be still viable irradiated cancer glands (bottom panels) (courtesy of Dr. Lawrence True).

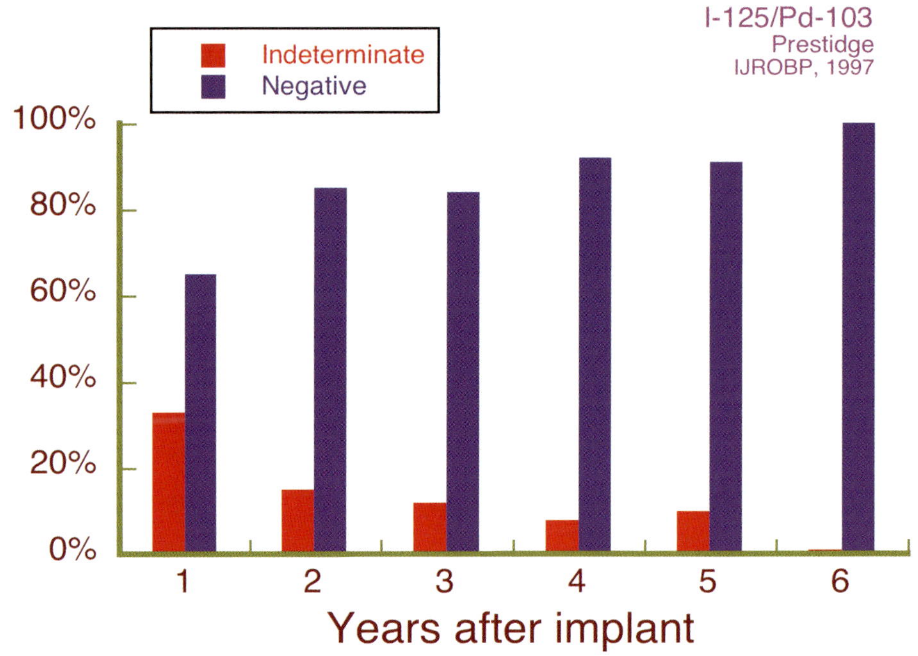

Figure 16-21. The percentage of indeterminate biopsies decreases (top panel) and the percent of negative biopsies increases (lower panel) as time passes after implantation.(PRESTIDGE)

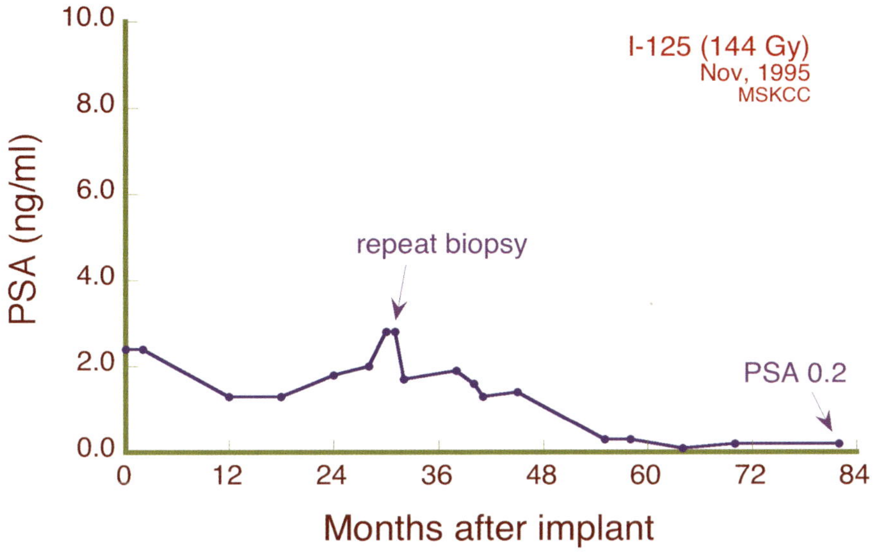

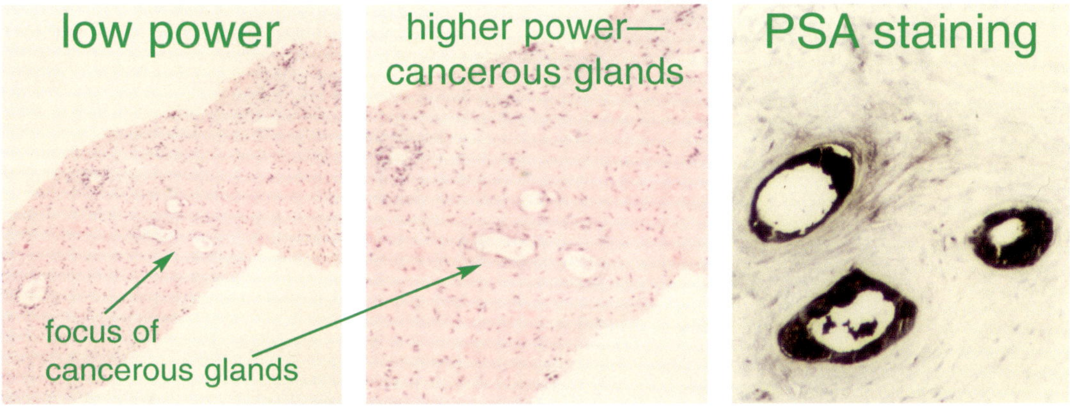

Figure 16-22. Post-implant PSA patterns and corresponding repeat biopsies can be doubly confusing. In this patient, a PSA rise two years after treatment for Gleason 3+3 cancer prompted a repeat biopsy, showing a single focus of histologically viable cancer. PSA staining was positive for cancer. In conjunction with the rising PSA, the patient's urologist strongly urged him to have a salvage prostatectomy. At K. Wallner's urging, the patient waited and his PSA subsequently fell to below 0.5 ng/ml. While further follow-up is needed, the point here is that even an apparently "positive" biopsy and a rising PSA are insufficient to make a definitive diagnosis of cancer persistence.

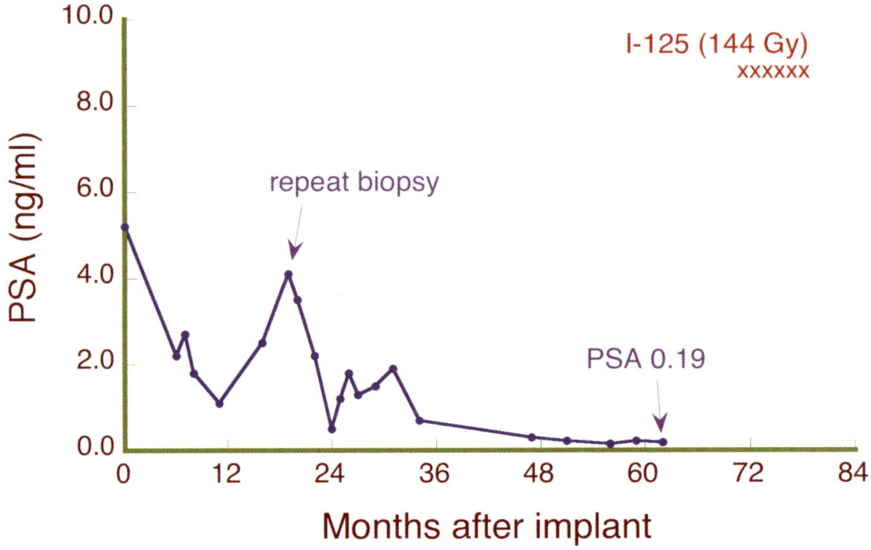

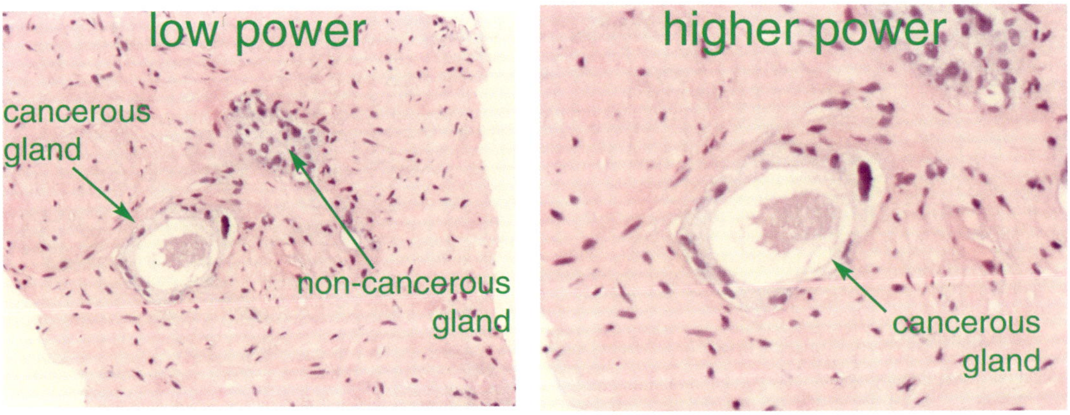

Figure 16-23. This patient, with Gleason score 3+3 and pre-treatment PSA of 5.2 ng/ml, underwent I-125 implantation (144 Gy) at age 61. Eight months after implantation he developed a rising PSA, which fell concomitantly with antibiotic administration (top panel). A second PSA rise between 18 and 24 months after implantation prompted a repeat biopsy, which showed a single cancerous gland. He declined the advice to have a salvage prostatectomy. Subsequently, his PSA fell to below 1.0 ng/ml, 38 months after brachytherapy.(SMATHERS)

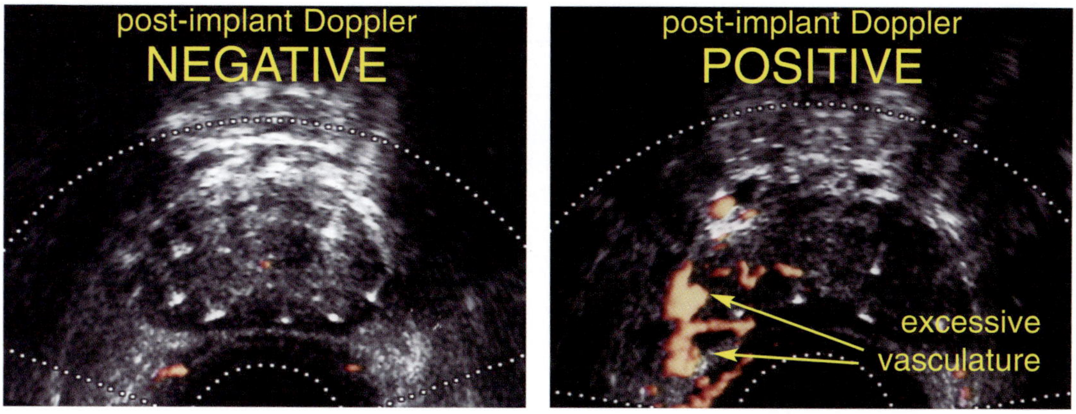

Figure 16-24. Follow-up prostate TRUS-Doppler images. The image on the right shows excessive vasculature in the right base. Repeat biopsy showed persistent cancer.

be to make a call about continuing to watch a PSA bounce or jumping in to recommend a salvage procedure.

BONE SCANS

Routine follow-up bone scans in the absence of a rising PSA are not warranted. At initial diagnosis, bone scans are rarely positive with a PSA of less than 20 ng/ml. After prostatectomy, it has been clearly established that follow-up bone scans are not necessary in the absence of biochemical failure.(CHER) The same probably holds true for brachytherapy. Routine repeat bone scan, as part of follow-up, should be performed only if the PSA is greater than 10 ng/ml (or higher?) or if there is clinical suspicion of bone metastases. Newer imaging modalities and serum markers may improve the detection of micrometastases (see Figure 15-38).(DE LA PIEDRA, THURAIRAJA, MORRIS, KWEE)

IS BIOCHEMICAL FAILURE RELEVANT?

PSA has emerged as the most sensitive indicator of residual disease, making routine post-implant digital rectal exams or repeat biopsies almost obsolete.(TRALINS) But while a high nadir PSA or a rising PSA are statistically associated with a high likelihood of subsequent clinically evident failure, many patients with a rising post-treatment PSA will remain symptom-free for many years.(POUND 99, KUPELIAN) It has been argued that we're getting too concerned about a biochemical parameter that often has little practical relevance. Some would go so far as to argue that a rising post-

What would *you* do?...

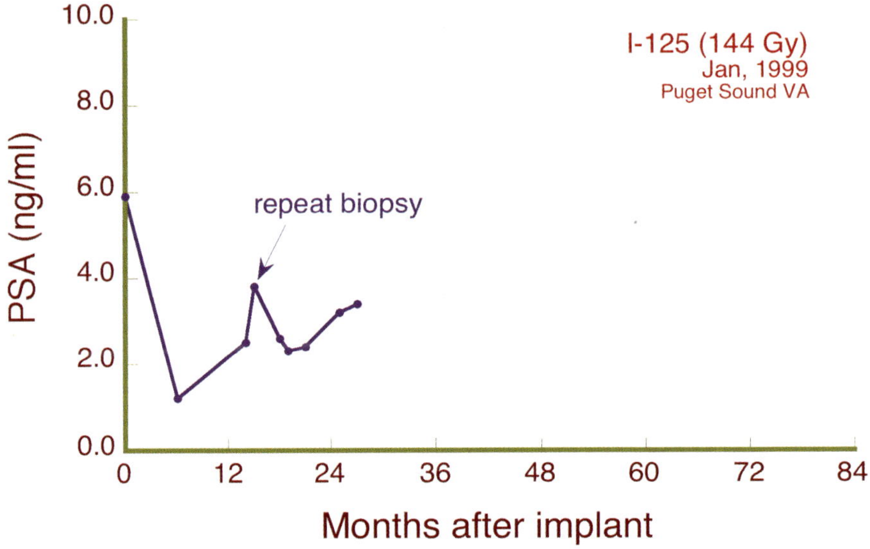

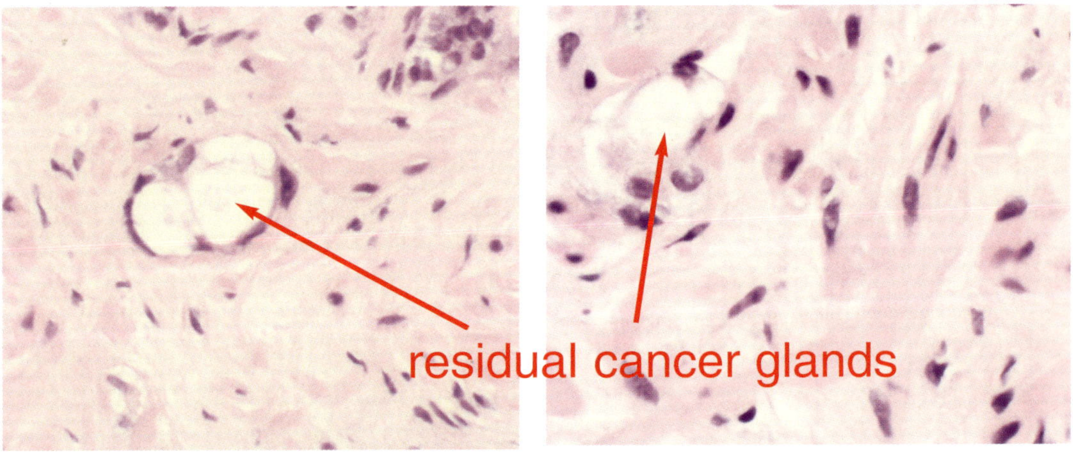

Figure 16-25. This 44-year-old patient had a I-125 (144 Gy) implant for a T1c cancer, with a pretreatment PSA of 5.9 and Gleason score 3+3. His PSA fell to 1.2, and then rose to 3.8 at 13 months postimplant. A repeat biopsy shows residual cancer glands with radiation effect (arrows) and he was strongly urged by his urologist to have a salvage prostatectomy. Instead, the patient has elected to wait... What would you advise? (See Figure 16-26 for outcome in this case)

treatment PSA is therefore not necessarily an indication of failed therapy. Ridiculous. Patients who remain asymptomatic for many years in the face of a slowly rising post-treatment PSA probably are the ones who didn't need treatment in the first place!(ADOLFSSON) There is increasing evidence that biochemical failure is associated with a higher risk of dying from metastastic disease, with a lag time of approximately 10-15 years.(FREEDLAND, D'AMICO) There is no reason to expect that the lag times from biochemical failure to death will differ among brachytherapy, prostatectomy and beam radiation patients.

REFERENCES

1. Adolfsson J, Cartensen J. Natural Course of Clinically Localized Prostatic Carcinoma in Men Less that 70 Years Old. J Urol 1991; 146:96-98.
2. ASTRO. Guidelines for PSA following radiation therapy. Int J Rad Oncol Biol Phys 1997; 37:1035-1041.
3. Aykol F, Ozyigit G, Selek U, Karabulut E. PSA boucning after short term androgen deprivation and 3D-conformal radiotherapy for localized prostate adenocarcinoma and the relationship with the kinetics of testosterone. European Urology 2005; 48:40-45.
4. Brawer MK, Nagle RB, Pitts W, Freiha F, Gamble SL. Keratin immuoreactivity as an aid to the diagnosis of persistent adenocarcinoma in irradiated human prostates. Cancer 1989; 63:454-460.
5. Cavanagh W, Blasko JC, Grimm PD, Sylvester JE. Transient elevation of serum prostate-specific antigen following I-125/Pd-103 brachytherapy for localized prostate cancer. Seminars in Urol Oncol 2000; 18:160-165.
6. Cesaretti J, Stone NN, Stock RG. Urinary symptom flare following I-125 prostate brachytherapy. Int J Rad Oncol Biol Phys 2003; 56:1085-1092.
7. Cher ML, Bianco FJ, Lam JS, al e. Limited role of radionuclide bone scintigraphy in patients with prostate specific antigen elevations after radical prostatectomy. J Urol 1998; 160:1387-1391.
8. Cox JD, Kline RW. Do prostatic biopsies 12 months or more after external irradiation for adenocarcinoma, Stage III, predict long-term survival? Int J Radiat Oncol Biol Phys 1983; 9:299-303.
9. Critz F, Levinson K. 10-year disease-free survival rates after simultaneous irradiation for prostate cancer with a focus on calculation methodology. J Urology 2004; 172:2232-2238.

...what happened

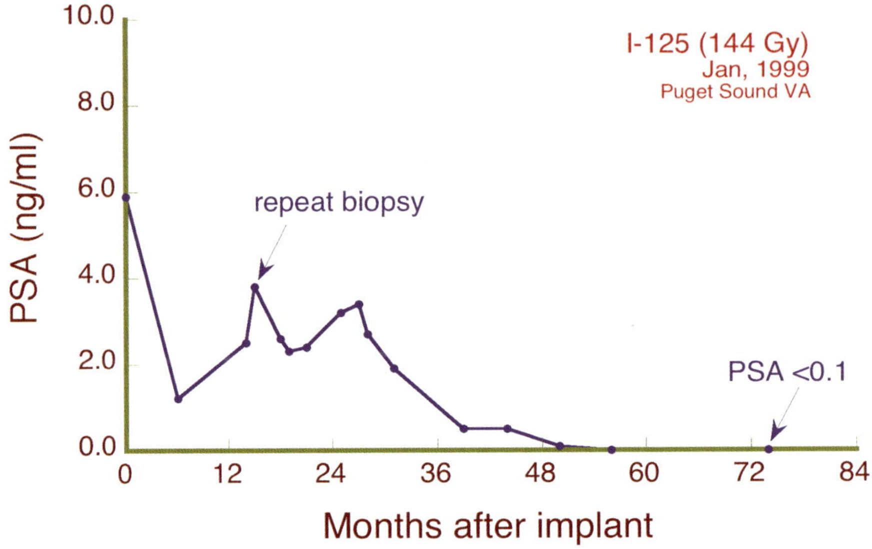

Figure 16-26. K. Wallner advised the patient in Figure 16-xx to hold of on salvage prostatectomy. The patient's PSA subsequently fell to <0.1 ng/ml. This pattern of late PSA fall is typical of patients with a slight to moderate PSA rise in the first 2 years after implantation.

10. Critz FA, Williams H, Holladay CT, Levinson AK, al e. Post-treatment PSA ″0.2 ng/ml defines disease freedom after radiotherapy for prostate cancer using modern techniques. Urol 1999; 54:968-971.

11. Critz FA, Williams WH, Benton JB, Levinson AK, Holladay CT, Holladay DA. Prostate specific anitgen bounce after radioactive seed implantation followed by external beam radiation for prostate cancer. J Urol 2000; 163:1085-1089.

12. Crook J, Malone S, Perry G, Bahadur Y, Robertson S, Abdolell M. Postradiotherapy prostate biopsies: What do they really mean? Results for 498 patients. Int J Rad Oncol Biol Phys 2000; 48:355-367.

13. D'Amico A, Moul J, Carroll P, Sun L, Lubeck D, Chen M. Prostate specific antigen doubling time as a surrogate end point for prostate cancer specific mortality followin radical prostatectomy or radiation therapy. J Urol 2004; 172:S43-S47.

14. Dattoli M, Wallner K, True L, Cash J, Sorace R. Long-term prostate cancer control using Palladium-103 brachytherapy and external beam radiotherapy in patients with a high likelihood of extracapsular cancer extension. Urology 2007.
15. de la Piedra C, Castro-Errecaorde N, Traba M, et al. Bone remodeling markers in the detection of bone metastases in prostate cancer. Clinica Chimica Acta 2003; 331:45-53.
16. Freedland S, Humphreys E, Mangold L, et al. Risk of prostate cancer-specific mortality following biochemical recurrence after radical prostatectomy. JAMA 2005; 294:433-439.
17. Hanlon AL, Hanks GE. Scrutiny of the ASTRO consensus definition of biochemical failure in irradiated prostate cancer patients demonstrates its usefulness and robustness. Int J Rad Oncol Biol Phys 2000; 46:559-566.
18. Horwitz E, Levy L, Thames H, et al. Biochemical and clinical significance of the posttreatment prostate-specific antigen bounce for prostate cancer patients treated with external beam radiation therapy alone: a multiinstitutional pooled analysis. Cancer 2006; 107:1496-1502.
19. Kavadi VS, Zagars GK, Pollack A. Serum prostate-specific antigen after radiation therapy for clinically localized prostate cancer: prognostic implications. Int J Rad Oncol Biol Phys 1994; 30:279-287.
20. Kuban D, Levy L, Potters L, et al. Comparison of biochemical failure definitions for permanent prostate brachytherapy. Int J Rad Oncol Biol Phys 2006; 65:1487-1493.
21. Kuban DA, El-Mahdi AM, Schellhammer P. The significance of post-irradiation prostate biopsy with long- term follow-up. Int J Radiat Oncol Biol Phys 1992; 24:409-414.
22. Kupelian PA, Buchsbaum JC, Patel C, et al. Impact of biochemical failure on overall survival after radiation therapy for localized prostate cancer in the PSA era. Int J Rad Oncol Biol Phys 2002; 52:704-711.
23. Kwee S, Coel M, Lim J, Ko J. Prostate cancer localization with 18-Fluorine fluorocholine positron emission tomography. J Urology 2005; 173:252-255.
24. Lee WR, Hanks GE, Hanlon A. Increasing prostate-specific antigen profile following definitive radiation therapy for localized prostate cancer: Clinical observations. J Clin Oncol 1997; 15:230-238.
25. Merrick GS, Butler WM, Wallner KE, Galbreath RW, Anderson RL. Prostate specific antigen (PSA) spikes following permanent prostate brachytherapy. Int J Rad Oncol Biol Phys 2002; 54:450-456.

26. Morris M, Akhurst T, Osman I, et al. Fluorinated deoxyglucose positron emission tomography imaging in progressive metastatic prostate cancer. Urology 2002; 59:913-918.
27. Obek C, Neulander E, Sadek S, Soloway MS. Is there a role for digital rectal examination in the follow-up of patients after radical prostatectomy? J Urol 1999; 162:762-764.
28. Patel C, Elshaikh M, Angermeier K, et al. PSA bounce predicts early success in patients with permanent Iodine-125 prostate implant. Urology 2004; 63:110-113.
29. Perez CA, Pilepich MV, Zivnuska F. Tumor control in definitive irradiation of localized carcinoma of the prostate. Int J Radiat Oncol Biol Phys 1986; 12:523-531.
30. Pollack A, Zagars GK, Kavadi VS. Prostate specific antigen doubling time and disease relapse after radiotherapy for prostate cancer. Cancer 1994; 74:670-678.
31. Pound CR, Christens-Barry OW, Gurganus RT, Partin AW, Walsh PC. Digital rectal examination and imaging studies are unnecessary in men with undetectable prostate specific anitgen following radical prostatectomy. J Urol 1999; 162:1337-1340.
32. Pound CR, Partin AW, Eisenberger MA, Chan DW, Pearson JD, Walsh PC. Natural history of progression after PSA elevation following radical prostatectomy. JAMA 1999; 281:1591-1597.
33. Prestidge BR, Hoak DC, Grimm PD, Ragde H, Cavanagh W, Blasko JC. Posttreatment biopsy results following interstitial brachytherapy in early-stage prostate cancer. Int J Radiat Oncol Biol Phys 1997; 37:31-39.
34. Reed D, Wallner K, Merrick G, Buskirk S, True L. Clinical correlates to PSA spikes and positive repeat biopsies after prostate brachytherapy. Urol 2003; 62:683-688.
35. Ritter MA, Messing EM, Shanahan TG, Potts S, Chappell RJ, Kinsella TJ. Prostate-specific antigen as a predictor of radiotherapy response and patterns of failure in localized prostate cancer. J Clin Oncol 1992; 10:1208-1217.
36. Rosser C, Kuban D, Levy L, et al. The prostate specific antigen bounce phenomenon after external beam radiation for clinically localized prostate cancer. J Urol 2002; 168:2001-2005.
37. Sartor CI, Strawderman MH, Lin X, Kish KE, McLaughlin PW, Sandler HM. Rate of PSA rise predicts metastatic versus local recurrence after definitive radiotherapy. Int J Rad Oncol Biol Phys 1997; 38:941-947.
38. Scardino PT, Wheeler TM. Prostatic biopsy after irradiation therapy for prostatic cancer. Urol 1985; 25:39-46.

39. Shipley WU. PSA following irradiation for prostate cancer: The upcoming ASTRO symposium. Int J Radiat Oncol Biol Phys 1996; 35:1115.
40. Smathers S, Wallner K, Sprouse J, True L. Temporary PSA rises and repeat prostate biopsies after brachytherapy. Int J Rad Oncol Biol Phys 2001; 50:1207-1211.
41. Stock RG, Stone NN, Cesaaretti J. Prostate-specific antigen bounce after prostate seed implantation for localized prostate cancer: descriptions and implications. Int J Rad Oncol Biol Phys 2003; 56:448-453.
42. Stock RG, Stone NN, Cesaaretti J, Rosenstein B. Biologically effective dose values for prostate brachytherrapy: Effects on PSA failure and posttreatment biopsy results. Int J Rad Oncol Biol Phys 2006; 64:527-533.
43. Thurairaja R, Iles R, Jefferson J, Persad R. Serum amino-terminal propeptide of Type 1 procollagen (P!NP) in prostate cancer: A potential predictor of bone metastases and prognosticator for disease progression and survival. Urologia Internationalis 2005; 76:67-71.
44. Tralins K, Wallner K. Follow-up costs after external beam irradiation for low risk prostate cancer. Int J Rad Oncol Biol Phys 1999; 44:323-326.
45. Vicini FA, Kestin LL, Martinez AA. The importance of adequate follow-up in defining treatment success after external beam irradiation for prostate cancer. Int J Rad Oncol Biol Phys 1999; 45:553-561.
46. Wallner K, Merrick G, True L, Sutlief S, Cavanagh W, Butler W. I-125 versus Pd-103 for low risk prostate cancer: Preliminary biochemical outcomes from a prospective randomized mulitcenter trial. Int J Rad Oncol Biol Phys 2003; 57:1297-1303.
47. Zelefsky MJ, Leibel SA, Gaudin PB, al e. Dose escalation with three-dimensional conformal radation therapy affects the outcome in prostate cancer. Int J Rad Oncol Biol Phys 1998; 41:491-500.
48. Zietman AL, Tibbs MK, Dallow KC, al e. Use of PSA nadir to predict subsequent biochemical outcome following external beam radiation therapy for T1-2 adenocarcinoma of the prostate. Radiother and Oncol 1996; 40:159-162.

17

Cure rates

With the widespread adoption of prostate brachytherapy during the last five years, the body of literature regarding tumor control rates has grown rapidly.(CRITZ, ZELEFSKY, MERRICK, KUPELIAN, SYLVESTER) Rather than present a detailed compilation of many published series, we'll summarize a few longer-term ones that have received the most attention.

Traditionally, brachytherapy has been believed to be best suited for patients most likely to have cancer limited to the prostate—those with a PSA less than 10 ng/ml and Gleason score of 6 or less. And there are now many series with minimum 5-year follow-up, showing biochemical cancer

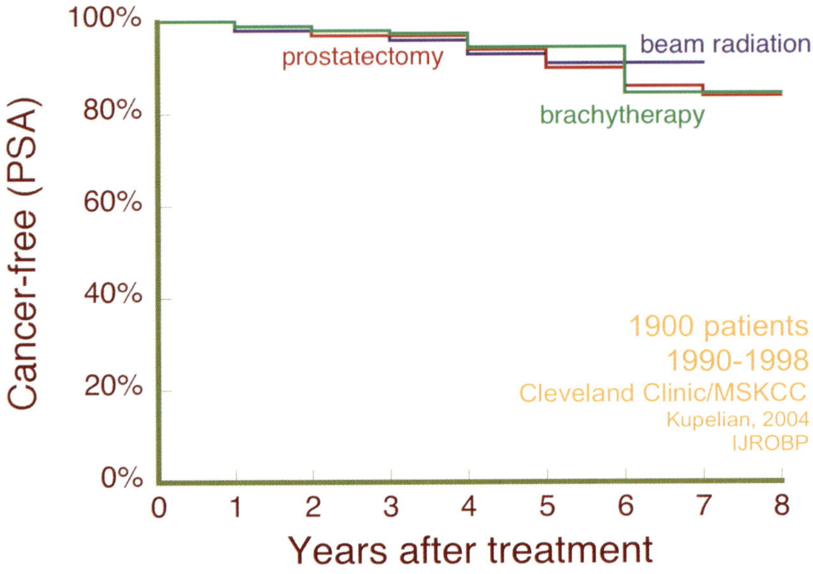

Figure 17-1. Freedom from biochemical failure in low-risk patients treated with surgery, beam or implant alone at Cleveland Clinic.(KUPELIAN)

control rates of 90% or greater in such low risk patients (**Figure 17-1**).(ZELEFSKY) At this point, few would argue that brachytherapy cure rates compare favorably with those achieved with prostatectomy.

COMPARING MODALITIES FOR LOW RISK PATIENTS

No modern controlled trials comparing surgery, external beam radiation, and brachytherapy have been performed, so we're left with retrospective uncontrolled comparisons. Before PSA, retrospective comparisons were nearly worthless, because patients grouped by clinical stage alone are so heterogeneous. With the advent of PSA categories, comparing outcome with different modalities for the same risk groupings likely gives a reasonably good idea of each modality's effectiveness.

In comparing brachytherapy with surgery, two concepts have been remarkably consistent. First, patients with low tumor burden (low PSA) do well with either modality when treated by capable physicians. With follow-up of approximately 10 years, each modality appears to eradicate cancer in 90% or more of such patients (**Figure 17-1**). If there is a cure rate advantage to any modalities, it's not apparent within the first ten years follow-up. This makes sense—if the cancer burden is small it can probably be eradicated with various approaches.

The major issues pertinant to comparison of brachytherapy with other modalities for low risk patients are the impact of treatment quality, length of follow-up, and morbidity. Most importantly, there is increasing appreciation that treatment quality varies widely from one physician to another, so that outcomes may be more dependent on who is performing the procedure than the choice of modality. (PAPAGIKOS)

Very important point

long-term outcomes may depend more on the quality of the procedure performed than the choice of modality

HIGHER RISK PATIENTS
High biochemical control rates for low-risk patients are pretty much routine. But the situation for patients with elevated PSA or higher Gleason scores is still filled with controversy. Because of greater heterogeneity among higher risk patients, comparing results among institutions is less meaningful than for patients with low risk factors. Rather than present a convoluted comparison between non-randomized retrospective series, we will simply discuss a couple of key studies.

Dattoli and colleagues have published some of the longest follow-up for more locally advanced cancers. They routinely used Pd-103 and supplemental beam radiation for patients with a pre-treatment PSA ≥10, Gleason score ≥7 or higher, or PAP ≥2.5 U (**Figure 17-3**).(DATTOLI) In their most recent update, for 243 patients treated from 1992 through 1996, freedom from biochemical failure was defined as a serum PSA less than 0.2 ng/ml at last follow-up. Due to concern regarding inter-observer variability in grading, the original biopsy slides for most patients were retrieved and re-reviewed by a single pathologist (L. True) at the University of Washington. The follow-up period for non-failing patients ranged from one to twelve years (median: nine years).

Biochemical failure developed in 41 patients. The overall actuarial freedom from biochemical progression at five years was 74%, with 198 patients followed beyond that time. These results are highly encouraging for patients with higher pre-treatment PSAs or Gleason scores (**Figure 17-**

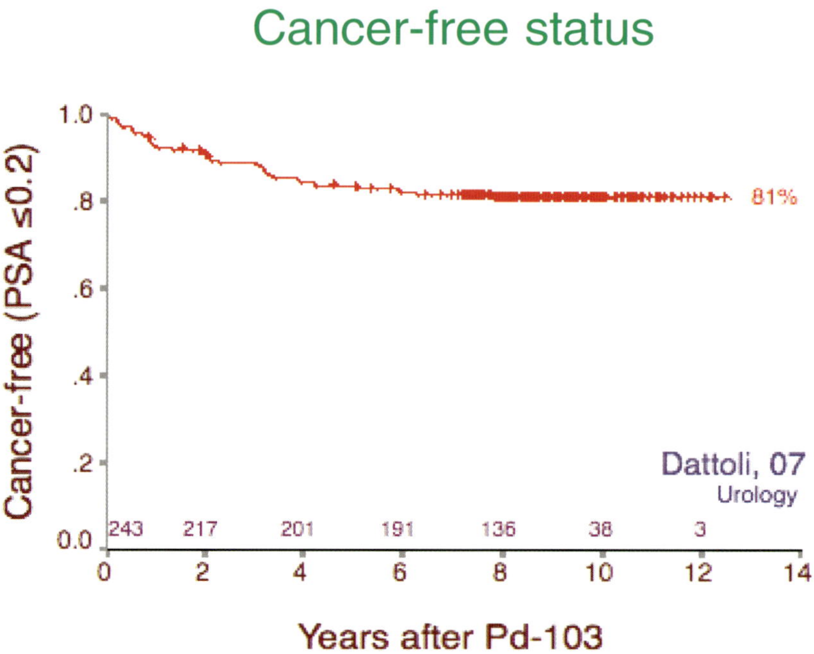

Figure 17-2. Freedom from biochemical progression for 243 patients with PSA >10 or Gleason score ≥7 treated with Pd-103 plus 41 Gy beam radiation. The curves level off at 74%, suggesting that a large percentage of patients with high risk features may be cured.

2). No clinically evident local failures occurred. Nearly all biochemical failures occurred within the first four years after treatment (**Figure 17-3**). The most encouraging aspect of these outcomes is the apparent leveling of the freedom-from-failure curves after 4 years in Figures 17-2 and 17-4, evidence that most of these higher risk patients can truly be cured. This levelling of the freedom from failure curve stands in sharp contrast to the persistent downward disease-free trend seen in most external beam series, and in many prostatectomy series.(HAN, D'AMICO 04) Cancer-specific survival was best predicted by pre-treatment PAP (**Figure 17-4**).

Higher pre-treatment PSA, Gleason score, or PAP were each associated with a progressively higher failure rate (**Figure 17-5**). In Cox proportional hazard multivariate analysis, considering each factor as a continuous variable, the strongest predictor of failure was elevated acid phosphatase (p=.02), followed by Gleason score (p=.1) and PSA (p=.14). There was lit-

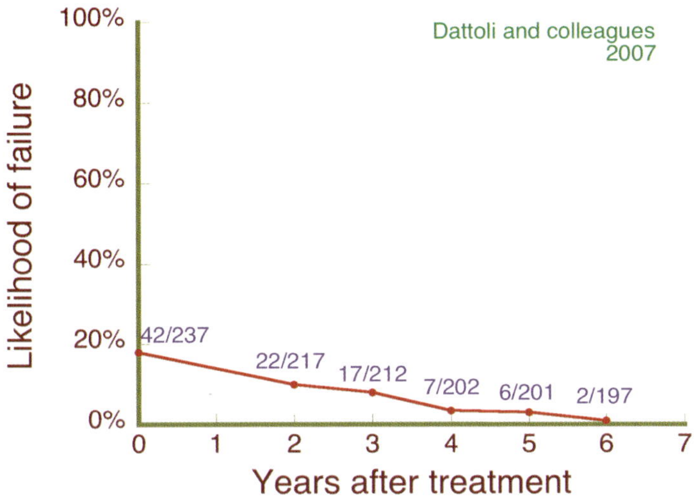

Figure 17-3. Likelihood of biochemcial failure and percent of failures occuring over time for higher risk patients treated with Pd-103 and supplemental beam radiation.(Dattoli 07)

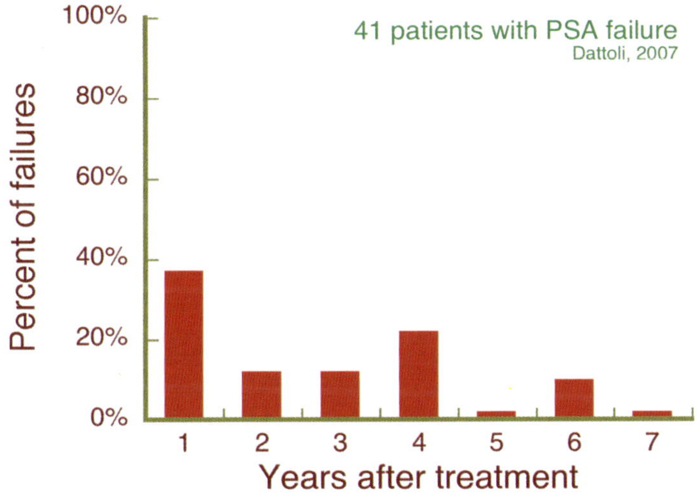

PSA

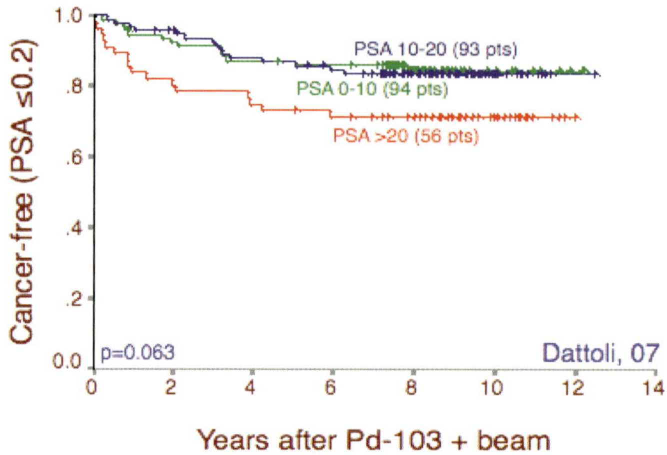

Figure 17-4. Freedom from biochemical failure for patients treated with Pd-103 + beam radiation, stratified by pretreatment PSA, Gleason score, or PAP.

Gleason

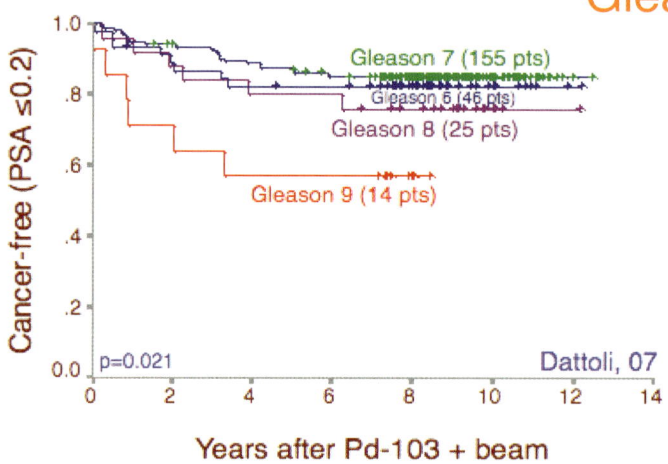

PAP

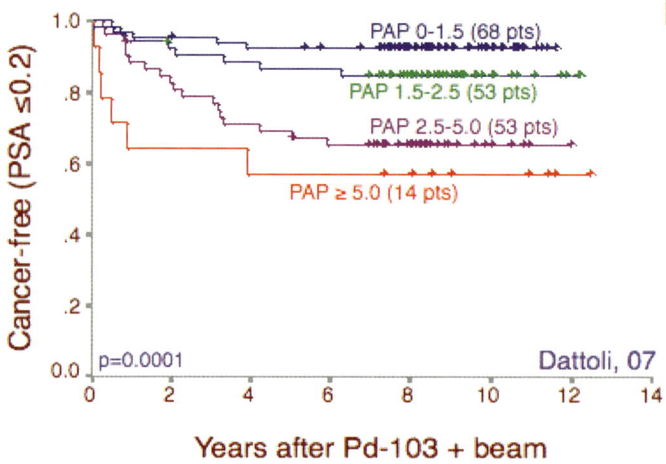

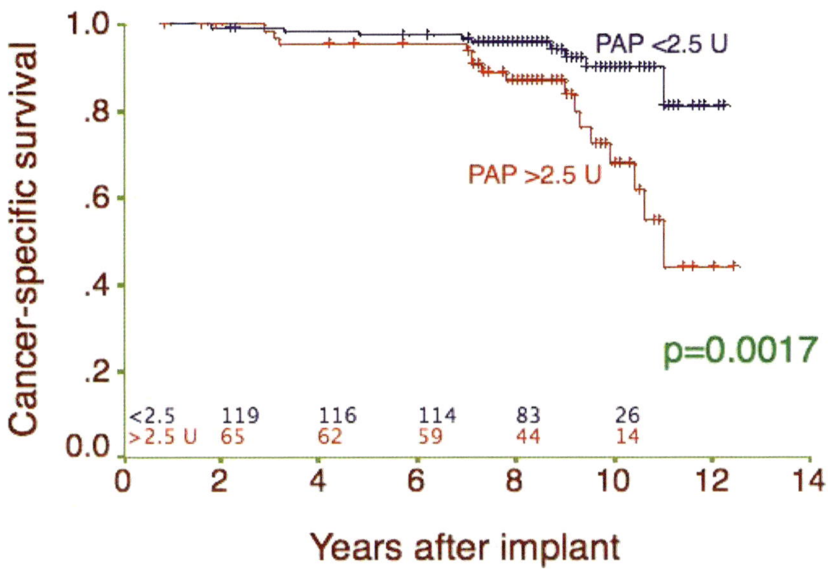

Figure 17-5. Cancer-specific survival for patients with pretreatment PAP below or above 2.5 U.

tle correlation among pretreatment PSA, Gleason score, or PAP, consistent with each factor being an independent outcomes predictor (**Figure 17-6**).(STAMEY, MOUL)

FOLLOW-UP BIOPSIES

Post-implant biopsy series have shown remarkably high rates of cancer elimination. Approximately half the patients treated at Northwest Tumor Institute (NWTI) with I-125 or Pd-103 alone had follow-up biopsies at one year or more.(PRESTIDGE) Of 201 patients biopsied, only 3% showed residual, apparently viable cancer on their last biopsy. An additional 17% were read as *indeterminate*, or residual cancer with profound radiation changes that could be consistent with dying cancer. With longer follow-up, most indeterminate biopsies were negative when repeated (**Figure 17-5**). Not all patients were biopsied. Those with a rising PSA or abnormal digital rectal exam were more likely to agree to a second biopsy, likely biasing the results toward evidence of cancer persistence.

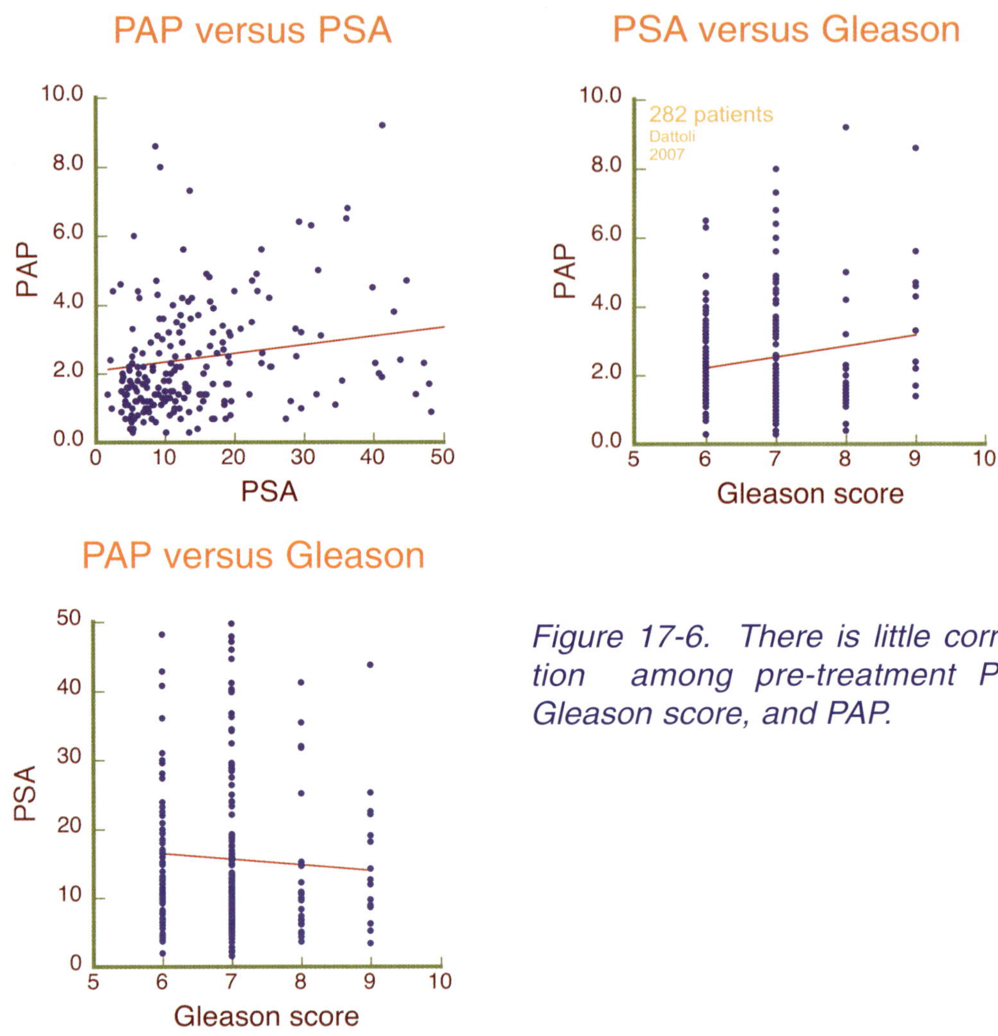

Figure 17-6. There is little correlation among pre-treatment PSA, Gleason score, and PAP.

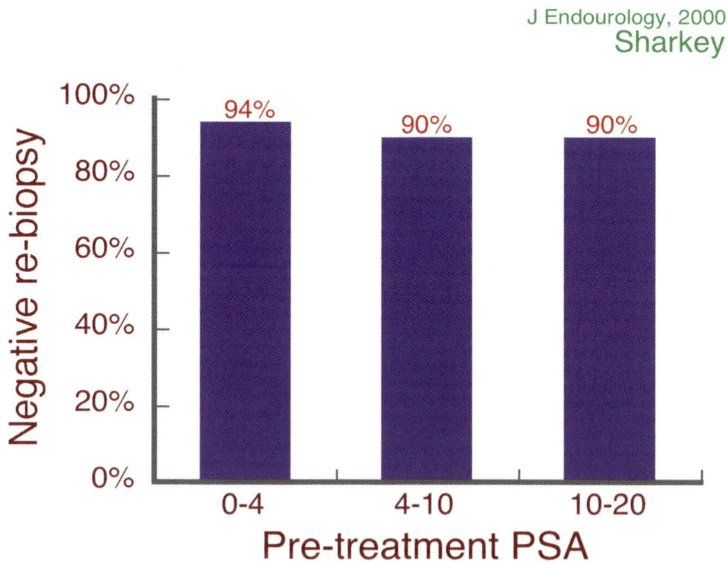

Figure 17-7. Percent of patients with negative biopsies after Pd-103 implantation, with or without adjuvant hormonal therapy.(SHARKEY)

Sharkey and colleagues obtained follow-up biopsies on 86% of 288 patients with two years follow-up after Pd-103. Their negative biopsy rate was 84% and 87%, respectively, for patients with or without adjuvant hormonal therapy. The high biopsy negativity rate was independent of pre-treatment PSA (**Figure 17-7**).(SHARKEY)

The lower rate of positive biopsy after contemporary series appears far better than that reported after conventional dose external beam radiation.(CROOK) However, we should pause before opening the champagne. Since introduction of PSA, cancers are being diagnosed at a far earlier stage, presumably with a much lower tumor burden than in earlier series. In fact, repeat biopsies in patients with prior positive biopsies, are frequently negative even in the absence of therapy—the tumor burden is frequently so low in PSA-screened patients that it is difficult to find cancer even in the untreated patient!(SVETEC, STROUMBAKIS)

CAUSE-SPECIFIC SURVIVAL

The major criticism of nearly all outcomes reports for early stage prostate cancer is the emphasis on biochemical control rather than cancer-specific survival, a state of affairs that reflects the long natural history of prostate

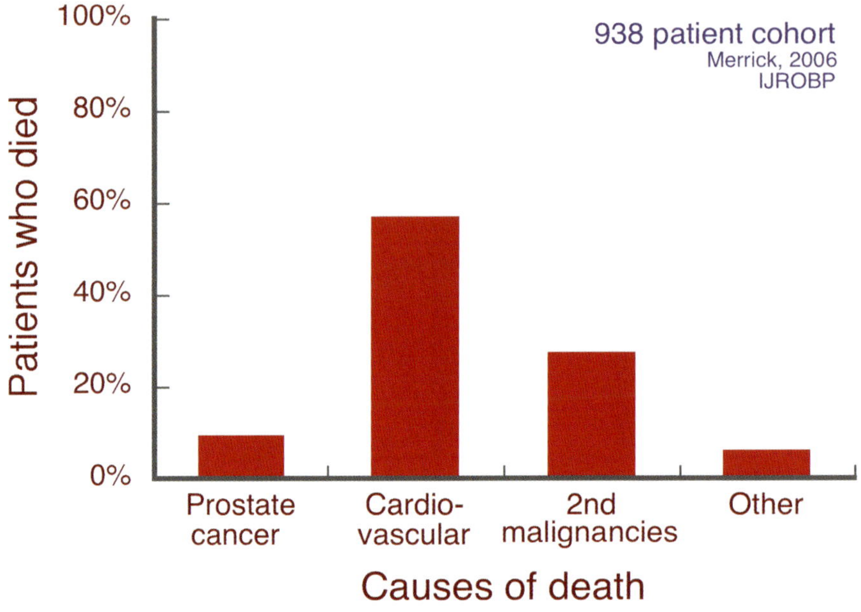

Figure 17-8. Causes of death among 102 deaths after imoplant-based therapy for prostate cancer.(MERRICK 06)

cancer. With longer follow-up of modern treatments, cause-specific outcomes are beginning to emerge. With the long natural history of the disease and high cure rates with good quality therapy, overall survival is reflective other death causes than prostate cancer. Cardiovascular disease is by far and away the biggest cause of death following high quality brachytherapy, even in prostate cancer patients with markedly elevated PSA or Gleason scores (**Figures 17-6, 17-8 and 17-9**).

POOR RESULTS

While outcomes reported by brachytherapy enthusiasts have generally compared favorably with those of surgery or external beam radiation, there are reports of remarkably poor brachytherapy results. Probably the most widely quoted are from D'Amico and colleagues, who have published extensively their low cure rates after all forms of prostate cancer therapy, including brachytherapy.(D'AMICO 98, HAN) Their poor results with all treatment modalities is still an enigma. One lesson to be learned from occasional poor outcome reports are that all forms of therapy require good qual-

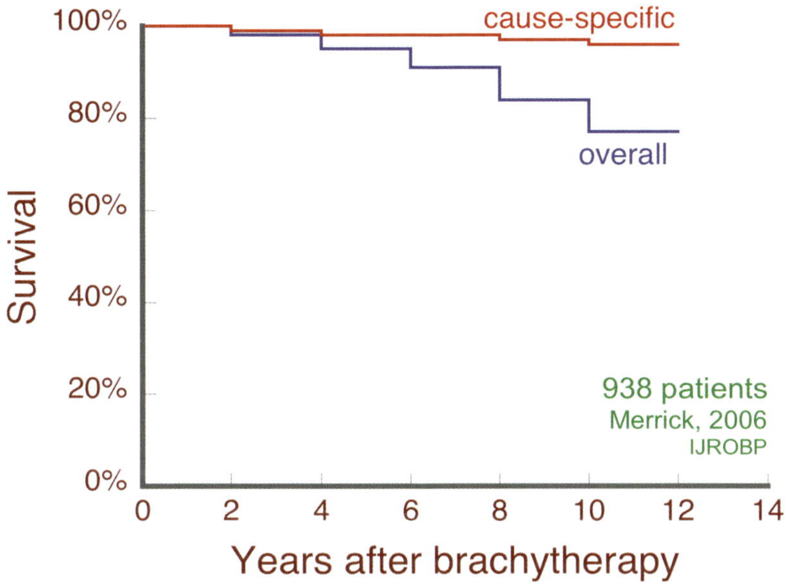

Figure 17-9. Overall and cause-specific survival following implat-based radiation.(MERRICK 06)

ity implementation to be effective. Isolated poor outcome reports may reflect misuse of a technique, rather than that the technique is inherently flawed. Fortunately, most prostate cancer investigators have not seen persistent late failure rates after brachytherapy, surgery or beam radiation.

MORE

The growing number of PSA-based follow-up reports is still dominated by a few select brachytherapists. Like the situation for nerve-sparing prostatectomy and conformal external beam radiation, the vast majority of published brachytherapy data come from a handful of subspecialist physicians, and may not be representative of the overall brachytherapy experience. In the next few years, more reports should emerge as other brachytherapy teams accumulate longer follow-up, making it clear just how generalizable the favorable results are.

REFERENCES

1. Critz F, Levinson K. 10-year disease-free survival rates after simultaneous irradiation for prostate cancer with a focus on calculation methodology. J Urology 2004; 172:2232-2238.

2. Crook J, Malone S, Perry G, Bahadur Y, Robertson S, Abdolell M. Postradiotherapy prostate biopsies: What do they really mean? Results for 498 patients. Int J Rad Oncol Biol Phys 2000; 48:355-367.

3. D'Amico A, Manola J, Loffredo M, Renshaw A, DellaCroce A, Kantoff P. 6-month androgen suppression plus radiation therapy alone for patients with clincally localized prostate cancer: A randomized controlled trial. JAMA 2004; 292:821-827.

4. D'Amico AV, Whittington R, Malkowicz SB, al e. Biochemical outcome after radical prostatectomy, external beam radiation therapy, or interstitial radiation therapy for clinically localized prostate cancer. JAMA 1998; 280:969-974.

5. Dattoli M, Wallner K, True L, Cash J, Sorace R. Long-term prostate cancer control using Palladium-103 brachytherapy and external beam radiotherapy in patients with a high likelihood of extracapsular cancer extension. Urology 2007; 69:334-337.

6. Han M, Partin AW, Pound CR, Epstein JI, Walsh PC. Long-term biochemical disease-free and cancer-specific survival following anatomic radical retropubic prostatectomy. Uro Clin N Am 2001; 28:555-565.

7. Kupelian P, Potters L, Khuntia D, et al. Radical prostatetomy, external beam radiotherapy ≥72 Gy, permanent seed implantation, or combined seeds/external beam radiotherapy for Stage T1-T2 prostate cancer. Int J Rad Oncol Biol Phys 2004; 58:25-33.

8. Merrick G, Butler W, Wallner K, Galbreath R, Allen Z, Adamovich E. Androgen-deprivation therapy dies not impact cause-specific or overall survival after permanent prostate brachytherapy. Int J Rad Oncol Biol Phys 2006; 65:669-677.

9. Merrick G, Wallner K, Butler W, et al. Brachytherapy in men aged ″54 years with clinically localized prostate cancer. BJU International 2006; 98:324-328.

10. Moul JW, Connelly RR, Perahia B, McLeod DG. The contemporary value of pretreatment prostatic acid phosphatase to predict pathological stage and recurrence in radical prostatectomy cases. J Urol 1998; 159:935-940.

11. Papagikos M, deGuzman AF, Rossi P, CMcCullough D, Clark P, Lee WR. Dosimetric quantifiers for low-dose-rate prostate brachytherapy: Is V100 superior to D90? Brachytherapy 2005; 4:252-258.

12. Prestidge BR, Hoak DC, Grimm PD, Ragde H, Cavanagh W, Blasko JC. Posttreatment biopsy results following interstitial brachytherapy in early-stage prostate cancer. Int J Radiat Oncol Biol Phys 1997; 37:31-39.
13. Sharkey J, Chovnick SD, Behar RJ, Perez R, al e. Minimally invasive treatment for localized adenocarcinoma of the prostate: Review of 1048 patients treated with ultrasound-guided palladium-103 brachytherapy. J Endourol 2000; 14:343-350.
14. Stamey TA, Kabalin JN, McNeal JE, et al. Prostate specific antigen in the diagnosis and treatment of adenocarcinoma of the prostate. II. Radical prostatectomy treated patients. J Urol 1989; 141:1076-1083.
15. Stroumbakis N, Cookson MS, Reuter VE, Fair WR. Clinical significance of repeat sextant biopsies in prostate cancer patients. Urol 1997; 49(S 3A):113-118.
16. Svetec D, McCabe K, Peretsman S, et al. Prostate rebiopsy is a poor surrogate of treatment efficacy in localized prostate cancer. J Urol 1998; 159:1606-1608.
17. Sylvester J, Grimm P, Blasko J, et al. 15-year biochemical relapse free survival in clinical stage T1-T3 prostate cancer followin combined external beam radiotherapy and brachytherapy: Seattle experience. Int J Rad Oncol Biol Phys 2007; 67:57-64.
18. Wallner K, Merrick G, Blasko J, Dattoli M. Prostate brachytherapy made complicated (third edition). Seattle: SmartMedicine Press, 2007.
19. Zelefsky MJ, Kuban D, Levy L, et al. Mulit-institutional analysis of long-term outcome for stages T1-T2 prostate cancer treated with permanent seed implantation. Int J Rad Oncol Biol Phys 2007; 67:327-333.

18

Salvage after implant

Intra-prostatic cancer persistence after brachytherapy is an uncommon event. Because of the small number of patients with residual intra-prostatic cancer, clinical data regarding salvage treatment for unsuccessful brachytherapy is even more scarce than that for external beam failures (see Chapter 23).

SALVAGE BEAM

Using external beam radiation to salvage failed implant patients is not practical—if an implant failed to eradicate a cancer, it is highly unlikely that external beam radiation could. If the implant was technically poor, a re-

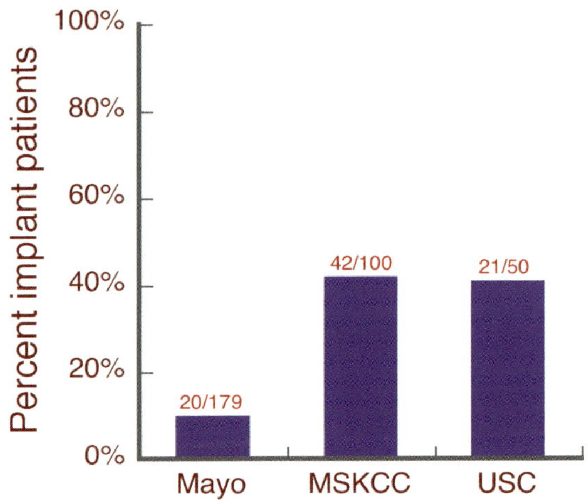

Figure 18-1. Percent of brachytherapy patients in three prospectively maintained databases of salvage prostatectomy for failed radiation.(SANDERSON, WARD, BIANCO)

implant would probably be preferable to salvage external radiation (see Chapter 11).

SALVAGE PROSTATECTOMY

There are three long-running salvage prostatectomy series for failed radiation. The three series, from Mayo, Baylor/MSKCC and USC, all deal predominantly with external beam failures, but have a substantial minority of failed implant patients (**Figure 18-1**). All three series all show a moderate risk of urinary incontinence (**Figure 18-2**). The likelihood of serious rectal damage appears to be small. Bladder neck contractures were common, but readily correctable. As expected, sexual dysfunction after salvage prostatectomy was the rule, but amenable to correction with a penile prosthesis.(SANDERSON)

The freedom from second cancer recurrence rates have been moderately encouraging, especially for patients with a PSA below 10 ng/ml at the time

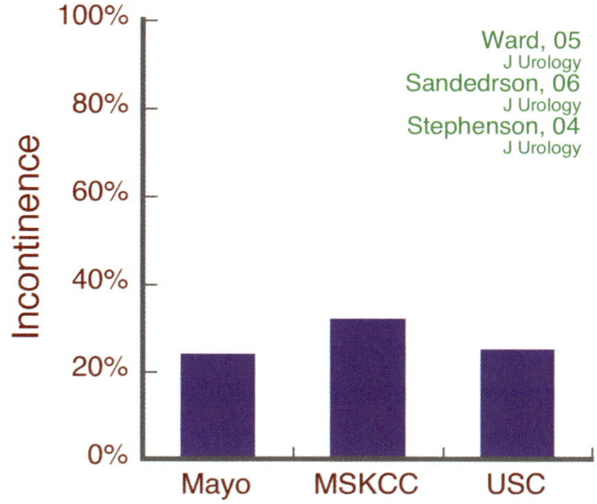

Figure 18-2. Urinary incontinence after salvage prostatectomy for locally recurrent cancer after failed external beam radiation or brachytherapy.(SANDERSON, WARD, BIANCO)

of salvage (**Figure 18-3**). Unfortunately, it is impossible to tease the morbidities and cure rates for implant failures versus beam failures from these series.

The most important caveat to all of the surgical salvage series is that they are probably heavily contaminated with implant patients who underwent salvage surgery for a PSA spike. It was not until 1997 that Wallner, Blasko and Merrick first reported the PSA spike phenomenon. And it was not until the early 2000's that Reed and colleagues warned that patients with a PSA spike and residual cancer on repeat biopsy might still be cancer-free with longer follow-up. Until these false cancer recurrence scenarios were recognized, it is likely that patients were prematurely labeled implant failures. To the extent that they are included in the salvage prostatectomy series, they would make the "cure" rates look artificially high.

Surgical salvage of implant failures

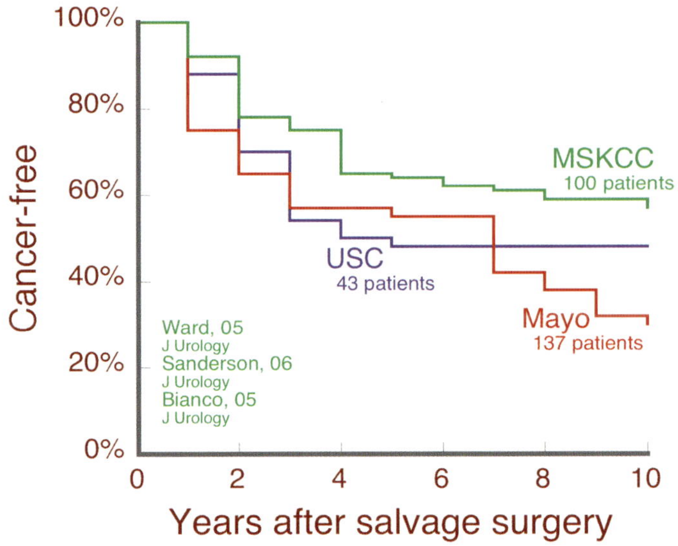

Figure 18-3. Freedom from second biochemical failure after salvage prostatectomy for failed external beam radiation or brachytherapy. The cure rates appear higher for patients operated on before the PSA reaches 10 ng/ml.(SANDERSON,, BIANCO, WARD)

Surgical salvage if PSA <10 ng/ml

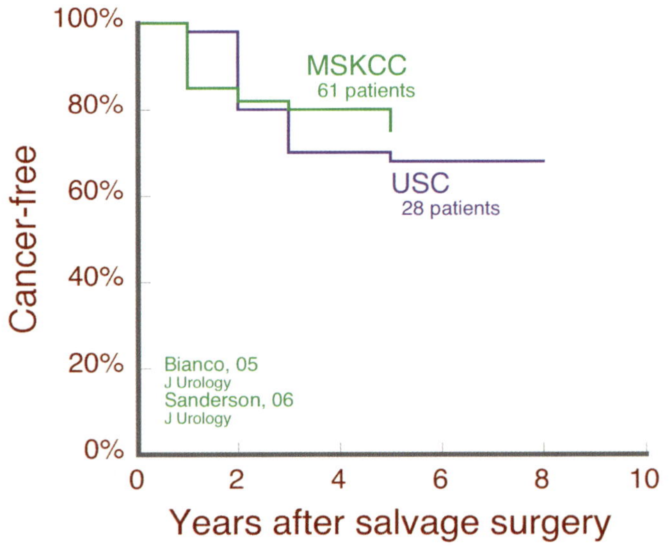

SALVAGE CRYOTHERAPY

There is little meaningful data published regarding cryotherapy as salvage for failed implant. The limited series published regarding cancer control with cryo include few, if any, brachytherapy patients.(PREPELICA, PERROTTI) The cancer control rates and incontinence rates with primary or salvage cryo have varied markedly between investigators, so that any estimates of success should be viewed skeptically.(MERRICK) There is a relatively high rate of incontinence from cryo for external beam failures, and we are concerned that it would be even higher after brachytherapy.

GOOD NEWS AND BAD NEWS

The good news regarding salvage therapy is that persistent cancer after brachytherapy is uncommon. The bad news is that for the few patients with persistent cancer, little clinical data is available to guide a choice regarding salvage options. Considering that implant quality will only get better, with even fewer local failures expected in the future, we suspect that it will take a long time to amass a meaningful database of salvage outcomes.

REFERENCES

1. Bianco F, Scardino PT, Stephenson A, DiBlasio C, Fearn P, Eastham J. Long-term oncologic results of salvage radical prostatectomy for locally recurrent prostate cancer after radiotherapy. Int J Rad Oncol Biol Phys 2005; 62:448-453.
2. Merrick G, Wallner K, Butler W. Prostate cryotherapy: More questions than answers. Urology 2005; 66:9-15.
3. Perrotti M, Litwin MS, McGuire E, Scott S, Von Eschenbach A. Quality of life after salvage cryotherapy: The implant of treatment parameters. J Urology 1999; 162:398-402.
4. Prepelica K, Okeke Z, Murphy A, Katz A. Cryosurgical ablation of the prostate: High-risk patient outcomes. Cancer 2005; 103:1625-1630.
5. Sanderson K, Penson D, Cai J, et al. Salvage radical prostatectomy: Quality of life outcomes and long-term oncological control of radiorecurrent prostate cancer. J Urology 2006; 176:2025-2032.
6. Stephenson A, Scardino PT, Bianco F, DiBlasio C, Fearn P, Eastham J. Morbidity and functional outcomes of salvage radical prostatectomy for locally recurrent prostate cancer after radiation therapy. J Urology 2004; 172:2239-2243.

7. Ward J, Sebo T, Blute M, Zincke H. Salvage surgery for radiorecurrent prostate cancer: Contemporary outcomes. J Urology 2005; 173:1156-1160.

19

Short-term morbidity

Many physicians and prospective patients believe that prostate brachytherapy has fewer side effects and complications than external beam radiation, a perception derived in part from the seemingly logical assumption that the more localized radiation of an implant should lead to fewer problems. Wrong. Brachytherapy typically causes *more* marked and *more* prolonged radiation-related urinary symptoms, at least in the first few post-implant months. Fortunately, nearly all implant-related problems resolve spontaneously.

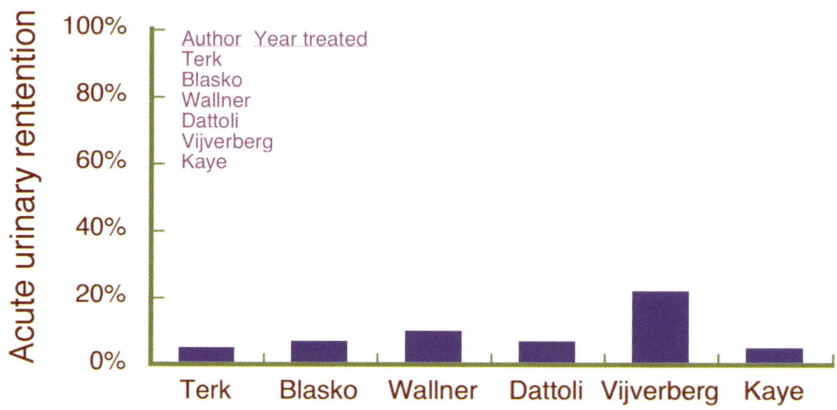

Figure 19-1. Likelihood of acute, post-implant urinary retention reported by various investigators.(TERK, BLASKO, WALLNER 96, DATTOLI, VIJVERBERG, KAYE)

Radiation-related morbidity is generally considered as early (short-term) or late (longer-term). With prostate brachytherapy, we generally considered the first 12 months to be the *short-term*.

URINARY RETENTION

Post-implant urinary retention is the most common serious acute morbidity of prostate brachytherapy, occurring in about 2% to 10% of patients (**Figures 19-1 and 19-2**). In most cases, retention lasts only a few days and is of no long-term consequence.(LANDIS, SHERERTZ) The management of acute retention is discussed in detail in Chapter 12.

URINARY FUNCTION

While the likelihood of acute retention is small, nearly all patients experience varying degrees of radiation-related prostatitis and proctitis in the first few months after implant. If given the choice, approximately half of patients use medication (alpha-blockers) for several months or longer.(WALLNER 96) Fortunately, radiation prostatitis is rarely incapacitating and typically resolves spontaneously within three to twelve months (see chapter 10).(KLEINBERG, MERRICK 00) Most patients return to their baseline AUA scores (**Figure 19-3, bottom**). Somewhat surprisingly, long-term AUA scores are not influenced by such pre-treatment parameters as prostate volume, age, pre-implant AUA scores, or urinary flow parameters (see Chapter 15).(LANDIS, MERRICK)

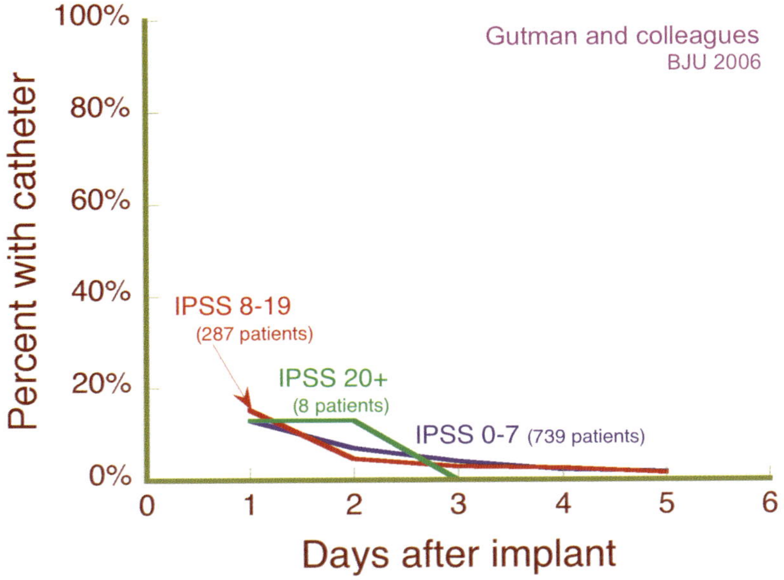

Figure 19-2. Days to catheter removal, for patient groups with increasing pre-implant IPSS.(GUTMAN)

FROM COMMON SENSE TO SCIENCE

Medical morbidity reporting has gone through a metamorphosis over the past 20 years. Before that time, it was standard to report the frequency and severity of specific problems like urinary incontinence, rectal bleeding, impotence, etc.(KLEINBERG, GELBLUM) In the early 1990's there was an realization that quantification of life-style effects could be made far more complex, using extensive patient-administered questionnaires. Summary scores, based on combinations of responses, were calculated and translated into concepts like *urinary bother*. Acronyms like FACT-G, Q-TWiST, CARES-SF, EPIC, EORTC QLQ-C30 proliferated. The reporting of morbidity was transformed into a *science*. Unfortunately, in converting complex questionnaires into summary scores, the link between the scores and simple questions like "do you leak urine?" was lost to most readers.(TESTA) In 2007, there has been widespread loss of interest in complex QOL scoring, due to the fact that they are difficult for patients and physicians to relate to.(BRUNER, TALCOTT)

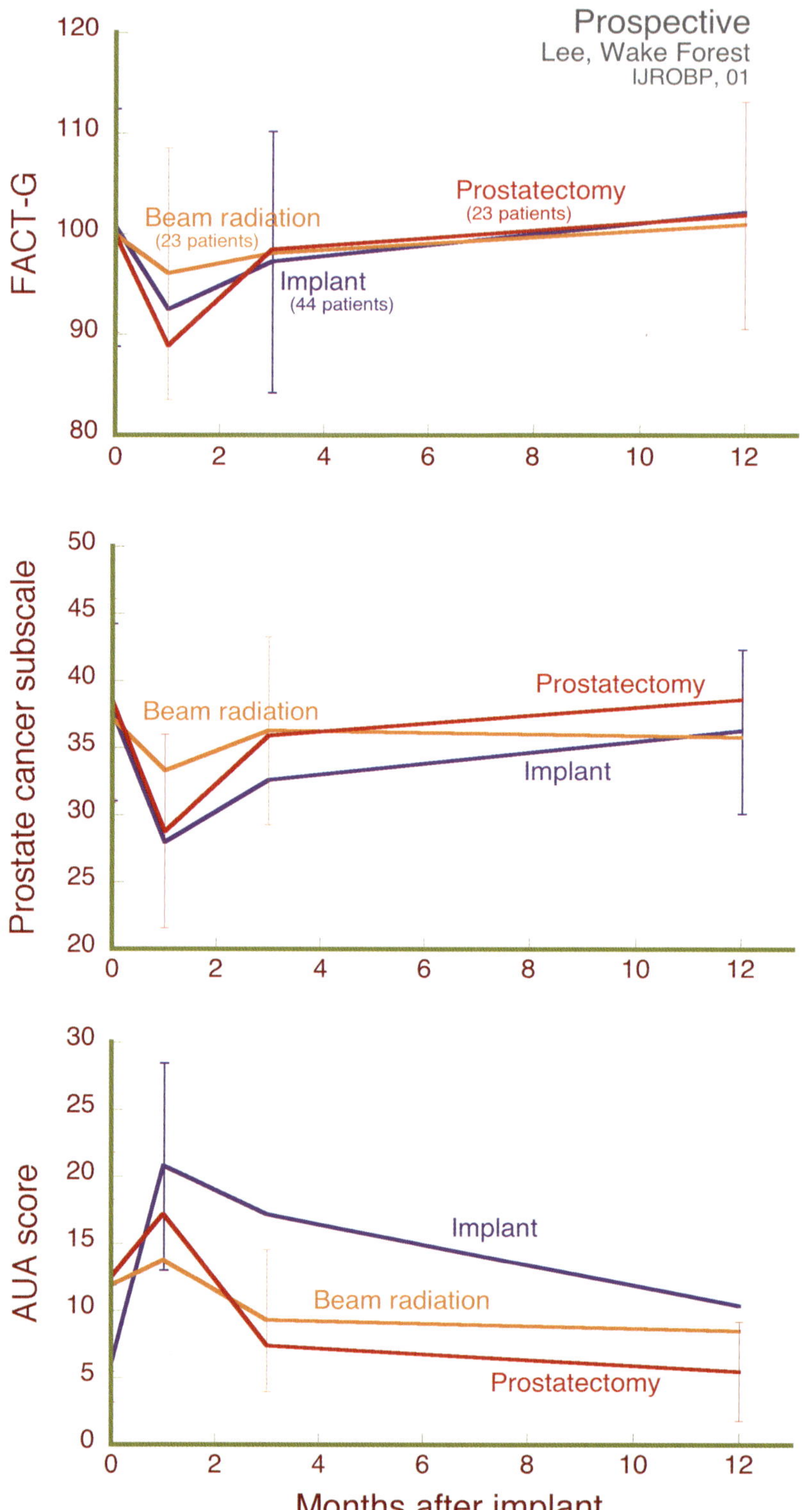
Prospective
Lee, Wake Forest
IJROBP, 01
FACT-G
120
110
100
90
80
Beam radiation
(23 patients)
Prostatectomy
(23 patients)
Implant
(44 patients)
0
2
4
6
8
10
12
Prostate cancer subscale
50
45
40
35
30
25
20
Beam radiation
Prostatectomy
Implant
AUA score
30
25
20
15
10
5
0
Implant
Beam radiation
Prostatectomy
Months after implant

Figure 19-3 (opposite page). Various QOL indices for patients treated with I-125 implant, external beam radiation, or prostatectomy.(LEE)

PAIN

Dysuria is a common problem during the first few months after implantation.(MERRICK) It typically responds to alpha blockers, and is not generally considered a *pain* issue. However, vague pelvic or low back pain is experienced by some patients, sometimes with an unclear connection to the brachytherapy. While often difficult to explain, such pain problems generally seem to resolve spontaneously. In unusual cases, more severe prostatic pains may be related to excessive peri-urethral doses.(WALLNER) Persistent rectal pain, possibly related to seeds in the pelvic diaphragm or peri-rectal muscles, occurs occasionally (see Chapter 21).

SEED EMBOLI

Also to be included in short-term morbidity is the potential for complications related to seed migration. Migration to the pulmonary vasculature, which occurs in 2-25% of patients, has no known clinical effect.(NAG) Rare cases of migration to vital organs has been reported (**Figure 19-4**).(DAVIS, ZHU)

WE'VE PROBABLY SEEN THE WORST

Modern prostate brachytherapy, using TRUS and CT guidance, has been widely practiced for almost twenty years. The first few years' experience, on which much of the published morbidity data is based, almost certainly indicates a higher complication rate than should currently be expected, given what we have learned about radiation tolerance and the technical experience we've gained. The substantial short-term and long-term morbidity in the early experiences of Wallner, Blasko, and others in the early 1990s is not representative of current implants. Morbidity in more recently treated patients, whose urethral and rectal doses were better controlled,

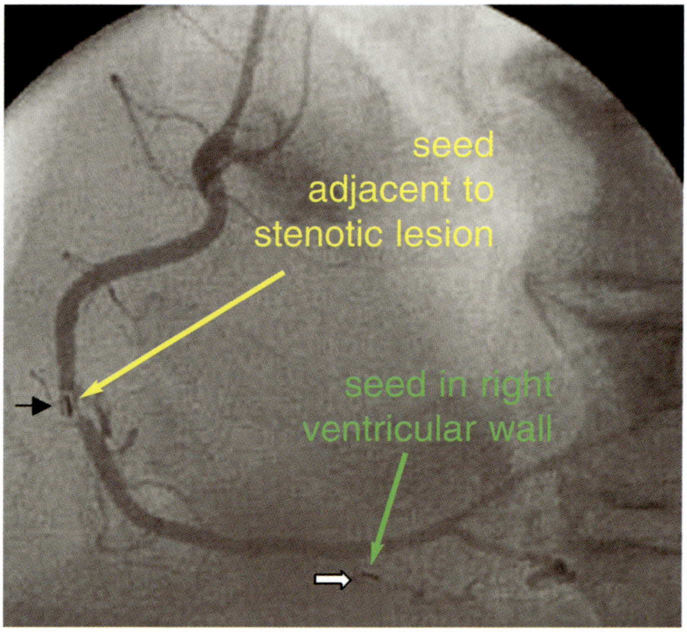

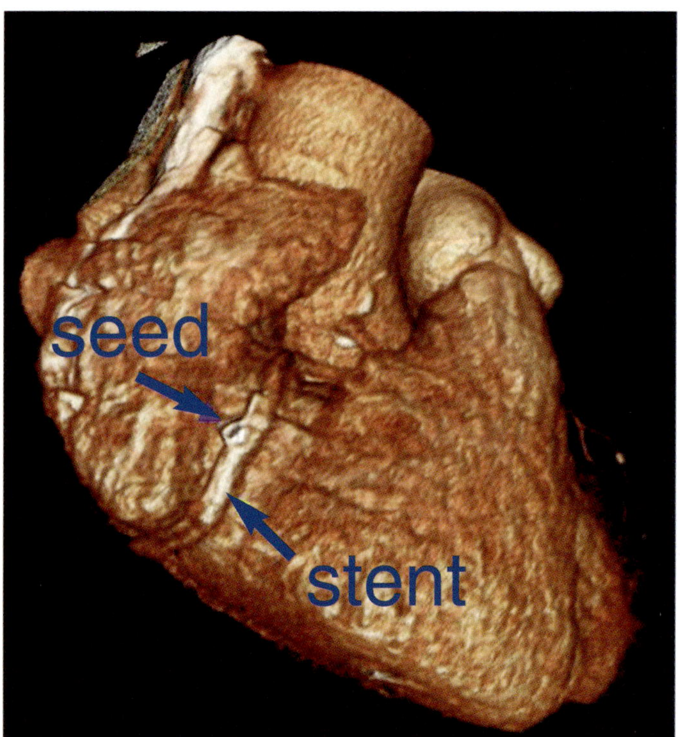

Figure 19-2. I-125 seeds adjacent to the site of a stenotic lesion of mid-right coronary artery. A second seed is noted within the right ventricular wall. After percutaneous coronary intervention, a cardiac CT demonstrated the stent in mid-right coronary artery with the adjacent seed.(ZHU)

has been much lower.(MERRICK 03, BROWN, HAN) In experienced hands, short-term morbidities are probably lower than previously described. Keeping the peri-urethral and rectal doses low has helped minimize both short-term and long-term morbidities (see Chapters 7 and 11).

REFERENCES

1. Blasko JC, Ragde H, Grimm PD. Transperineal Ultrasound-Guided Implantation of the Prostate: Morbidity and Complications. Scand J Urol Nephrol Suppl 1991; 137:113-118.

2. Brown D, Colonias A, Miller R, Benoit R, al e. Urinary morbidity with a modified peripheral loading technique of transperienal 125-I prostate implantation. Int J Radiat Oncol Biolo Phys 2000; 47:353-360.

3. Davis B, Bresnahan J, Stafford S, Karon B, King B, Wilson T. Prostate brachytherapy seed migration to a coronary artery found during angiography. J Urol 2002; 168:1103.

4. Gelblum DY, Potters L. Rectal complications associated with transperineal interstitial brachytherapy for prostate cancer. Int J Rad Oncol Biol Phys 2000; 48:119-124.

5. Gelblum DY, Potters L, Ashley R, Waldbaum R, Wang X, Leibel S. Urinary morbidity following ultrasound-guided transperineal prostate seed implantation. Int J Rad Oncol Biol Phys 1999; 45:59-67.

6. Gutman S, Merrick G, Butler W, et al. Temporal relationship between prostate brachytherapy and the diagnosis of colorectal cancer. Int J Rad Oncol Biol Phys 2006; 66:48-55.

7. Han BH, Demel KC, Wallner KE, Young L. Patient reported short-term complications after prostate brachytherapy. J Urol 2001; (in press).

8. Kaye KW, Olson DJ, Payne JT. Detailed preliminary analysis of 125 iodine implantation for localized prostate cancer using percutaneous approach. J Urol 1995; 153:1020-1025.

9. Kleinberg L, Wallner K, Roy J, et al. Treatment-related symptoms during the first year following transperineal I-125 prostate implantation. Int J Radiat Oncol Biol Phys 1994; 28:985.

10. Landis D, Wallner K, Locke J, et al. Late urinary morbidity after prostate brachytherapy. Brachytherapy 2002; 1:21-26.

11. Lee WR, Hall M, McQuellon R, Case L, McCullough D. A prospective quality-of-life study in men with clinically localized prostate carcinoma treated with radical prostatectomy, external beam radiotherapy, or interstitial brachytherapy. Int J Rad Oncol Biol Phys 2001; 51:614-623.

12. Merrick G, Butler W, Wallner K, et al. Dysuria following permanent prostate brachytherapy. Int J Rad Oncol Biol Phys 2003; 55:979-985.
13. Merrick G, Wallner K, Butler W. Minimizing prostate brachytherapy-related morbidity. Urol 2003; 62:786-792.
14. Merrick GS, Butler WM, Lief JH, Dorsey AT. Temporal resolution of urinary morbidity following prostate brachytherapy. Int J Radiat Oncol Biolo Phys 2000; 47:121-128.
15. Sherertz T, Wallner K, Wang H, Sutlief S, Russell K. Long-term urinary function after transperineal brachytherapy for patients with large prostate glands (submitted) 2002.
16. Talcott J, Clark J, Manola J, Mitchell S. Bringing prostate cancer quality of life reserach back to the bedside: Translating numbers into a format that patients can understand. J Urol 2006; 176:1558-1564.
17. Terk MD, Stock RG, Stone NN. Identification of patients at increased risk for prolonged urinary retention following radioactive seed implantation of the prostate. J Urol 1998; 160:1379-1382.
18. Testa M, Simonson D. Assessment of quality-of-life outcomes. N Eng J Med 1996; 334:835-840.
19. Vijverberg PLM, Kurth KH, Blank LECM, Dadhoiwala NF, de Reijke THM, Koedooder K. Treatment of localized prostatic carcinoma using the transrectal ultrasound guided transperineal implantation technique. European Urology 1992; 21:35-41.
20. Wallner K, Elliott K, Merrick G, Ghaly M, Maki J. Chronic pelvic pain following prostate brachytherapy: A case report. Brachytherapy 2004; 3:153-158.
21. Wallner KE, Roy J, Harrison L. Dosimetry guidelines to minimize urethral and rectal morbidity following transperineal I-125 prostate brachytherapy. Int J Radiat Oncol Biol Phys 1995; 32:465-471.
22. Wallner KE, Roy J, Harrison L. Tumor control and morbidity following transperineal I-125 implantation for Stage T1/T2 prostatic carcinoma. J Clin Oncol 1996; 14:449-453.
23. Zhu A, Wallner K, Frivold G, Ferry D, Jutzy K, Foster G. Prostate brachytherapy seed migration to the right coronary artery associated with an acute myocardial infarction. Brachytherapy 2006; 5:262-265.

20

Urinary morbidity

Radiation prostatitis and its accompanying obstructive symptoms are nearly universal after brachytherapy (see Chapter 12). While most patients return to their baseline urinary patterns within four to twelve months, some are left with long-term urinary changes causing chronic bother. Additionally, there a possibility of more serious complications, including superficial urethral necrosis, incontinence and urethral strictures.

Predicting the likelihood of long-term urinary troubles for individual patients has proven very difficult. Somewhat surprisingly, long-term AUA score changes appear to have little relationship to pre-treatment parameters

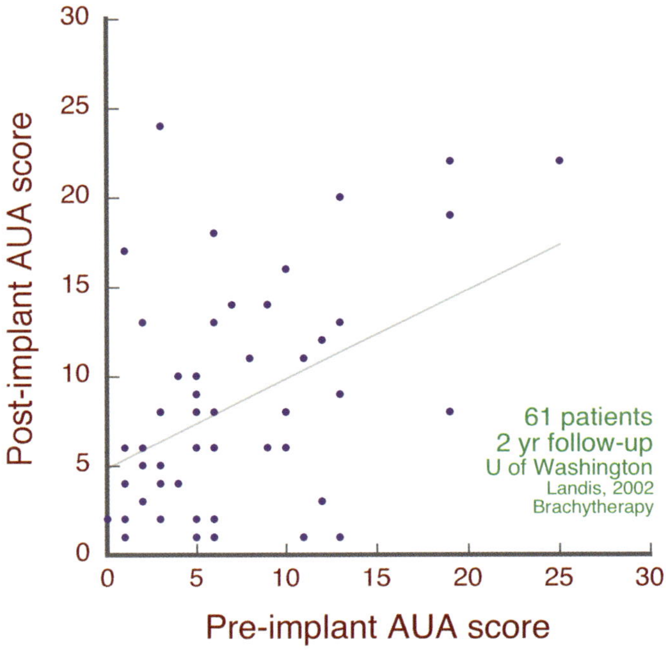

Figure 20-1. Change in AUA score at two years following brachytherapy in 62 patients treated at the University of Washington in 1998. There was little correlation between pre-implant AUA scores patients' AUA scores two years after therapy.(LANDIS)

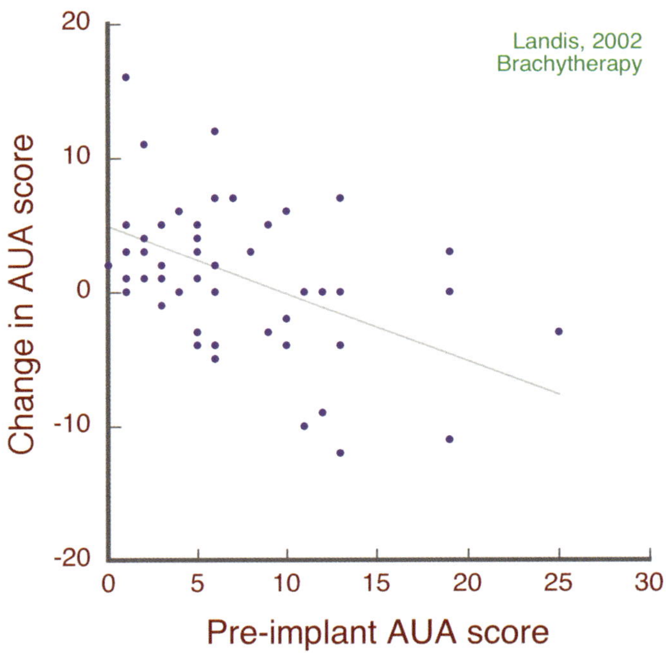

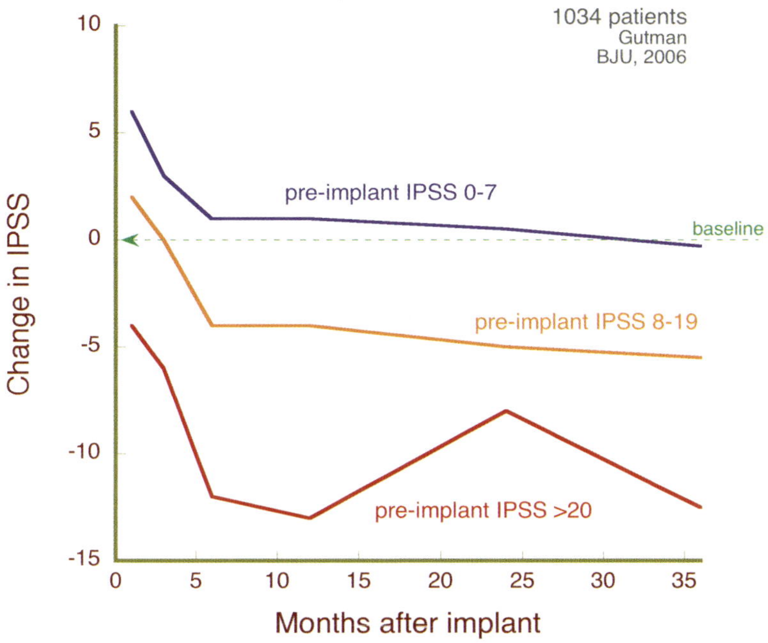

Figure 20-2. Long-term IPSS score changes for patients with various categories of pre-implant scores. Note that on average, patients with higher pre-implant scores actually had lower scores after brachytherapy, due to routine institution of alpha-blockers.(GUTMAN)

including prostate volume, age, pre-implant AUA scores, and urinary flow parameters (**Figure 20-1 and20-2**).(LANDIS, GUTMAN) This is why the use of such parameters for patient selection is so suspect (see Chapter 15).

Superficial urethral necrosis
Probably the most severe late urinary complication, seen primarily in the early days of TRUS-based prostate brachytherapy, was superficial urethral necrosis (SUN). Associated with severe dysuria and urinary incontinence, it was reported to occur in up to 4% of patients treated by Blasko and colleagues in the late 1980s and early 1990s (**Figure 20-3**).(BLASKO) Its occurrence among patients treated in the early TRUS experience probably reflected astronomical urethral doses from homogeneous seed placement

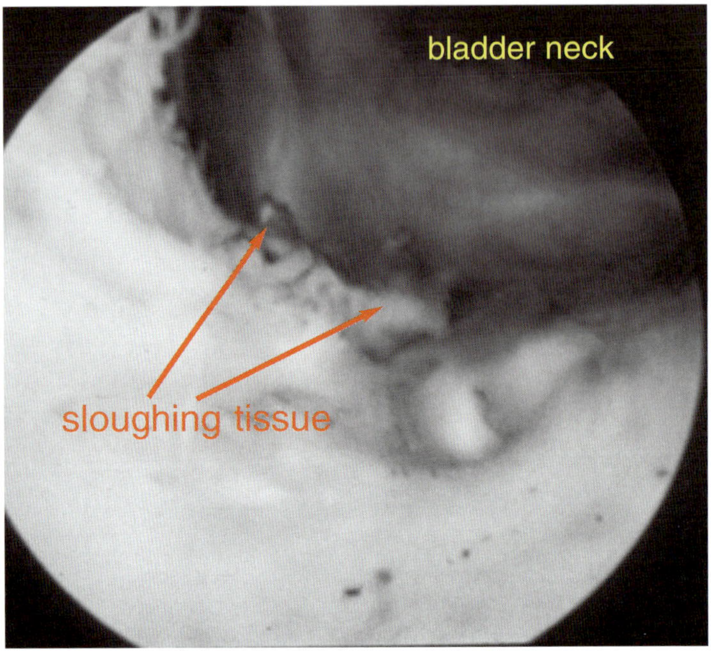

Figure 20-3. Cystoscopic view of superficial urethral necrosis with sloughing tissue. SUN is rarely seen since peripheral source placement was widely adopted.

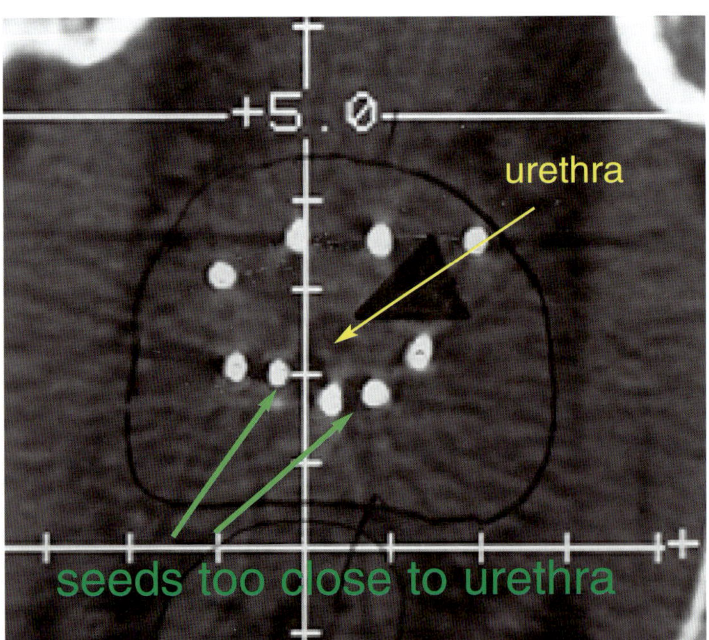

Figure 20-4. Example of posterior seeds mistakenly placed too close to the urethra.

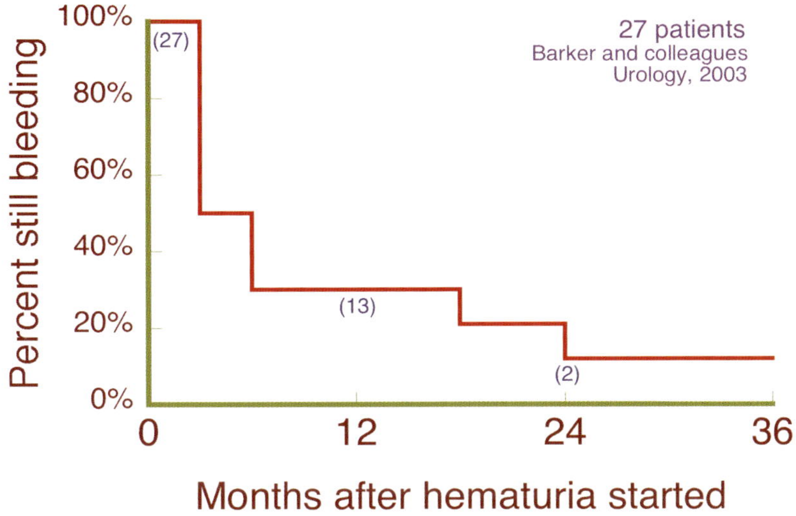

Figure 20-5. Resolution of clinically apparent bleeding in 27 patients with late gross hematuria.(BARKER)

patterns typically used at that time (**Figure 20-4**). With the current peripheral loading patterns, urethral necrosis is rare.

HEMATURIA

While variable hematuria and passage of small clots is common in the first few post-implant days, late hematuria occurs in only about 10% of patients.(BARKER) It typically starts 6-18 months after implant, and usually resolves spontaneously within a few days or months (**Figure 20-5**). Cystoscopy at the time of late bleeding nearly always shows urethral erythema.

The biggest clinical dilemma in the setting of late post-implant hematuria is deciding whether to pursue a work-up for other causes of hematuria. We typically wait a couple of weeks, and proceed with a general hematuria work-up only if the bleeding persists. Urethral bleeding leading to hemodynamic compromise has never been reported.

URINARY INCONTINENCE

Reports regarding the incidence of post-implant urinary incontinence are mixed. With short-term follow-up, none of 184 Northwest Tumor Institute (NWTI) patients who had not undergone TURP developed incontinence.

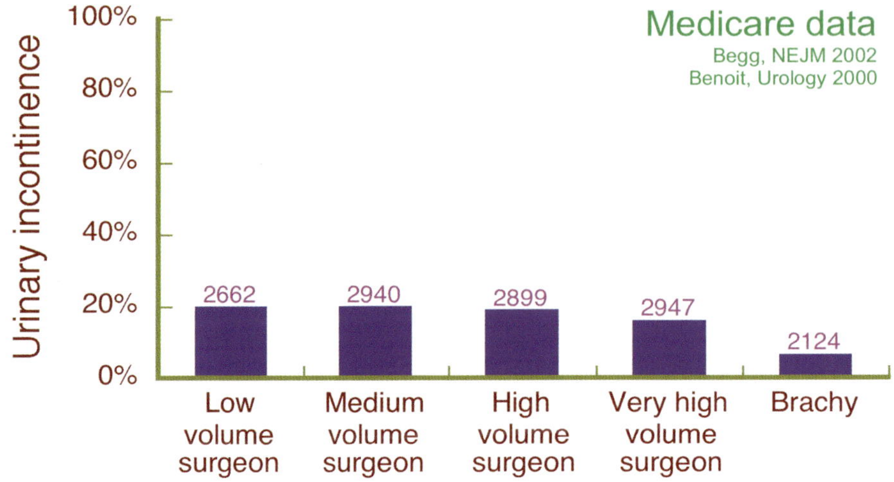

Figure 20-6. Incidence of urinary incontinence based on Medicare claims. Numbers on top of bars represent paitent denominator in study group.(BEGG, BENOIT)

However, incontinence was more common in patients who had had a TURP before or after(especially) implantation.(TALBOTT,BLASKO)

The homogeneous seed loading pattern that led to a relatively high incidence of SUN in some early patients likewise resulted in an increased risk of long-term incontinence. With longer follow-up of the early NWTI patients, a relatively high rate of incontinence was seen even in patients without prior TURP, likely secondary to excessive urethral doses from homogeneous seed loading patterns used at the time.(TALCOTT)

In contrast to the excessive urethral morbidity reported in some early series, more recently urinary incontinence has been unusual with peripheral seed loading patterns. Large Medicare databases show that incontinence is substantially lower with brachytherapy than even in highly experienced surgical hands (**Figure 20-6**). The low incontinence rates in more recent series almost certainly reflect a better appreciation of the importance of keeping central doses relatively low. Doses 110% to 150% of the prescription dose are routinely achievable (**Figure 20-7**). In more recent reports, with better control of central prostatic doses, permanent incontinence is unusual.(ALLEN) One group of investigators showed a stronger relationship between urinary incontinence and pre-implant AUA scores and

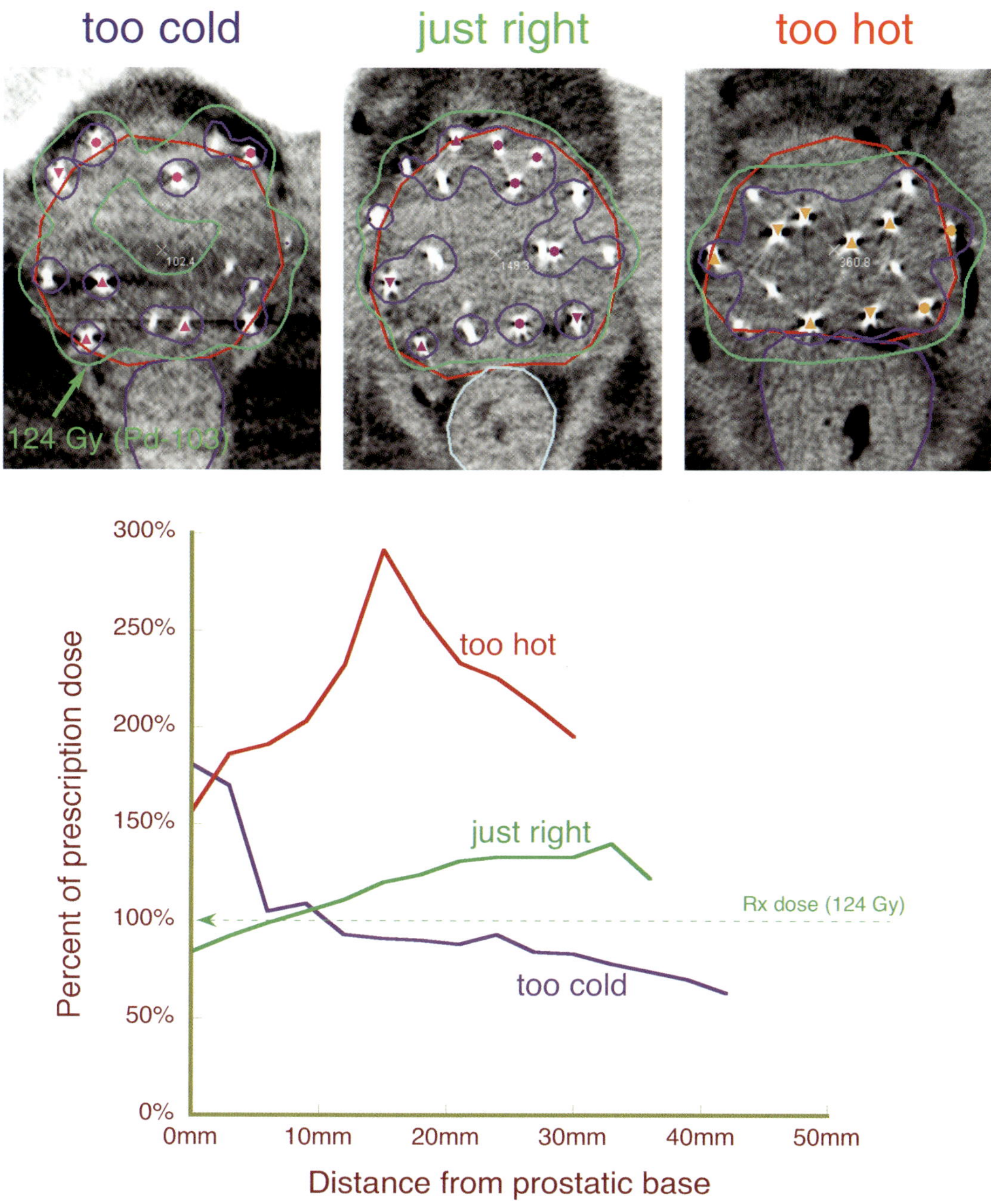

Figure 20-7. Urethral dose examples at mid prostate (upper panels) and along prostatic urethra (lower panel). Note that the urethral dose can vary significantly along the urethra, depending on proximity of seeds to the urethra along its course.

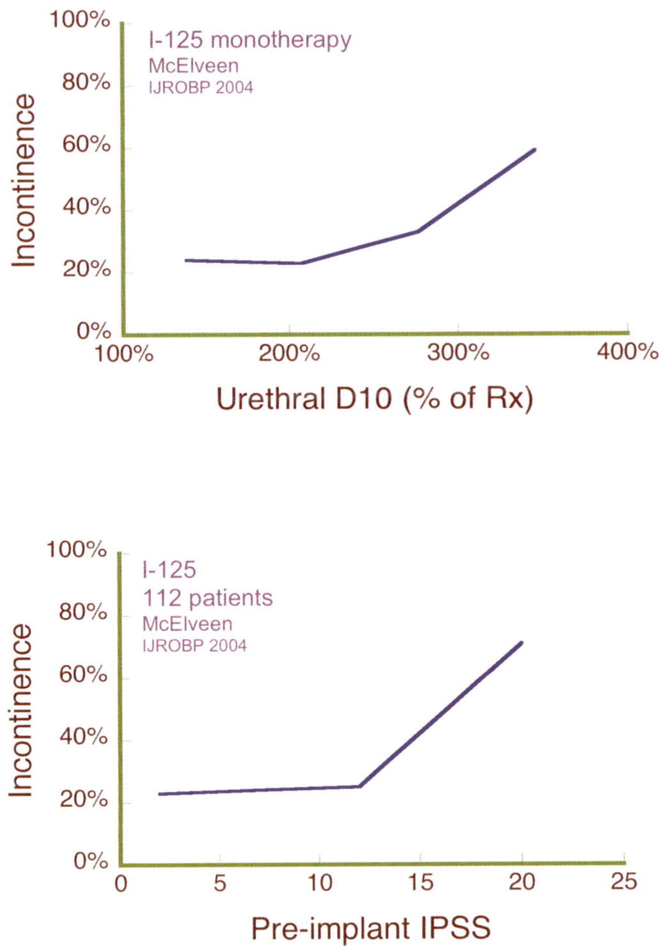

Figure 20-8. Incidence of post-implant urinary incontinence in relation to urethral D10 or pre-implant IPSS. (MCELVEEN) *This relationship between late incontinence and IPSS has not been seen in larger contemporary series, in which the central prostatic doses have been kept relatively low.*

urethral doses. However, their report contained only a small number of patients, treated with what are today considered excessive doses (**Figure 20-8**).(MCELVEEN)

BRACHYTHERAPY AFTER A TURP

There are conflicting reports regarding the risk of urinary incontinence in patients with prior TURP (see chapter 12). Both TURP and radiation can impair urinary continence and their combination may have additive adverse effects. TURP may predispose patients to radiation-related incontinence by compromising the urinary sphincters or by denuding the urethral lining. Blasko, Grimm, and Ragde were the first to draw attention to the higher risk of incontinence in men with prior TURP.(BLASKO) Of 90 patients with pre-

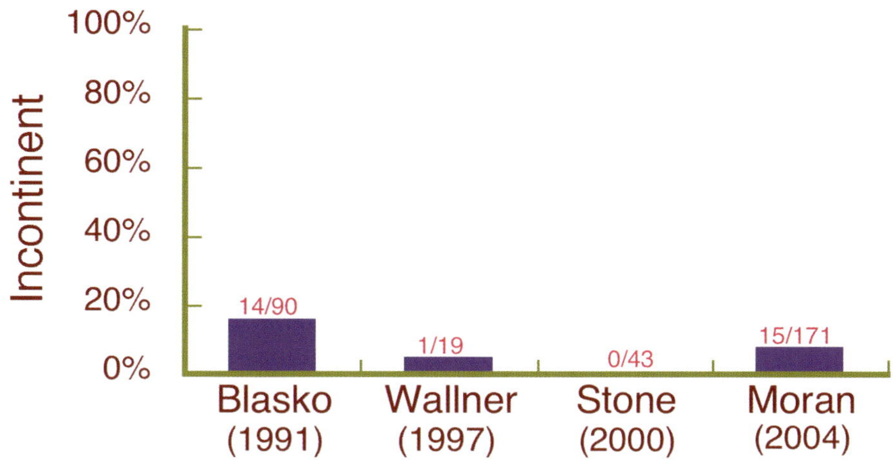

Figure 20-9. Incidence of post-implant urinary incontinence in patients with a prior TURP.(BLASKO, WALLNER 97, STONE, MORAN)

or post-implant TURP, there was a 17% likelihood of incontinence, usually associated with superficial urethral necrosis. And the likelihood of incontinence increased with longer follow-up (unpublished data).

Fortunately, the early brachytherapy experience in patients with prior TURP has not been representative of later series. In a more recent report, only two of twenty-four patients developed post-implant urinary incontinence (one mild and one severe), with the lower incidence attributable to a more peripheral seed placement pattern (see chapter 6).(WALLNER 97) Since adopting a more peripheral seed loading as of 1994, Blasko and colleagues have also noted a lower incidence of urinary incontinence (unpublished data). Other investigators have confirmed a low incidence of incontinence in patients with a prior TURP, provided that a peripheral seed loading pattern is used (**Figure 20-9**).

TURP AFTER BRACHYTHERAPY

Patients who undergo TURP to relieve refractory urinary retention after implantation are at some increased risk of developing urinary incontinence. Hu and Wallner reviewed ten patients who underwent TURP or TUIP (transurethral incision of the prostate) to relieve urinary obstruction, from 1 to 22 months following brachytherapy.(HU 98) Seven of the ten patients

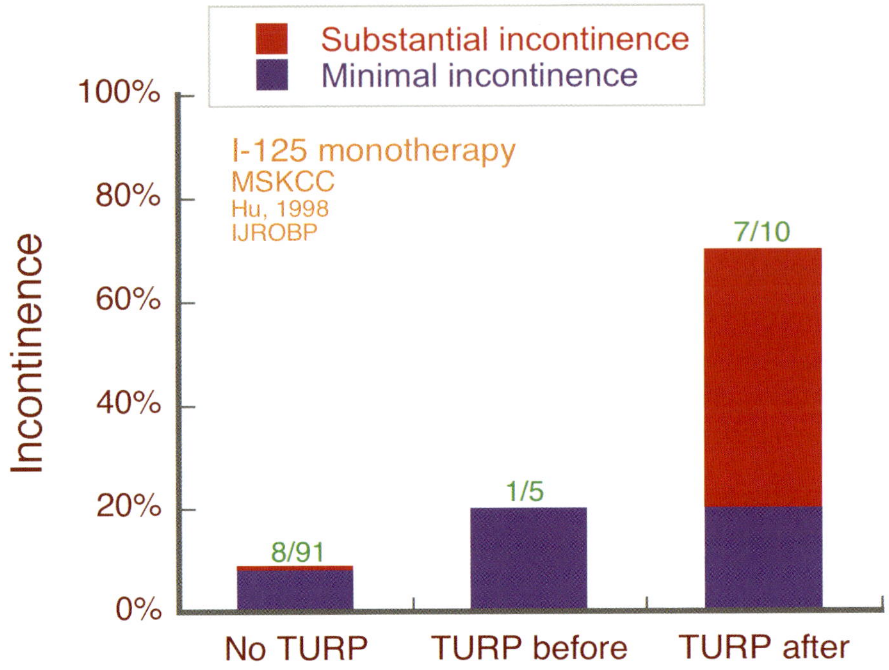

Figure 20-10. Incidence of urinary incontinence in patients treated with I-125 alone by Wallner and colleagues. Six of the eight patients who developed incontinence without having had a TURP before or after implant described urgency, that would occasionally lead to slight leakage if they could not get to a bathroom, symptoms that would not be considered incontinent by the LENT scoring system.(LEE, LAWTON)

developed some degree of permanent urinary incontinence (**Figure 20-10**). Three had minimal stress incontinence and four developed severe incontinence. There was no obvious relationship between the extent of the surgical procedure (TURP versus TUIP) and the likelihood of incontinence. Equally perplexing, there was no obvious relationship between the development of incontinence and the amount of tissue resected at the time of TURP, or between the time from implant to TURP. In five of the patients for whom urethral dose calculations were done, the maximal dose exceeded the prescription dose by 2.5-fold, the level at which the risk of urinary morbidity may rise.(WALLNER 95)

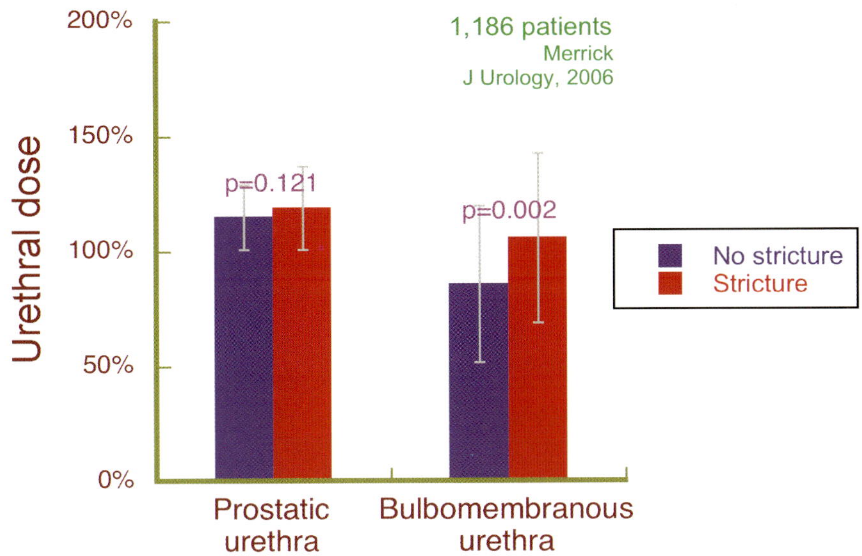

Figure 20-11. Implant doses to the prostatic and bulbomembranous urethra in patients with or without urethral stricture.(MERRICK)

The high incidence of incontinence in post-implant TURP patients reported by Hu and Wallner is likely higher than would be expected in today's patients, because more effort is being taken to keep the urethral doses within acceptable levels.(MERRICK) However, because of the risk of incontinence, patients with refractory post-implant urinary retention should be managed conservatively, with prolonged self-catheterization if necessary. Post-implant resections should be postponed much longer, if not indefinitely, to allow spontaneous resolution of urinary obstruction (see chapter 11). Not surprisingly, patients who undergo both pre-implant and post-implant TURP are at especially high risk for urinary problems.(MERRICK 04)

URETHRAL STRICTURE

Urethral stricture is an occasional complication of modern brachytherapy, probably related to excessive apical radiation doses (**Figure 20-11**).(MERRICK 02) The low incidence of stricture in more recent series likely reflects better adherence to modified peripheral loading patterns (**Figure 20-12**). One early case the authors identified was associated with multiple seeds dragged down to the prostatic apex (**Figure 20-13**). Strictures are typically

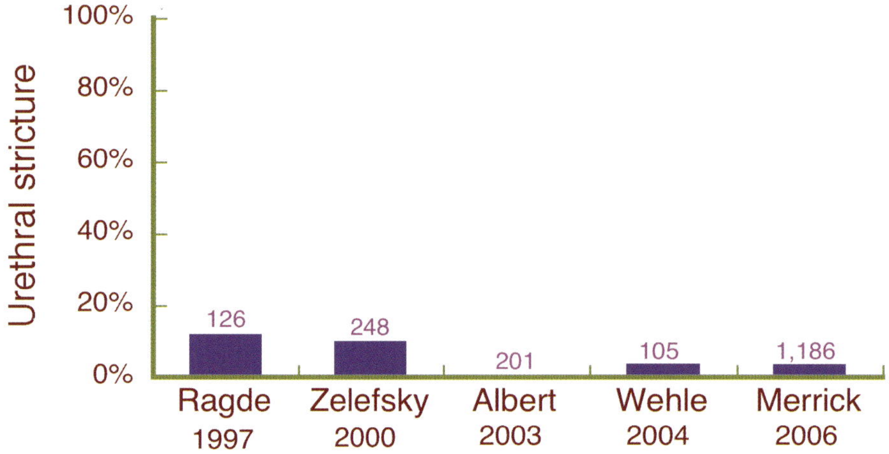

Figure 20-12. Incidence of urethral stricture in various series. Numbers on top of bars represent the study denominators.

relieved with one or more urethral dilations. Internal urethral urethrotomy is generally safe. More invasive procedures should be avoided, if possible.

WE'VE PROBABLY SEEN THE WORST

The first few years' experience, on which much of the early published morbidity data was based, almost certainly indicates a higher urinary complication rate than is currently seen, due to widespread adoption of peripheral seed loading and the technical experience that has been gained. The substantial short-term and long-term morbidity in the early experiences of 1980s and 1990s is not representative of current implants. With good quality implants, serious urinary complications are now surprisingly infrequent.

REFERENCES

1. Albert M, Tempany C, Schultz D, Chen M, Cormack R, Kumar S. Late genitourinary and gastrointestinal toxicity after magnetic resonance image-guided prostate brachytherapy with or without neoadjuvant external beam radiation therapy. Cancer 2003; 98:949-.

2. Allen Z, Merrick G, Butler E, et al. Detailed urethral dosimetry in the evaluation of prostate brachytherapy-related urinary morbidity. Int J Rad Oncol Biol Phys 2005; 62:981-987

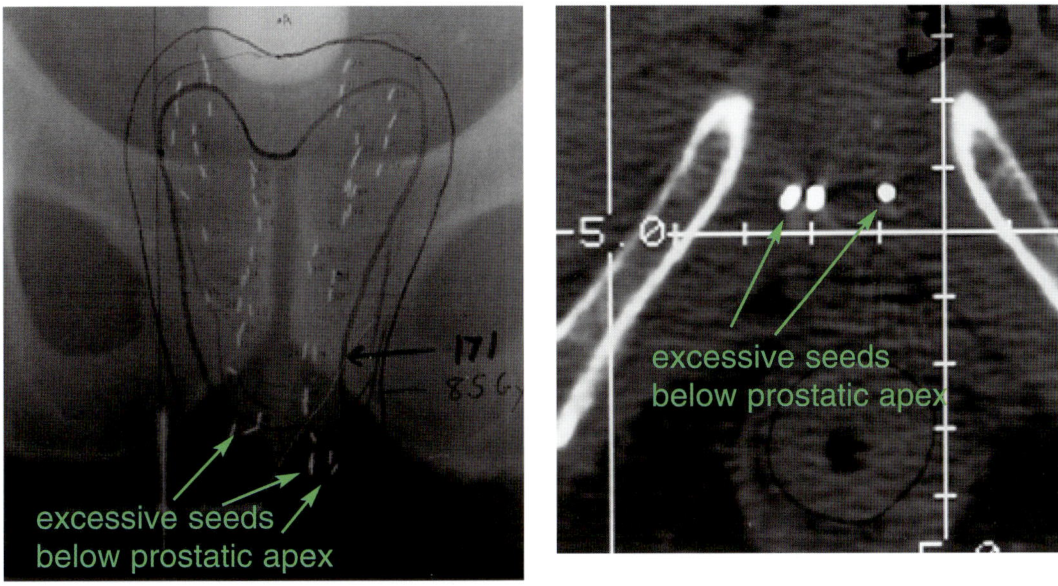

Figure 20-13. Postimplant radiograph and CT scan of a patient who developed an apical urethral stricture 18 months after I-125 implant. An excessive number of sources were placed at prostatic apex, probably contributing to late stricture formation.

3. Barker J, Wallner K, Merrick G. Gross hematuria after prostate brachytherapy. Urol 2003; 61:408-411.

4. Benoit RM, Naslund MJ, Cohen JK. Complications after prostate brachytherapy in the Medicare population. Urol 2000; 55:91-96.

5. Blasko JC, Ragde H, Grimm PD. Transperineal Ultrasound-Guided Implantation of the Prostate: Morbidity and Complications. Scand J Urol Nephrol Suppl 1991; 137:113-118.

6. Gutman S, Merrick G, Butler W, et al. Temporal relationship between prostate brachytherapy and the diagnosis of colorectal cancer. Int J Rad Oncol Biol Phys 2006; 66:48-55.

7. Hu K, Wallner KE. Urinary incontinence in patients who have a TURP/TUIP following prostate brachytherapy. Int J Radiat Oncol Biol Phys 1998; 40:783-786.

8. Landis D, Wallner K, Locke J, et al. Late urinary morbidity after prostate brachytherapy. Brachytherapy 2002; 1:21-26

9. Lawton CA, Won M, Pilepich MV. Long-term Treatment Sequelae Following External Beam Irradiation for Adenocarcinoma of the Prostate: Analysis of RTOG Studies 7506 and 7706. Int J Radiat Oncol Biol Phys 1991; 21:935-939.

10. Lee WR, Schultheiss TE, Hanlon AL, Hanks GE. Urinary incontinence following external beam radiotherapy for clinically localized prostate cancer. Urol 1996; 48:95-99.

11. McElveen TL, Waterman FM, Kim H, Dicker AP. Factors predicting for urinary incontinence after prostate brachytherapy. Int J Rad Oncol Biol Phys 2004; 59:1395-1404.

12. Merrick G, Butler W, Wallner K, Galbreath R. Effect of transurethral resection on urinary quality of life after permanent prostate brachytherapy. Int J Rad Oncol Biol Phys 2004; 58:81-88.

13. Merrick G, Butler W, Wallner K, et al. Risk factor for the development of prostate brachytherapy related urethral strictures. J Urol 2006; 175:1376-1381.

14. Moran B, Stutz M, Gurel M. Prostate brachytherapy can be performed in selected patients after transurethral resection of the prostate. Int J Rad Oncol Biol Phys 2004; 59:392-396.

15. Ragde H, Blasko J, Grimm P, et.al. Interstitial Iodine-125 radiation without adjuvant therapy in the treatment of clinically localized prostate carcinoma. Cancer 1997; 80:442-453.

16. Stone NN, Ratnow ER, Stock RG. Prior transurethral resection does not increase morbidity following real-time ultrasound-guided prostate seed implantation. Techniques in Urology 2000; 6:123-127.

17. Talcott JA, Clark JC, Stark P, Nadir B, Ragde H. Long-term treatment-related complications of brachytherapy for early prostate cancer: A survey of treated patients. Proceedings of ASCO 1999; 18:311a.

18. Wallner K, Lee H, Wasserman S, Dattoli M. Low risk of urinary incontinence following prostate brachytherapy in patients with a prior TURP. Int J Radiat Oncol Biol Phys 1997; 37:565-569.

19. Wehle M, Lisson S, Buskirk S, Broderick G, Young P, Igel T. Prediction of genitourinary tract morbidity after brachytherapy for prostate adenocarcinoma. Mayo Clin Proc 2004; 79:314.

20. Zelefsky MJ, Hollister T, Raben A, Matthews SM, Wallner KE. Five-year biochemical outcome and toxicity with transperineal CT-planned permanent I-125 prostate implantation for patients with localized prostate cancer. Int J Rad Oncol Biol Phys 2000; 47:1261-1266.

21

Proctitis

The potential for rectal problems have been at the top of the list of concerns with dose escalation by external beam radiation or brachytherapy, due to proximity of the prostate and rectum and the potentially serious nature of rectal complications.

Some degree of post-implant radiation proctitis is almost inevitable, given the proximity of the prostate to the rectum. Patients commonly develop more frequent bowel movements and urgency (**Figure 21-1**). Diarrhea is unusual. They may also experience an urge to defecate when urinating—some will actually sit down to urinate, out of concern that they may also

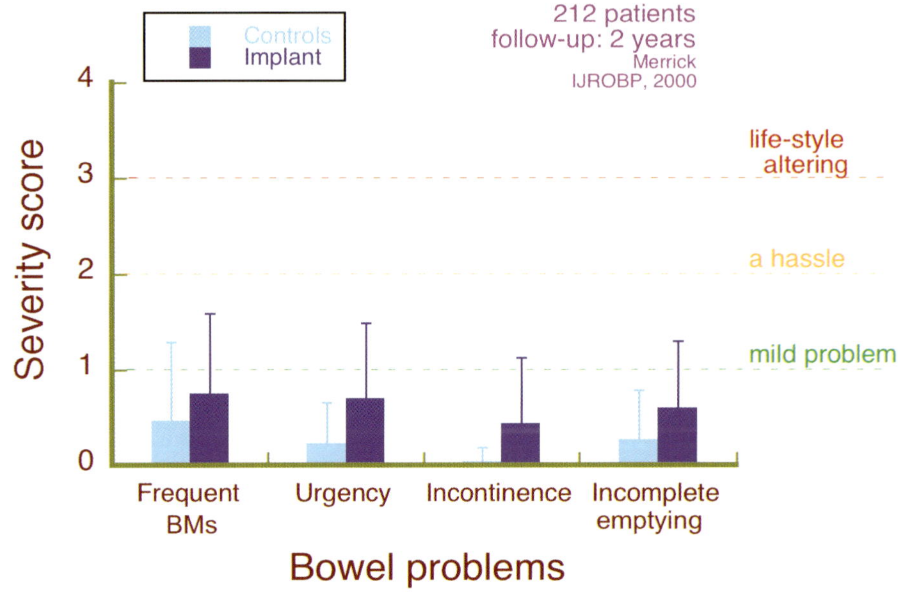

Figure 21-1. Specific bowel changes, at an average of two years following brachytherapy.(MERRICK)

pass stool. Although radiation-related rectal symptoms are common, rectal incontinence is unusual.

Proctitis symptoms usually resolve within a few months. Nearly all patients' rectal function returns to the pre-implant level by one to two years (**Figure 21-2 and 21-3**).(MERRICK 99)

Rectal bleeding

Radiation proctopathy with bleeding has been reported to occur in 2% to 10% of patients, usually appearing between 6 and 18 months after implantation (**Figures 21-4**).(GELBLUM, HAN, MERRICK 99) The incidence has varied substantially from one series to the next, probably due to differences in reporting criteria and differences in the typical R100s achieved by the brachytherapist. The occurrence of proctitis is probably decreasing as more brachytherapists become familiar with and adhere to published dose guidelines.(TRAN)

Endoscopy usually reveals a circumscribed area of intense erythema, telangiectasias and friability on the anterior rectal wall, overlying the

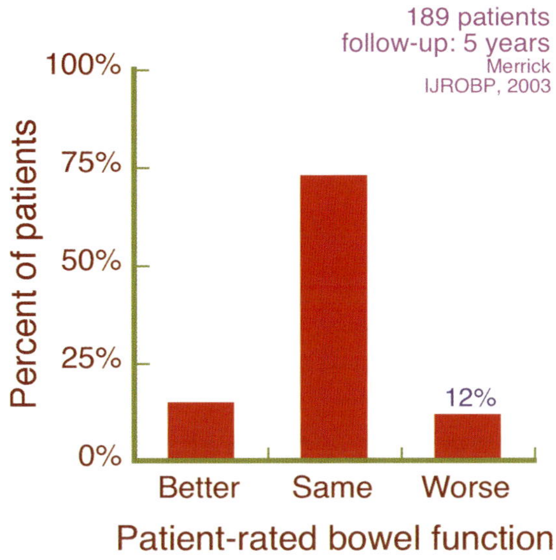

Figure 21-2. Long-term rectal function compared with pre-implant function.(MERRICK)

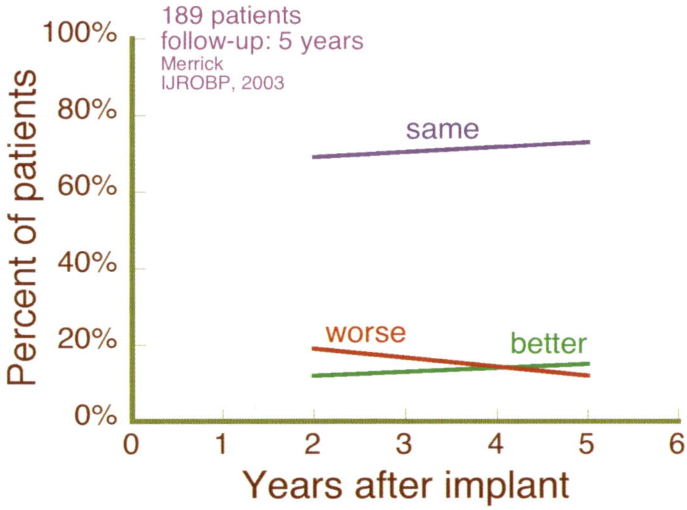

Figure 21-3. Rectal function appears to continue to gradually improve from 2 to 5 years following brachytherapy.(MERRICK)

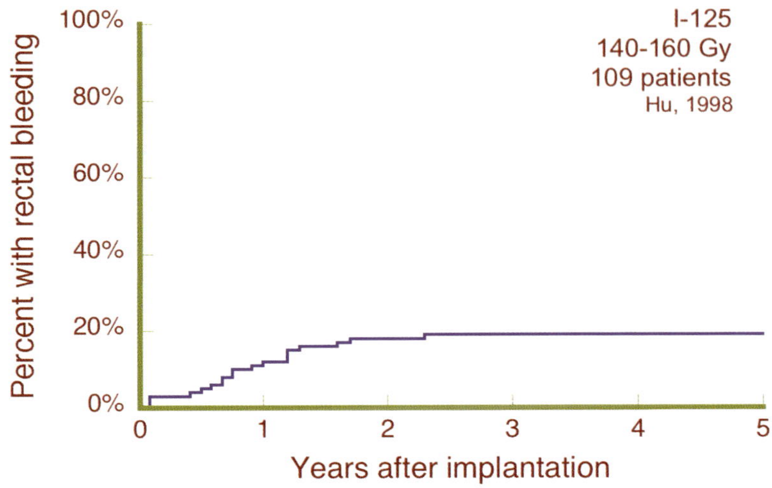

Figure 21-4. Incidence of rectal bleeding over time—nearly all cases manifest in the first six to twenty-four post-implant months.(HU)

prostate (**Figures 21-5 through 21-7**). Blood loss is typically minimal, rarely requiring transfusions.

In some cases of proctitis, misplaced seeds are obvious on post-implant CT scan (**Figure 21-8**). Most of the time, however, errors are not obvious and rectal doses are only mildly higher in patients with clinically apparent proctitis (see Chapter 11). The loose correlation between dosimetry and rectal complications might be explained by a predisposition of some patients to rectal complications due to inherent radiation sensitivity, diabetes, or microvascular damage from other causes. Mueller and colleagues showed that a limited number of errant peri-rectal sources does not, in itself, place patients at increased risk of rectal bleeding, providing that the overall rectal wall doses are within acceptable values (see Chapter 11).(MUELLER).

Three teams have shown a consistent relationship between rectal doses and the likelihood of proctitis.(SNYDER, WATERMAN, MUELLER) Their work has lead to verified, achievable dose limit recommendations that minimize the likelihood of serious rectal complications while maintaining very high cure rates (see Chapter 11).

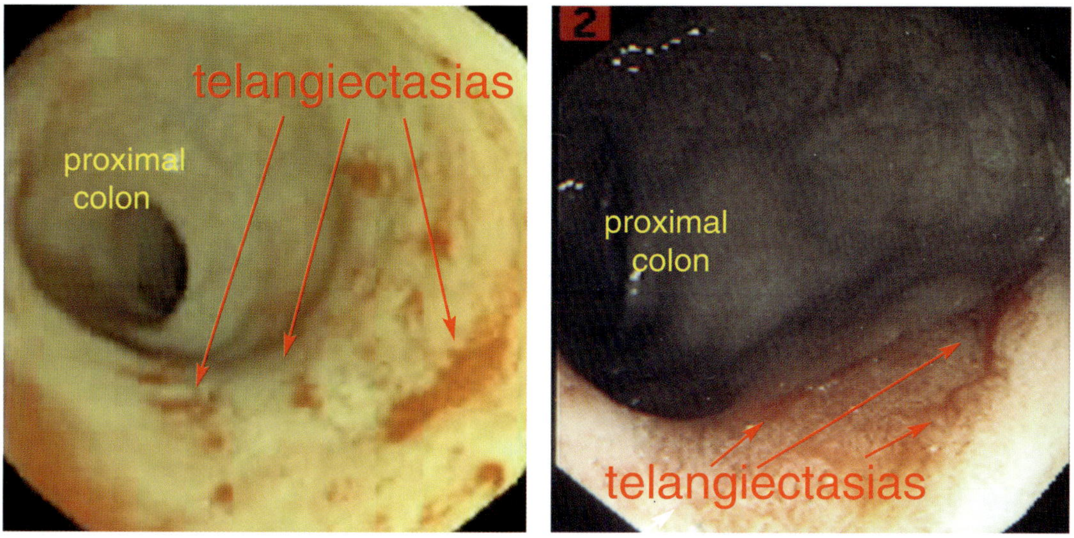

Figure 21-5. Post-implant proctitis with telangiectasias (arrows) in patients who developed painless rectal bleeding. The erythema is well localized to the anterior rectal wall.

Supplemental beam and proctitis

Reports regarding the effects of supplemental external beam radiation on rectal morbidity are mixed. Iversen and colleagues treated patients with a full dose (160 Gy) I-125 implant followed by 47 Gy whole-pelvic irradiation at 220 cGy/day.(IVERSEN) Severe late complications, including rectal ulceration, colostomy, and severe radiation cystitis, were reported in 14 of 33 patients. This toxicity would be unacceptable by any standard, and likely resulted from their use of whole pelvic irradiation at high daily fractions, preceded by a full dose implant. Although the report by Iversen and colleagues was frightening, the incidence of significant proctitis with combined implant plus external beam radiation is low with current techniques.(HAN) In most series, the addition of supplemental beam radiation has increased the likelihood of rectal bleeding, but has not clearly been associated with more severe complications, such as ulceration or fistula (**Figure 21-10**).(TRAN) Some authors report higher rates of severe rectal complications with supplemental beam radiation performed *after* brachytherapy, but this issue is unsettled.(ZEITLIN, PATEL)

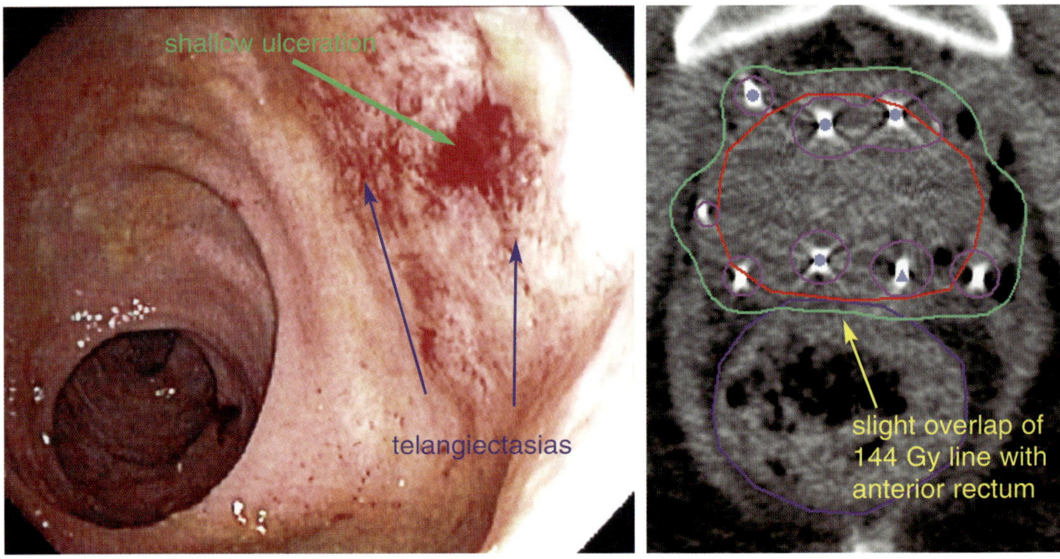

Figure 21-6. Example of post-implant proctitis in patient with relatively low V100 of 0.56 cc. Note minimal overalap between 144 Gy Rx isodose and the anterior rectal wall.

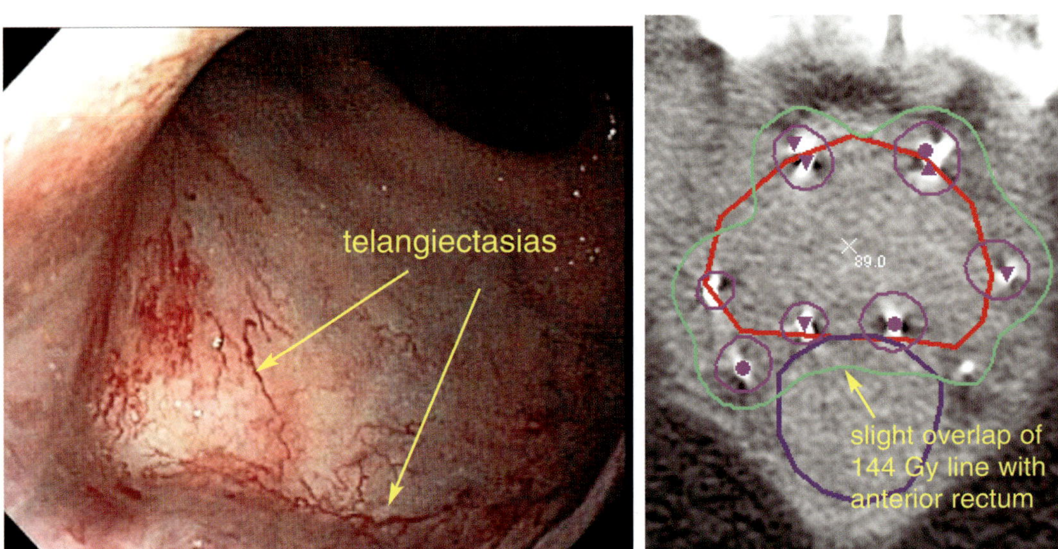

Figure 21-7. Example of post-implant telangiectasias three years after Pd-103 and supplemental beam in patient with slightly high V100 of 1.27 cc Note moderate overlap of the 86 Gy Rx isodose with the anterior rectal wall.

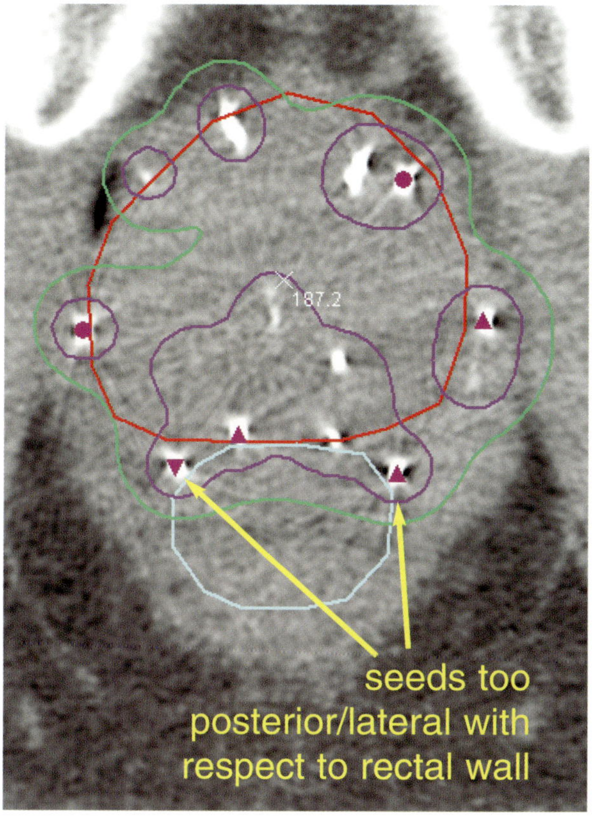

Figure 21-8. Seeds placed too posteriorly can lead to excessive R100 values.

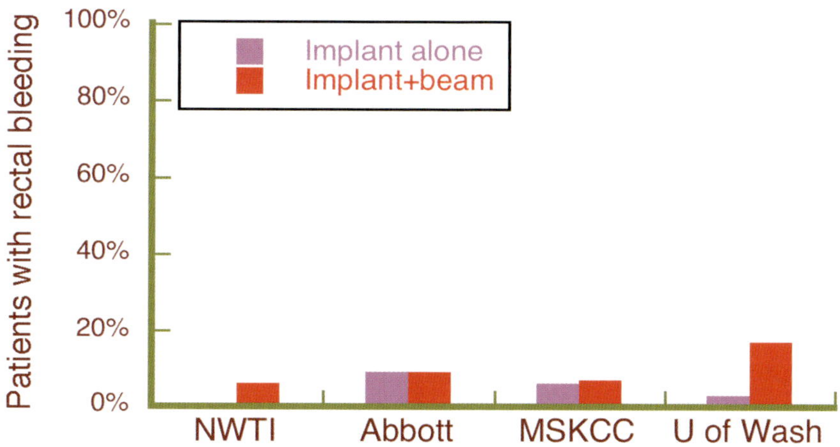

Figure 21-9. Incidence of implant-related rectal bleeding after brachytherapy, with or without supplemental external beam radiation.(BLASKO, KAYE, GELBLUM, HAN)

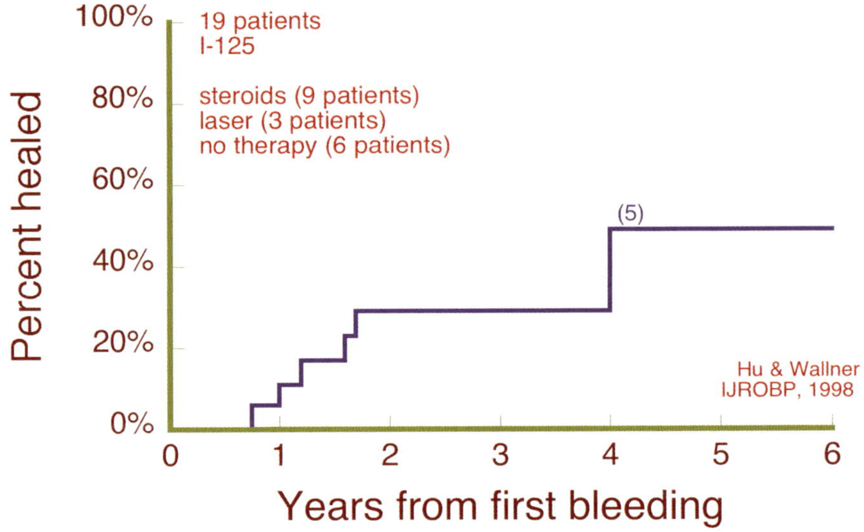

Figure 21-10. Long-term resolution of rectal bleeding.(HU)

Treatment of proctitis

If and when to intervene for rectal bleeding is often a difficult decision. Given enough time, most will heal spontaneously (**Figure 21-10**).(CROOK, SHIPLEY, TESHIMA, HU) However, healing is typically slow. In the meantime, persistent bleeding can be a substantial nuisance for patients—repeated soiling of the underwear is especially distressing. Medical therapies, including mesalamine or steroid enemas, are commonly prescribed, with mixed results (**Table 21-1**).(BABB, KOCHBAR) Nonetheless, such therapies are seldom harmful and a therapeutic trial seems reasonable. Of eighteen I-125 patients reported by Hu and Wallner, nine were treated with steroid enemas, three had laser coagulation, and six had no intervention. Although the series was retrospective and uncontrolled, there was no obvious difference in the resolution rate between treatment groups.(HU)

Table 21-1. Probably effective treatment for proctitis.

- topical formalin
- argon plasma coagulation
- time
- hyperbaric oxygen(?)

Table 21-2. Probably ineffective remedies.

- rowasa
- topical steroids
- high/low fiber diet

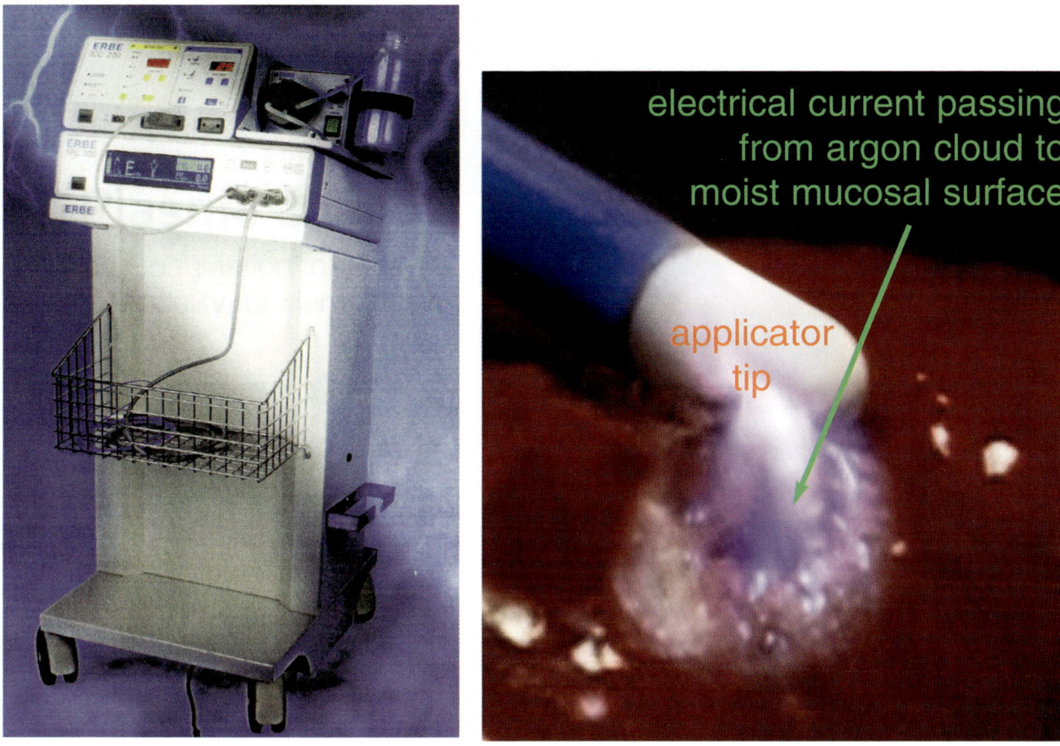

Figure 21-11. ERBE APC unit.

In contrast to medical therapies, more invasive therapies with argon plasma coagulation (APC) or topical formalin are highly effective, with what appears to be a low likelihood of complications (**Figure 21-11 through 21-14**).(VIGGIANO, KAASSIS, ROCHE, BISWAL) At the Puget Sound Health Care System VA hospital, patients with radiation-related proctitis have generally responded well to one or more treatment sessions with argon plasma laser coagulation.(SMITH) However, we are aware of cases, at other institutions, in which laser therapy may have exacerbated bleeding followed by fistualization. Such interventions should be undertaken cautiously.

PAIN

Rectal bleeding from radiation proctitis is typically painless. When pain does occur, it may indicate involvement of the sphincter muscles (**Figure 21-15**). It may also result from rectal spasms, which may respond to dicyclomine (Bentyl) or belladonna/opium suppositories.

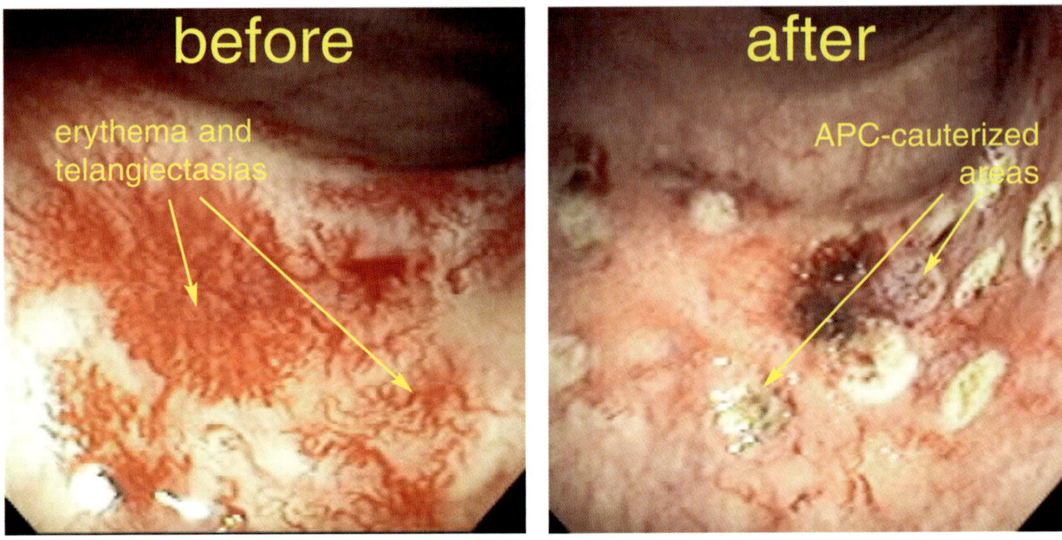

Figure 21-12. Example of argon plasma coagulated (APC) in a patient treated by Dr. Jason Dominitz at the Puget Sound Health Care System VA Hospital.(SMITH)

Pain in itself does not appear to portend a worse outcome.(HU 98) Management of rectal pain can present a dilemma. We are reluctant to start patients on long-term narcotics. Fortunately, patients nearly always improve spontaneously with time.

ULCERATION AND FISTULAS

While persistent rectal bleeding is a nuisance and may adversely impact patients' lifestyles, it is the progression of proctitis to a rectal ulcer or rectal-prostatic fistula that is most devastating (**Figures 21-16 through 21-18**). The only good thing that can be said about brachytherapy-related rectal fistulas is that they have been very uncommon, even in the early days of TRUS-guided implants. Brachytherapy-related fistulas occurred with about the same frequency as peri-prostatic death in large sugical series (**Figure 21-19**).

In general, prostatic tissue has been remarkably resistant even to the ultra-high doses near seed clusters. However with a combination of proctitis from typical intra-prostatic doses and even a moderately high R100, there is a small risk of fistualization. The low numbers of fistulas meant that a

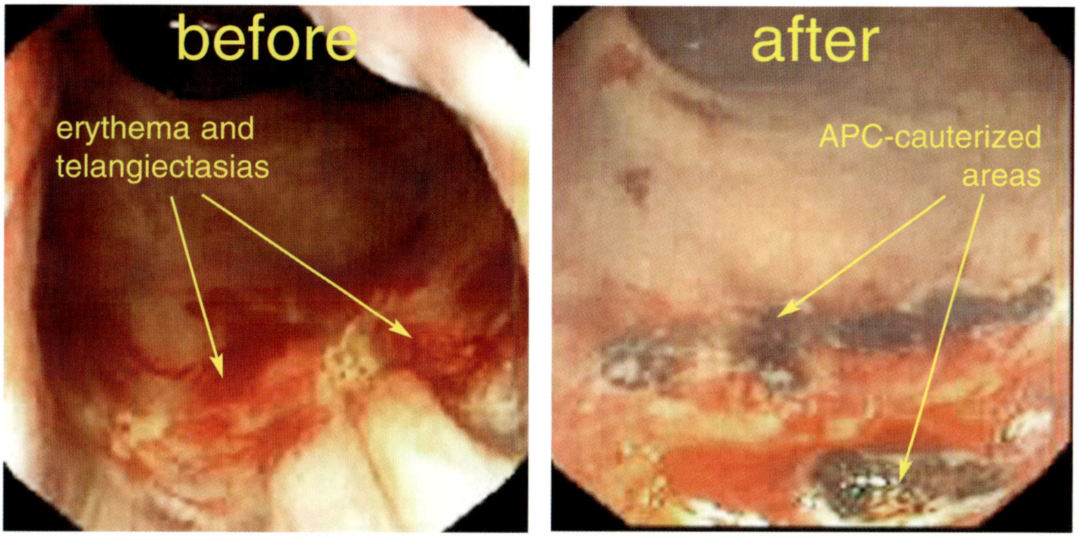

Figure 21-13. Another example of argon plasma coagulated (APC) in a patient treated by Dr. Jason Dominitz at the Puget Sound Health Care System VA Hospital.(SMITH)

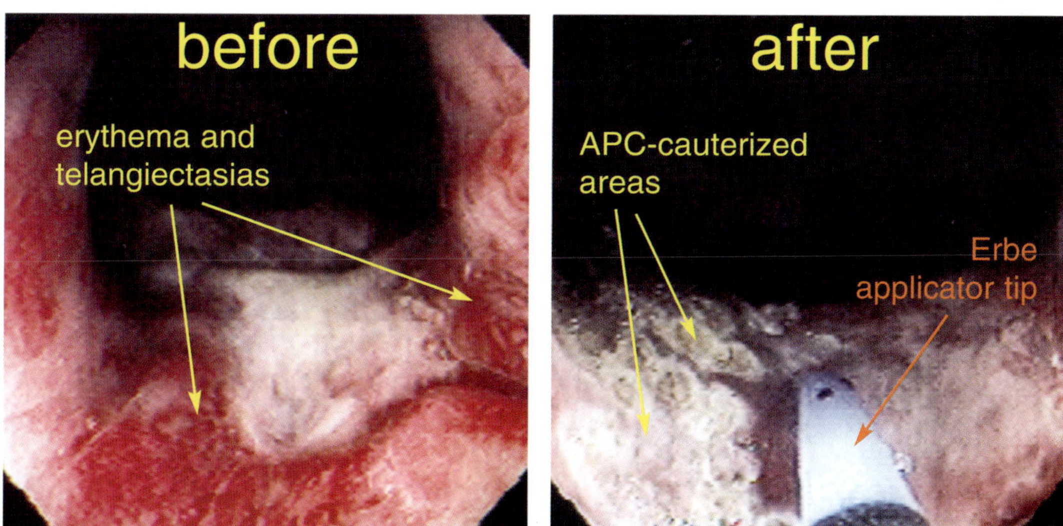

Figure 21-14. Another example of argon plasma coagulated (APC) in a patient treated by Dr. Jason Dominitz at the Puget Sound Health Care System VA Hospital.(SMITH)

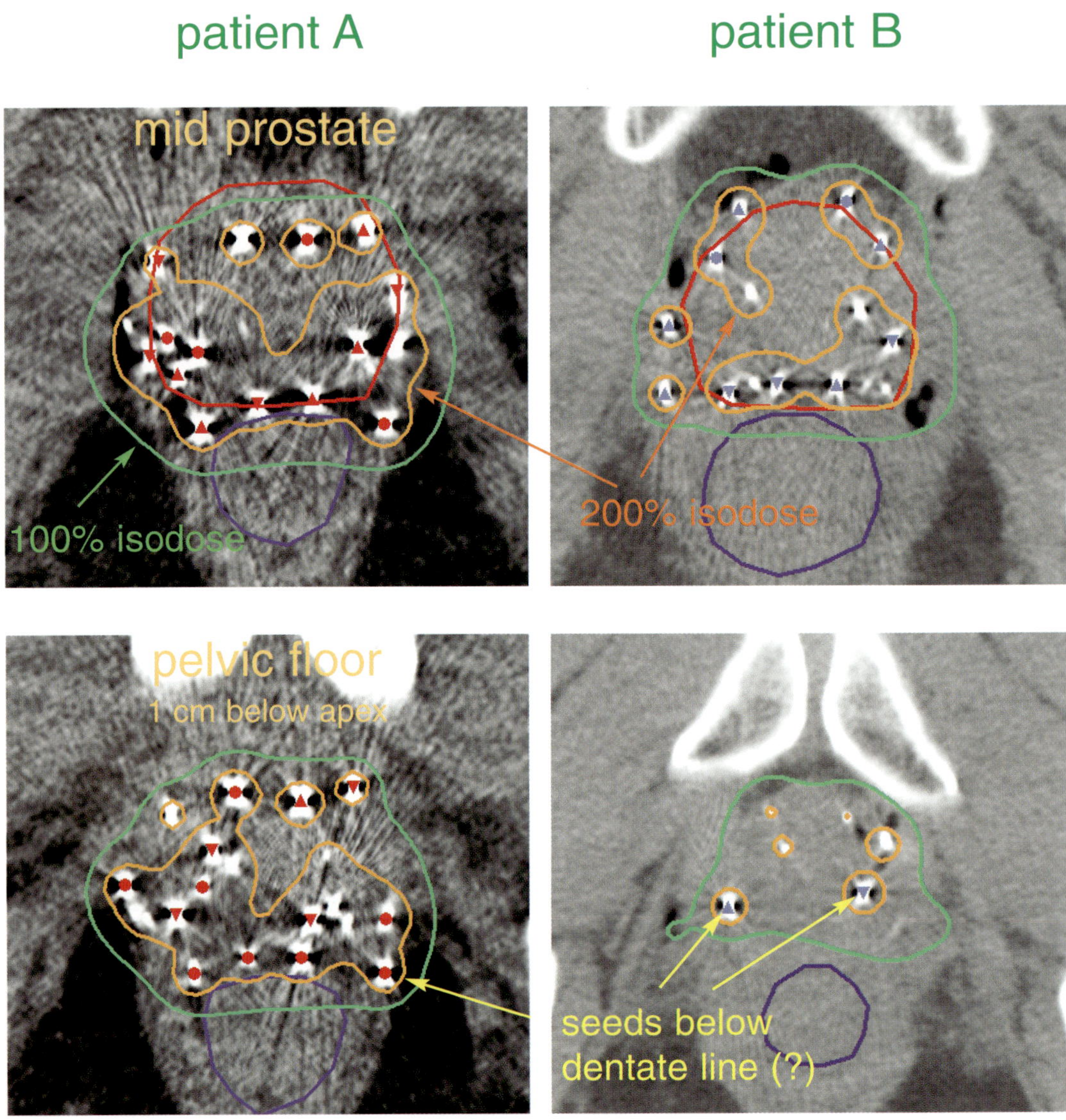

Figure 21-15. Both of these patients developed rectal bleeding and rectal pain. Pain from rectal radiation damage is atypical. Their pain may have been due to mucosal destruction from excessive seeds below the dentate line.

superficial rectal ulcer   deep rectal ulcer

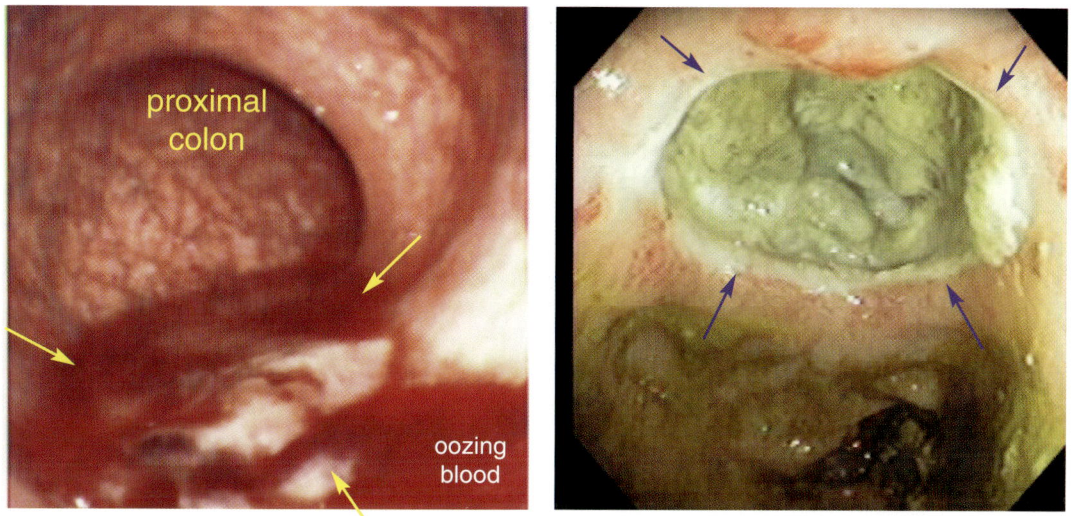

Figure 21-16. Post-implant rectal ulcerations (arrows) overlying the prostate, a much less common occurrence.

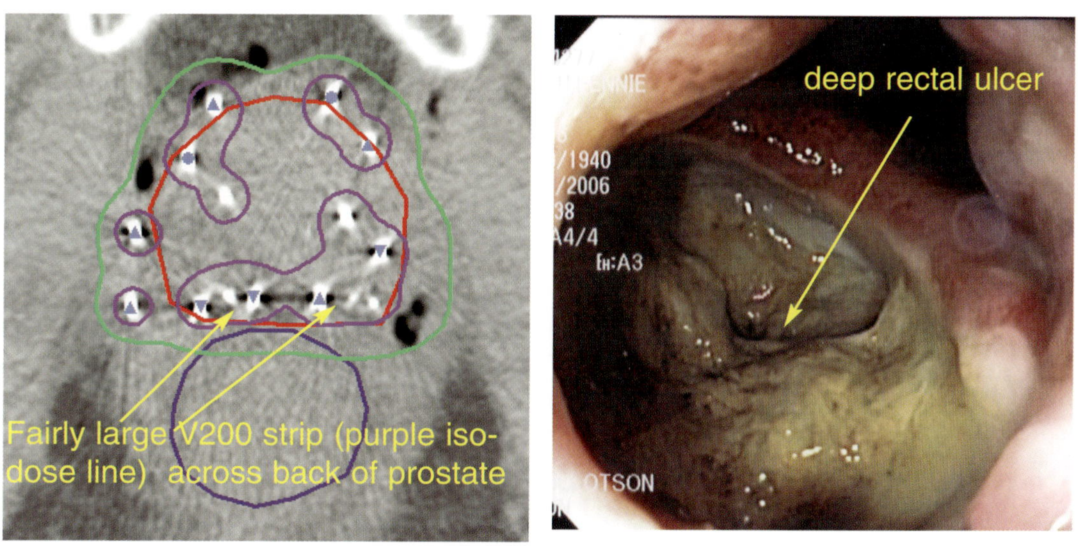

Figure 21-17. Example of a deep rectal ulcer following I-125 monotherapy. The R100 was only 0.51 cc. The R200 was 0.0 cc. It is possible, however, that the V200 strip along the back of the prostate lead to the ulcer. But we've had many patients with a similar posterior V200 strip who did not go on to form an ulcer....

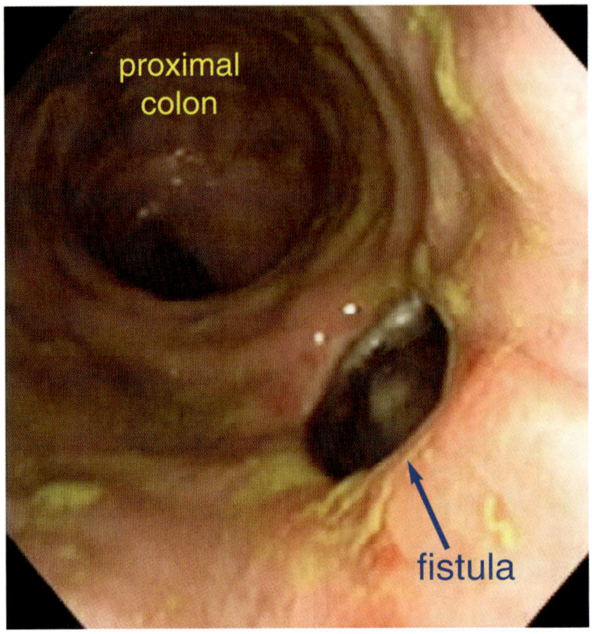

Figure 21-18. Endoscopic view of 62-year-old patient who developed a rectal ulcer and then fistula 18 months after a 144 Gy I-125 implant. The ulcer measured about 10 mm across. CT scan (below) shows gas between the outer rectal wall and the posterior prostate, leaking through the fistula.

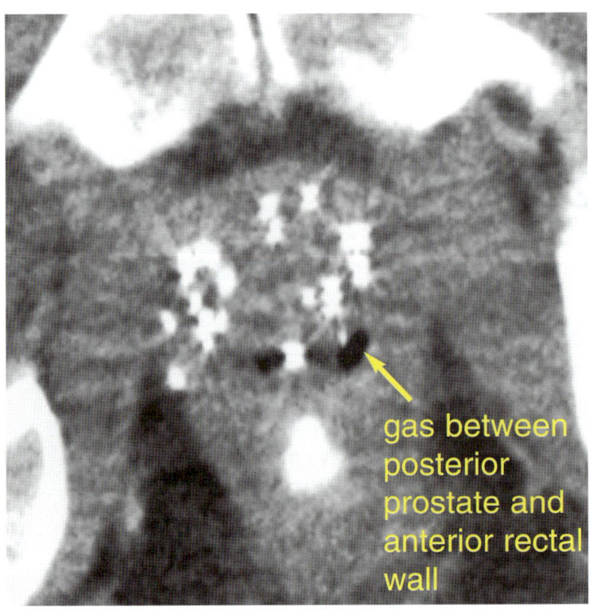

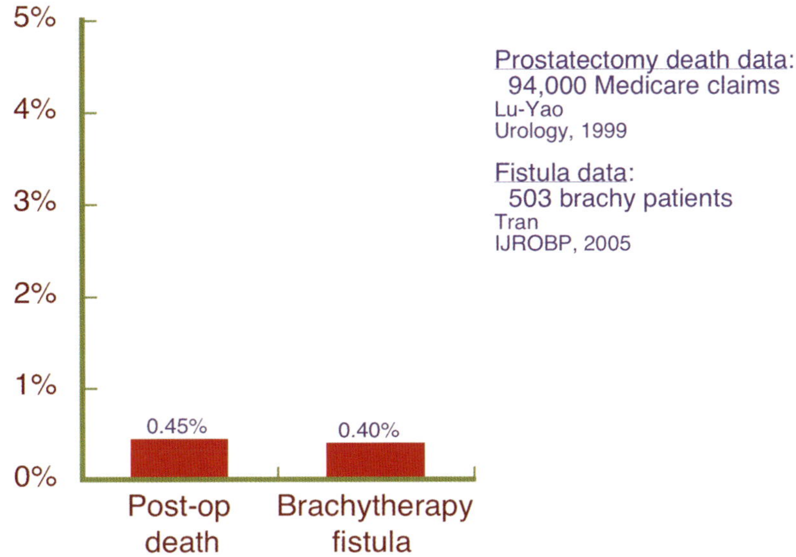

Figure 21-19. Incidence of a rectal fistula after brachytherapy versus peri-operative death from prostatectomy. Fistulas are serious complications that frequently lead to lawsuits. But most would consider prostatectomy-related death to be even worse.

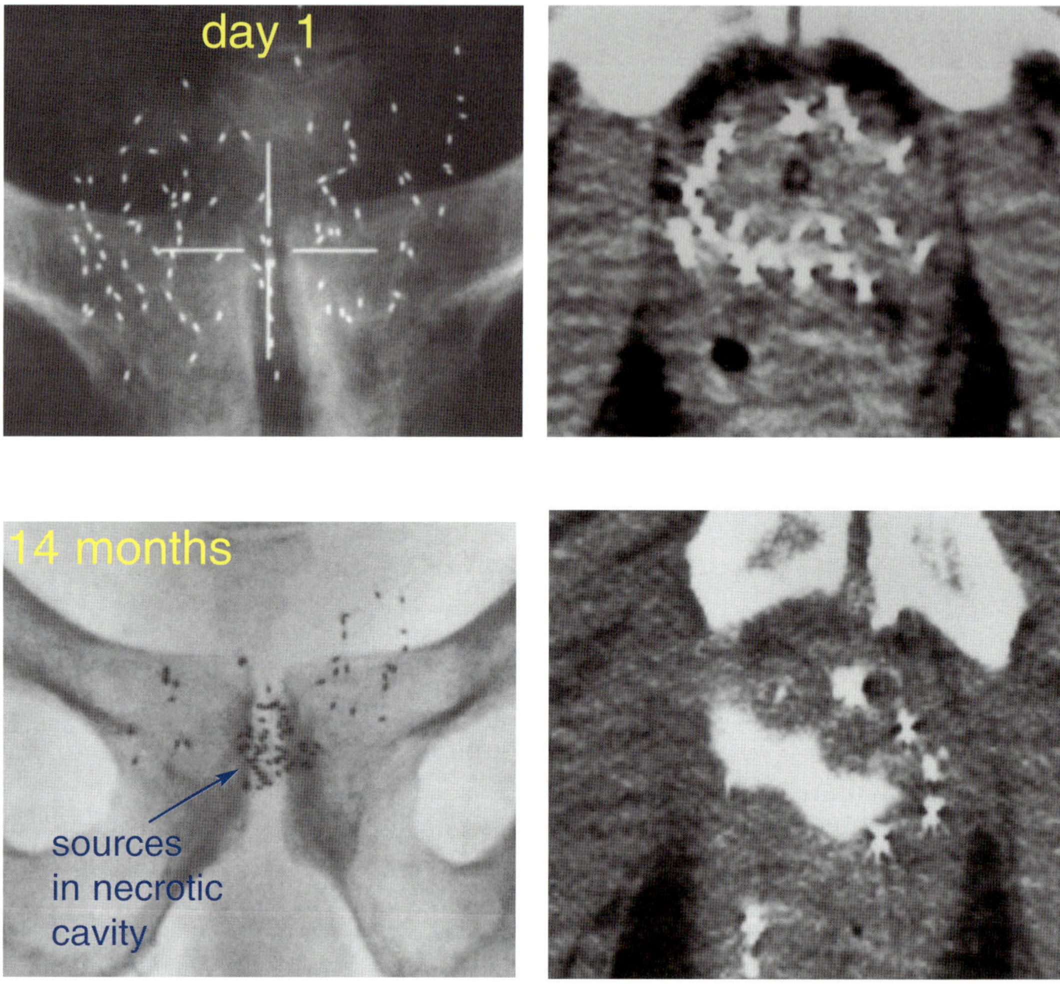

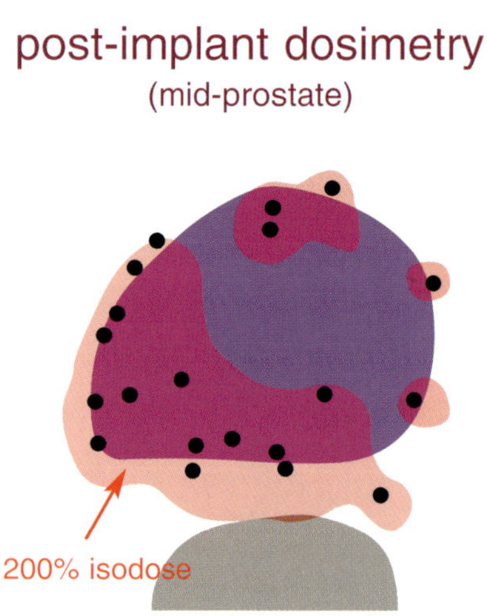

Figure 21-20. Day 1 anterior film (top) and CT of patient who developed diffuse prostatic necrosis one year after a 115 Gy Pd-103 implant. The middle photos show diffuse source loss and clumping within a central necrotic cavity. The post-implant dose reconstruction showed a fairly large V200 region corresponding to the necrotic cavity (bottom, left). Complications like this have been rare.

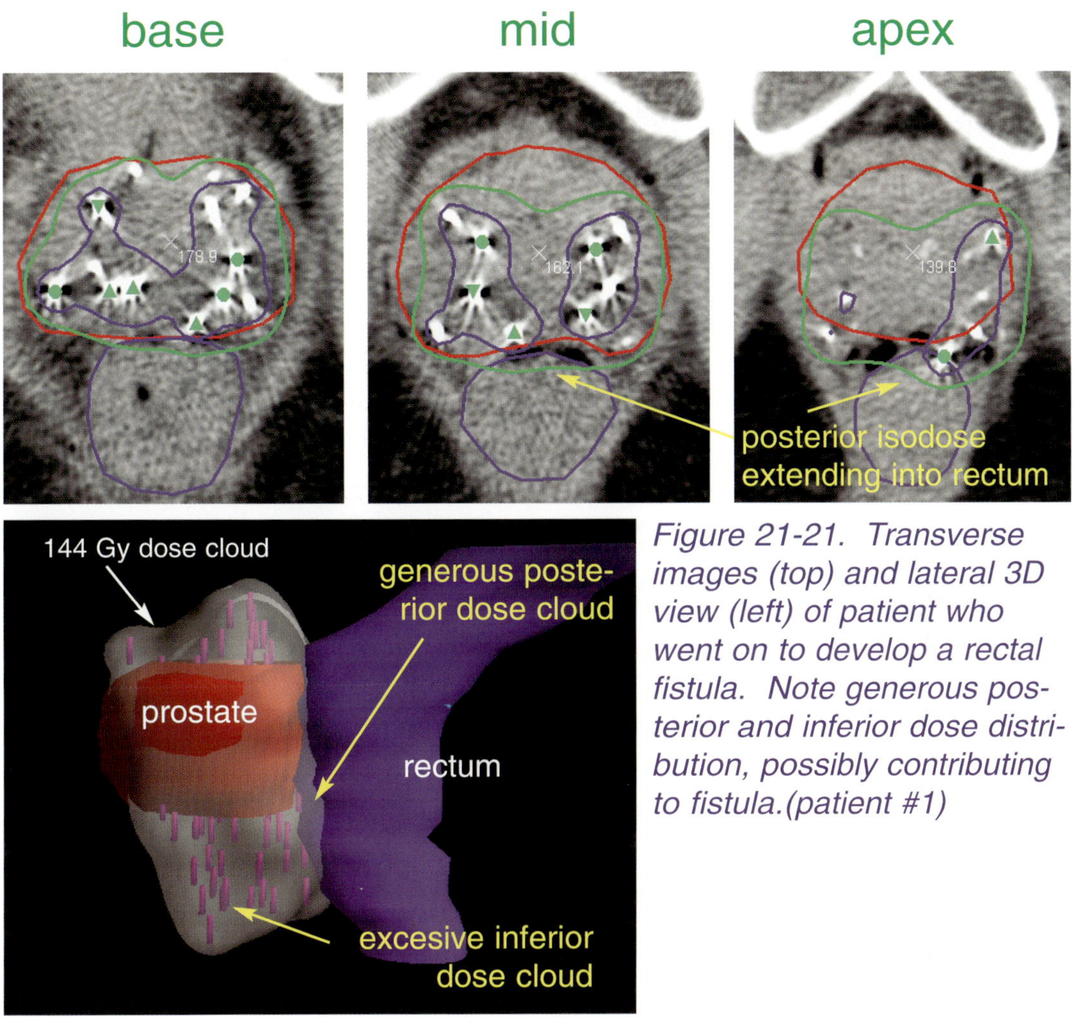

Figure 21-21. Transverse images (top) and lateral 3D view (left) of patient who went on to develop a rectal fistula. Note generous posterior and inferior dose distribution, possibly contributing to fistula.(patient #1)

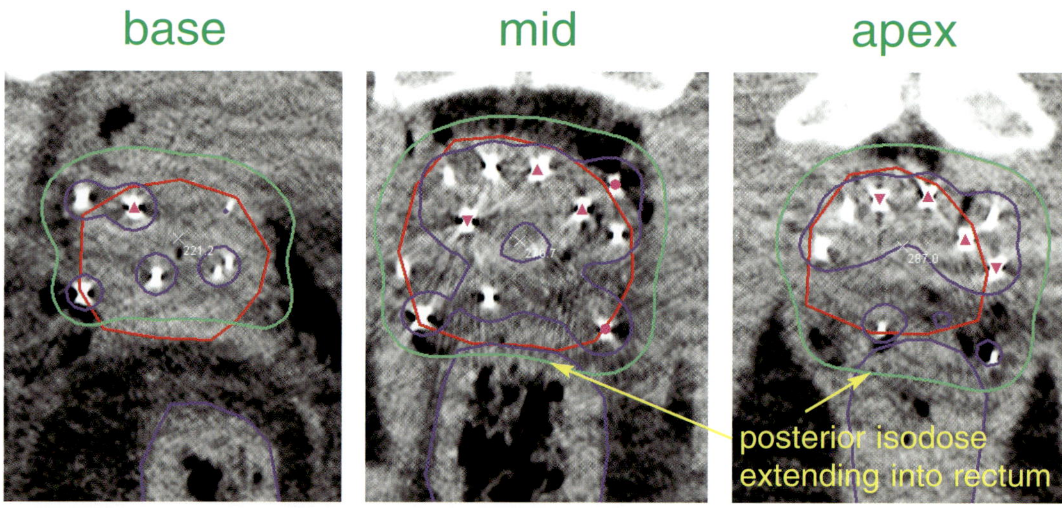

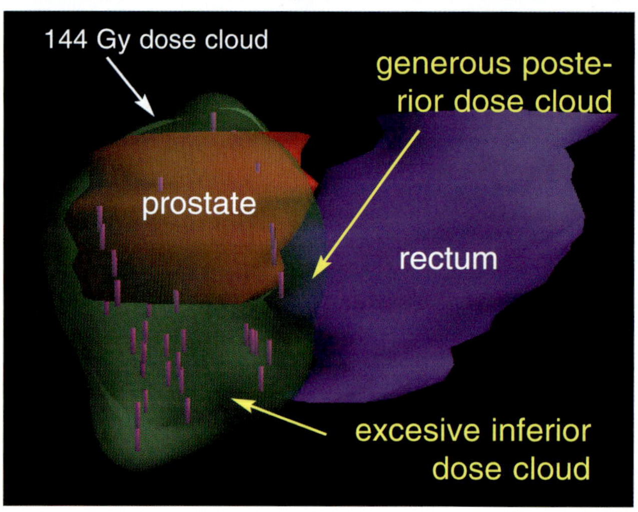

Figure 21-22. Transverse images (top) and lateral 3D view (left) of patient who went on to develop a rectal fistula. Note generous posterior and inferior dose distribution, presumably responsible for fistula.(patient #2)

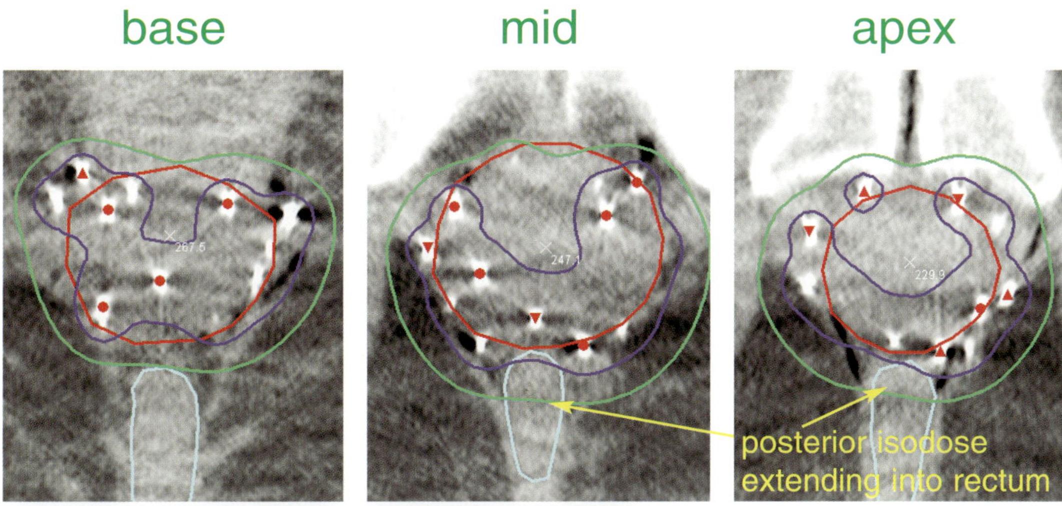

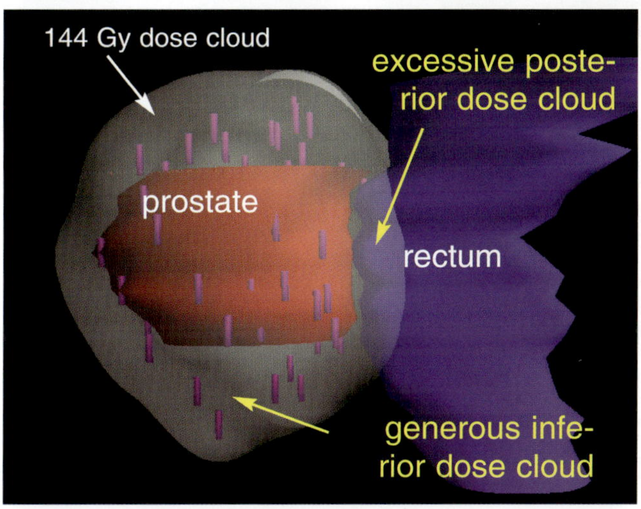

Figure 21-23. Transverse images (top) and lateral 3D view (left) of patient who went on to develop a rectal fistula (white arrows). Note generous posterior and inferior dose distribution, presumably responsible for fistula.(patient #3)

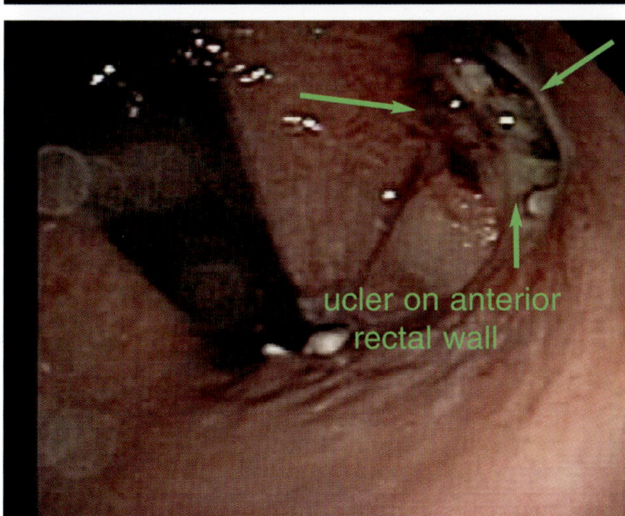

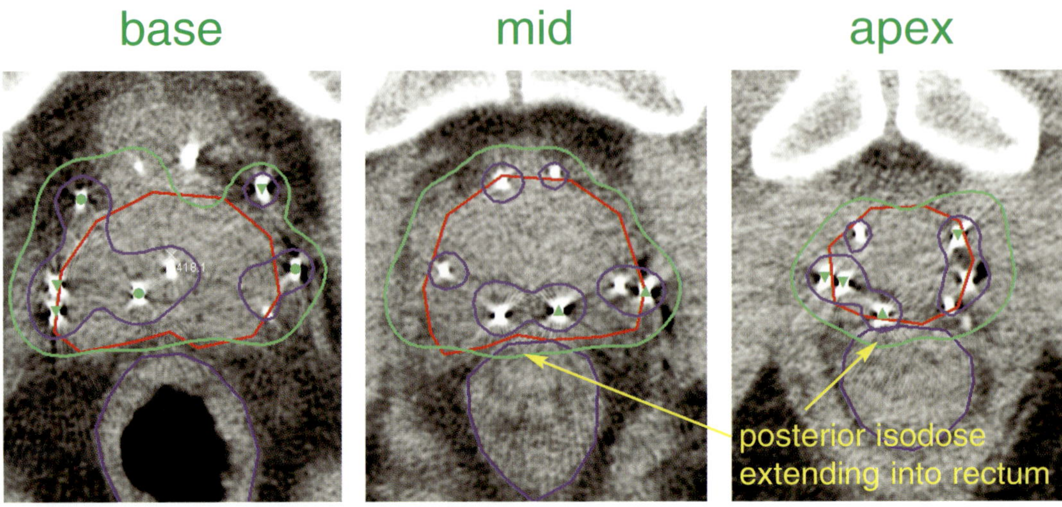

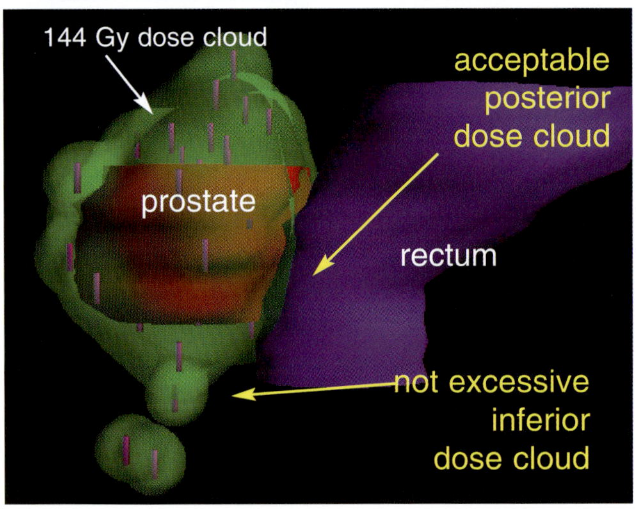

Figure 21-24. Transverse images (top) and lateral 3D view (left) of patient who went on to develop a rectal fistula. Posterior and inferior dose distribution was not obviously excessive in this case.(patient #4)

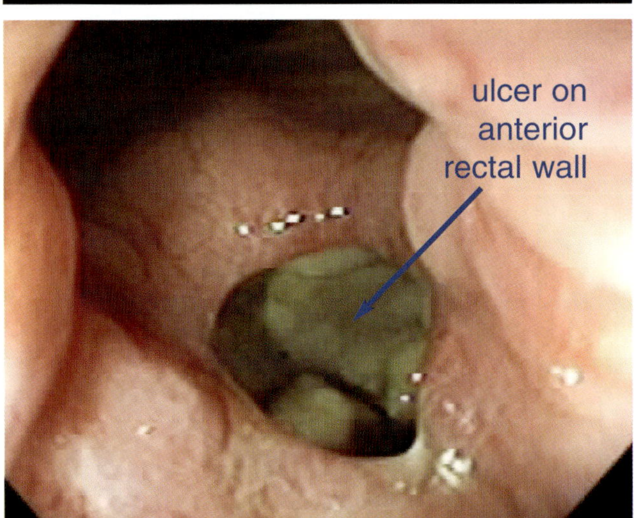

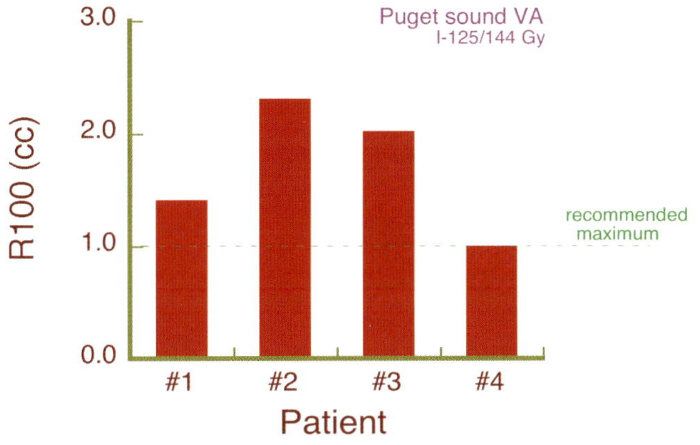

Figure 21-25. R100s and V200s in the four VA patients in Figures 21-19 through 21-23 who developed rectal fistulas.

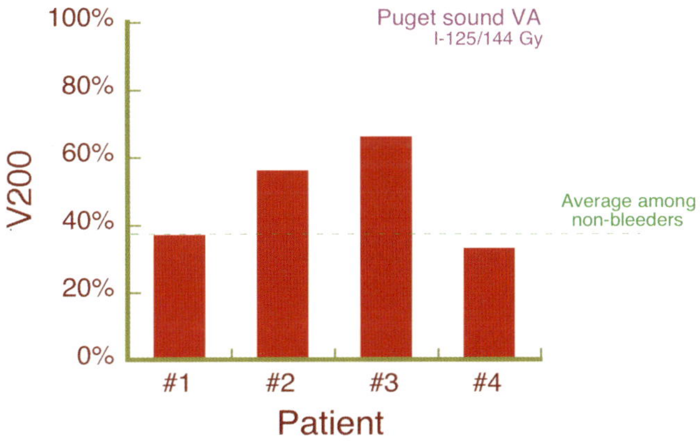

number of years passed before enough occurred to be able to study them. The first report correlating fistuals with dosimetry appeared in 1990. Howard and colleagues, based on only three cases, concluded that "serious rectal complications appear to occur in an unpredictable manner, typically unrelated to known dosimetric parameters."(HOWARD)

The next report regarding dose and fistulas appeared in 2004.(TRAN) Based on their own two cases and review of other experience, Tran wrote that "although the occurrence of a fistula does not necessarily reflect grossly high rectal wall doses, cases almost never occur if the R100 was kept below 1.0 cc." The authors concluded that although there was no R100 beyond which patients were at high risk of ulceration, "High rectal radiation doses should be avoided a priori, to minimize the likelihood of

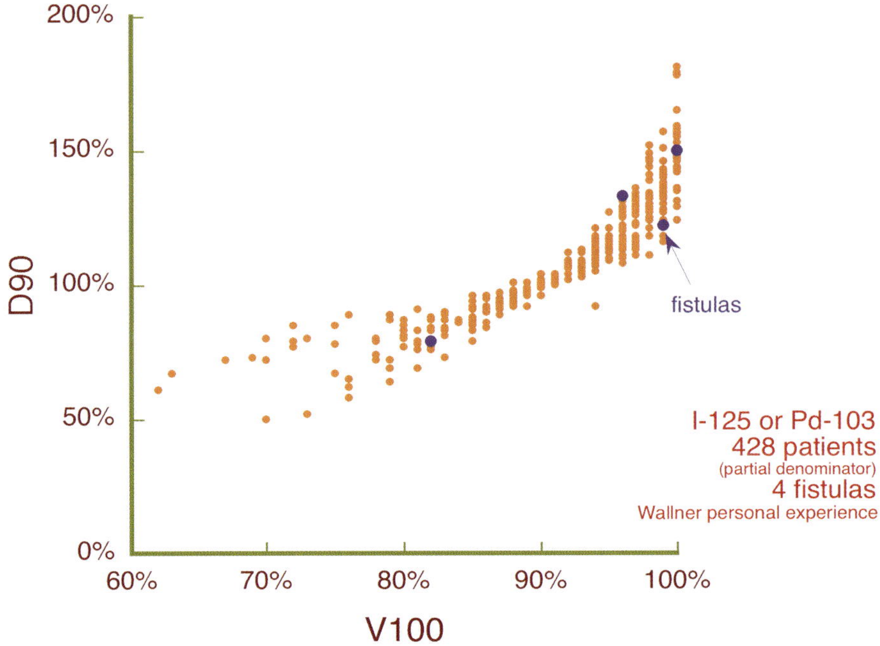

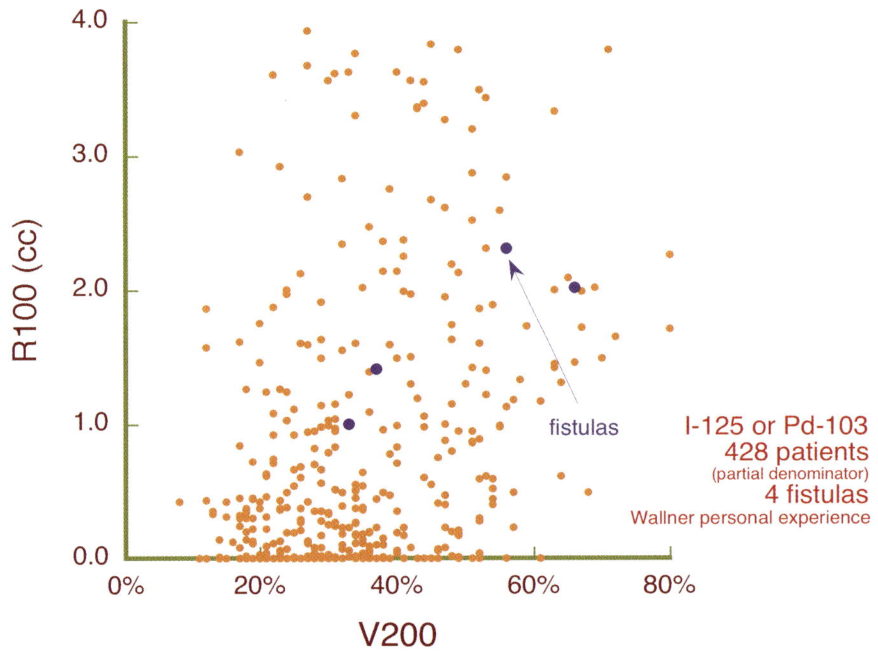

Figure 21-26. R100s vs V200s in I-125 or Pd-103 monotherapy patients implanted by KW. Four patients with rectal fistulas are denoted by blue circles.

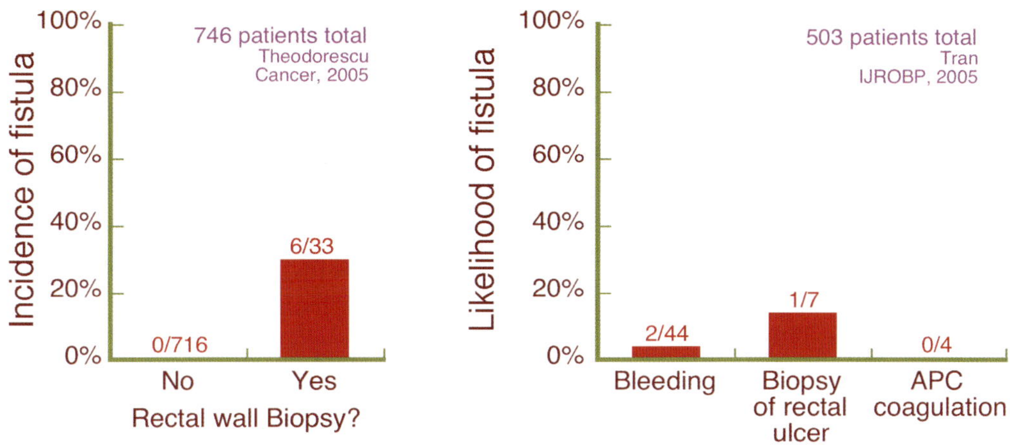

Figure 21-27. Incidence of rectal fistula formation by whether or not a post-implant rectal wall biopsy had been performed. (THEODORESCU) Likelihood of fistula formation after rectal bleeding, rectal biopsy or argon plasma laser coagulation (TRAN)

rectal bleeding, and hence the likelihood that invasive procedures will be performed."

Figures 21-20 through 21-24 illustrate four patients with fistulas, for which detailed dosimetric information is available. It is worthwhile to review their images, dosimetric details and isodose patterns. These patients' R100s were all on the high side, but not outragiously so. We believe that their cases are consistent with the conclusions that while fistulas appear in a somewhat unpredictable manner, they should be a rarity if the R100 is kept below 0.5 cc. In fairness, however, it is also important to keep in mind that even in the most experienced hands, R100s will sometimes exceed 1.0 cc due to vagaries of seed placement or tissue changes in the weeks after implantation.(TRAN) The R100s, V100s, V200s and D90s from the four patients illustrated in Figures 21-21 through 21-24 were higher than usual, but not inordinately so (**Figures 21-25 and 21-26**).

INVASIVE PROCEDURES AND RECTAL DAMAGE

One of the more controversial areas in the management of implant-related irradiated proctitis has been the inclination of gastroenterologists to biopsy the rectal wall. In a large series from the University of Virginia, patients who underwent rectal wall biopsy in the course of evaluation for implant-related proctitis were clearly at higher risk of fistula formation.(THEODORESCU) In fairness, however, it should be pointed out that the majority of patients in the Virginia series, and all three in the series by Howard and colleagues, did *not* have a biopsy prior to developing a fistula (**Figure 21-27**). Similarly, Tran and colleagues showed that only one of seven patients biopsied for proctitis went on to develop a fistula (**Figure 21-27, right**). Accordingly, it seems that while biopsy may predispose patients to further damage, most cases of fistualization are due to the implant rather than subsequent procedures.

Treatment options for rectal ulcerations are very limited. There is no clearly effective therapy. A diverting colostomy seems reasonable, but supporting data is lacking. Hyperbaric oxygen has been advocated by some, but it is expensive and of limited benefit for patients with more severe damage.(DALL'ERA, PASQUIER, JONES, GIRNIUS) The only randomized hyperbaric trials, for head and neck patients, showed minimal efficacy.(ANNANE)

Proper management of the tiny fraction of patients who progress to fistula or clinically significant blood loss is unclear. Cases of spontaneous healing after suprapubic catheterization, diverting colostomy, or both have been reported.(HOWARD, THEODORESCU) However, spontaneous healing of fistulas is unlikely. To date, there are limited data regarding the surgical repair of rectal fistulas.(JORDAN, THEODORESCU, MORIERA) Published reports have typically been authored by surgeons, who have not provided detailed surgical or dosimetric information, so that making any conclusion regarding specifically effective procedures is impossible. Colo-anal anastomosis might be an alternative to more elaborate repair procedures, but has not been described.

PROBLEM GREATLY REDUCED, BUT NOT SOLVED. REMAIN VIGILANT!

Rectal complications plagued the first 15 years of TRUS-based prostate brachytherapy. With a better appreciation of the nuances of rectal dosimetry, their occurrence has been decreased, and the risk of fistualization minimized. However, it is essential to remain vigilant. Monitor rectal doses as part of your implant program quality assurance policies.

REFERENCES

1. Annane D, Depondt J, Aubert P, et al. Hyperbaric oxygen therapy for radionecrosis of the jaw: A randomized, placebo-controlled, double-blind trial from the ORN96 Study Group. J Clin Oncol 2004; 22:4893-4900.
2. Babb RR. Radiation proctitis: A review. American Journal of gastroenterology 2000; 91:1309-1311.
3. Biswal BM, Lal P, Rath GK, Shukla NK, Mohanti BK, Deo S. Intrarectal formalin application, an effective treatment for grade III haemorrhagic radiation proctitis. Radiother Oncol 1995; 35:212-215.
4. Crook J, Esche B, Futter N. Effect of pelvic radiotherapy for prostate cancer on bowel, bladder, and sexual function: The patient's perspective. Urology 1996; 47:387-394.
5. Dall'Era M, Hampson N, Hsi R, Madsen B, Corman J. Hyperbaric oxygen therapy for radiation induced proctopathy in men treated for prostate cancer. J Urol 2006; 176:87-90.
6. Gelblum DY, Potters L. Rectal complications associated with transperineal interstitial brachytherapy for prostate cancer. Int J Rad Oncol Biol Phys 2000; 48:119-124.
7. Girnius S, Cersonsky N, Gesell L, Cico S, Barrett W. Treatment of refractory radiation-induced hemorrhagic proctitis with hyperbaric oxygen therapy. Am J Clin Onc 2006; 29:588-592.
8. Han B, Wallner K. Dosimetric and radiographic correlates to prostate brachytherapy-related rectal complications. International Journal of Cancer 2002; 96:372-378.
9. Howard A, Wallner K, Han B, Schneider B, al e. Clinical course and dosimetry of rectal fistulas after prostate brachytherapy. JBI 2001; 17:37-42.
10. Hu K, Wallner K. Clinical course of rectal complications following I-125 prostate brachytherapy. Int J Rad Oncol Biol Phys 1998; 41:263-265.
11. Iversen P, Nielsen L, Bak M, et al. Ultrasonically guided 125Iodine seed implantation with external radiation in management of localized prostatic carcinoma. Urol 1989; 34:181-186.
12. Jones K, Evans A, Bristow R, Levin W. Treatment of radiation proctitis with hyperbaric oxygen. Radiother and Oncol 2006; 78:91-94.
13. Jordan GH, Lynch DF, Warden SS, McGraw JD, Hoffman GC, Schellhammer PF. Major pelvic complications following interstitial implantation of Iodine-125 for carcinoma of the prostate. J Urol 1985; 134:1212-1214.

14. Kaassis M, Oberti F, Burtin P, Boyer J. Argon plasma coagulation for the treatment of hemorrhagic radiation proctitis. Endoscopy1 2000; 32:673-676.

15. Kaye KW, Olson DJ, Payne JT. Detailed preliminary analysis of 125 iodine implantation for localized prostate cancer using percutaneous approach. J Urol 1995; 153:1020-1025.

16. Kochbar R, Patel F, Dhar A, et al. Radiation-induced proctosigmoiditis: Prospective, randomized, double-blind controlled trial of oral sulfasalazine plus rectal steroids versus rectal sucralfate. Digestive diseases and sciences 2000; 36:103-107.

17. Lu-Yao GL, Albertsen P, Warren J, Yao S-L. Effect of age and surgical approach on complications and short-term mortality after radical prostatectomy*A population-based study. Urol 1999; 54:301-307.

18. Merrick GS, Butler WM, Dorsey AT, Galbreath RW, Blatt H, Lief JH. Rectal function following prostate brachytherapy. Int J Rad Oncol Biol Phys 2000; 48:667-674.

19. Merrick GS, Butler WM, Dorsey AT, Lief JH, Walbert HL, Blatt HJ. Rectal dosimetric analysis following prostate brachytherapy. Int J Rad Oncol Biol Phys 1999; 43:1021-1027.

20. Merrick GS, Butler WM, Wallner K, Hines AL, Allen Z. Late rectal function after prostate brachytherapy. Int J Rad Oncol Biol Phys 2003; 57:42-48.

21. Moreira S, Seigne J, Ordorica R, Marceet J, Pow-sang J, Lockhart J. Devastating complications after brachytherapy in the treatment of prostate adenocarcinoma. Br J Urol 2004; 93:31-35.

22. Mueller A, Wallner K, Merrick G, Cavanagh W, Butler W. Peri-rectal seeds as a risk factor for prostate brachytherapy-related rectal bleeding. Int J Rad Oncol Biol Phys 2004; 59:1047-1052.

23. Pasquier D, Hoelscher T, Schmutz J, et al. Hyperbaric oxygen therapy in the treatment of radio-induced lesions in normal tissues: A literature review. Radiother and Oncol 2004; 72:1-13.

24. Patel J, Worthen R, Abadir R, Weaver DJ, Weinstein S, Ross G. Late results of combined Iodine-125 and external beam radiotherapy in carcinoma of prostate. Urol 1990; 36:27-30.

25. Roche B, Chautems R, Marti MC. Application of formaldehyde for treatment of hemorrhagic radiation-induced proctitits. World J Surg 1996; 20:1092-1095.

26. Shipley WU, Zietman AL, Hanks GE, et al. Treatment related sequelae following external beam radiation for prostate cancer: A review with an update in patients with Stages T1 and T2 tumor. J Urol 1994; 152:1799-1805.

27. Smith S, Wallner K, Han B, et al. Argon plasma coagulation for rectal bleeding following prostate brachytherapy Int J Rad Oncol Biol Phys 2001; 51:636-642.

28. Snyder KM, Stock RG, Hong SM, Lo YC, Stone NN. Defining the risk of developing grade 2 proctitis following 125-I prostate brachytherapy using a rectal dose-volume histogram analysis. Int J Rad Oncol Biol Phys 2001; 50:335-341.

29. Teshima T, Hanks GE, Hanlon AL, Peter RS, Schultheiss TE. Rectal bleeding after conformal 3D treatment of prostate cancer: Time to occurrence, response to treatment and duration of morbidity. Int J Radiat Oncol Biol Phys 1997; 39:77-83.

30. Theodorescu D, Gillenwater JY, Koutrouvelis PG. Prostatourethral-rectal fistula after prostate brachytherapy: Incidence and risk factors. Cancer 2000; 89:2085-2091.

31. Tran A, Wallner K, Merrick G, Seeberger J, Armstrong J, Mueller A. Rectal fistulas following prostate brachytherapy. Int J Rad Oncol Biol Phys 2005; 63:150-154.

32. Viggiano TR, Zighelboim J, Ahlquist DA, Gostout CJ, Wang KK, Larson MV. Endoscopic Nd:YAG laser coagulation of bleeding from radiation proctopathy. Gastrointestinal endoscopy 2000; 39:513-517.

33. Waterman FM, Dicker AP. Probability of late rectal morbidity in I-125 prostate brachytherapy. Int J Rad Oncol Biol Phys 2003; 55:342-353.

34. Zeitlin SI, Sherman J, Raboy A, Lederman G, Albert P. High dose combination radiotherapy for the treatment of localized prostate cancer. J Urol 1998; 160:91-96.

22

Sexual (dys)function

Potency loss is the most common permanent sequela of treatment for early-stage prostate cancer. Brachytherapy is generally believed to offer some advantage over surgery or external radiation in regards to potency preservation, but the true magnitude of its advantage is less than previously believed.

DEFINITION

Quantification of treatment effects requires a working definition of sexual potency. The one used typically in mainstream surgical literature is *the ability to maintain an erection sufficient for intercourse*. The most widely quoted potency figures, by the most widely known surgeons, are based on this simple, practical definition.(CATALONA, QUINLAN) Unfortunately, this definition leaves considerable room for interpretation on the part of the patient and the investigator. An NIH consensus definition of erectile dysfunction is "the inability to attain and/or maintain penile erection sufficient for satisfactory sexual performance," another simple and practical definition.(NIH)

Critics of simple definitions called for more detailed criteria.(ZINREICH, BANKER) Quality-of-life experts have introduced increasingly sophisticated measures of sexual function—quantifiers such as "sexual bother" or "SFIQ scores" are commonplace.(KRUPSKI, BRANDEIS) The problem with these more sophisticated but more nebulous measures is that they make it difficult for physicians and patients to relate to the findings.

Probably the most widely used sexual potency assessment tool is the IEFF—International Index of Erectile Function. It is a 15-item validated questionnaire. A score of ≥26 is generally considered as "no ED." Various abridged versions have been used. The score cut-off for considering patients potent also varies between series, making comparisons difficult.(MERRICK 03)

SPONTANEOUS POTENCY LOSS

Analysis of the effect of treatment on potency is clouded by the fact that prostate cancer occurs in an age group for which there is a substantial incidence of impotence prior to treatment. As many as 50% of men are already impotent by the time they are diagnosed with prostatic carcinoma.(ZINREICH) The Massachusetts Male Aging Study summarized the incidence of impotence versus age in normal men.(FELDMAN) Based on personal interviews, men between the ages of 40 and 80 spontaneously lose potency at a rate of approximately 1.5% per year (**Figure 22-1**). In the short term, gradual, "natural" potency loss should not substantially affect treatment-related potency changes. However, with increasing follow-up time, age-related potency changes should be taken into consideration.

COLLECTING POTENCY INFORMATION

Collecting potency data is frequently an exercise in frustration. Patients sometimes are surprisingly inconsistent in their responses, for a variety of reasons. Many are simply not sexually active at this time of their life and others are reluctant to admit potency loss. Most vexing are substantial fluctuations in sexual function in the first few years after brachytherapy,

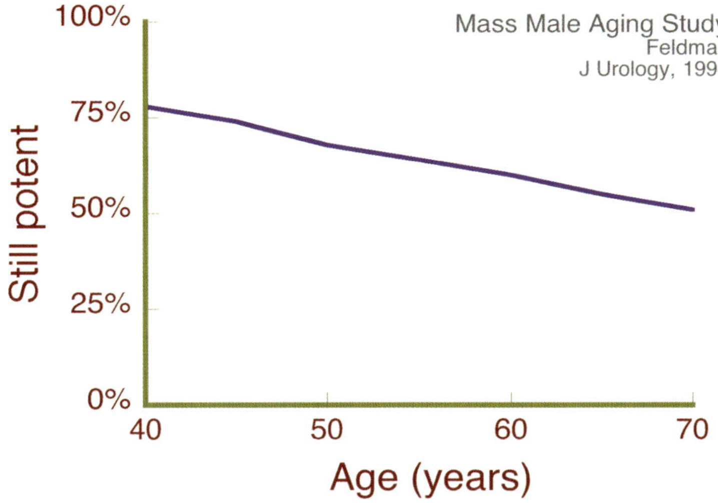

Figure 22-1. Sexual potency versus age in the general population. Data are based on personal interviews.(FELDMAN)

probably related to development and resolution of radiation-related inflammation.

Another common assumption regarding analysis of potency status is that spouses should be interviewed separately, because patients may not be realistic or honest in reporting their erectile capacity. On the contrary, patients and spouses generally report similar function.(ZINREICH, CHINN) Another commonly raised concern has been that potency data should be verified with physiologic testing, in order to be more objective. But considering that patients and spouses are generally consistent in their answers when interviewed separately, physiologic testing may not shed much additional light.

It has also become important that reports of potency preservation specify whether or not patients are reliant on pharmacologic support. While phospodesterase inhibitors (PDEIs) are almost standard issue, their use needs to be taken into account when comparing potency preservation between modalities.

ACUTE SEXUAL SEQUELAE

Most reports of treatment-related dysfunction have focused exclusively on erectile function. However, it is important to realize that impotence is only

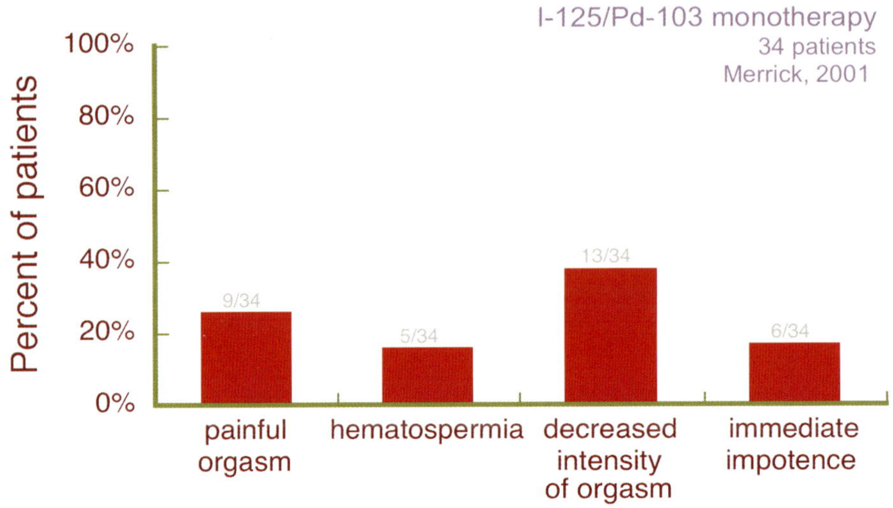

Figure 22-2. Sexual symptomatology among patients randomized to I-125 or Pd-103.(MERRICK 02)

the most outward change. There are a variety of subtle and not-so-subtle changes in sexual function following prostate cancer treatment, most of which have only recently been described.(MERRICK 02)

Patients commonly experience burning with orgasm (orgalmasia) in their first six to twelve post-implant months, probably related to inflammation of the terminal portion of the ejaculatory ducts and the urethra. In retrospective surveys, approximately one-third to one-half of patients report painful ejaculation for several months or longer, necessitating temporary abstinence (**Figure 22-2 & 22-3**).(MERRICK 02) Bloody ejaculate is very common in the first several weeks after implantation, without apparent significance. Patients commonly report a diminished volume of ejaculate and a change in its consistency in the first few years following brachytherapy. Dry ejaculate occurs in approximately one-fourth of patients. Intermittent bloody semen (hematospermia) occurs commonly, as both an early and late phenomenon, probably due to radiation-induced capillary fragility and seems to be of no clinical significance. Patients likely are sterile sooner or later, but post-implant impregnation has been reported.(MYDLO, GROCELA)

These various sexual dysfunctions, apart from impotence, are not unique to brachytherapy, but also occurs commonly after beam radiation. Similar

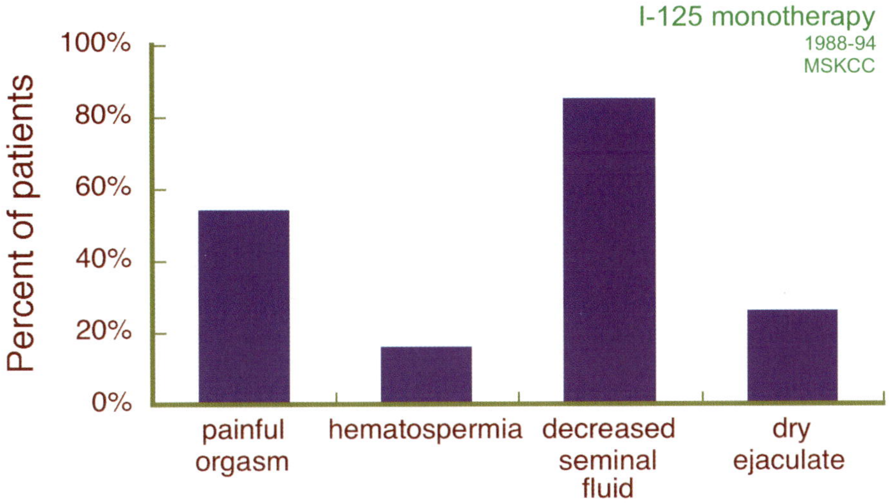

Figure 22-3. Incidence of painful ejaculation, bloody seminal fluid, or dry ejaculate in patients treated with I-125 implant at MSKCC.

dysfunctions are also known to occur after prostatectomy, but have received scant attention from investigators.(LEE, MATTHEWS) Apart from Merrick and colleagues, the myriad dysfunction have been virtually ignored by clinical investigators. None of the quasi-scientific, commonly used quality of life scales adequately address surgery-related or radiation-related ejaculatory symptoms.

ERECTILE DYSFUNCTION

About 15% of patients develop impotence immediately after their implant procedure, presumably due to needle trauma to the neurovascular bundles or venous bodies (**Figure 22-2**).(MERRICK) Patients with acute post-implant impotence often spontaneously improve over time, but the likelihood of recovery has not yet been well documented.

There has been wide discrepancy among investigators regarding the likelihood of potency preservation after brachytherapy, for several reasons. First, it has become apparent that potency rates are highly dependent on

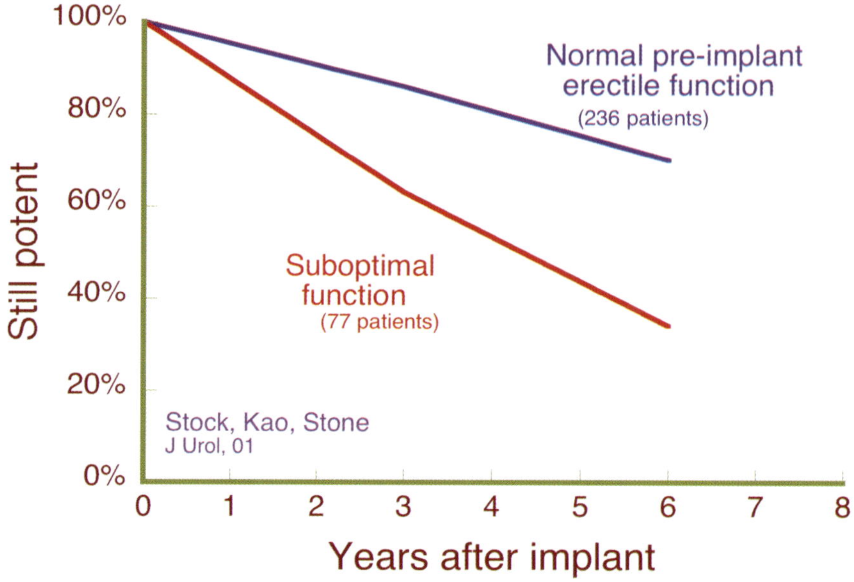

Figure 22-4. Increased potency loss in patients with diminished pre-implant function.(STOCK 01)

follow-up times. Favorable reports of high potency rates after brachytherapy were almost uniformly based on short-term follow-up of a couple of years. Unfortunately, the likelihood of impotence increases in the years after radiation, a phenomenon first described by Bagshaw and colleagues in the 1980s.(BAGSHAW)

A second reason for the discrepancy regarding post-implant potency preservation is that rates vary depending on the degree of compromise prior to therapy. Stock and colleagues have shown that patients with compromised pre-implant erectile function are at higher risk of complete impotence than are patients with full potency (**Figure 22-4**). More recently, Merrick and colleagues showed a clear separation in the likelihood of potency preservation based on pre-implant IIEF score (**Figure 22-5**). This variability in potency with the level of pre-therapy functioning is exacerbated by potency fluctuation in the post-implant period, a phenomenon that hasn't been adequately addressed to date.

A third reason for discrepancies in post-implant potency rates has been the (mis)use of statistical methods—the use of crude percentages can grossly

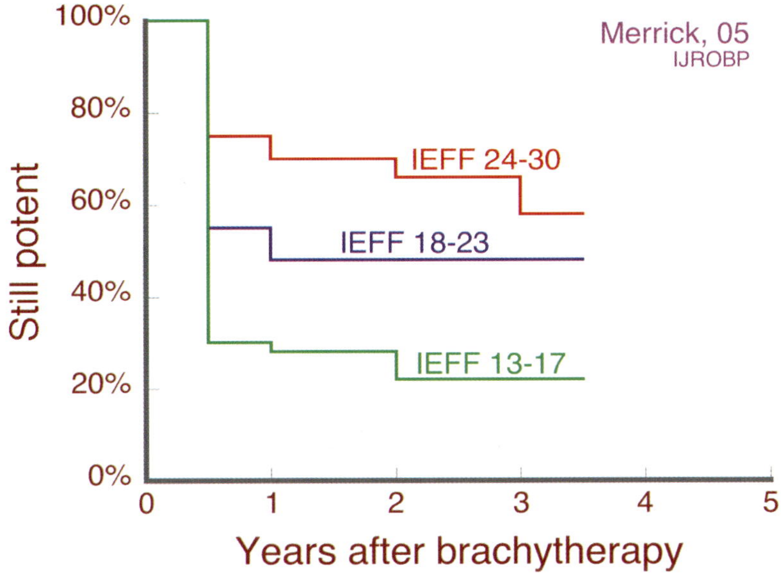

Figure 22-5. Potency preservation based on pre-implant IEFF score.(MERRRICK 05)

inflate the potency preservation rates. Because potency rates decline over time, actuarial statistics, which account for length of time patients have been followed since treatment, give a much more realistic potency rate calculation (**Figure 22-6**). Surprisingly, most published series from mainstream academicians have used crude rates and short follow-up times.

The effect of pre-treatment patient characteristics on potency loss has varied somewhat from one series to another.(STOCK, POTTERS, MERRICK) In some series, younger patients do better (**Figure 22-7**). Merrick and colleagues have shown greater potency loss in patients who receive supplemental external beam radiation (**Figure 22-8**). Diabetes likely exacerbates brachytherapy-related impotence.(MERRICK) In contrast, in multivariate analysis of patients treated to 70–80 Gy with conformal external beam radiation or brachytherapy at MSKCC, anti-androgen use and patient age were not associated with diminished potency preservation. (ZELEFSKY 99) Differences from one series to the next in regards to exacerbating factors likely results from subtle variance in patient characteristics, and possibly variable technical factors (see below).

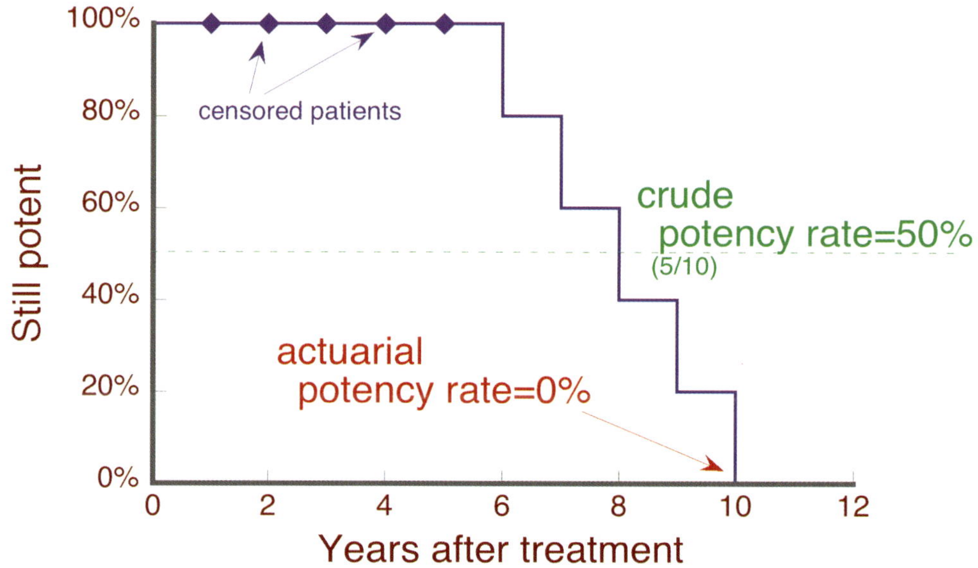

Figure 22-6. Example of crude versus actuarial potency rates. Assume that one patient is treated per year from 1985 through 1995 and that the first five patients become impotent in 1995, the year that the potency rate is calculated. Actuarial calculation gives a potency rate of 0% at 10 years, while the crude rate is 5 of 10, or 50%!

Very important point

The use of crude versus actuarial calculations can lead to very, very different statistical conclusions. Make sure that you understand how misleading the use of raw percentages can be

MECHANISM OF IMPOTENCE

The mechanism of radiation-related impotence is probably multi-factorial, with radiation damage to the neurovascular bundles and to the penile venous system being the most obvious candidates for the blame.(ZELEFSKY 98).

An early report of radiation-induced arterial occlusion of the internal iliac, internal pudendal, and penile arteries, based on only two patients, has never been confirmed.(GOLDSTEIN) Pelvic neural testing after external beam radiation has been unremarkable—not surprising considering that peripheral nerves

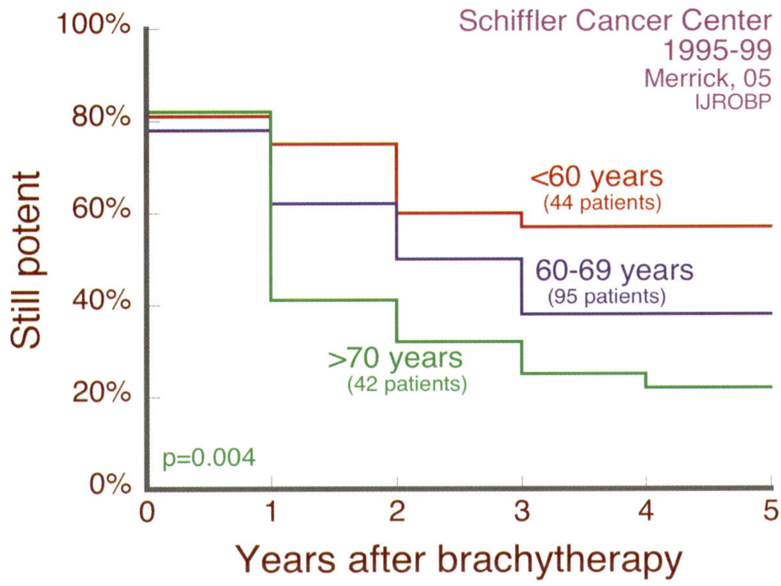

22-7. Potency preservation by age group (MERRICK).

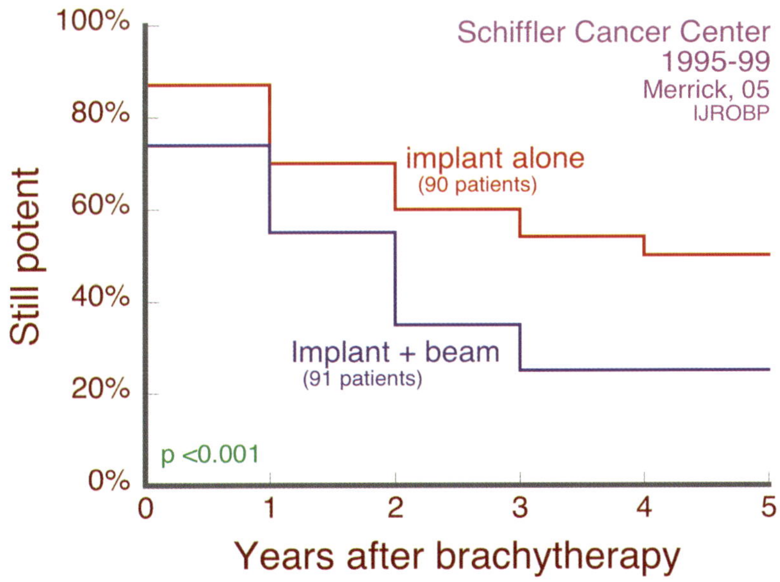

Figure 22-8. Potency preservation following implantation with or without supplemental beam radiation (MERRICK).

readily tolerate high doses in the course of radiation for extremity sarcomas and other pelvic tumors.(GOLDSTEIN) Radiation-induced impotence generally responds to intracavernosal papaverine or PGE1 injection or to sildenafil (Viagra™).(PIERCE, MERRICK 99, ZELEFSKY 99) The relationship between a response to pharmacologic agents and the mechanism(s) of impotence is unclear. Whether impotence is due to arterial, venous, neural, or some other type of damage, pharmacologic agents may work simply by virtue of bolstering one among several compromised components of a complex system.

Neurovascular bundles

Walsh and colleagues have attributed post-prostatectomy impotence to neurovascular bundle (NVB) trauma.(LEPOR, WALSH) Similarly, excessive radiation doses to vascular or neural components of the NVBs might account for brachytherapy-related impotence. The typical onset of radiation-related impotence, months or years after treatment, is more consistent with delayed radiation damage as the cause of impotence, rather than to needle trauma.

DiBiase and colleagues first investigated the role of NVB radiation doses in brachytherapy-related impotence. They estimated the doses in brachytherapy because the NVBs cannot be visualized consistently on CT, TRUS or MR (**Figure 22-9**), Calculation points were taken posterior-laterally, 2.0 mm from the prostatic capsule, according to the anatomic description of Lepor and colleagues (**Figure 22-10 & 22-11**).(LEPOR)

In contrast to popular perception, NVB doses were usually far higher than the prescription dose, because of the 3–6 mm treatment margins that typically lie beyond the NVBs (see chapter 6). Doses varied widely between the right and left side of the same patient and among patients (**Figures 22-12 and 22-13**). Average NVB doses along the course of the NVB ranged from 150% to 200% of the prescription dose and were similar for Pd-103 and I-125 (**Figure 22-14**).

Merrick and colleagues did not find a relationship between NVB doses and impotence among patients followed up to four years post-implantation (**Figure 22-15**).(MERRICK 00) But this is not the final word on NVB dosimetry! Because the onset of impotence is often delayed by several years, longer follow-up might show some relationship between dose and treat-

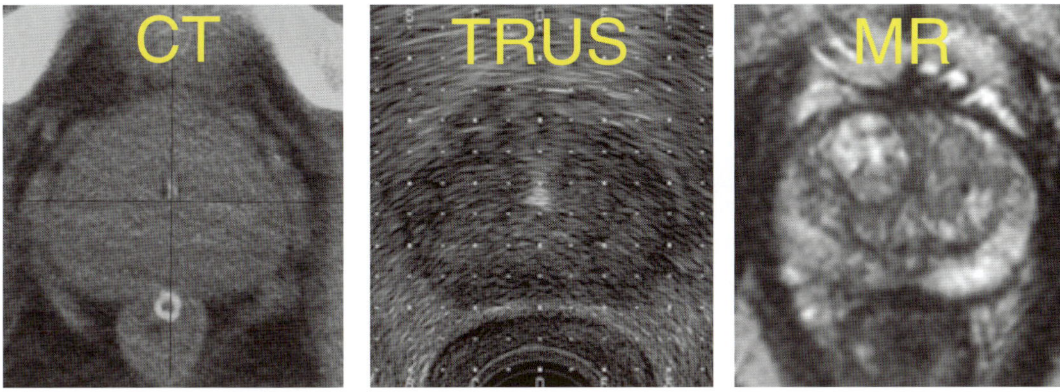

Figure 22-9. Transverse mid-prostate on CT, TRUS, and MR. Contrary to some claims in the literature, the NVBs are not typically well visualized with any modality. Published studies of NVB doses have instead relied on arbitrary NVB location estimates.(DIBIASE, MERRICK 01)

ment-related sexual dysfunction. And dosimetric computations may need to be more complex, because the NVB is really a neurovascular *plexus*, for which point calculations may be too simplistic.

The lack of an effect of NVB radiation doses is consistent with growing evidence that NVBs are not as crucial to potency as alleged by investigators at Johns Hopkins University Hospitals.(KIM) Also keep in mind that the two classic reports regarding NVB location were each based on a single autopsy study, and that more sophisticated intra-operative investigations are raising considerable doubt about their location and function.(WALSH, LEPOR, MICHL) In the next few years, the role that NVB doses have on potency impairment should be clarified, by correlating more sophisticated NVB dose calculations with larger numbers of patients with longer follow-up.

PENILE BULB

A second possible mechanism of radiation-induced impotence is venous insufficiency from damage to the proximal corpus spongiosum (*bulb)* or proximal corpus cavernosum of the penis (**Figure 22-16**). Separated from the prostate by the striated urethral sphincter, the bulb typically lies 0.5–1.0 cm below the prostatic apex and is fairly well visualized on CT, TRUS, or MR (**Figures 22-17 & 16-18**). It typically has a volume of 5–7 cc and usually receives a maximal radiation dose of about 50% of the brachytherapy

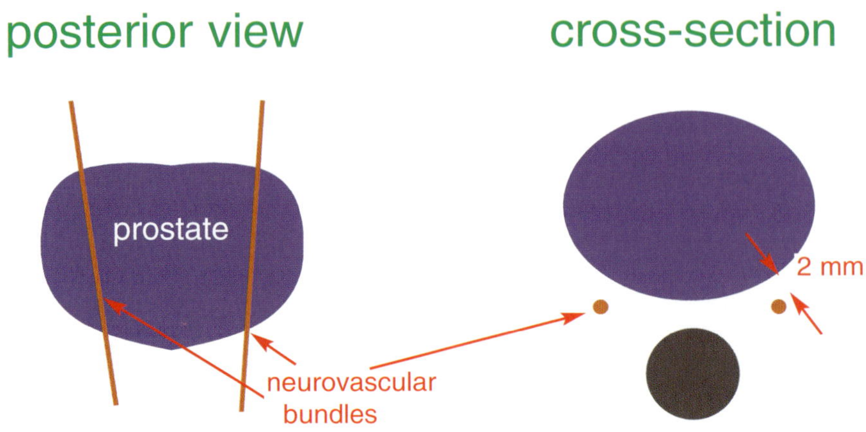

Figure 22-10. The neurovascular bundles are allegedly located approximately 2 millimeters from the posterior prostatic capsule.(LEPOR) The problem with using this description is that it is based on only two cases.(WALSH, LEPOR) There is remarkably little other published information regarding the actual location of the NVBs.(SOKOLOFF)

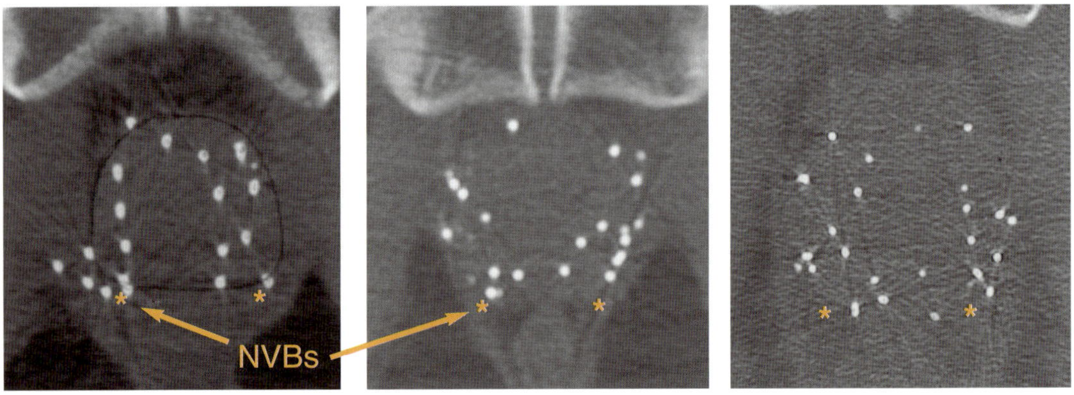

Figure 22-11. Typical post-implant CT images showing seeds near or even behind the neurovascular bundles. Contrary to some claims, brachytherapy is not *a NVB-sparing therapy. (STOCK 96)*

NVB dose (Gray)

NVB dose as percentage of prescription dose

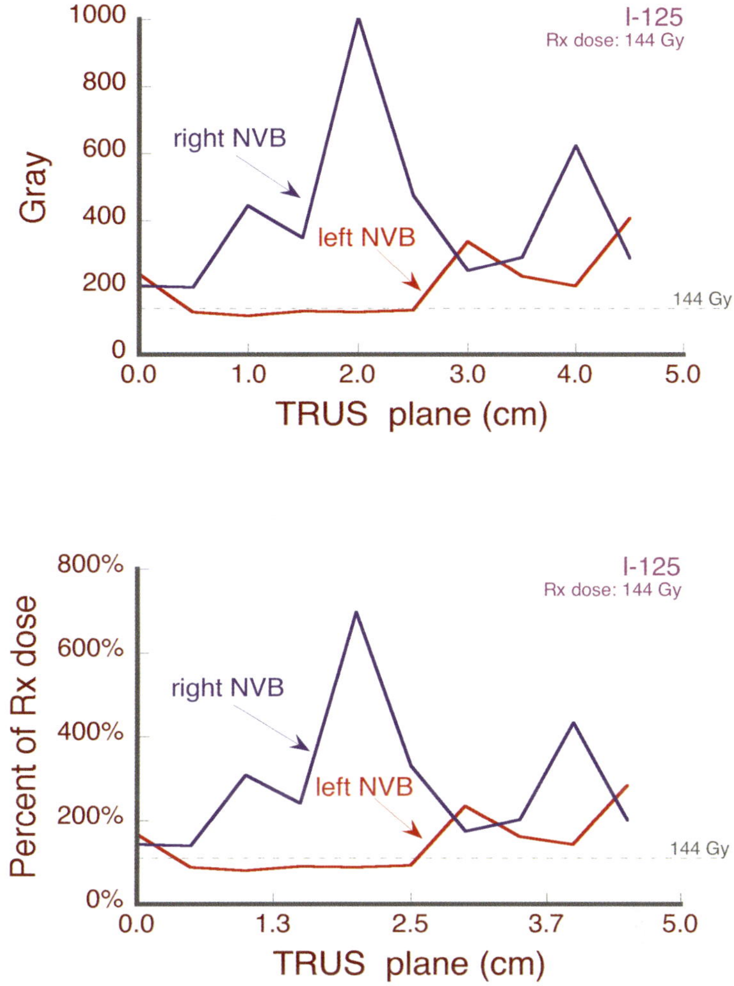

Figure 22-12. NVB doses from base to apex of the prostate expressed in Gy (top panel) or as the percentage of the prescription dose (lower panel). Note the substantial difference from one side to the next, a typical finding among patients.

I-125

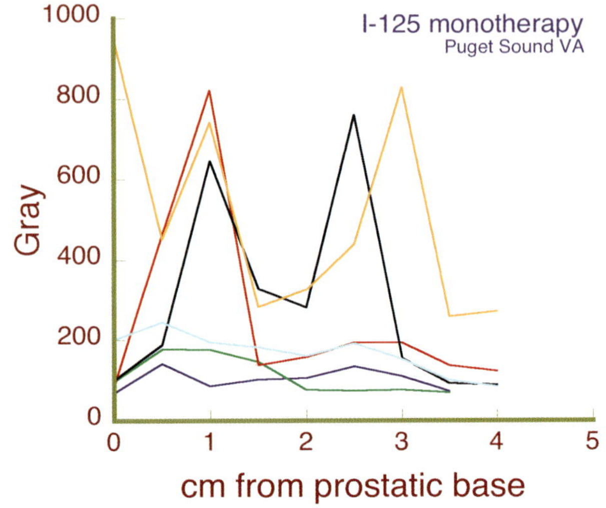

Pd-103

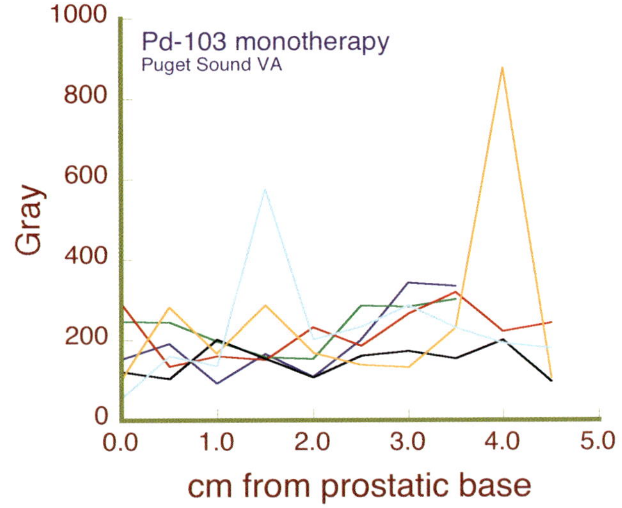

Figure 22-13. Composite NVB doses from three unselected I-125 (top) and Pd-103 (lower panel) patients. Note the remarkable variability among patients, due to very rapid dose fall-off in the region of the NVBs.

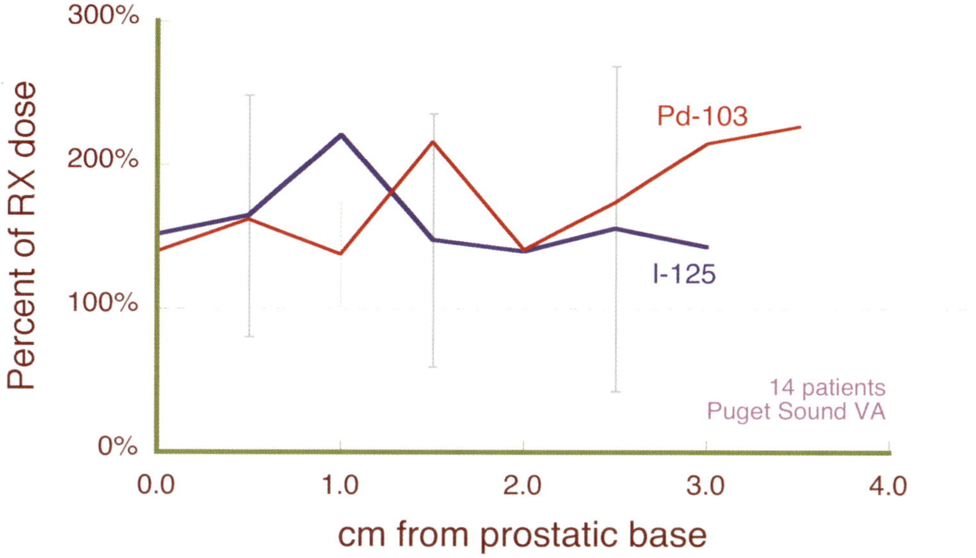

Figure 22-14. Average NVB doses expressed as the percentage of the prescription dose from base to apex of the prostate for full dose I-125 or Pd-103 implants. Note the similarities in the averages between the two isotopes.(DIBIASE)

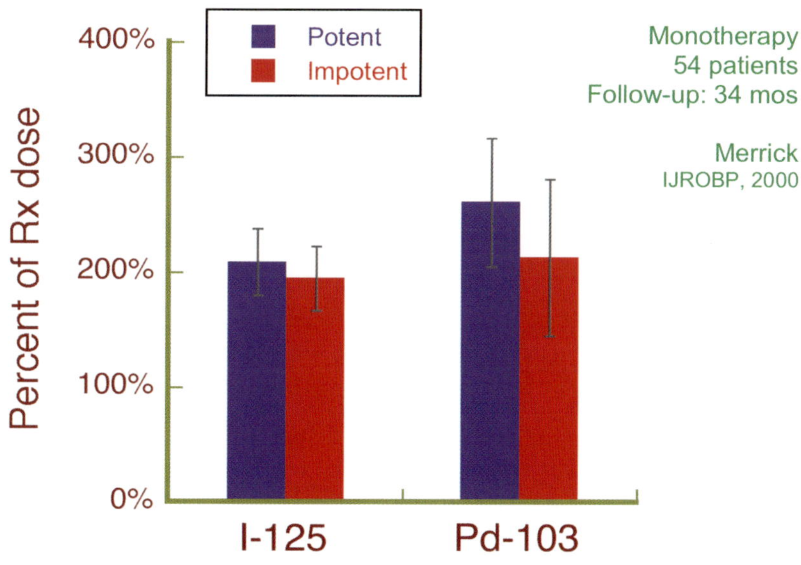

Figure 22-15. NVB doses among patients with or without post-implant impotence.(MERRICK 00)

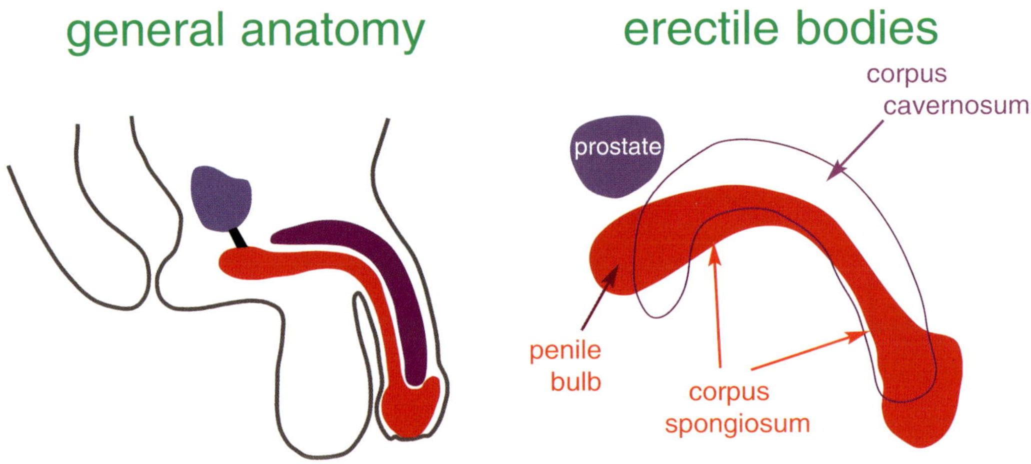

Figure 22-16. General anatomy and erectile bodies of the penis.

prescription dose (**Figure 22-19 & 22-20**). Pickett, Roach, and colleagues showed that bulb doses from external beam radiation correlate well with post-therapy impotence (**Figure 22-21**).(PICKETT, ROACH)

Brachytherapy doses to the penile bulb depend on the distance between the prostatic apex and bulb, as well as the magnitude of the planning treatment margins. Because of the proximity of the bulb to the prostatic apex and the tendency to use generous treatment margins at the the apex, it was fairly common that seeds were adjacent to or even inside the bulb (**Figures 22-22 & 22-23**). Cases of excessive peri-bulbar seeds are not difficult to find in the authors' early experience (**Figures 22-24 & 22-25**).

Using post-implant CT to identify the bulb, Merrick and colleagues showed a strong correlation between proximal crura and penile bulb doses and post-implant impotence (**Figure 20-26**).(MERRICK 05) Doses to both the proximal crura and the penile bulb may be important. These doses should be taken into consideration in order to maximize tumor control while minimizing treatment-related morbidity. Better appreciation of penile bulb and corpus spongiosum doses may lead to less impotence after brachytherapy (**Figure 22-27**).(MERRICK 05)

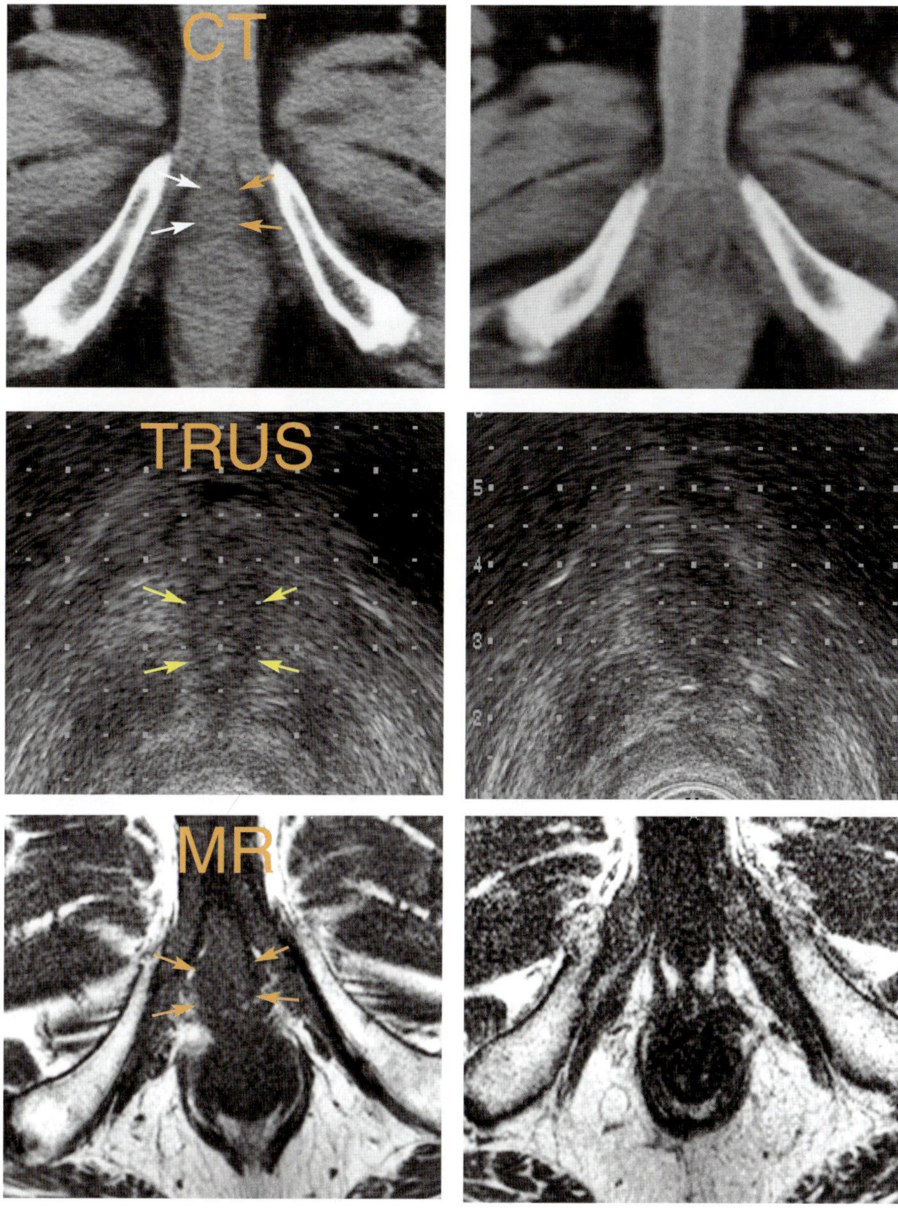

Figure 22-17. Typical CT, TRUS, or MR images through the midbulb (arrows). The bulb shows up surprisingly well on preimplant scans, but not as clearly in the post-implant setting (see Figures 16-12 and 16-13).

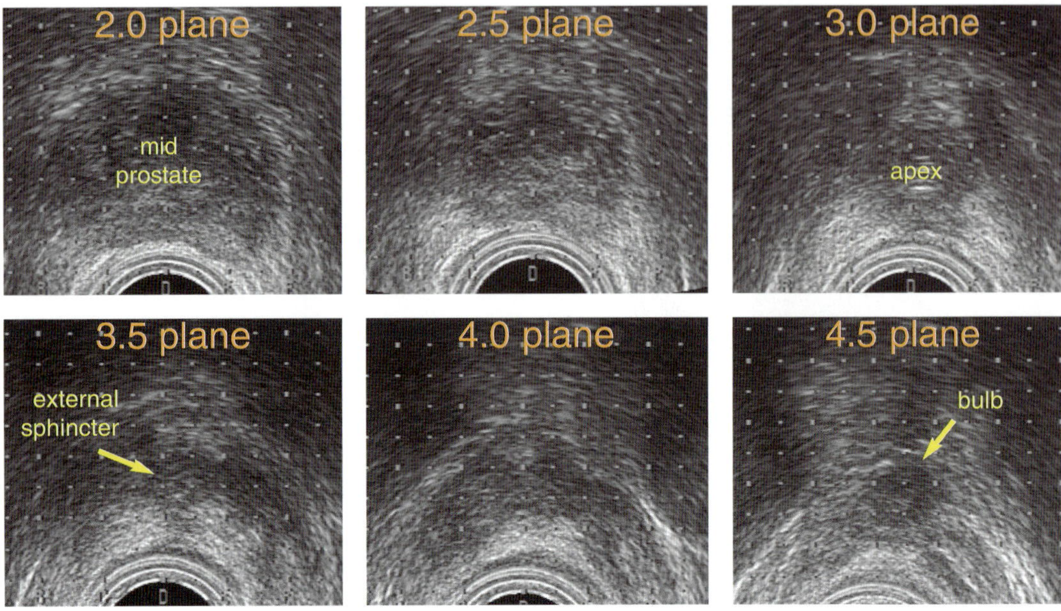

Figure 22-18. The bulbous spongiosum is typically separated from the prostatic apex by 5–10 mm of the striated external sphincter/pelvic floor. In this series of TRUS images, the prostatic apex ends at the 3.0 plane, and the top of the bulb is seen at the 4.5 plane.

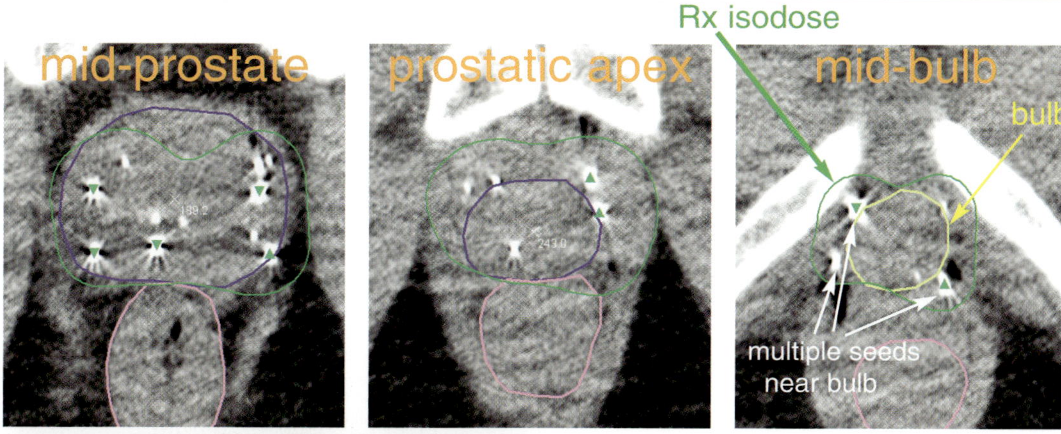

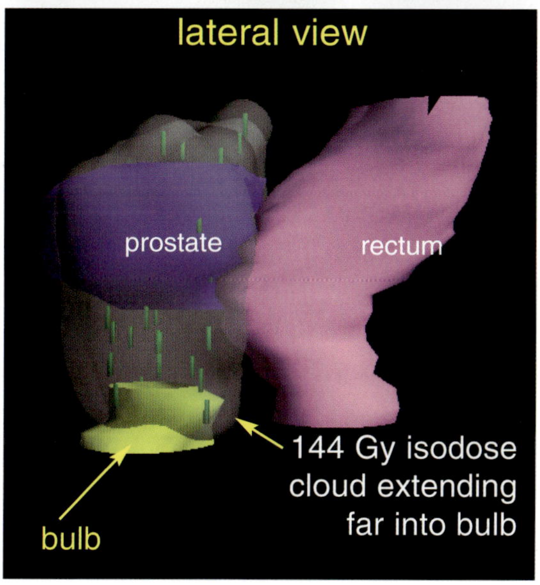

Figure 22-19. Example of CT scans, lateral view, and dose volume histogram of prostate and penile bulb doses from a 144 Gy I-125 implant. Note that in this patient, several sources were placed distal to the prostatic apex, resulting in excessive bulb doses. 51% of the 6 cc bulb received a dose in excess of the prescription, which is high even by external beam radiation standards (see DVH below).

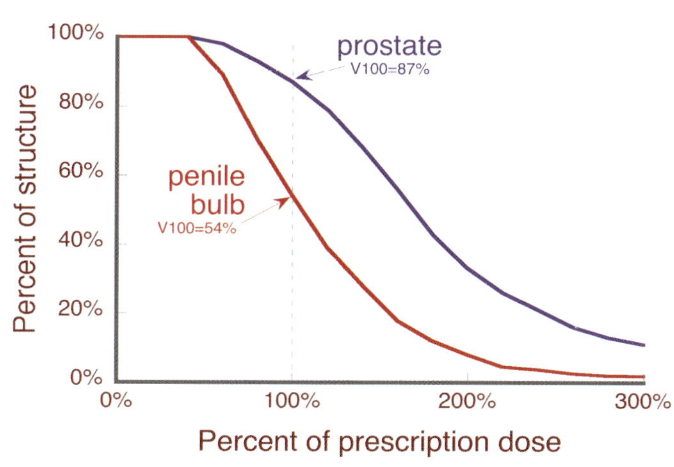

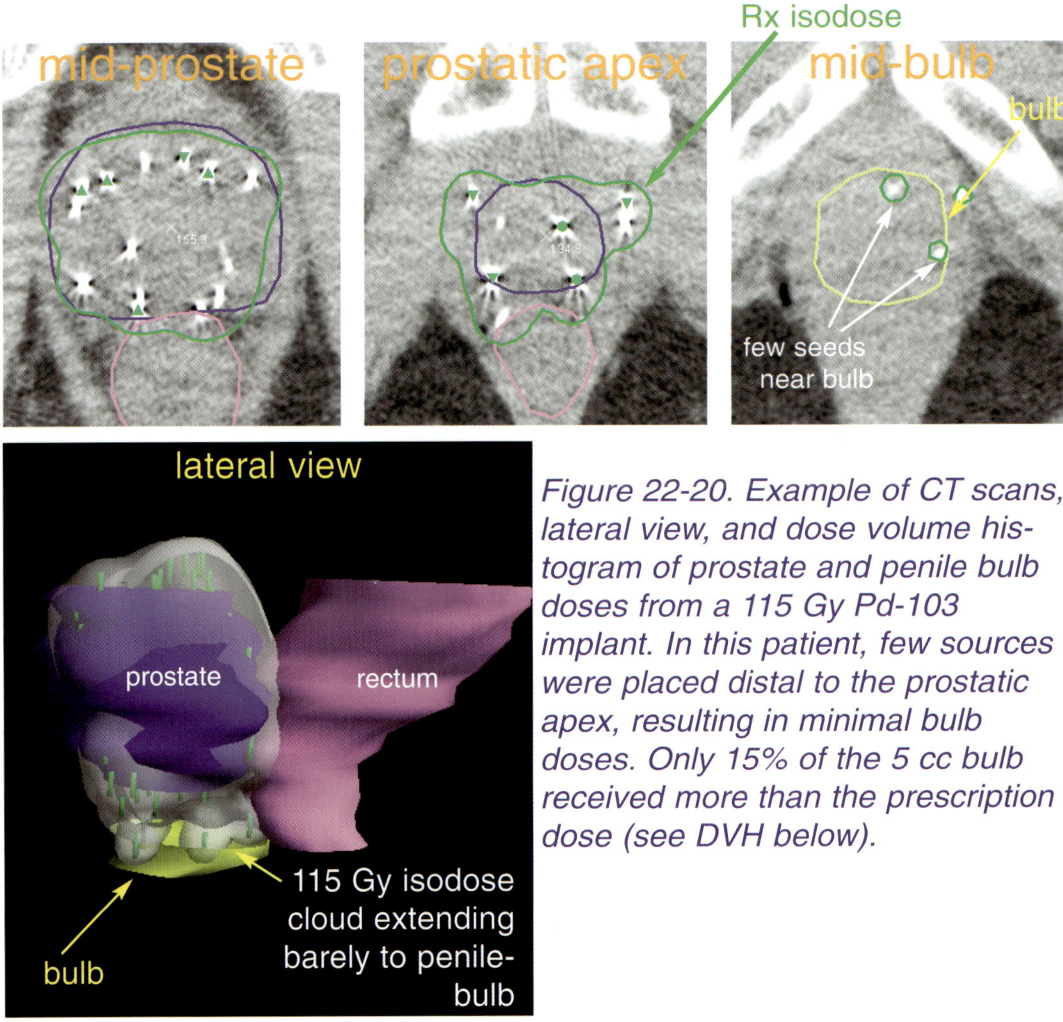

Figure 22-20. Example of CT scans, lateral view, and dose volume histogram of prostate and penile bulb doses from a 115 Gy Pd-103 implant. In this patient, few sources were placed distal to the prostatic apex, resulting in minimal bulb doses. Only 15% of the 5 cc bulb received more than the prescription dose (see DVH below).

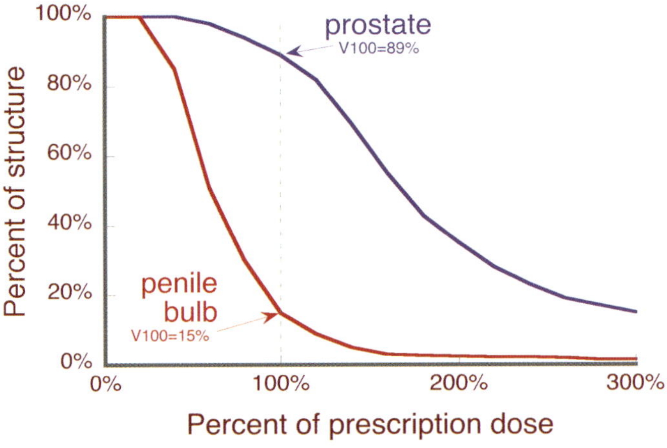

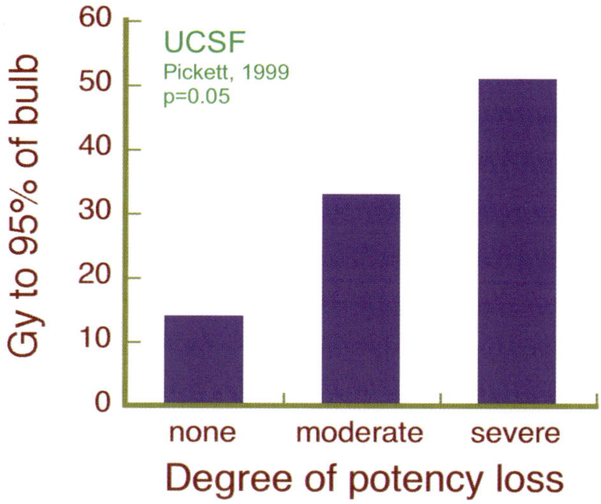

Figure 22-21. Bulb doses from external beam radiation correlate with post-treatment impotence.(PICKETT)

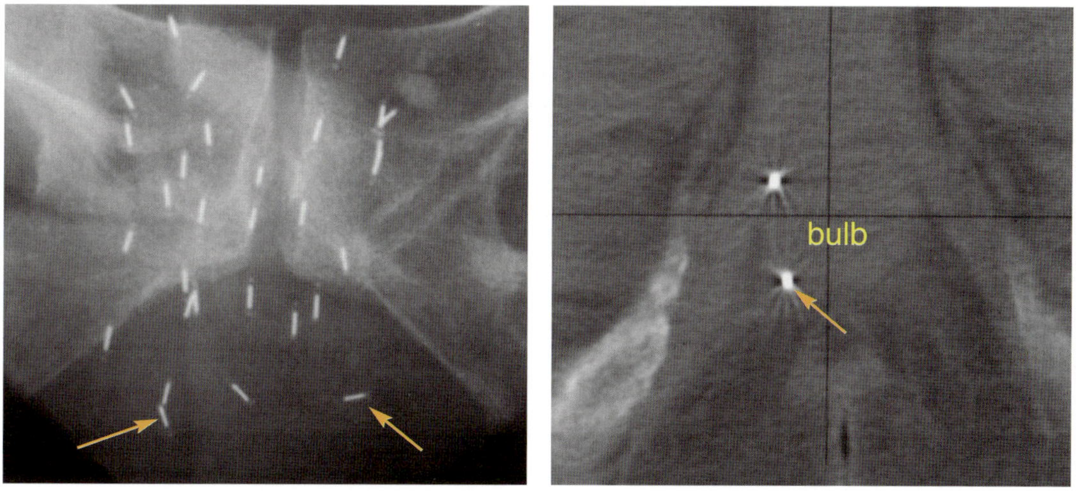

Figure 22-22. One cause of excessive penile bulb brachytherapy doses is that four seeds are pulled too far inferiorly (orange arrows). In this example, several seeds were deposited too distal. Stray seeds may contribute to brachytherapy-related impotence. As we learn more about where not to place sources, it should be possible to decrease the adverse potency effects of brachytherapy.

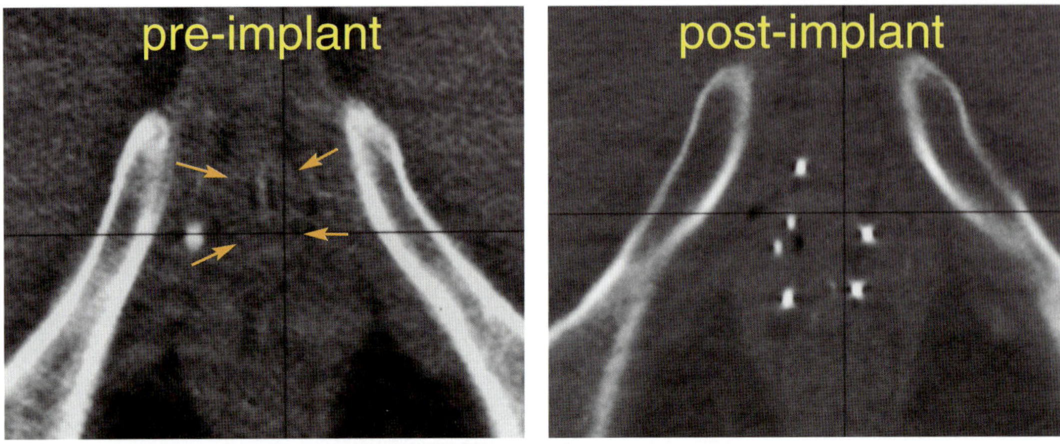

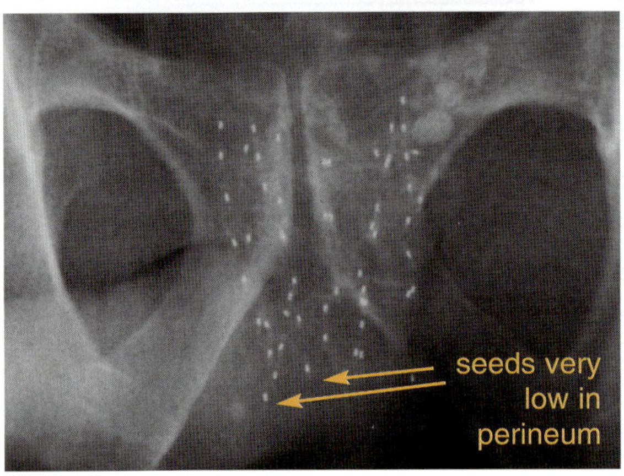

Figure 22-23. Another example of excessive sources around the penile bulb (arrows), a result of overly generous treatment planning margins at the prostatic apex. Notice how low the implant extends on the anterior view (left).

COMPARING MODALITIES

Despite the huge number of patients treated for early stage prostate cancer every year, long-term reports regarding potency preservation are amazingly few, a red flag suggesting that outcomes are much worse than commonly acknowledged. The largest series regarding the effect of external beam radiation on potency is from Stanford, based on a simple mailed questionnaire.(BAGSHAW) Potency was preserved in 86% of patients at fifteen months after treatment, but only in 50% at 5 years (**Figure 22-28**). The loss of potency decelerated at 30% at approximately ten years after treatment. Drs. Bagshaw, Cox and Ray should be congratulated on their early interest and statistical prowess but their results should be interpreted cautiously, because they are based on an anonymous survey of a small proportion of patients treated, with no mention of how potency was defined. More recently, Zelefsky and colleagues reported longer-term actuarial potency preservation rates following 3D conformal external beam radiation, and their rates are similar to those reported by Bagshaw (**Figure 22-**

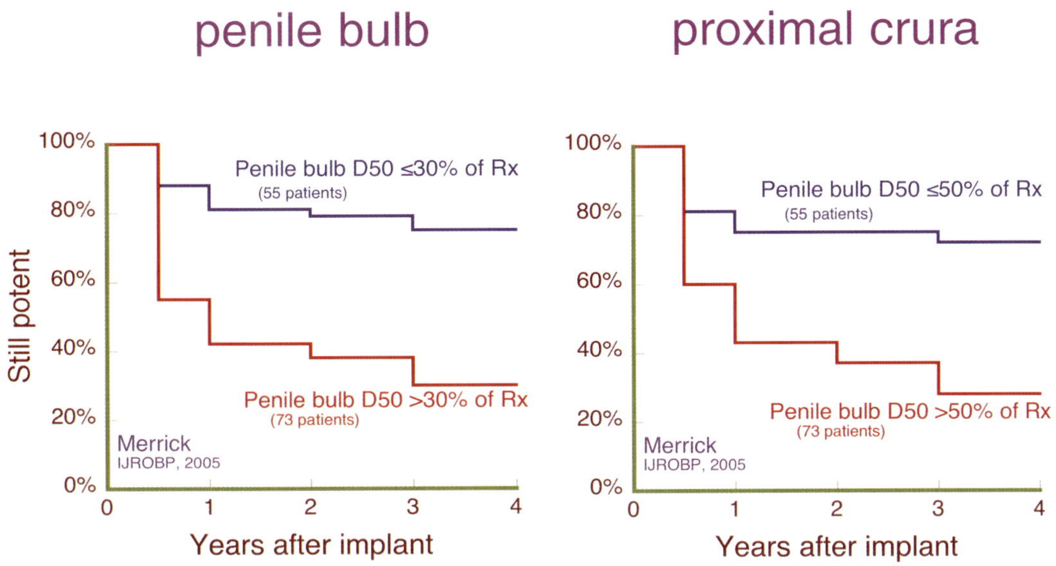

Figure 22-24. Mean penile bulb doses (left) and volumes (right) in patients with or without post-implant impotence. (MERRICK 05)

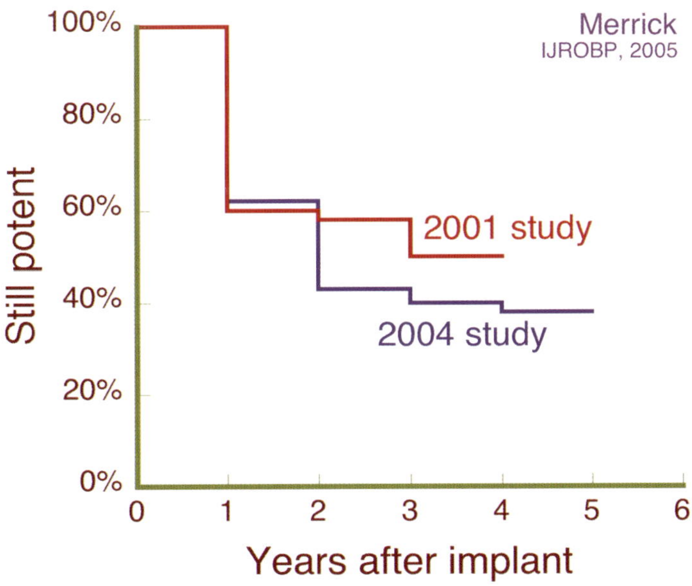

Figure 22-27. Potency data in older versus more recent review.(MERRICK 05)

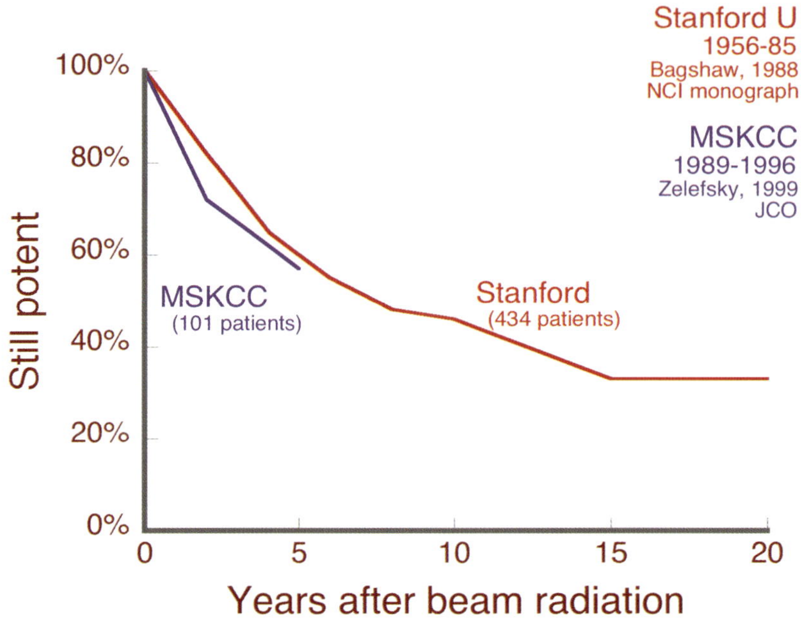

Figure 22-28. Longer-term potency preservation in external beam patients treated at Stanford with conventional external beam radiation or at Memorial Sloan-Kettering (MSKCC) with conformal radiation.(BAGSHAW, ZELEFSKY 99)

28). The relationship between potency loss and radiation volume, patient age, field size, or radiation dose has not been rigorously examined.

In the early 1980s, Walsh and colleagues demonstrated that potency could often be preserved after radical prostatectomy if the pelvic splanchnic nerves were identified and preserved.(WALSH) In the most favorable report by Dr. Walsh at Johns Hopkins University, maintenance of potency was achieved in approximately 60% of patients, with markedly better results in younger patients. Patients younger than 60 years of age had a 68% likelihood of maintaining potency, versus 55% in patients 60 years or older.(QUINLAN)

While the potential for potency-sparing surgery was quickly parroted by urologists around the world, giddy reports by surgeons at Johns Hopkins should be viewed skeptically, at best—they have not been widely reproduced by other surgeons. In fact, potency rates by other experienced sur-

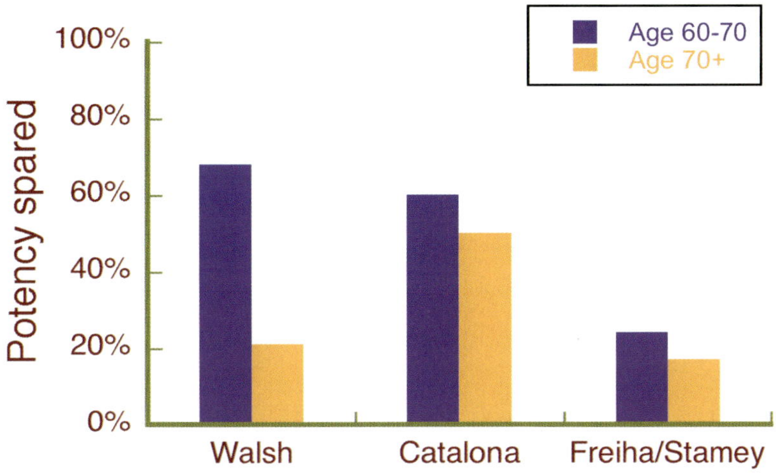

Figure 22-29. More examples of the tremendous variability in reported potency preservation rates following nerve-sparing prostatectomy.(QUINLAN, GEARY, CATALONA)

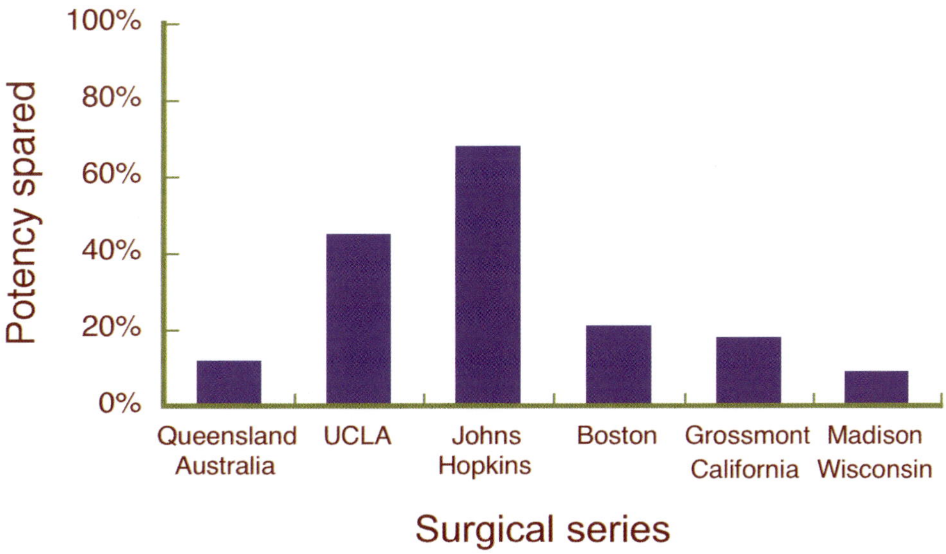

Figure 22-30. There is a large, perplexing variation in reported potency preservation rates following nerve-sparing prostatectomy.(TALCOTT, RITCHIE, QUINLAN, HEATHCOTE, GAYLIS, JONLER) Either some surgeons are a lot better than others, or some are particularly adept at massaging their data. Chances are that both factors may be at work!

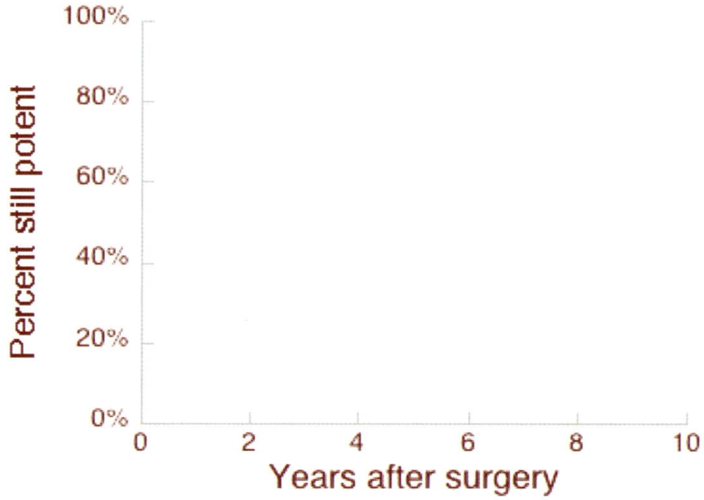

Figure 22-31. Compilation of long-term potency follow-up reports after nerve-sparing prostatectomy. (No mistake here—there are none!)

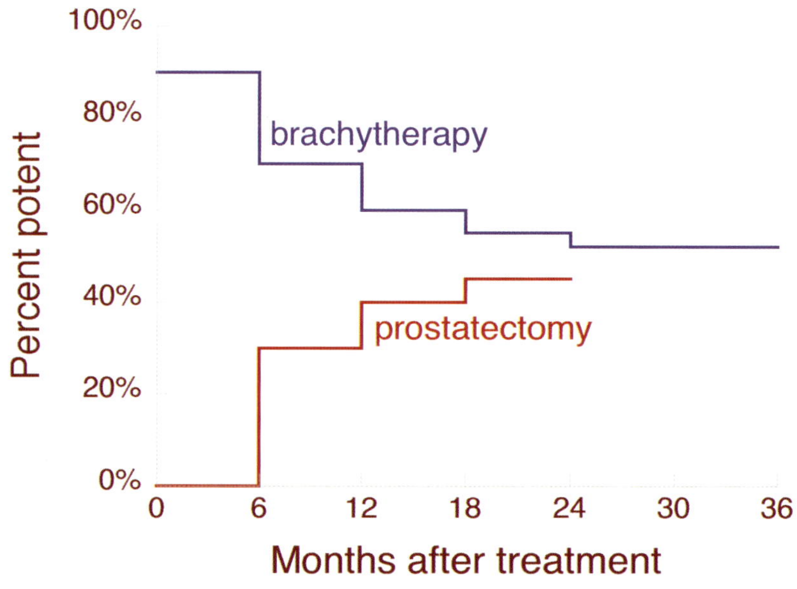

Figure 22-32. Schematic approximatlon of potency preservation after prostectomy, after brachytherapy.

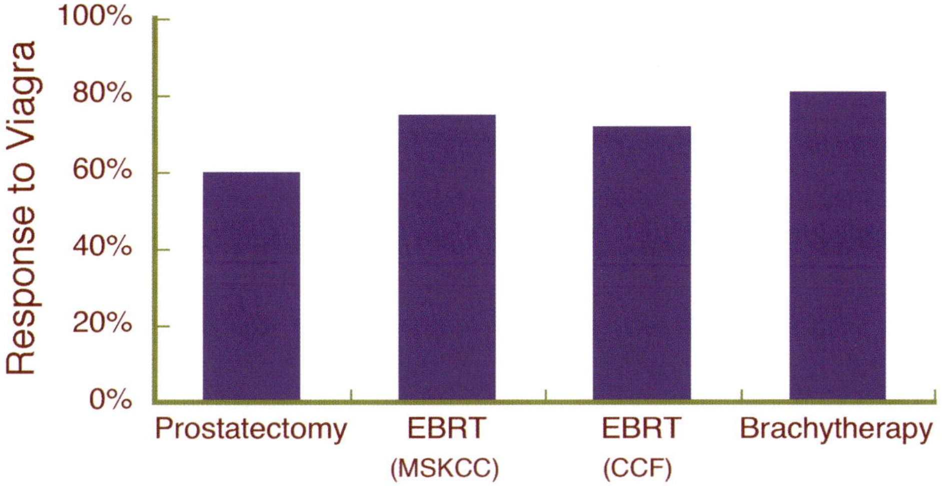

Figure 22-33. Approximate response to Viagra' (sildenafil) after prostatectomy, external beam radiation (EBRT), or brachytherapy. (LOWENTRITT, ZELEFSKY 99, KEDIA, MERRICK 99)

geons have typically been far, far lower (**Figures 22-29 & 22-30**). And like most external radiation series, surgical series have rarely included actuarial calculations, which would substantially decrease the stated rates of potency preservation. Furthermore, no investigator has reported longer-term follow-up of post-nerve-sparing prostatectomy potency preservation, numbers that would seem to be of prime interest given the frequent recommendation that "young patients should be treated by prostatectomy rather than radiation" (**Figure 22-31**).

The precise effect that different treatment modalities have on potency is still far from clear. In general, reported potency rates following brachytherapy have been higher than those following prostatectomy or external beam radiation. However, comparisons between modalities should be made with caution and qualification, considering the dearth of good quality actuarial long-term data for any modality. Brachytherapy offers some advantage over prostatectomy in the first two year after treatment. But in the longer term, as prostatectomy patients recover function, brachytherapy's advantage diminishes **(Figure 20-32**).

Table 22-1. Oral potency drugs.

brand name	Viagra™	Levitra™	Cialis™
generic name	sildenafil	vardenafil	tadalafil
peak action	1 hour	1 hour	2 hours
effect duration	4+ hours	4+ hours	24+ hours
food interaction?	yes	yes	no

TREATMENT

Patients who develop radiation-related impotence generally respond to corrective measures. Treatment with vasoactive agents after external beam radiation is usually successful.(PIERCE) Patients with treatment-related impotence after surgery or any form of radiation are likely to respond favorably to Viagra™/sildenafil (**Figure 22-33**). There is no clear correlation with clinical or implant parameters and the response to sildenafil.(MERRICK 99) The optimal choice among phosphodiesterase type 5 inhibitors is still unclear (**Table 22-1**).(CARSON)

Penile implants typically are highly effective and well tolerated in radiation patients.(DUBOCQ) However, considering that brachytherapy patients commonly recover some erectile function with time, mechanical implants should be recommended cautiously, because their placement usually destroys any remaining erectile function.

While the success of therapies for brachytherapy-related impotence has been a pleasant surprise, enthusiasm for corrective measures should be tempered by reports of high attrition rates for potency therapies in general.(MULHALL, VARDI)

THE FUTURE OF POTENCY PRESERVATION

Two major developments have improved the outlook for sexually active patients treated with brachytherapy. The first has been the introduction of PDEIs. As the choice and effectiveness of pharmacologic agents improves, erectile dysfunction will become a less important side effect. Secondly, the identification of the proximal penis as an important site of dysfunction has allowed us to be more cognizant of it's level of irradiation. Sophisticated efforts to limit excessive radiation to normal structures should help decrease sexual dysfunction.

REFERENCES

1. Bagshaw MA, Cox RS, Ray GR. Status of Radiation of Prostate Cancer at Stanford University. NCI Monogr 1988; 7:47-60.
2. Banker RL. The preservation of potency after external beam irradiation for prostate cancer. Int J Radiat Oncol Biol Phys 1988; 15:219-220.
3. Carson CC, Robertson CN. Late hematogenous infection of penile prosthesis. J Urol 1988; 139:50-52.
4. Catalona W, Carvalhal G, Mager D, Smith D. Potency, continence and complication rates in 1,870 consecutive radical prostatectomies. J Urol 1999; 162:433-438.
5. Chinn DM, Holland J, Crownover RL, Roach M. Potency following high-dose three-dimensional conformal radiotherapy and the impact of prior major urologic surgical procedures in patients treated for prostate cancer. Int J Radiat Oncol Biol Phys 1995; 33:15-22.
6. DiBiase SJ, Wallner KE, Tralins K, Sutlief S. Brachytherapy radiation doses to the neurovascular bundles. Int J Rad Oncol Biol Phys 2000; 46:1301-1307.
7. Dubocq FM, Bianco FJ, Maralani SJ, Forman JD, Dhabuwala CB. Outcome analysis of penile implant surgery after external beam radiation for prostate cancer. J Urol 1997; 158:1787-1790.
8. Feldman HA, Goldstein I, Hatzichristou DG, al e. Impotence and its medical and psychosocial correlates: Results of the Massachusetts Male Aging Study. J Urol 1994; 151:54-61.
9. Gaylis FD, Friedel WE, Armas OA. Radical retropubic prostatectomy outcomes at a community hospital. J Urol 1998; 159:167-171.
10. Geary ES, Dendinger TE, Freiha FS, Stamey TA. Nerve sparing radical prostatectomy: A different view. J Urol 1995; 154:145-149.
11. Goldstein I, Feldman MI, Deckers PJ, al e. Radiation-associated impotence: A clinical study of its mechanism. JAMA 1984; 251:903-910.
12. Heathcote PS, Mactaggart PN, Boston RJ, James AN, Thompson LC, Nicol DL. Health-related quality of life in Australian men remaining disease-free after radical prostatectomy. Medical Journal of Australia 2001; 168:483-486.
13. Jonler M, Messing EM, Rhodes PR, Bruskewitz RC. Sequelae of radical prostatectomy. Br J Urol 1994; 74:352-358.
14. Kedia S, Zippe CD, Agarwal A, Nelson DR, Lakin MM. Treatment of erectile dysfunction with sildenafil citrate (Viagra) after radiation therapy for prostate cancer. Urol 1999; 54:308-312.

15. Lee J, Hersey K, Lee C, Fleshner N. Climacturia following radical prostatectomy: prevalence and risk factors. J Urol 2006; 176:2562-2565.
16. Lepor H, Gregerman M, Crosby R, al e. Precise localization of the autonomic nerves from the pelvic plexus to the corpora cavernosa: A detailed anatomical study of the adult male pelvis. J Urol 1985; 133:207-212.

17. Lowentritt BH, Scardino PT, Miles BJ, et al. Sildenafil citrate after radical retropubic prostatectomy. J Urol 1999; 162:1614-1617.
18. Matthew A, Goldman A, Trachtenberg J, et al. Sexual dysfunction after radical prostatectomy: Prevalence, treatments, restricted use of treatments and distress. J Urol 2005; 174:2105-2110.
19. Merrick G, Bulter W, Wallner K, et al. The importance of radiation doses to the penile bulb vs. crura in the development of postbrachytherapy erectil dysfunction. Int J Rad Oncol Biol Phys 2002; 54:1055-1062.
20. Merrick G, Butler WM, Wallner K, et al. Erectile function after prostate brachytherapy. Int J Rad Oncol Biol Phys 2005; 62:437-447.
21. Merrick G, Wallner K, Butler W. Sexual dysfunction after prostate brachytherapy. Oncol 2003; 17:52-62.
22. Merrick GS, Butler WM, Dorsey AT, Lief JH, Donzella JG. A comparison of radiation dose to the neurovascular bundles in men with and without prostate brachytherapy induced erectile dysfunction. Int J Rad Oncol Biol Phys 2000; 48:1065-1070.
23. Merrick GS, Wallner KE, Butler WM, Lief JH, Sutlief S. Short-term sexual function after prostate brachytherapy. Radiat Oncol Invest 2001; 96:313-319.
24. Michl U, Dietz R, Huland H. Is intraoperative electrostimulation of erectile nerves possible? J Urol 1999; 162:1610-1613.
25. Mulhall JP, Jahoda AE, Cairney M, al e. The causes of patient dropout from penile self-injection therapy for impotence. J Urol 1999; 162:1291-1294.
26. Mydlo J, Lebed B. Does brachytherapy of the prostate affect quality and/or fertility in younger men? Scan J Urol Nephrol 2004; 38:221-224.
27. NIH. NIH consensus conference: Impotence. JAMA 1993; 270:83-90.
28. Pierce LJ, Whittington R, Hanno PM, al e. Pharmacologic erection with intracavernosal injection for men with sexual dysfunction following irradiation: A preliminary report. Int J Radiat Oncol Biol Phys 1991; 21:1311-1314.

29. Quinlan DM, Epstein JI, Carter BS, Walsh PC. Sexual Function Following Radical Prostatectomy: Influence of Preservation of Neurovascular Bundles. J Urol 1991; 145:998-1002.
30. Ritchie AWS, James K, deKiernion JB. Early post-operative morbidity of total prostatectomy. Br J Urol 1989; 64:511-515.

31. Roach M, Winter K, Michalski J, Bosch W, Lin X. Mean dose to the bulb of the penis correlates with risk of impotence at 24 months: preliminary analysis of Radiation Therapy Group (RTOG) phase I/II dose escalation trial 9406. Int J Rad Oncol Biol Phys 2000; 48:#2104.
32. Sokoloff M, Brendler. Indications and contraindications for nerve-sparing radical prostatectomy. Uro Clin N Am 2001; 28.
33. Stock RG, Kao JK, Stone NN. Penile erectile function after permanent radioactive seed implantation for the treatment of prostate cancer. J Urol 2001; 165:436-439.
34. Stock RG, Stone NN, Iannuzzi C. Sexual potency following interactive ultrasound-guided brachytherapy for prostate cancer. Int J Radiat Oncol Biol Phys 1996; 35:267-272.
35. Talcott JA, Rieker P, Propert KJ, Clark JA, al e. Patient-reported impotence and incontinence after nerve-sparing radical prostatectomy. J National Cancer Inst 1997; 89:1117-1123.
36. Vardi Y, Sprecher E, Gruenwald I. Logistic regression and survival analysis of 450 impotent patients treated with injection therapy: long-term dropout parameters. J Urol 2000; 163:467-470.
37. Walsh PC, Donker PJ. Impotence following radical prostatectomy: Insight into etiology and prevention. J Urol 1982; 128:492-497.
38. Wilson J, Clarke M, Ewings P, Graham J, Macdonagh R. The assessment of patient life-expectancy: how accurate are urologists and oncologists? BJU International 2004; 95:794-798.
39. Zelefsky MJ, Eid JF. Elucidating the etiology of erectile dysfunction after definitive therapy for prostatic cancer. Int J Rad Oncol Biol Phys 1998; 40:129-133.
40. Zelefsky MJ, McKee AB, Lee H, Leibel SA. Efficacy of oral sildenafil in patients with erectile dysfunction after radiotherapy for carcinoma of the prostate. Urol 1999; 53:775-778.
41. Zinreich ES, Derogatis LR, Herpst J, Auvil G, Piantadosi S, Order SE. Pre and posttreatment evaluation of sexual function in patients with adenocarcinoma of the prostate. Int J Radiat Biol Phys 1990; 19:729-732.

23

Seeds as salvage therapy

There are two aspects with regard to salvage therapy and brachytherapy—the use of implants as salvage, and salvage for a failed implant. Data regarding either situation are limited. This chapter will cover what little is known regarding the use of implants as salvage therapy.

With conventional dose external beam radiation, the likelihood of persistent intra-prostatic cancer has been relatively high in most series, and the number of patients potentially eligible for brachytherapy salvage is huge—approximately 20% of the 40,000 patients treated with external beam radiation annually in the United States. The biggest question regarding sal-

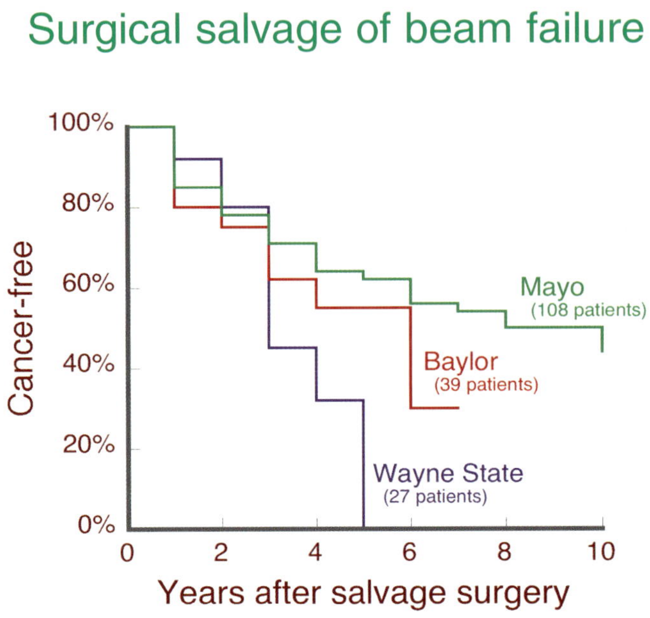

Figure 23-1. Freedom from second biochemical failure after salvage prostatectomy or salvage brachytherapy for locally recurrent cancer after external beam radiation failure.(AMLING, ROGERS, TEFILLI, BEYER, GRADO, WONG)

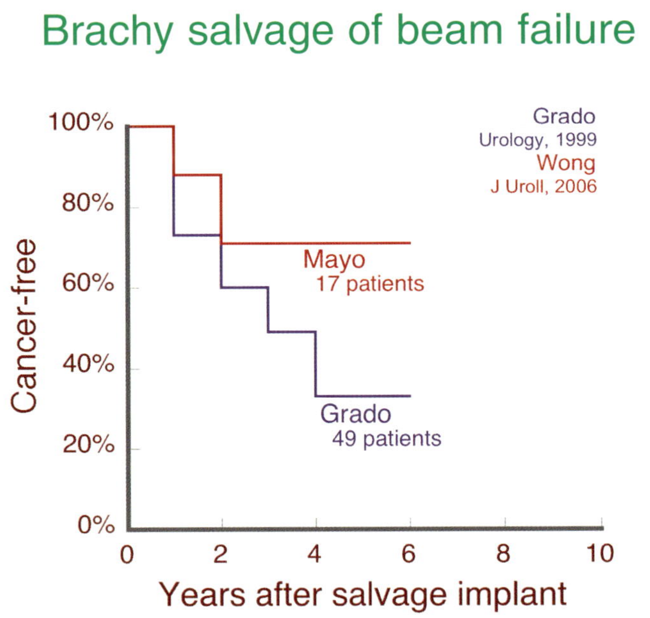

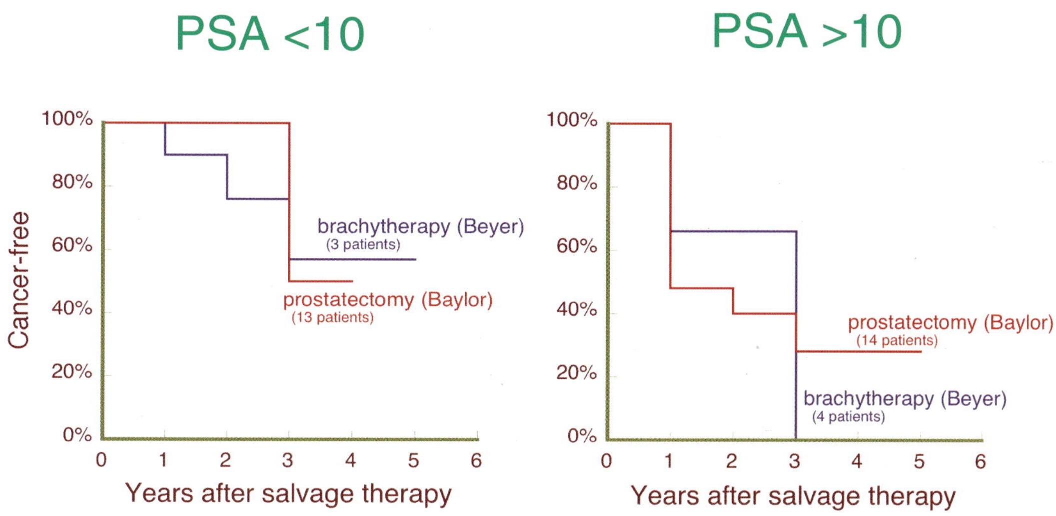

Figure 23-2. Freedom from second biochemical failure after salvage brachytherapy or salvage prostatectomy for locally recurrent cancer after external beam radiation (the Beyer series line for PSA less than 10 ng/ml excludes patients with a PSA of 0–4).(BEYER, ROGERS)

vage of external beam failures is how many are really salvageable with *any* local therapy. Some patients already have micrometastatic disease by the time intra-prostatic tumor persistence is demonstrated, and local therapy is unlikely to have an impact on their survival or improve their quality of life.

The limited number of salvage prostatectomy series published to date are unanimous in showing that the surgical salvage rates are low (**Figure 23-1, top**). While the biochemical control rates are acceptable in the first couple of post-salvage years, the number of second failures continues to climb with longer follow-up, so that the ultimate salvage rates appear very low.

Two investigators have reported results with salvage brachytherapy for failed external beam patients. Grado reported on 49 patients salvaged with either I-125 or Pd-103 between 1990 and 1996.(GRADO) At five years, the biochemical freedom from failure in salvaged patients was 33%, similar to that reported in surgical salvage series (**Figure 23-1, bottom**). Six percent of patients developed urinary incontinence and one patient required a colostomy for rectal bleeding.

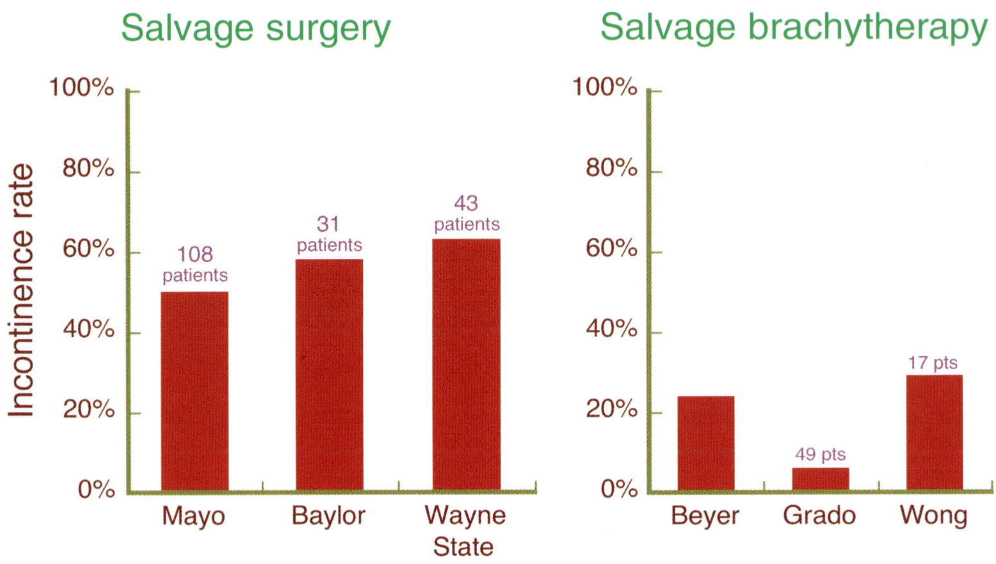

Figure 23-3. Urinary incontinence after salvage implant or salvage prostatectomy for locally recurrent cancer after external beam radiation.(AMLING, ROGERS, TEFILLI, BEYER, GRADO, WONG)

Beyer reported 17 patients treated with reduced dose I-125 or Pd-103 salvage implants.(BEYER) At five years, the overall freedom from second relapse was 53%, with 24% of patients developing urinary incontinence.

The chance for successful salvage brachytherapy could be predicted in part by the pre-treatment PSA. For patients with a PSA below 10 there may be a leveling off of the biochemical freedom-from-failure curves at about 50% after salvage surgery or brachytherapy, suggesting that a substantial percentage of such patients might still be cured. Patients with a PSA above 10 at the time of salvage fare poorly (**Figure 23-2**).

In contrast to salvage prostatectomy, the risk of incontinence has been relatively low after salvage brachytherapy (**Figure 23-3**). However, the incidence may rise with longer follow-up. Also, a substantial minority of patients may have other urinary morbidities.(WONG)

While these limited results are mildly encouraging, it should be remembered that the number of patients studied is low, and the few that were reported may not be representative of what we'd see if salvage implants were done on a widespread basis. What is missing from the reports are the details of how the implants were actually done. Implant doses used by Dr. Grado, for instance, varied during the study period. And it's likely that both Drs. Grado and Beyer varied their implant techniques during the study periods. Simply stating the prescription dose of a salvage implant does not tell enough about the implant technique to safely duplicate it at another center (see Chapter 11). The treatment margins used in the planning process, in particular, can have a substantial impact on the true dose to the prostate and adjacent normal tissues. For instance, Dr. Beyer was careful to avoid over-radiating the prostatic apex by ensuring that seeds were not placed outside of the prostate apex, a limitation that he does not use for previously untreated patients (personal communication). More information on how salvage doses and treatment margins can affect the complication rates is needed.(BICE)

Keeping in mind the myriad caveats, both salvage brachytherapy reports suggest that it may be effective in a sizable percentage of failed external beam radiation patients. But more detailed scrutiny of the techniques used and longer-term outcomes are called for before widespread adoption of salvage brachytherapy for beam radiation failures.

In the absence of objective data regarding dosimetry and outcomes for salvage implants, we have included some of our own examples (**Figures 23-4 and 23-5**). None of us have enough salvage cases to perform a statistical analysis of the relationship between dosimetry and outcomes. These examples are shown only to give the reader an idea of what *we* do.

POTENTIAL FOR LAWSUITS

The use of prostate brachytherapy for salvage of failed beam radiation is of particular concern from a medicolegal point (see Chapter 26). Although good data is lacking, one must assume that the likelihood of a rectal fistula is increased, even though the only two publications on the subject state that it is relatively safe.(GRADO, BEYER) Faced with the lack of data demonstrating a substantially increased complication risk in the salvage setting, plaintiff attorneys have been hesitant to pursue such cases. But salvage brachytherapy should be undertaken under the assumption that there is a

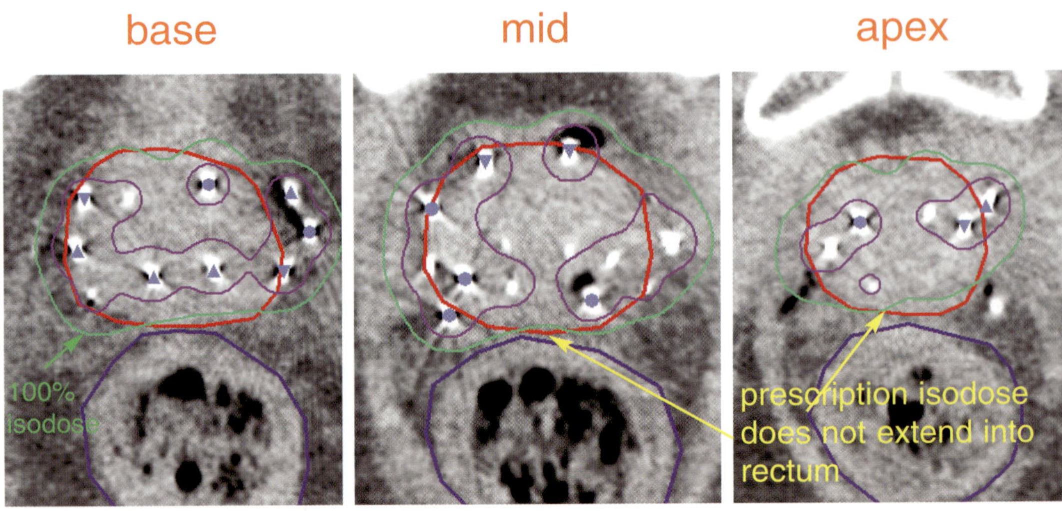

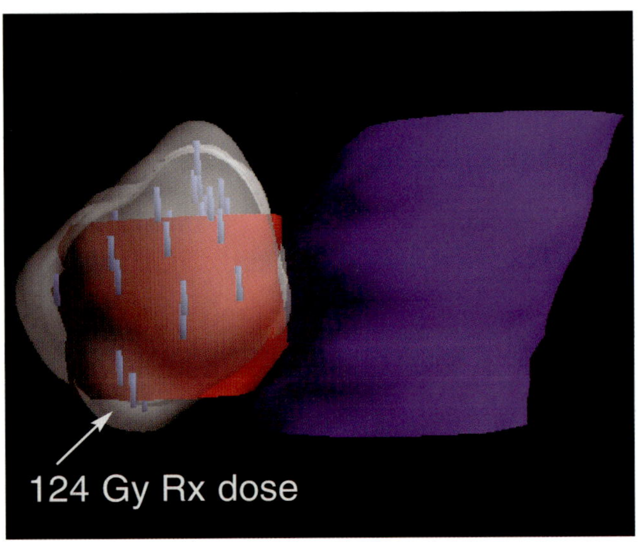

Figure 23-4. Example of 124 Gy Pd-103 salvage implant for cancer persistance after 70 Gy beam radiation (K. Wallner). Note full coverage of prostate with generous treatment margins, except posteriorly. The R100 was 0.0 cc. Wallner chose to use a full Pd-103 prescription dose.

higher than recognized fistula and incontinence risk, and that patients are likely to consider a suit if they develop a major complication.

Figures 23-4 and 23-5 show the post-implant dosimetry from salvage implants performed by two authors of this book. Neither of the patients shown has developed a serious complication from their salvage procedures. But to emphasize the legal risk in performing salvage implants, **Figure 23-6** shows a salvage implant performed three years after biochemical failure. The patient developed a fistula and sued, claiming that he was not fully appraised of the severity of the possible complications.

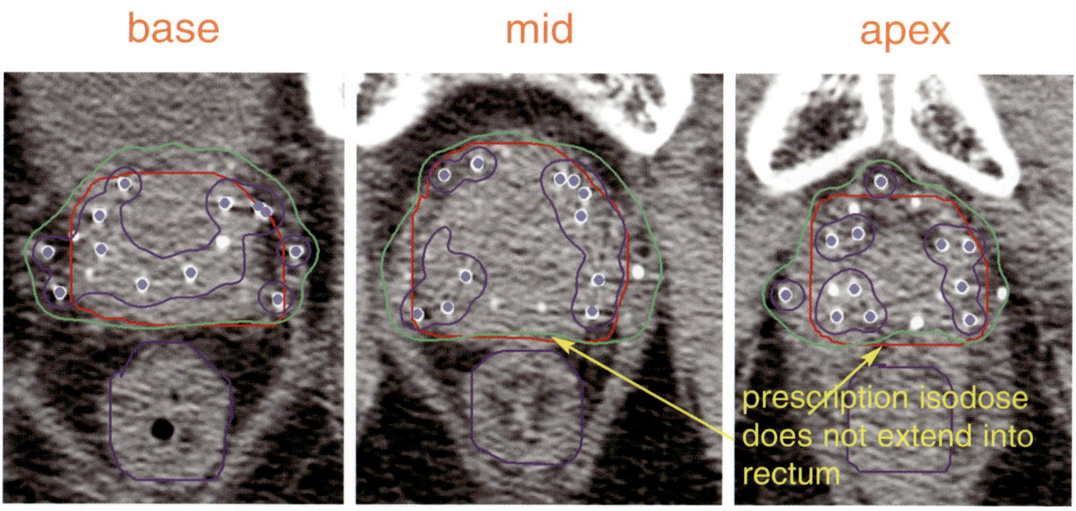

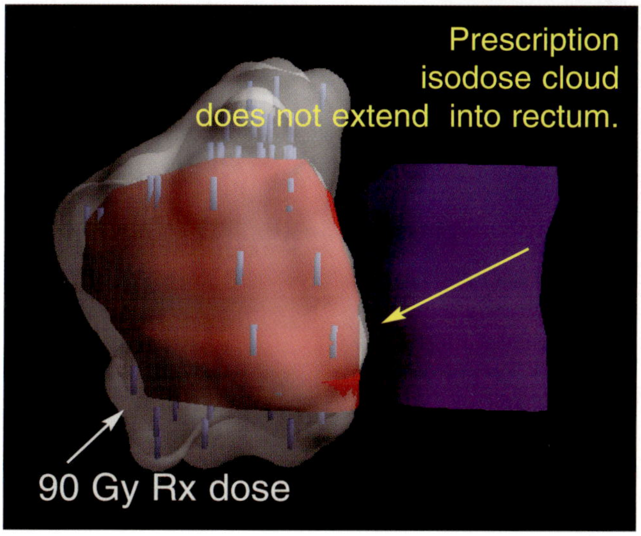

Figure 23-5. Example of 90 Gy Pd-103 salvage implant for cancer persistance after 68 Gy beam radiation.(by Merrick) The R100 was 0.0 cc. Note that Merrick used a lowered prescription dose.

Although the implant appeared within standard practice, the brachytherapist's insurer insisted on a settlement rather than risk a monstrous monetary award by a sympathetic jury. This example should serve as a warning that salvage implants are risky endeavors, both for the patient and the brachytherapist!

Because of the potential for a lawsuit, even with an ideal salvage implant, all authors of this textbook are leery of them. If you choose to provide this service, you must make a great effort to document that patients have been

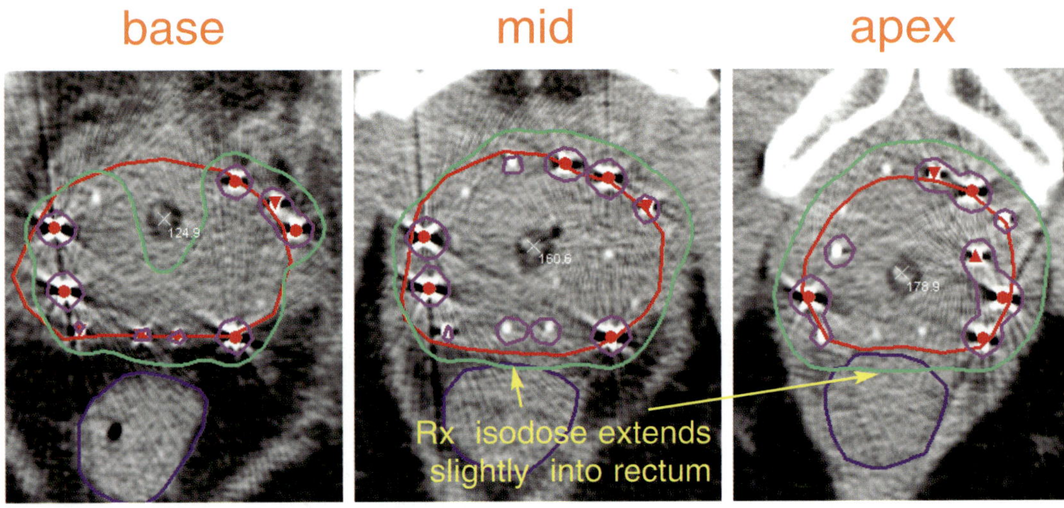

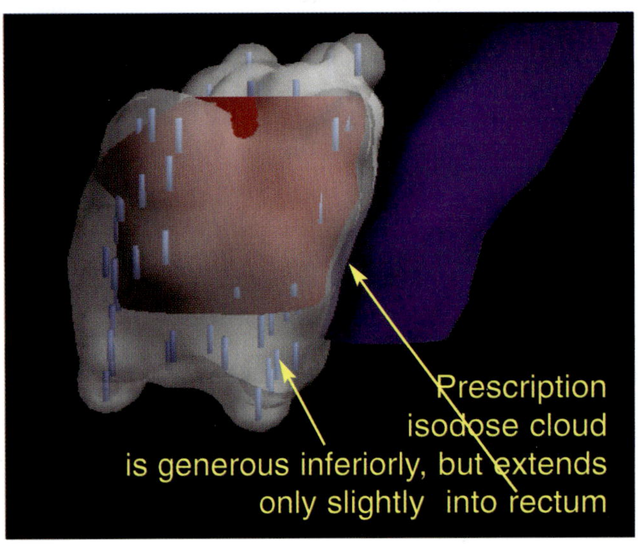

Figure 23-6. Example of salvage implant after 70 Gy beam radiation (J. Sheldon). Note full coverage of prostate with generous treatment margins. The R100 was only 0.32 cc. The patient developed a rectal fistula and sued. The case was settled at the insurer's insistence. The patient claimed to not be fully informed about the severity of the potential complications.

made aware of the controversy about the role of salvage brachytherapy, and the potential for severe complications.

SALVAGE FOR FAILED CRYO

Another potentially important use of brachytherapy is for cancer persistence after cryotherapy. We are unaware of data specifically regarding failed cryo. One report of salvage external beam for six patients showed no predisposition to excessive complications.(MCDONOUGH) Our guess is that salvage brachytherapy is safe in the setting of failed cryo, but there is no published data in this regard.

SALVAGE FOR FAILED PROSTATECTOMY

Use of salvage brachytherapy for biochemical recurrence after prostatectomy has not been reported. While the limited published data suggests that it is safe, we are aware of at least one unpublished case of fistula in this setting. In the absence of data to the contrary, one must assume that brachytherapy for post-surgical biochemical recurrence is risky and without good precedent. We question the rationale for brachytherapy in a setting where the ability to accurately define the area at risk for microscopic disease is limited. There is more rationale for adding brachytherapy to boost a tumor mass after prostatectomy, with some clinical outcomes data.(LOSA) However, even in the setting of a tumor mass one should be mindful of the potential for rectal damage, that appears to be minimal with adjuvant or salvage beam radiation alone.

REFERENCES

1. Amling CL, Lerner SE, Martin SK, al e. Deoxyribonucleic acid ploidy and serum prostate specific antigen predict outcome following salvage prostatectomy for radiation refractory prostate cancer. J Urol 1999; 161:857-863.

2. Beyer DC. Permanent brachytherapy as salvage treatment for recurrent prostate cancer. Urol 1999; 54:880-883.

3. Bice WS, Freeman JE, Russell LF, al e. Use of image coregistration in salvage prostate brachytherapy. Techniques in Urology 2000; 6:151-156.

4. Grado GL, Collins JM, Kriegshauser JS, al e. Salvage brachytherapy for localized prostate cancer after radiotherapy failure. Urol 1999; 53:2-10.

5. Losa A, Nava L, Di Muzio N, et al. Salvage brachytherapy for local recurrence after radical prostatectomy and subsuquent external beam radiotherapy. Urology 2003; 62:1068-1072.

6. Rogers E, Ohori M, Kassabian VS, al e. Salvage radical prostatectomy: Outcome measured by serum prostate specific antigen levels. J Urol 1995; 153:104-110.

7. Tefilli MV, Gheiler EL, Tiguert R, al e. Salvage surgery or salvage radiotherapy for locally recurrent prostate cancer. Urol 1998; 52:224-229.

8. Wong W, Buskirk S, Schild S, Prussak K, Davis B. Combined prostate brachytherapy and short-term androgen deprivation therapy as

salvage therapy for locally recurrent prostate cancer after external beam irradiation. J Urology 2006; 176:2020-2024.

24

Randomized trials

As prostate brachytherapy matures, there is increasing interest in higher quality, prospective randomized clinical trials. There are many questions that can only be answered definitively with randomization. Researchers at the Cleveland Clinic have worked on single institution trials, including the prophylactic use of the alpha-blocker, tamsulosin.(ELISHAIKH) Canadian investigators from Princess Margaret and the University of British Columbia have also been notably active.

Table 24-1. Completed prospective, randomized brachytherapy trials (2007)

Title	Institution	Patient #
Prophylactic tamsulosin (Flomax) in patients undergoing prostate 125I brachytherapy for prostate carcinoma: final report of a double-blind placebo-controlled randomized study(ELSHAIKH)	Cleveland Clinic	118
Randomized trial of high- and low-source strength 125I prostate seed implants (NARAYANA)	Michigan	40
A prospective randomized comparison of stranded versus loose iodine-125 seeds for prostate brachytherapy (REED)	Wheeling/ Seattle	63
High versus low dose supplemental external radiation with Pd-103 for prostate cancer (WALLNER)	Wheeling/ Seattle	587
I-125 versus Pd-103 for low risk prostate cancer (WALLNER)	Wheeling/ Seattle	602
Role of prophylactic tamsulosin±dexamethasone in patients undergoing prostate I125 seed implants for prostate carcinoma: A randomized double-blind study (CARLSON)	Cleveland Clinic	100

ONGOING TRIALS

The number of prospective randomized brachytherapy-related trials is growing. Most of those listed in **Tables 24-1 and 24-2** are described in www.clinicaltrials.gov as of January, 2007. Not all listed trials will be completed, and more trials will be started by the time you read this book. We included these tables to give you an idea of the things investigators are interested in. TRUS-guided prostate brachytherapy is a relatively young field, and randomized trials to objectively test new (or old) ideas are still sparse. Many more trials are in progress as opposed to completed (**Table 24-2**). We hope that more investigators will employ scientific methods to advance the field, moving beyond the retrospective, uncontrolled studies that have dominated much of radiation oncology to date.

Probably the most ambitious brachytherapy trial has been the RTOG test of the effect of supplemental beam radiation for intermediate risk patients. The design calls for 1,520 patients to be randomized between implant

Table 24-2. Ongoing prospective, randomized brachytherapy trials (2007).

Title	Institution	Patient #
Interstitial brachytherapy with or without external-beam radiation therapy in treating patients with prostate cancer	RTOG	1,520
Prophylactic Vs. therapeutic use of Uroxatrol in men undergoing brachytherapy	NY Prostate Institute	150
Selenium in treating patients who are undergoing brachytherapy for Stage I or Stage II prostrate cancer	Roswell Park	160
Long acting LHRH versus short acting LHRH in the treatment of prostate cancer	U of British Columbia	100
Androgen suppression combined with elective nodal and dose escalated radiation therapy	U of British Columbia	400
Mobicox: Study of meloxocam to reduce prostate swelling in permanent seed prostate brachytherapy	Princess Margaret	100
Study of tamsulosin and/or dutasteride to relieve urinary symptoms after brachytherapy for localized prostate cancer	Cleveland Clinic	348
Prostate seed implant with or without external beam radiation	Wheeling/ Seattle	600
I-125 versus Pd-103 for medium risk prostate cancer	Wheeling/ Seattle	600
Fine-tuning the prostate seed implant radiation dose	Wheeling/ Seattle	2,000
Implant and external radiation for prostate cancer, with or without hormonal therapy: A prospective, randomized trial	Wheeling/ Seattle	350
Long acting LHRH versus short acting LHRH in the treatment of prostate cancer	U British Columbia	100
Randomized trial of tamsulosin and/or dutaseride versus placebo to relieve urinary symptoms after brachytherapy for the treatment of localized prostate cancer	Cleveland Clinic	348
Androgen suppression combined with elective nodal and dose escalated radiation therapy	U of British Columbia	400
Randomized Prospective Study Comparing Prophylactic and On Demand Sildenafil Citrate Usage Administered During and After Radiotherapy in Combination with or without Hormone Therapy versus Radiotherapy Alone for the Preservation of Erectile Function in Potent Patients with Clinically Localized Prostate Cancer	Memorial Sloan-Kettering	285

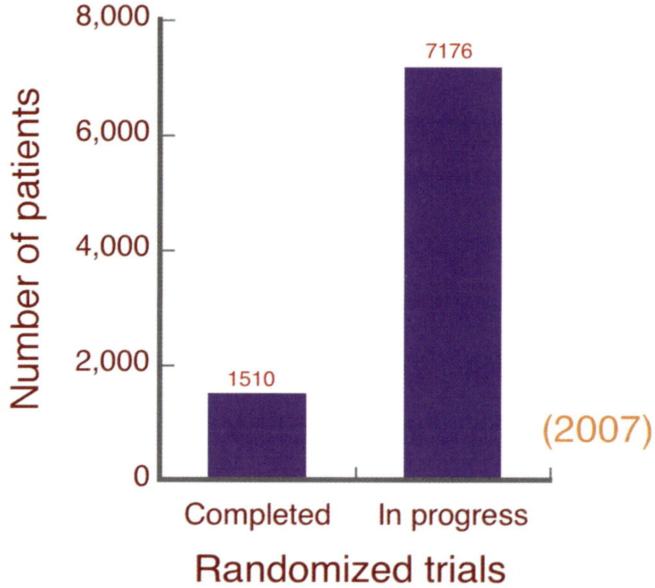

Figure 24-1. Total patients entered on completed trials compared with trials-in-progress (patient numbers taken from Tables 24-1 and 24-2).

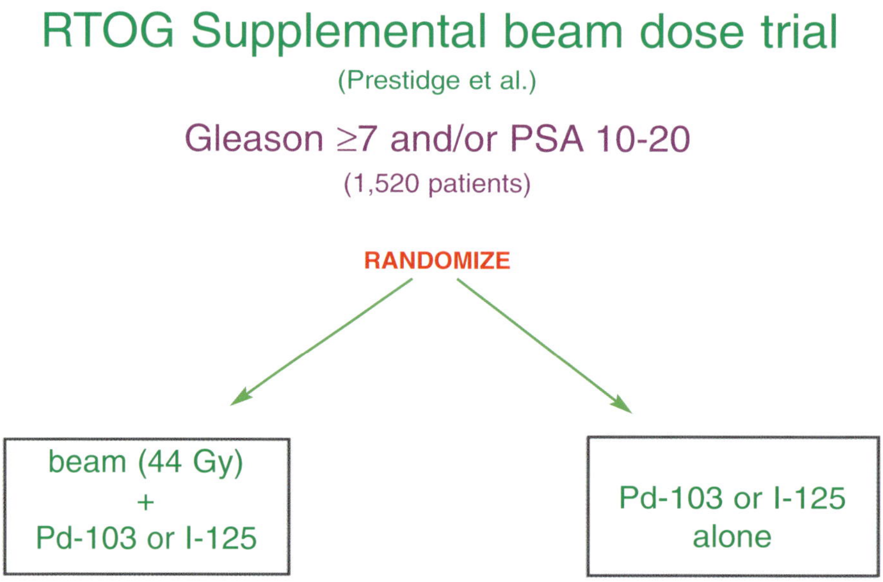

Figure 22-2. Design of ongoing RTOG trial to compare moderate- versus low-dose supplemental external beam radiation (135 patients randomized as of October, 2006).

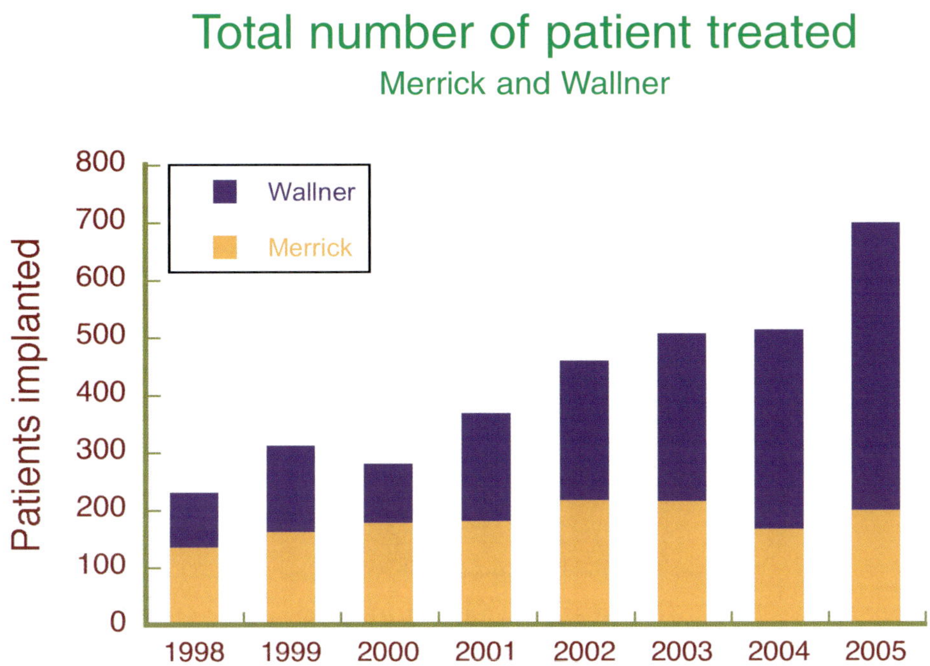

Figure 24-2. Total patients implanted annually in combined practices of G. Merrick and K. Wallner, from 1998 through 2005.

alone versus implant plus 45 Gy supplemental beam radiation (**Figure 24-2**). This trial tests a central tenet of brachytherapy, and is of great importance. Unfortunately, accrual has been slow, with approximately 100 patients entered as of September, 2006.

MERRICK AND WALLNER

Drs. Gregory Merrick and Kent Wallner have also made a notable contribution to the clinical science of prostate brachytherapy. Using their large practice bases, they have moved aggressively into prospective, randomized trials, most with cancer control rates as endpoints. They have completed enrollment for separate trials of I-125 versus Pd-103 for low-risk or intermediate risk patients (**Tables 24-1 and 24-2**).(WALLNER) They are in the midst of prospectively randomizing patients to progressively lower doses of supplemental beam radiation, with the second phase randomizing between 20 Gy versus no supplemental beam radiation. And they currently are accruing to randomizations testing the effect of neoadjuvant hor-

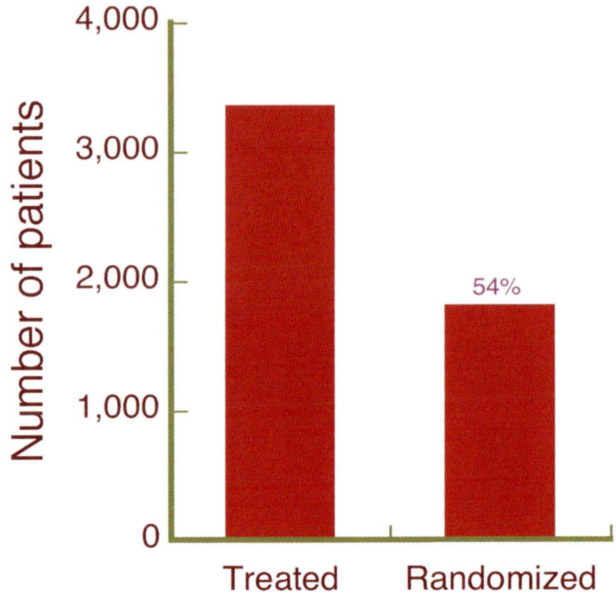

Figure 24-3. Total patients treated versus those entered onto randomized trials in the combined practices of G. Merrick and K. Wallner, from 1998 through 2005.

monal ablation, and Pd-103 dose reduction. Together, the prospective randomized trials organized by Merrick and Wallner have enrolled over 2,000 patients, and will reach 5,000 by the time their current trials are completed (**Figure 24-2 and 24-3**). Their success has been due, in part, to picking questions that are answerable, and randomizations that are palatable to patients.

REFERENCES

1. Elshaikh M, Ulchaker J, Reddy C, et al. Prophylactic tamsulosin (Flomax) in patients undergoing prostate I-125 brachytherapy for prostate carcinoma: Final report of a double-blind placebo-controlled randomized study. Int J Rad Oncol Biol Phys 2005; 62:164-169.

2. Wallner K, Merrick G, True L, Sutlief S, Cavanagh W, Butler W. I-125 versus Pd-103 for low risk prostate cancer: Preliminary biochemical outcomes from a prospective randomized mulitcenter trial. Int J Rad Oncol Biol Phys 2003; 57:1297-1303.

25

Really Bad Mistakes

Prostate brachytherapy has come a long way, thanks to good quality, easy-to-use TRUS equipment and sophisticated but user-friendly treatment planning systems. And we've learned, sometimes the hard way, what *not* to do to avoid complications. If you follow basic guidelines printed here and elsewhere, you should get good tumor control rates and acceptable complication rates. But you still have to pay attention to what you're doing, while you're doing it. Even though guidelines are fairly well worked out and should keep you out of serious trouble, there's always the possibility of making a really stupid mistake. Unfortunately, even the smartest, most conscientious people make one once in a while.

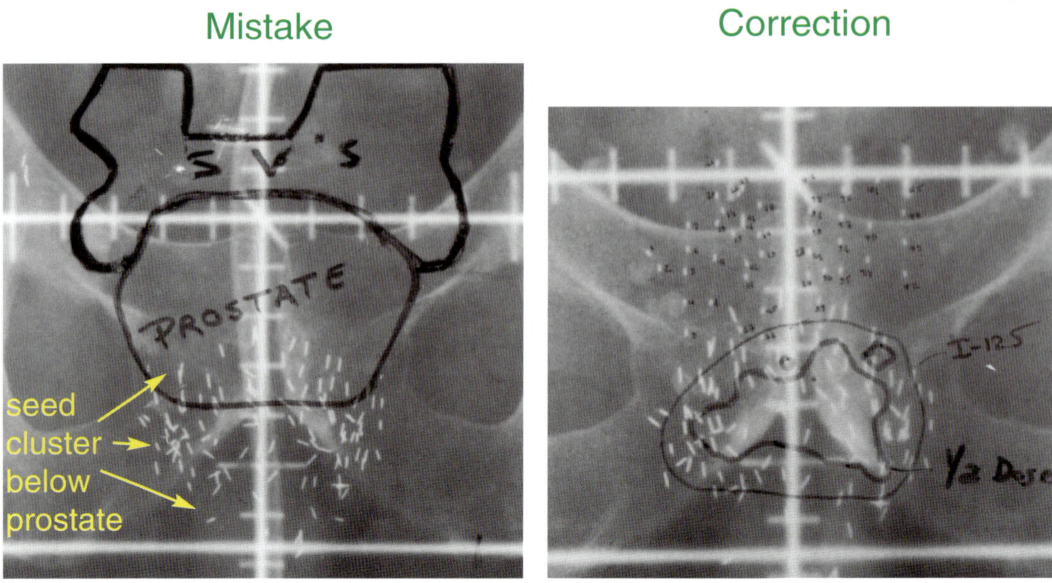

Figure 25-1. In this case, the brachytherapist somehow didn't visualize the prostate correctly. Perhaps the probe was oriented backward toward the sacrum or the external sphincter was mistaken for prostatic tissue. We don't know exactly what went wrong in this case, but when consulted about the patient, Michael Dattoli elected to go back and implant the prostate as it should have been in the first place. The patient did well, and has not developed rectal complications in the two years after his "patch-up" implant.

Whatever the reason—you weren't feeling well, you were distracted, or you simply blew it—disasters *can* occur. And if you do enough procedures, one probably *will* occur at some point in your practice. Just to get you in the proper frame of mind to handle disaster, we've collected a number of them that we've seen over the years.

MISSING THE PROSTATE

One of the most embarrassing mistakes you could make is to miss the prostate (**Figure 25-1**). It happens—we know of several instances, probably related to mis-interpreting the TRUS images at the time of initial setup. Unfortunately, you can't go back and remove the misplaced sources, short of resecting the prostate.

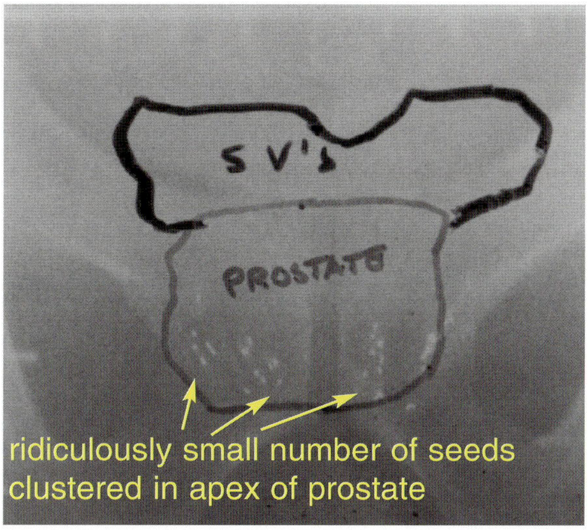

Figure 25-2. This is another miss-the-prostate mistake, partly due to gross under-planning. It may have resulted from a faulty pre-implant volume study suggesting a prostate volume much smaller than it really was. When consulted about the patient after this implant, Michael Dattoli elected to go back and implant the rest of the prostate. Like the patient in Figure 25-1, the patient has done well after his "patch-up" implant.

The prostate should appear obvious on TRUS. If you're setting up and not sure whether you're looking at the prostate, something is *very* wrong—stop and reposition the probe or take it out and start again. Either the probe setup is wrong (backward, looking at the sacrum, for instance) or you're not in far enough. A quick anterior fluoroscopic view with a catheter in place is the surest way to prevent mistakes like the one in **Figure 25-1**. If you *really* goof up and miss the prostate altogether, often the best remedy is to go back and re-implant (correctly), providing the patient isn't going to wind up with excessive rectal doses.

GROSS UNDER-DOSE

More common than outright missing the prostate is grossly under-dosing it. Mistakes like this probably result from a brachytherapy team not fully understanding what they're doing. And we're talking about the *whole team* here. A gross under-treatment like the one shown in **Figure 25-2** can be avoided if even one member of the brachytherapy team pays appropriate

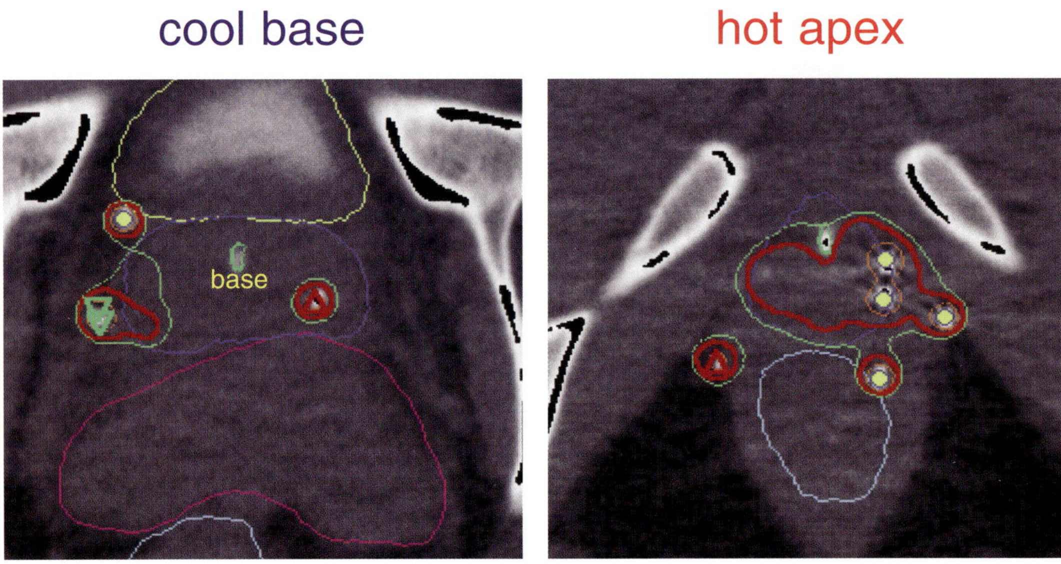

Figure 25-3. This is a less egregious, but still fairly bad error. The implant was planned properly, but somehow the implant seed cluster was misplaced, approximately one cm inferiorly from the base. The result is inadequate coverage of the base and excessive coverage of peri-apical tissue, an error that typically results from under-inserting the needles. It can be prevented by over-insertion of the needles and then pulling them back to their proper position before ejecting the seeds. Over-insertion creates a track for the seeds to rest in (see Chapter 10).

attention—the radiation oncologist should know from simple inspection of the planning images and treatment plan that something is wrong, the dosimetrist should know that the target is going to be grossly under-dosed, and even the urologist, without formal training, should see that this kind of seed distribution could not *possibly* be adequate to treat a patient's prostate. The saving grace for blunders like this is that they are relatively easy to fix—it's pretty straightforward to run the post-implant dosimetry and go back and add seeds to bring coverage of the prostate up to where it should be. The chance for complications (apart from severe embarrassment) should be minimal.

More common than the egregious under-dosage in Figure 25-2 is missing the prostatic base by a centimeter or two (**Figure 25-3 and 25-4**). We've

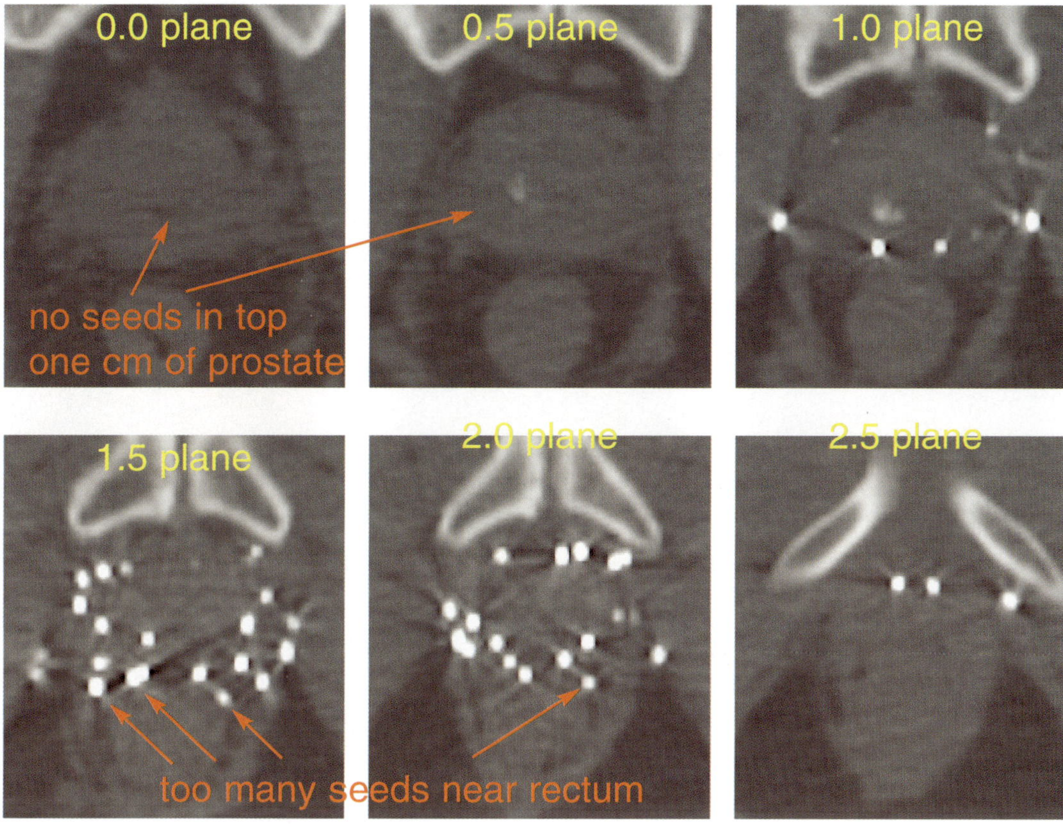

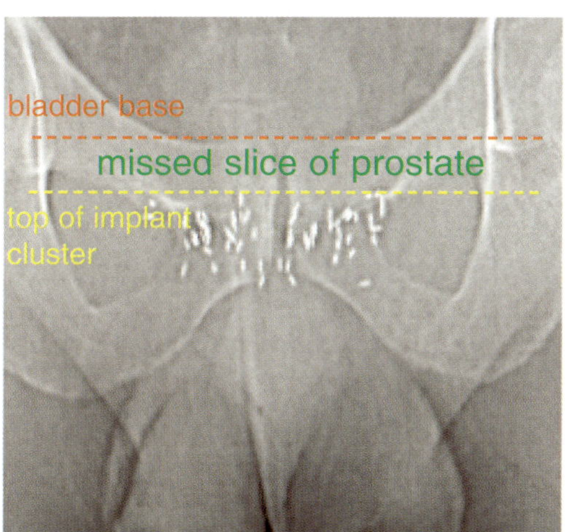

Figure 25-4. another example of seeds placed too low in the prostate. This one is doubly vexing, since there are multiple posterior seeds near the rectum.

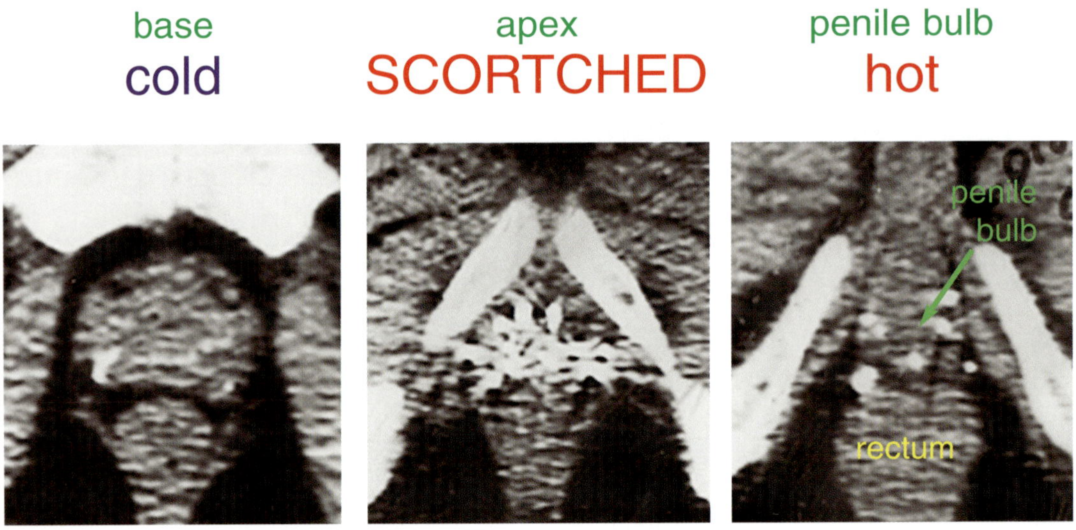

Figure 25-5. Yet another example of missed base and over-radiated apex. The plan for a fix is to add seeds to the base. It's too soon to say, but we suspect that this patient would be at risk of distal urethral stricture and apical urethral necrosis. An increased risk of impotence due to excessive penile bulb seeds is probably the least of his potential problems.

seen a number of these over the years. They are typically due to technical errors involving needle tip depth. The prostate might be pushed cephalad during needle insertion, and no corrective measure used (see Chapter 10).

Probably the worst thing to do with an under-dosage mistake is to ignore it—the patient will likely develop cancer recurrence and possibly die from your mistake. And the proof of your ineptness is obvious to anyone taking even a cursory look at the films!

OVERDOSE

The bad mistakes in Figures 25-1 through 25-5 were related to under-dosing the prostate, the primary clinical result being a missed chance at cure. The other type of really bad mistake is *over*dosing. Overdosing the prostate itself is typically not the issue; the real problem is overdosing the urethra or rectum. And remember, there are overdoses, and there are *over*doses—the second type is the one we're talking about here.

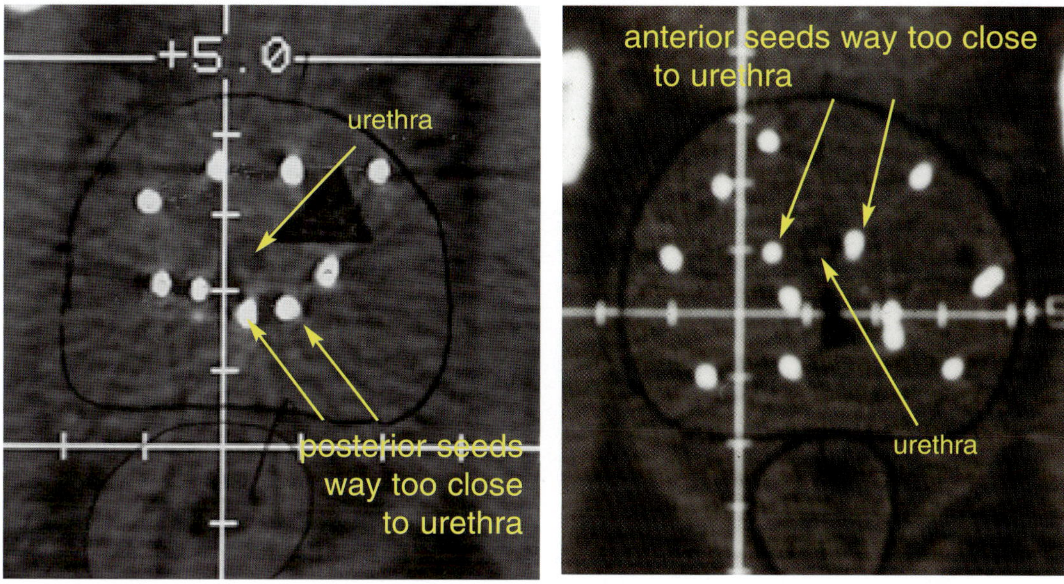

Figure 25-6. The mistake on the left was committed in the early 1990s. For some reason, the posterior sources were too anterior, resulting in an excessive urethral dose and inadequate dose to the back of the prostate. If this occurred today, we'd probably go back and add a few sources in the posterior prostate, to make sure of an adequate cancercidal dose posteriorly, even if it meant overdosing the urethra—a problem from which patients usually recover spontaneously.

The excessive number of peri-urethral seeds in the patient on the right is not as egregious as that on the left, but we consider the placement of 3 peri-urethral seeds to be a mistake. This may have resulted from a planning error or an implantation error.

Gross urethral overdose
Following typical peripheral seed placement patterns, urethral doses are easily kept below the recommended maximum of 1.5 to 2.5 times the prescription dose. Deviations from the peripheral pattern, however, can lead to huge urethral doses, a problem that could come from a faulty plan, seed placement error, or a lack of appreciation of a markedly asymmetric urethra, leading to gross overdosage despite a peripheral loading pattern. The patient in **Figure 25-6** had several high activity I-125 seeds placed too

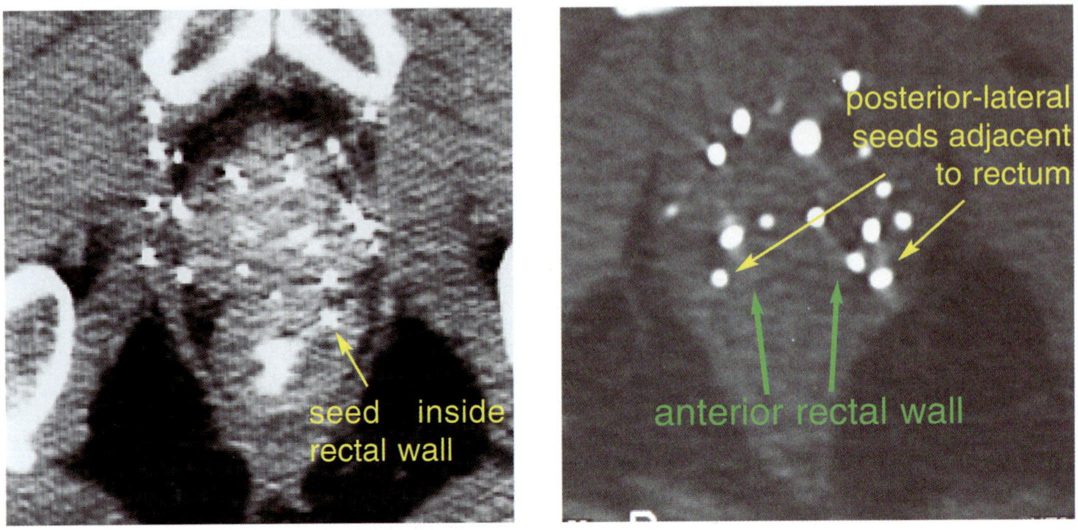

Figure 22-7. These examples show two classic errors in peri-rectal seed placement. The case on the left shows one seed in the middle of the rectal wall. The case on the right shows two seeds placed too posterio-laterally along the rectal wall. Although not as hazardous as the rectal seed in the example on the left, these posterior seeds can result in an excessive R100 (see Chapter 11).

close to his urethra, resulting in excessive urethral doses and prolonged urinary morbidity. Fortunately, his symptoms resolved spontaneously without long-term complications.

The second patient in **Figure 25-5** had several seeds placed near the center of the gland, within a mm or two of the urethra. We don't know how this happened; it could have been a faulty plan or faulty execution. Whatever the explanation, multiple seeds so close to the urethra would never be needed to achieve cancercidal central doses.

Gross rectal overdose

While serious rectal complications are infrequent and not typically a product of *really* bad mistakes, it is possible to place several seeds too posteriorly, resulting in grossly excessive rectal doses (**Figures 25-7 and 25-8**). There are two potential serious sequelae from this kind of mistake. The first is that such patients are at higher risk of a rectal complication. The sec-

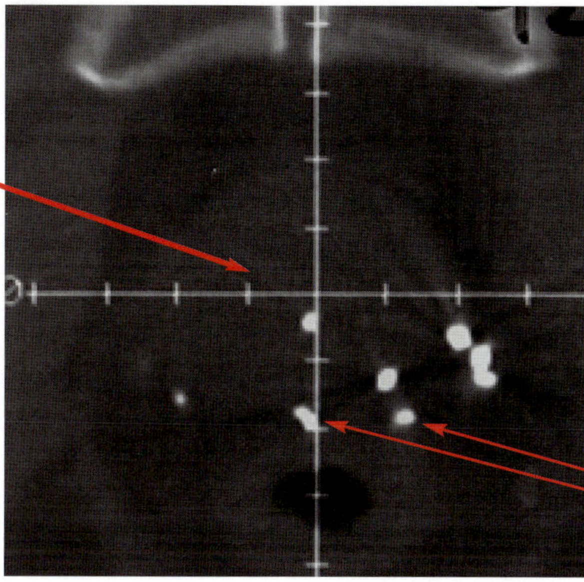

Figure 25-8. This error was committed in the early days of transperineal implants—we're not sure how it happened. The patient developed a severe rectal ulcer, but no fistula. If the prostatic dose were up to what it should have been, a fistula would likely have developed. The patient's ulcer gradually healed spontaneously, but he developed local tumor progression.

It's tough to know what would have been the proper action at the time the error was detected. One reasonable option might have been to proceed with a prostatectomy, in the hope of curing him and preventing over-radiation of the rectum. Another option, going back to implant additional seeds to achieve an adequate cancericidal dose to the prostate, might have pushed him over the edge to fistualization.

ond, equally serious problem is that such patients are at substantial risk of cancer progression, since many of the seeds that were supposed to contribute to their prostatic irradiation are instead contributing only to their rectal dose.

WRONG SEEDS, WRONG PATIENT, WRONG PLAN, ETC.

Perhaps the most common really bad mistake is mixing up patients' intended therapy (**Figure 25-9**). Especially in a high-volume practice, it's

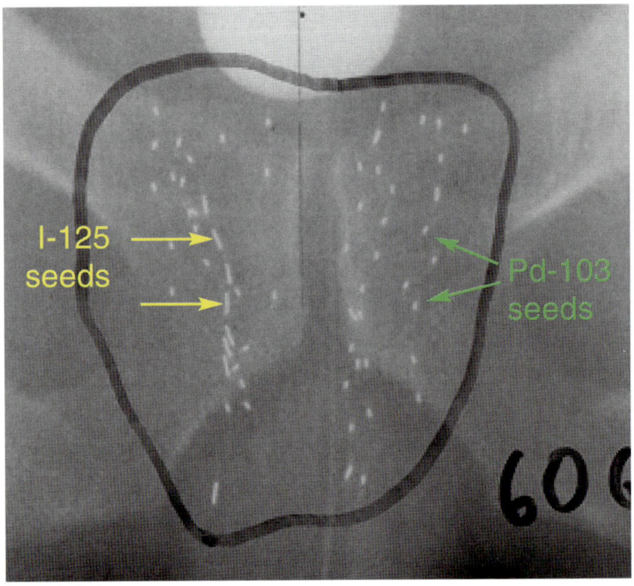

Figure 25-9. This is our best illustration of what is probably the most common mistake—a mix-up. This patient's sources were mixed up with another's at the time of sterilization. The mistake was caught early on fluoroscopy when a few I-125 sources (arrows) were apparent instead of the intended Pd-103 sources. There are a variety of source mix-ups that can occur. So when you discover a source mix-up error, make sure you're not about to make the reciprocal error in the next patient.

not surprising that such errors occasionally occur. The best safeguard is to have a system of checks in place, whereby multiple people involved in the planning and implementation re-check that everything is consistent, from the prescription to the actual seeds taken to the operating room. But if NASA researchers can use the wrong units in calculating the distance to Mars, you can be sure that a small brachytherapy team can use the wrong seeds or wrong dose for an implant patient.

WHEN YOU DISCOVER A MISTAKE

As we said earlier, no matter how smart you are, if you do enough procedures, you're likely to make a bad mistake at some point, probably when you least expect it. When it happens, it's important not to panic. Most of what you initially think are bad mistakes will likely turn out to be only *sort of bad* ones, or even within the range of accepted practice. For instance, if you mix up the seeds between two patients, the target coverage could easily still be well within acceptable treatment guidelines. Take time to asses the situation. First, do the dosimetry and assess whether your error makes any clinical difference. Remember, any corrective action likely won't be taken immediately anyhow.

If you're in the middle of the implant when you discover the mistake, try to call another expert to assess the mistake in real-time and determine what, corrective measure might be done intra-operatively. Again, even an egregious error may prove to be medically unimportant. Determine the clinical significance.

LAWSUITS
Finally, keep in mind that none of the really bad errors shown here have resulted in lawsuits (yet). Among the many malpractice suits that the authors *have* been involved with to date have instead involved complications from technically acceptable implants. As painful as it may be, be open with staff and the patient about a significant error. Be readily available to answer questions. Honesty is the best policy.

26

Malpractice

written with
Kathryn Elliott, JD, MD and Paul Herstein, MD

Medical malpractice is considered to be a *tort*, or personal injury. It is defined as the provision of medical care that falls below the prevailing standard of practice, resulting in physical or emotional damage.(GARNER). In most states, the cost of medical malpractice insurance is increasing faster than the cost of living (**Figure 26-1**). The cause of these rate increases is multi-factorial, including more suits filed, larger payouts, and higher insurance company profits (**Figure 26-2**).

Physician groups contend that increasing malpractice premiums are largely due to an increase in frivolous suits and sympathetic juries who

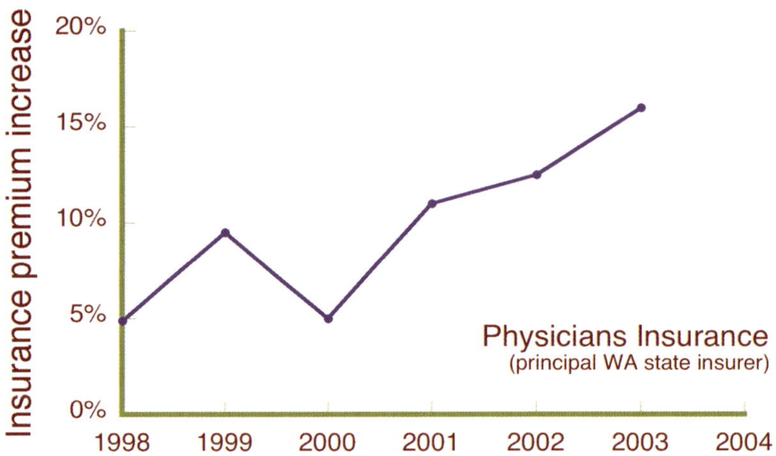

Figure 26-1. Washington state malpractice insurance premium increases.

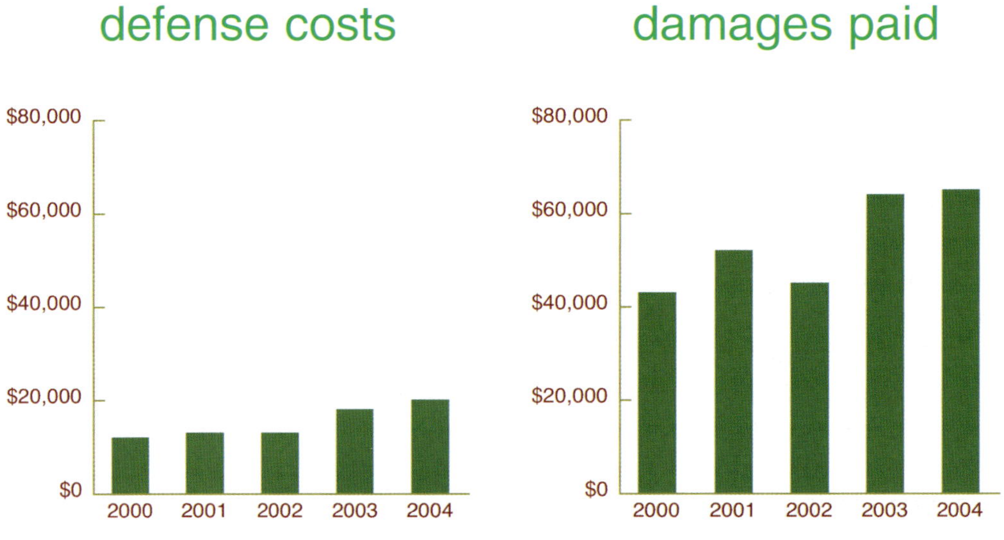

Figure 26-2. Washington state per case malpractice damages and defense costs.

Table 26-1 Reasons patients sue their doctors.(VINCENT)

- to hold the offending caregiver accountable
- to seek a more complete or satisfying explanation for the adverse event
- to stop similar events from occurring to other patients
- to obtain financial compensation

choose to compensate patients for bad outcomes that often are not directly related to medical error. Legal and patient advocacy groups prefer to blame insurance companies' business decisions and poor quality care for large malpractice premium increases. The true mix of causes is complex and includes partial truths from each camp.(MELLO) The precise contribution of various aspects also varies state-to-state, depending on the malpractice laws and how they are applied by the courts. Insurance business practices also vary by state.

WHY PATIENTS SUE

Many patients suffer unintentional harm in the course of their care.(ZHAN) There are several reasons why certain injured patients choose to sue (**Table 26-1**).(VINCENT) Financial gain is obviously an important motivator. In the United States health care system, pursuing a malpractice suit is often the only option some patients have to pay to care for a treatment-related injury.

In the fragmented, largely private medical care system of the United States, accurate malpractice statistics are not fully available. Information regarding the size of settlements are largely unavailable to the public. The national physicians database summarizes the number of cases settled or tried, but offers no details on financial sums (www.npdb-hipdb.com).

Malpractice statistics within specialties are especially scarce. Radiation oncology is not included in reports of high-risk specialties like anesthesia, obstetrics, orthopedic and neurosurgery, in part due to the small number of radiation oncologists. In fact, there is no published detailed information

Table 26-2. Establishing malpractice

- Define the standard of care
- Show that the defendant violated that standard
- Show that the violation proximately resulted in the plaintiff's injury

regarding specific causes of radiation-related suits in radiation oncology, apart from that reported for prostate brachytherapy.(ELLIOTT) This lack of specific, published information is especially surprising considering how prominent the issue is in the popular media.

Because of the relative rarity of serious complications and the lag time of one or more years for complications to manifest themselves, it has taken several years of widespread use for brachytherapy-related malpractice cases to appear in significant numbers. Prostate brachytherapy malpractice mirrors the experience of Lasik eye surgery; the incidence of serious complications is low, so that many thousands of patients had to be treated before enough complications occurred to become a prime target for plaintiff attorneys.

ESTABLISHING MALPRACTICE IN THE COURTROOM

The criteria for establishing medical malpractice are simple and logical (**Table 26-2**). The plaintiff's team must establish for the jury the standard of care, show how the accused violated that standard, and demonstrate that the violation resulted in the adverse outcome. While each of these three steps seems straightforward, there is a lot of room for argument at each step.

Establishing the standard of care for a relatively new procedure can be problematic, in that there will be few published standards. And the ones that are published may be of dubious value; a good example would be the ABS prostate brachytherapy recommendations published in 2001.(NAG) They contained multiple recommendations regarding patient selection and dose parameters that were unfounded in clinical data and ultimately proved to be questionable, at best (see Chapter 15).

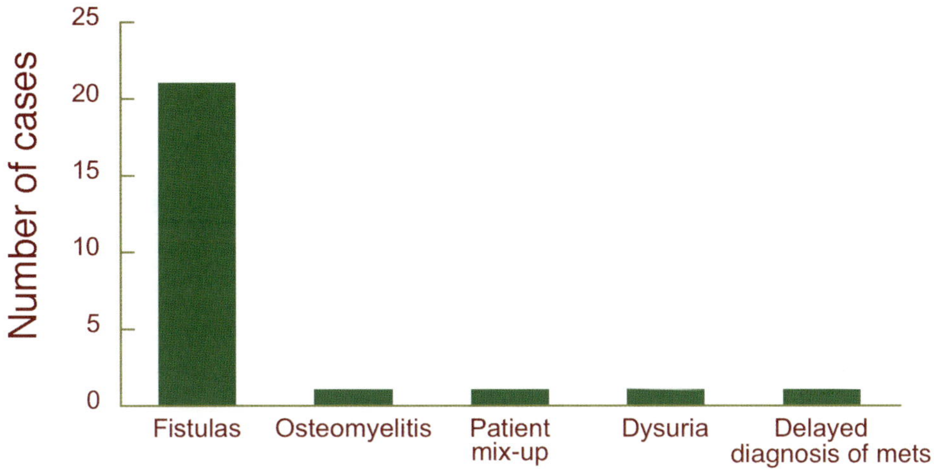

Figure 26-3. Primary damages leading to prostate brachytherapy malpractice suits.

Showing that a defendant violated a standard of care can also be problematic, partly because the standard of care itself is often arguable. Also, juries typically will allow for reasonable human error.

Finally, showing that a violation of standard of care resulted in an adverse outcome can be problematic in that adverse outcomes can have multi-factorial causes. For instance, a case of post-implant incontinence could be due to excessive urethral dose, a post-implant TURP, or perhaps to a patient's predisposition to incontinence that would have developed even in the absence of his implant.

CT SCANS AS EVIDENCE

Brachytherapy has a particular vulnerability with respect to malpractice litigation—the post-implant CT scan. The scan gives a fairly accurate objective summation of the implant, from which doses to the prostate, rectum and urethra are readily derived. The ability to image seeds in relation to the regions of interest offers an unprecedented opportunity to objectively study the relationships between dose, cure and complications. However, it also opens physicians to second-guessing by plaintiffs who experience a poor outcome. Even a single seed adjacent to the rectum or urethra could be alleged to have caused a complication, and could be portrayed to a jury as a breach of the standard of care.

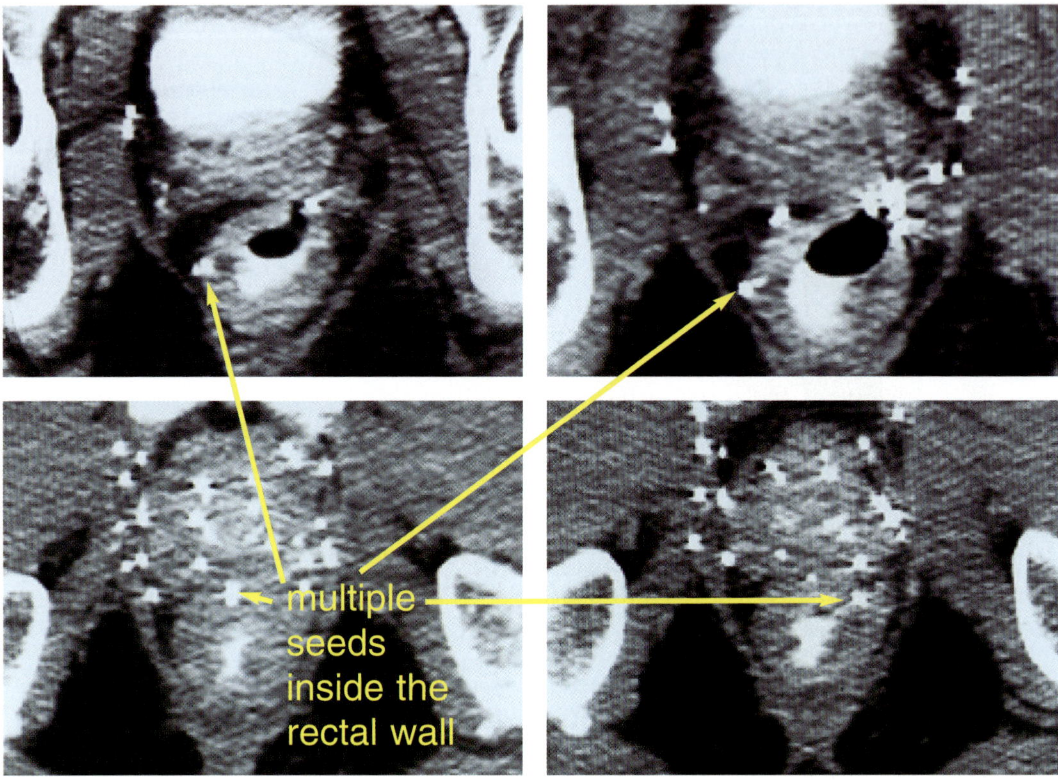

Figure 26-4. This sort of implant is almost impossible to defend. Even without rectal dose calculations, it looks obvious to a lay person that too many seeds were placed in the rectal wall. Even the most sympathetic defense expert would have trouble explaining this one away! The case was settled without going to trial.

PUBLISHED DATA

The only published data regarding prostate brachytherapy malpractice come from the efforts of Elliott and colleagues to summarize K. Wallner's personal experience as an expert witness or a defendant. Elliott summarized the complaint and principle issues of the first 13 such cases. The personal experience now includes 24 cases, including patients implanted from 1992 through 2005 (**Figure 26-3**) KW was the defendant in six cases, and an expert witness in the remaining 18 cases. Those cases were dominated by rectal fistulas, and a handful of miscellaneous adverse outcomes.

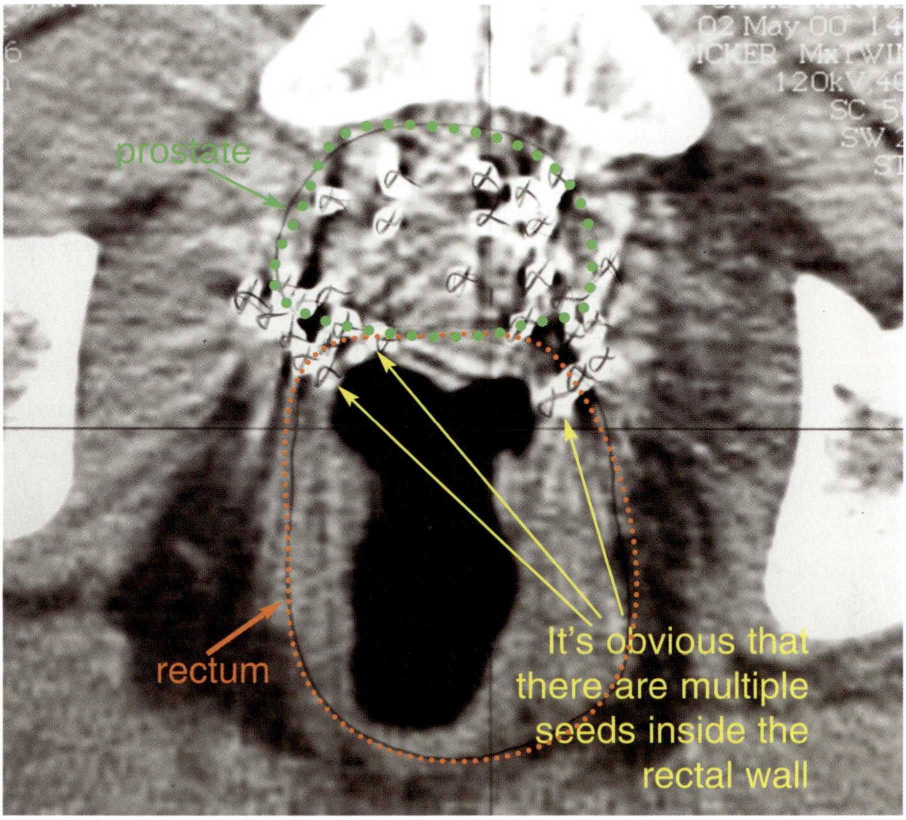

Figure 26-5. This sort of implant is also difficult to defend. It appears obvious that way too many seeds were inserted in the rectal wall. Perhaps this could have been defended in the past, but not in 2007!

Fistulas

Rectal fistulas have long been a feared complication of pelvic radiation. They allow spontaneous urine leakage from the prostate into the rectum and contamination of the urinary tract by fecal bacteria, typically requiring a colostomy and a urinary diversion. Even with rectal and urinary diversion, they heal in only a minority of cases.(MOREIRA) The sequelae can be physically, emotionally and financially devastating. Although uncommon, rectal fistulas have been far and away the dominant problem in prostate brachytherapy malpractice.

Most of the rectal fistula cases summarized by Elliott and colleagues did not involve an egregious seed placement error. Instead, plaintiff attorneys

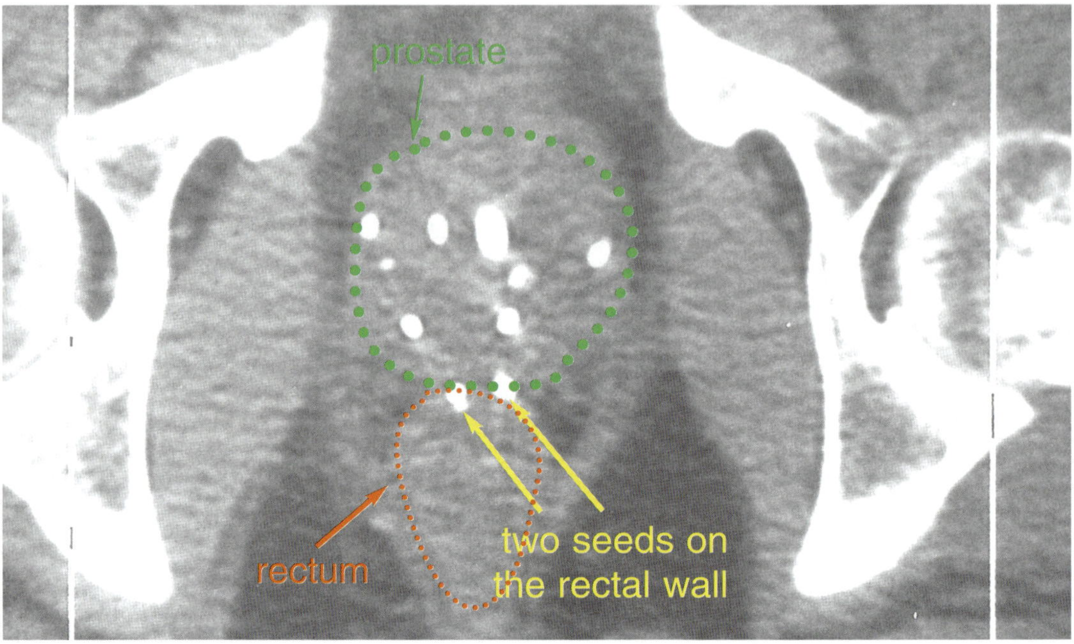

Figure 26-6. Example of seed placement allegedly responsible for post-implant rectal complication. In this patient, two seeds were on the rectal wall. An occasional peri-rectal seed is not, in itself, harmful.(MUELLER) However, a sincere-sounding plaintiff expert might convince a jury that this was the cause of a fistula.

typically claimed breach of standard of care for what most physicians would likely consider to be variations within the standard of care at the time of the implant. For example, one alleged breach of standard of care was the presence of several peri-rectal seeds, even though the overall rectal radiation dose was relatively low.(MUELLER) The plaintiff hoped that a lay jury could be convinced that even a limited number of errant seeds could be directly responsible for a serious rectal complication. In another case, a plaintiff alleged that his large prostate was the cause of his rectal fistula, even though the rectal radiation doses were not high. While these plaintiff claims were not well supported by the medical literature, there was concern that a sympathetic jury would vote a large settlement, and the cases were settled rather than tried.

While most of the fistula cases reviewed by Elliott did not involve egregious seed placement errors, they involved excessive rectal doses by today's

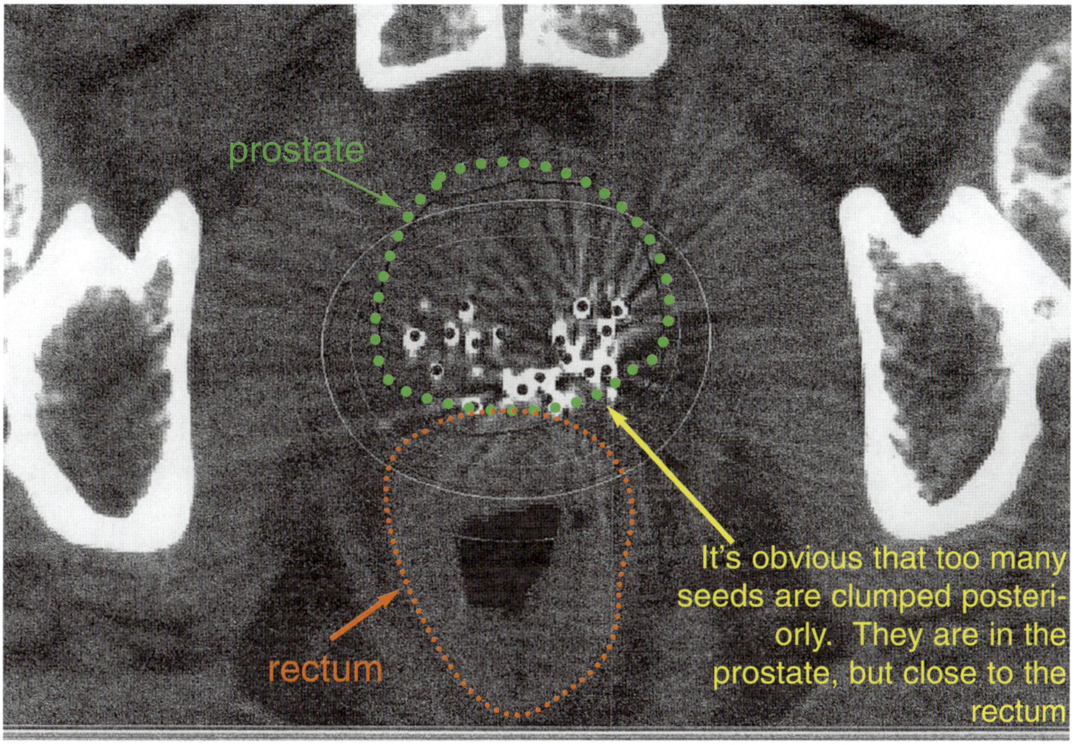

Figure 26-7. This patient developed a rectal fistula. Like many of these cases that have gone to settlement or trial, it is obvious to a layman that too many seeds are too posteriorly placed.

standards (**see Figures 26-4 through 26-8**). Many of the cases were defensible by virtue of the fact that so little data regarding proper rectal doses was available until the early 2000's.(TRAN, SNYDER) Having so little data available made it difficult for plaintiffs to establish a standard of care to support their contention of a deviation from same. However, it became clear by 2006 that more effort must be made to limit the rectal radiation dose in order to minimize the possibility of a fistula.(TRAN) The examples in Figures 24-3 to 24-7, if performed after 2006, would be very difficult to defend.(TRAN) We expect to see far fewer fistula-related cases, given what has been published more recently. Other than rectal fistulas, causes for prostate brachytherapy malpractice suits have been mostly isolated problems.

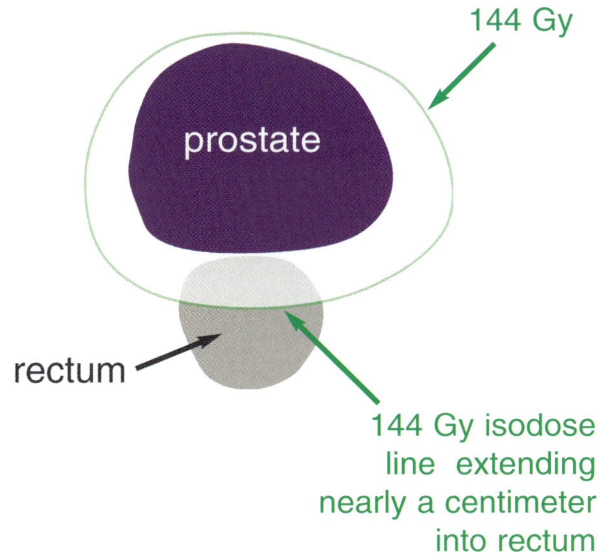

Figure 26-8. This patient developed a rectal fistula two years after a 144 Gy I-125 implant. His seed placement looks superficially acceptable, but the R100 would be high by today's standards.

Prophylactic antibiotics
One patient in the Elliott series developed osteomyelitis after an implant without prophylactic antibiotics. Even though data regarding the necessity of prophylactic antibiotics is non-existent, the plaintiff will argue that anti-bacterial prophylaxis is the standard of care.(WALLNER, DICKER) The case is ongoing.

Dysuria
One patient in the Elliott series sued over persistent dysuria. The case was dropped when no dosimetric irregularities were apparent.

Patient mix-ups
The only patient mix-up in the Elliott series was a patient who discovered in the recovery room that the plan of a different patient with the same name had been used. Fortunately for the defendant, the patients had similar sized prostates, so that the implant itself was technically appropriate. The

case was settled for a small amount, with the plaintiff claiming emotional duress.

Dose prescription errors

Patient mix-ups or mistaken dose prescriptions are hard to defend. We have seen several cases of wrong prescription doses. Fortunately, such events have usually not resulted in bad outcomes, primarily because of the range of acceptable degrees of prostate coverage. However, an obvious dose prescription error will almost always be blamed for a bad outcome, and it is hard to convince a jury otherwise. The cases we've seen to date typically involve full dose implants mistakenly prescribed with supplemental external beam radiation.

WHAT MOTIVATES PROSTATE BRACHYTHERAPY PLAINTIFFS

Rectal fistulas, in particular, entail significant morbidity, lifestyle effects and financial cost. As such, it is understandable that injured patients seek redress, even if they believe that their physicians were acting with the best intention and within the standard of care. Also likely to figure prominently is patients' desire to learn whether or not their poor outcomes were the result of malpractice, or simply bad fortune. The desire to learn the causes of therapy-related injury is understandable. In fact, little is known about the causes of unusual complications after brachytherapy; if the causes are a mystery to brachytherapy specialists, it is easy to understand that patients with poor outcomes are suspicious of a breach of standard of care. Unfortunately, filing a malpractice claim may be the only way to get a thorough airing of the quality of care delivered.(VINCENT)

FRAGMENTED CARE

One factor in the incidence of brachytherapy-related sequelae has been fragmented follow-up care. The most common cross-specialty issue has been development of a fistula after a gastroenterologist biopsies the rectal wall of a patient with proctitis. While it would seem that biopsying or cauterizing a radiation burn may make the injury worse, gastroenterologists typically claim that they felt compelled to rule out malignancy. There have been lengthy arguments over who is at fault. However, in most states the radiation oncologist is held liable, the rationale being that it was the radiation injury that lead to other damaging procedures. There have also been instances of TURPs preceding fistula development. It is possible that the urologist would be targeted as the defendant, but such cases have to be assessed individually.

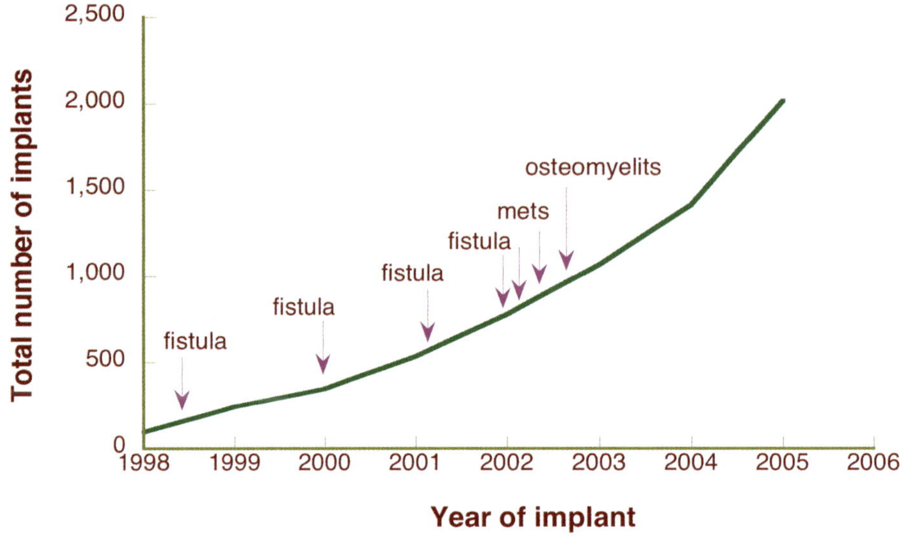

Figure 26-9. Events leading to malpractice claims against K Wallner.

Blaming other doctors for complicated post-implant management can get messy. Radiation oncologists must strive to minimize the risk of radiation-related injuries in the first place.

RADIATION ONCOLOGIST VERSUS UROLOGIST

In the Elliott series, the radiation oncologist alone was named in eight cases and the radiation oncologist and the urologist in five cases. In no case was a urologist named as a defendant without the radiation oncologist. Whatever the relationship between urologist and radiation oncologist may be in usual practice, when a complication occurs, the urologist will nearly always blame the radiation oncologist for a bad outcome, since it is the latter who prescribes the radiation dose and who should have final say intra-operatively regarding proper needle placement. Even in situations were urologists are intimately involved with seed placement, both parties must realize that it is the radiation oncologist who will likely face the brunt of a legal action. Urologists typically claim that they depend on the radiation oncologist, as the radiation expert, to assure that the doses and implementation were optimal. This defense usually successfully shields the urologist from legal exposure.

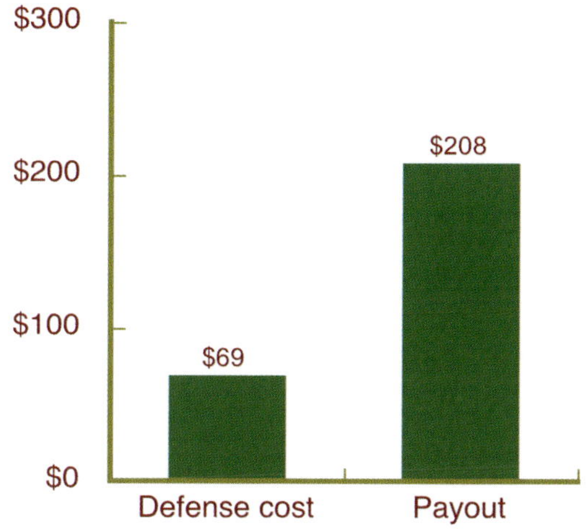

Figure 26-10. Calculated per patient legal costs for 2016 patients treated from 1998 through 2005, assuming Washington state average of $20,000 to defend each case, and average payout of $60,000 per case. The total estimated legal costs for the seven plaintiffs were averaged over the entire 2016 patients treated.

PROSPECTIVE SERIES

The retrospective work of Elliott and colleagues was the first to identify causes for brachytherapy malpractice claims. However, a more enlightening database is drawn from Kent Wallner's personal experience as a defendant. From 1998 through 2005, he implanted a total of 1940 patients at the University of Washington, the Puget Sound VA and Group Health Cooperative. To date, a total of 7 patients have filed malpractice claims against Wallner. Five of the seven claims involved rectal fistulas. A sixth case was post-operative osteomyelitis in patient who did not receive prophylactics antibiotics. The seventh case arose from failure to diagnose early metastatic disease after treatment (**Figure 26-9**). To date, three cases has been dropped, one was settled out of court, two are ongoing, and the last was settled without blame attributed to K Wallner.

A unique feature of this medico-legal series is the availability of both the number and type of complaints, and the total number of patients treated, allowing some simple calculations of the legal costs per patient treated.

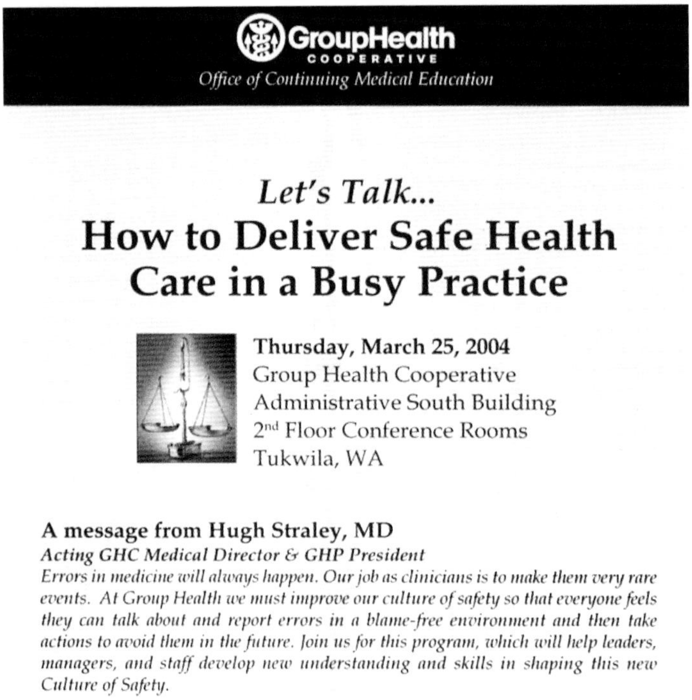

Figure 26-11. Risk management course advertisement from Group Health Cooperative in Puget Sound. There is an increasing emphasis on patient safety and risk management in corporate medicine.

While the actual costs of each case are not readily available, the typical cost to defend a case in Washington State is $20,000. Assuming $20,000 for each of the seven plaintiffs averaged over 1940 patients treated, the defense cost per patient was $69 (**Figure 26-10**). Likewise, assuming an average Washington state payout of $60,000 for each of the seven patients, the average over the 1940 patients was $208.

While the legal cost calculations are only estimates, they give a rough idea of the per patient legal costs. Of course the costs could vary dramatically depending on the particulars of each case, but even with a relatively high number of claims, the per patient costs seem relatively small. And the per patient cost should be much lower in the future, with the current minimization of rectal complications.(TRAN)

PREVENTING LAWSUITS

With most adverse situations, the best way to fix them is to avoid them. There is a growing interest, especially in corporate medicine, in managing risk (**Figure 26-11**). Most advice is of a general nature, including timely record-keeping and good patient rapport. Another common suggestion is to maintain good patient-doctor communication, even in the face of an adverse event. While no one would argue against good communication, our impression is that it does little good in the setting of a catastrophic event like a rectal fistula.

Another common piece of legal advice is to keep of detailed records. In the case of prostate brachytherapy, most record keeping revolves around the post-implant CT, since suboptimal seed placement is the basis of most claims. Analysis of a post-implant CT is standard, and the lack of one would be viewed as sloppy practice.

It seems inherently obvious that the first step to minimize legal exposure is to identify the causes and fixes for adverse events. Identification and analysis of adverse events has long been the rule for the automobile and airline industries, where mistakes can have catastrophic repercussions.(HELMREICH) Unfortunately, little published data exists regarding specific causes of suits in medical care. Instead, the specifics of medical malpractice are largely hidden from publication. How stupid. Hiding mistakes is the best way to keep them happening again and again.

The work of Elliott and colleagues serves as a model of how radiation oncologists should address malpractice risk. Had Elliott not made the effort to summarize and publicise cases, there would still be no published guidance regarding the importance of fistulas in the malpractice arena. Now that their central role in prostate brachytherapy malpractice has been analyzed and publicized, practitioners can focus on avoiding them, thereby minimizing their own exposure to litigation risk.

CONSENT FORMS

There is remarkably little objective data to guide the content and scope of informed consent documents. General advice is to make consents detailed, and document that all forseeable risks were discussed between practitioner and patient. The reality, however, is that a patient who experiences a bad outcome can *always* claim insufficient medical knowledge to truly understand the consent form. Additionally, regardless of discussion beforehand, plaintiff attorneys can argue that an informed consent does not include consent to malpractice. So a deviation from standard of care will most likely not be excused based on informed consent for the procedure.

Table 26-3. Specifics of Puget Sound VA consent form

<u>Potential complications from prostate seed implants</u>
temporary use of tube (catheter) in penis to allow urination
(1 out of 20 patients)

permanent urine leakage, requiring pads
(1 out of 20 patients)

permanent impotence (loss of erections) and/or loss of semen
(1 out of 2 patients)

radiation burn to rectum, requiring major surgery
(1 out of 500 patients)

movement of seeds to the heart or brain, causing serious damage
(1 out of 2,000)

movement of seeds to the lungs, with no known ill effects
(1 out of 4)

I have read these potential complications and have had a chance to clarify my questions

Patient Initials: X__________

Written informed consent is not as protective as one might like, but omitting it can be a problem. Lack of it can be used to bolster an otherwise marginal case. The consent form used by K Wallner at the Puget Sound VA is very specific regarding the likelihood of myriad complications (**Table 26-3**).

TORT REFORM

Another reason why the medical tort system is unlikely to change is that the players, both attorneys and experts, find it very profitable. Defense and plaintiff attorneys stand to collect large fees, mostly in cases that are settled without a court appearance. Expert witnesses make a lot money, too. Plaintiff witnesses, especially, may be paid thousands of dollars simply to sign a statement that a case is medically legitimate. There are multiple

Table 26-4. Commonly advocated strategies to improve the malpractice system.

Better self-policing
Of course it would be nice if doctors would self-police more effectively, but we've not done well in this regard. The closest we've come to this in is peer-review. But peer-review has been plagued by financial undertones that make the whole process suspect. Doctors, especially bad ones, are too arrogant and litigious for this to work well. **Won't work**.

Special health courts
This is a nice idea, and it has a precedent in tax courts, where specially trained judges are better qualified to make fair decisions. But it is unlikely to work with medical malpractice, partly because the number of cases is too small to warrant a whole new court system. **Unlikely**.

Policing of experts
Yes, this seems reasonable, but plaintiff attorneys would not tolerate infringement on their right to seek experts willing to make their case. This policy sounds good, but would be contentious in action. **Won't work**.

Dispute resolution
This would essentially require that patients give up their right to a jury trial. **Unlikely**. **Unconstitutional.**

No fault system
This could work well, and would likely direct monies from legal personnel back to injured patients. But putting it in place would require a monumental, sustained political effort. Insurers would fight it. **Unlikely**. **Massive cost.**

Limit lawyer fees
This is tantamount of limiting citizens' right to representation. **Good luck**!

Caps on damages
This has been partially effective, but the caps are still high enough to make malpractice judgements painful for the defense. **Mildly helpful, at best**.

Table 26-5. Real-life deposition exchange between plaintiff attorney and a prostate brachytherapist. This should give you an idea of how degrading the deposition process can get.

attorney: are you surprised, based on the medical school training and internship,residency, chief resident and a fellowship, with all those credentials and experience, are you surprised that you cannot pass the Board certification?

doctor: I think there are other factors involved in passing the exams.

attorney: Do you tell your patients that you haven't passed this Board certification?

doctor: It doesn't come up.

attorney: Do you think that's something a patient should be informed about?

doctor: I don't think so.

attorney: Okay. Are you comfortable with putting on record today that in your opinion you have a special expertise in the area of radiation oncology?

proposals to improve the current malpractice environment. Most are somewhere between impractical and unconstitutional (**Table 26-4**).

ADVICE TO BRACHYTHERAPISTS FACING A LAWSUIT

Fortunately, only a minority of brachytherapists will face a serious lawsuit. For those that do, there a a few points to keep in mind:

First, you are not alone. Even the "experts" gets sued. Wallner is a poster child example of a practitioner who lives, eats and breaths prostate brachytherapy, and still has faced numerous suits. And there are other, not-to-be-named prominent brachytherapists who have faced multiple suits. So you're in good company.

Second, regardless of how your supporters want to downplay the significance, the outcome of a suit is important—it can substantially affect insur-

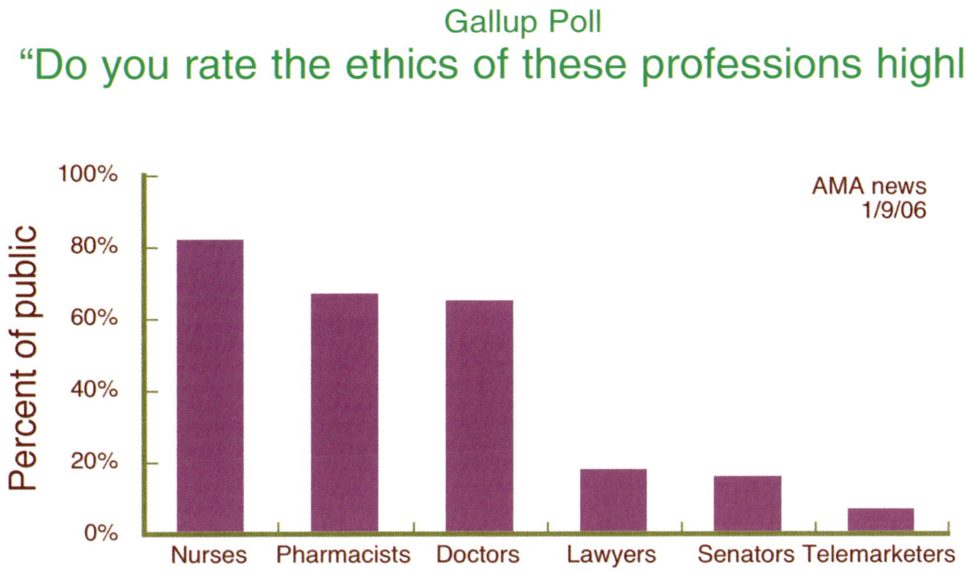

Figure 26-12. Public perception of the ethics of various professions.

ance rates and your reputation. So pay attention. It is imperative that the defense of a suit move to the top of your priority list. Review the case and be aware of the potential criticisms. Be ready to defend your actions in dealing with the patient. Don't get caught by surprise by a plaintiff attorney. Be humble. Be available to your defense team. Get an expert who is very familiar with the literature, and who can convey knowledge to a jury. (The authors of this text have faced a number of well-credentialed, famous experts who were obviously inadequately familiar with the literature, or were too arrogant.)

Third, understand that plaintiff attorneys are extremely skilled at making doctors look bad in a deposition or in front of a jury. Expect them to questions your credentials and every decision, often in a surprisingly derisive manner (**Table 26-5**). Doctors walk into a court room with a tremendous reputational advantage over plaintiff lawyers (**Figure 26-12**). But lawyers will work to chip away at that goodwill. When all else fails, they will ask how much money your experts are being paid—an effective strategy to diminish a jury's sympathy for doctors (**Figure 26-13**).

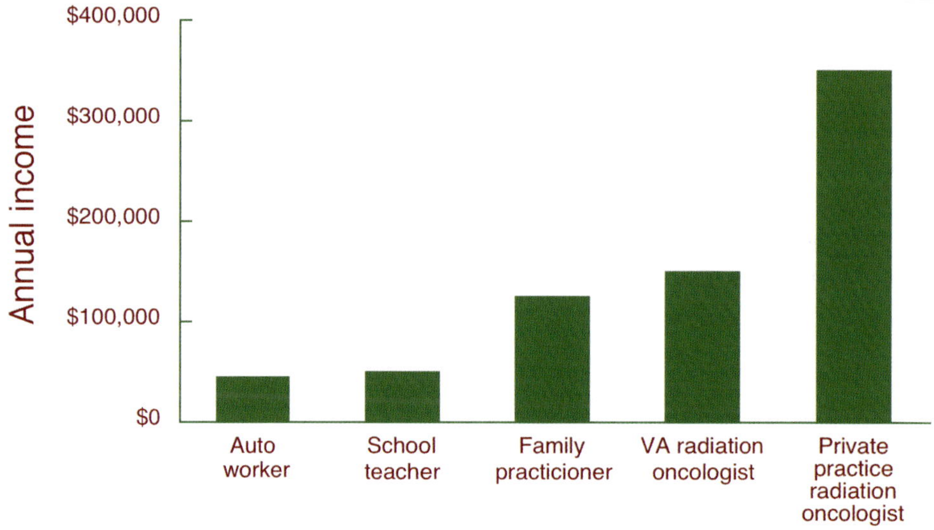

Figure 26-13. Sampling of typical physician incomes versus some other occupations. These disparities lessen a jury's sympathy for a physician, especially faced with a plaintiff who has incurred overwhelming medical bills. The huge disparity in physician income and that of a typical patient/juror is easily alluded to in the course of a trial. And a juror is much more likely to identify with an auto worker or school teacher than a private practice radiation oncologist.

THE FUTURE OF PROSTATE BRACHYTHERAPY LAWSUITS

Prostate brachytherapists should brace themselves for the likelihood of more lawsuits. First, the sheer number of implants continues to increase, so that the law of averages may result in more adverse outcomes. Even if we completely prevent fistulas, plaintiff attorneys are likely to identify more bases for lawsuits in the future.

One potential basis for future suits may be failure-to-cure. There is increasing evidence that cure rates are linked to achievement of minimal radiation dose parameter values (V100 or D90 and treatment margins).(HERSTEIN, ORIO, STOCK, POTTERS, PAPAGIKOS) It seems likely that future patients who are not cured may claim substandard care if their post-implant parameters were sub-optimal. Anyone performing prostate brachytherapy needs to keep up with the dosimetric literature and make sure that the CT-based dosimetry parameters stay within the standard of care.

REFERENCES

1. Dicker AP, Figura AT, Waterman FM, al e. Is there a role for antibiotic prophylaxis in transperineal interstitial permanent prostate brachytherapy? Techniques in Urology 2000; 6:104-108.
2. Elliott K, Wallner K, Merrick G, Herstein P. Medical malpractice claims in a prostate brachytherapy practice: Causes and legal costs. (submitted) 2006.
3. Garner B. Black's law dictionary. St. Paul, MN: West Group, 1999.
4. Helmreich RL. On error management: lessons from aviation. BMJ 2000; 320:781-785.
5. Mello MM, Studdert DM, Brennan TA. The new medical malpractice crisis. N Eng J Med 2003; 348:2281-2284.
6. Moreira S, Seigne J, Ordorica R, Marceet J, Pow-sang J, Lockhart J. Devastating complications after brachytherapy in the treatment of prostate adenocarcinoma. Br J Urol 2004; 93:31-35.
7. Mueller A, Wallner K, Merrick G, Cavanagh W, Butler W. Peri-rectal seeds as a risk factor for prostate brachytherapy-related rectal bleeding. Int J Rad Oncol Biol Phys 2004; 59:1047-1052.
8. Nag SN, Beyer D, Friedland J, Grimm P, Nath R. American Brachytherapy Society (ABS) recommendations for transperineal permanent brachytherapy of prostate cancer. Int J Radiat Oncol Biol Phys 1999; 44:789-799.
9. Orio P, Wallner K, Merrick G, et al. Dosimetric parameters as predictive factors for biochemical control in patients with higher risk prostate cancer treated with Pd-103 and supplemental beam radiation. Int J Rad Oncol Biol Phys 2007; 67:342-346.
10. Papagikos M, deGuzman AF, Rossi P, CMcCullough D, Clark P, Lee WR. Dosimetric quantifiers for low-dose-rate prostate brachytherapy: Is V100 superior to D90? Brachytherapy 2005; 4:252-258.
11. Potters L, Cao Y, Calugaru E, Torre T, Fearn P, Wang X. A comprehensive review of CT-based dosimetry parameters and biochemical control in patients treated with permanent prostate brachytherapy. Int J Rad Oncol Biol Phys 2001; 50:605-614.
12. Snyder KM, Stock RG, Hong SM, Lo YC, Stone NN. Defining the risk of developing grade 2 proctitis following 125-I prostate brachytherapy using a rectal dose-volume histogram analysis. Int J Rad Oncol Biol Phys 2001; 50:335-341.

13. Stock RG, Stone NN, Cesaaretti J, Rosenstein B. Biologically effective dose values for prostate brachytherrapy: Effects on PSA failure and posttreatment biopsy results. Int J Rad Oncol Biol Phys 2006; 64:527-533.
14. Tran A, Wallner K, Merrick G, Seeberger J, Armstrong J, Mueller A. Rectal fistulas following prostate brachytherapy. Int J Rad Oncol Biol Phys 2005; 63:150-154.
15. Vincent C, Young M, Phillips A. Why do people sue doctors? A study of patients and relative taking legal action. Lancet 1994; 343:1609-1613.
16. Wallner K, Merrick G, True L, Sutlief S, Cavanagh W, Butler W. I-125 versus Pd-103 for low risk prostate cancer: Preliminary biochemical outcomes from a prospective randomized mulitcenter trial. Int J Rad Oncol Biol Phys 2003; 57:1297-1303.
17. Wallner KE, Roy J, Harrison L. Low risk of perioperative infection without prophylactic antibiotics for transperineal prostate brachytherapy. Int J Radiat Oncol Biol Phys 1996; 36:681-683.
18. Zhan C, Miller M. Excess length of stay, charges, and mortality attributable to medical injuries during hospitalization. JAMA 2003; 290:1868-1874.

27

Cost

Treatment of prostate cancer is expensive. Of approximately 200,000 new cases diagnosed annually in the Unites States, 80% are clinically localized to the prostate. If all patients with localized disease are treated with definitive therapy, at an average charge of $25,000, the annual consumer cost of primary treatment alone would be almost $4 billion per year (**Table 27-1**). Initial treatment of all early-stage patients amounts to approximately 1% of the yearly Medicare budget (**Figure 27-1**). And the cost of treatment-related problems, cancer recurrence, and palliative care for patients with metastatic cancers is considerably higher.(CARLSSON, WILSON)

Table 27-1. Approximate annual cost of curative treatment of clinically localized prostate cancer in the United States.

New cases:	200,000
Clinically localized (80%):	160,000
Average cost per patient:	$25,000
Total cost, all patients:	$4,000,000,000

PRICES, CHARGES, AND COSTS

Prices, *charges,* and *costs* are relative terms, the proper choice of which depends on the context in which they are used. By definition, the *price* of a commodity is the market-based agreement between what the consumer is willing to pay and the provider is willing to accept. Thus, in a free-market system, price is arrived at efficiently. In contrast, the price of medical care is influenced by third-party payers (government, insurers, employers) who stand between the patient (consumer) and the medical industry (provider). Because they represent large numbers of patients, third-party payers have a remarkable influence on the market-derived price. *Charges* are the fees that providers (physicians and hospitals) bill for their services. In the past, charges were similar to prices. But prices of medical services currently are typically substantially lower than the charges, because of discounting demanded by third parties. And the prices, charges, and costs of medical care in the United States are constantly changing due to evolving governmental and managed care policies.

The best way around the vagaries of prices and charges would be to analyze medical care in terms of its *production cost*. Unfortunately, the production cost of medical care is even harder to determine than current charges or prices, due in part to the complexity of separating out the production cost of a service from the myriad overlapping activities of physician time and hospital services. In fact, most institutions don't know their production cost for a complex procedure like prostate brachytherapy. And if they do, they're typically not interested in publishing it.(CIEZKI)

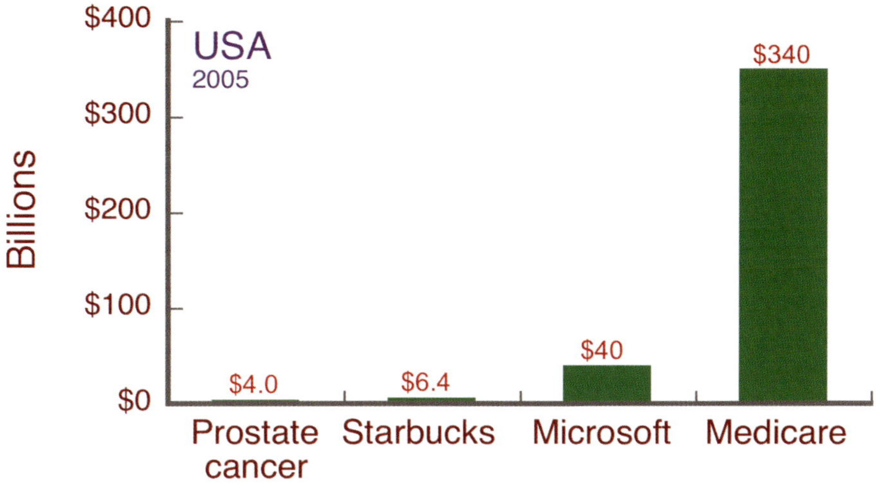

Figure 27-1. Total cost to provide primary, curative treatment for all U.S. patients with clinically localized prostate cancer, compared to net revenue for Starbucks coffee products, Microsoft or the annual Medicare budget.

To make matters worse, the definition of *cost* varies. For instance, a hospital bill for open-heart surgery is viewed as a "charge" by the local dominant HMO, only a starting point for negotiations in the final price. But the same hospital bill is clearly a *cost* to a private patient, paying out-of-pocket and legally obligated to pay in full. Any discussion regarding the specifics of medical costs is fraught with inconsistencies and ambiguities in how *costs* are cited.

WHO PAYS THE BILLS

Analysis of medical costs is complicated by the plethora of payer types within U.S. health care. There are four general categories of payers: individuals, government programs (Medicare and Medicaid), private fee-for-service (the "Blues" and other indemnity plans), and managed care (HMOs, PPOs, etc.) (**Table 27-2**). Medicare rates have a disproportionate effect on other pricing systems because they are used for guidance by non-governmental parties when setting the consumer price of medical care. The percent of patients in various payer categories has changed substantially, and the movement toward managed care probably will continue.

Table 27-2. Who pays the bills.

Type of payer	Source of money	Primary price-setter
Medicare	Federal tax	Centers for Medicare and Medicaid Services (CMS)
Medicaid	Federal/state tax	HCFA/state agencies
Managed care	Employer/individual	Market
Fee-for-service	Employer/individual	Physician/hospital

Of the four payer types, fee-for-service plans generally offer the highest reimbursements to providers, presumably the cost for patients to have their free choice of doctors and to be treated in the more prestigious institutions (perhaps) by the more prestigious doctors (perhaps). The cost of fee-for-service plans is inflated by cost-shifting, whereby fee-for-service patients are charged more because they are not organized to negotiate lower prices. Fee-for-service patients cannot negotiate down their costs, and are legally responsible for the amounts billed. Sporadic attempts to control fee-for-service charges through government-mandated price controls have failed. Cost-shifting will continue to some extent, as long as there is some element of fee-for-service in the system. However, as the percent of patients enrolled in managed care climbs, cost-shifting has become an increasingly impractical way for physicians and hospitals to cover costs or boost income.

THE COST OF FAILURE

Before delving into the cost of therapy, it's important to emphasize that cancer therapy costs are dwarfed by the cost of recurrence. Patients who are not cured may require palliative therapy and long-term hormonal ablation, and suffer substantial income loss. A patient who lives five years with recurrent, metastatic disease might lose five years of productive work time, valued at $250,000. He would typically receive five years of androgen ablation at an approximate total cost of $30,000. At the more advanced stage of metastatic disease, hospitalization and palliative treatment costs climb rapidly. A conservative estimate of the additional cost in this case would be $320,000, dwarfing the initial treatment charges of more than $35,000 for even the most costly therapy—combined implant plus supple-

Cost of recurrence versus therapy

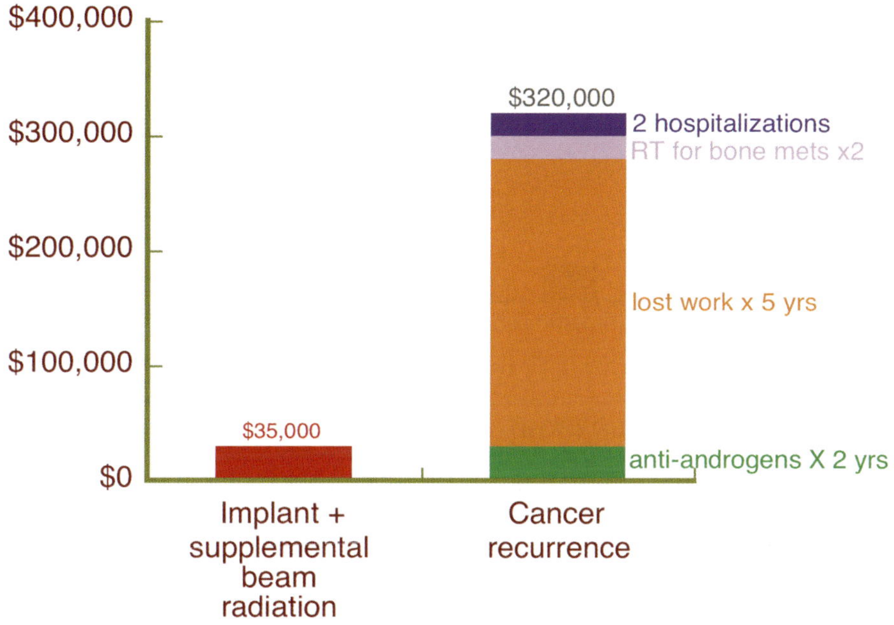

Figure 27-2. Even the most expensive therapy appears cheap compared to the cost of cancer recurrence.

mental external radiation (**Figures 27-2**). And the actual cost of cancer recurrence could rise to many times the $320,000 estimated in Figure 27-3, depending on whether salvage therapy is used and how much palliative care is required. The cost of palliative therapies are likely to increase substantially in the foreseeable future.(WILSON) And for younger patients especially, lost wages could far exceed direct medical costs.

COMPARING MODALITIES

There is still surprisingly little written about the cost of prostate cancer treatment. Earlier studies comparing external radiation, prostatectomy, and brachytherapy are outdated due to substantial changes in the way treatments are delivered.(HANKS, COTTER) In the next few pages, we'll summarize the limited number of more recently published series regarding prostate cancer treatment costs. Read all of this skeptically, because the published numbers may be outdated, or skewed by how a procedure is

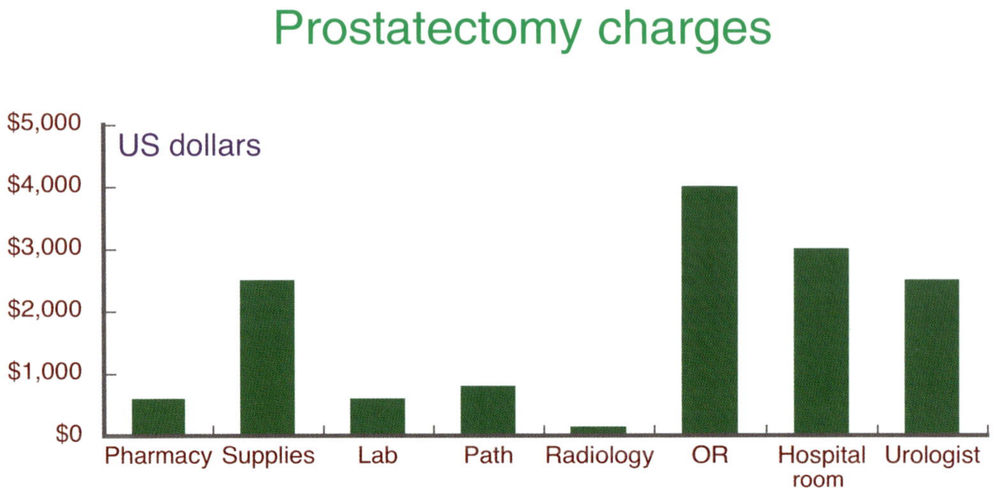

Figure 27-3. Breakdown of approximate charges for radical prostatectomy in 2006.

conducted at a particular institution. Overhead costs are especially difficult to accurately determine for a specific medical procedure.

Prostatectomy

Based on Medicare reimbursements, the total consumer cost of a prostatectomy is approximately $14,000, 80% of which represents hospital charges and 20% physician fees (**Figure 27-3**).(ONCOLOGY)

Since most of the surgical costs represent hospital charges, substantial savings can be achieved through early abdominal drain removal, early ambulation and oral feeding, early hospital discharge, and more judicious use of laboratory tests. These goals can be achieved through aggressive preoperative patient education and by continuous monitoring by a dedicated cost-control team. With a concerted effort, substantial savings have been achieved. University of Chicago surgeons were able to decrease the average hospitalization from five days to two days, with total treatment cost cut by 34%.(PALMER) Such cost savings require constant vigilance to maintain.

Robotic surgery can be substantially more expensive that open operations.(LOTAN) The US dollar approximations shown in Figure 27-3 do not reflect the $2,000 additional cost of robotic disposables per case, longer

External beam radiation charges

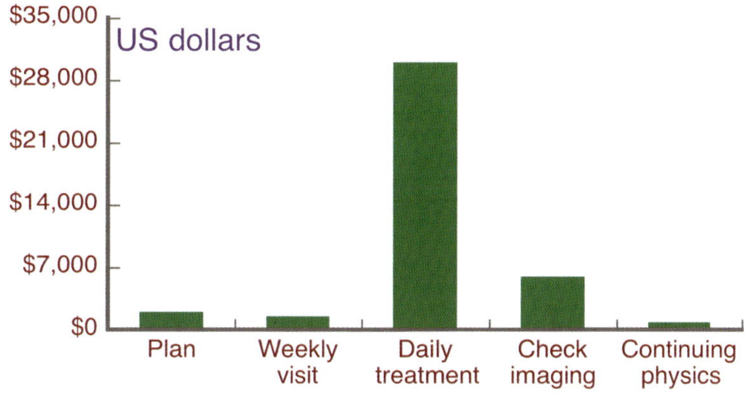

Figure 27-4. Approximate Medicare reimbursments for IMRT external beam radiation (75 Gy) in 2006.

operating room time or additional anesthesia. Nor do they include the $200,000 annual robot service agreement cost that should be spread out over the patients treated.

External beam radiation

Based on Medicare reimbursements, the cost of 76 Gy external beam radiation is approximately $35,000, 80% of which is due to hospital charges and 20% to physician fees (**Figure 27-4**). And IGRT (image guided) is driving these costs still higher.

In past analyses, charges for external beam radiation have been lower than that of a prostatectomy.(HANKS, COTTER) However, the provider cost to deliver external radiation has risen with increasingly sophisticated treatment plans and delivery systems, such that private charges for high-dose IMRT are approaching $100,000. While managed care plans currently may not reimburse at this charge level, if outcomes data show that better technical delivery and higher doses increase cure rates while decreasing complication rates, upward price pressure will persist.

The beam radiation figures quoted here are charges. Actual production cost figures are hard to come by. European investigators estimate exter-

Brachytherapy charges

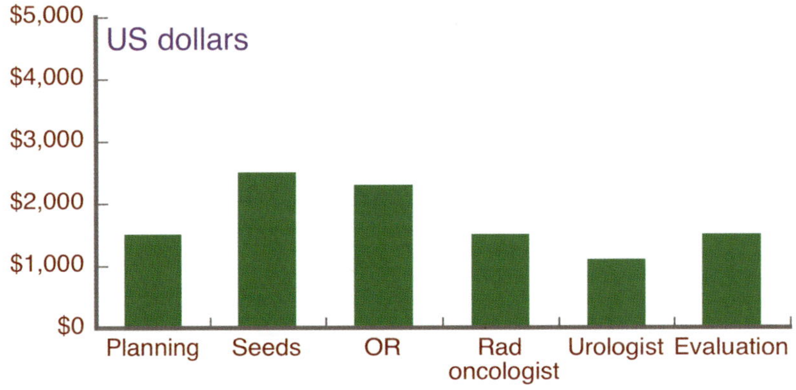

Figure 27-5. Approximate Medicare brachytherapy reimbursements in 2006.

nal beam production costs at about $220 per dose, pooling all departmental costs and dividing by the number of patients treated.(WODINSKY) And keep in mind that the cost of providing conformal therapy and IMRT is substantially higher.(HORWITZ)

Implant alone

Based on 1996 Medicare reimbursement rates, the charges for a prostate brachytherapy totals approximately $12,000, 80% of which represents hospital charges and 20% physician charges (**Figure 27-5**).

The cost of the seeds themselves is a substantial portion of the bill. The typical cost to the provider for I-125 or Pd-103 is about $2,500 to $5,000. Some hospitals mark up the seed price, bringing the charges to $6,000 or more.

Supplemental external beam radiation

Implant alone is a cost-competitive therapy relative to prostatectomy or external radiation. However, the addition of supplemental external beam radiation increases the cost substantially. The consumer cost of the supplemental radiation (40–50 Gy) is close to that of full-course radiation alone, since a simulation is still needed and the number of treatments is decreased by only 30%. The brachytherapy costs can be decreased from those of a full-dose implant if 30% fewer seeds are used. However, many practitioners use lower activity seeds for boost implants, so that just as many are required.

If the high cure rates reported by some investigators are truly representative, then the high up front costs of implant plus supplemental external radiation could be a bargain in the long-term by avoiding the costs of cancer recurrence. But in the short term, it's very expensive therapy.

COMPARING COSTS

Several reports regarding the charges for brachytherapy versus radical prostatectomy have appeared. Disregarding the cost of the radioactive seeds, brachytherapy is less costly than surgery, the primary cost components being operative room time and physician fees. But when the cost of seeds is included, brachytherapy charges are similar to surgery (**Figures 27-3 through 27-10**). Published studies, to date, compared only *charges*, as opposed to actual provider's cost to deliver therapy. But either way, probably the same conclusion would be reached—there is no clear cost advantage surgery versus brachytherapy. What is becoming clear is that external beam radiation is rapidly outpacing other modalities as being far and away the most expensive treatment option (**Figure 27-11**).(WILSON 07)

DIRECT, INDIRECT, AND INTANGIBLES

Using Medicare or private charges is the most common way to compare the cost of medical therapies. But the total cost of a medical therapy is far more complicated than simply tabulating the initial charges for the treatment itself. First of all, it is nearly impossible to calculate accurate production cost figures, which are difficult to separate from other services provided at a large medical center. Second, therapy charges quoted don't include the associated costs of treatment-related complications and accessory therapies. To get a more realistic cost estimate, medical costs can be divided into direct, indirect, and intangible costs (**Table 27-3**).

Direct costs

Direct costs include amounts paid to medical providers for medical goods and services. They can be divided into *primary* and *secondary* direct costs.

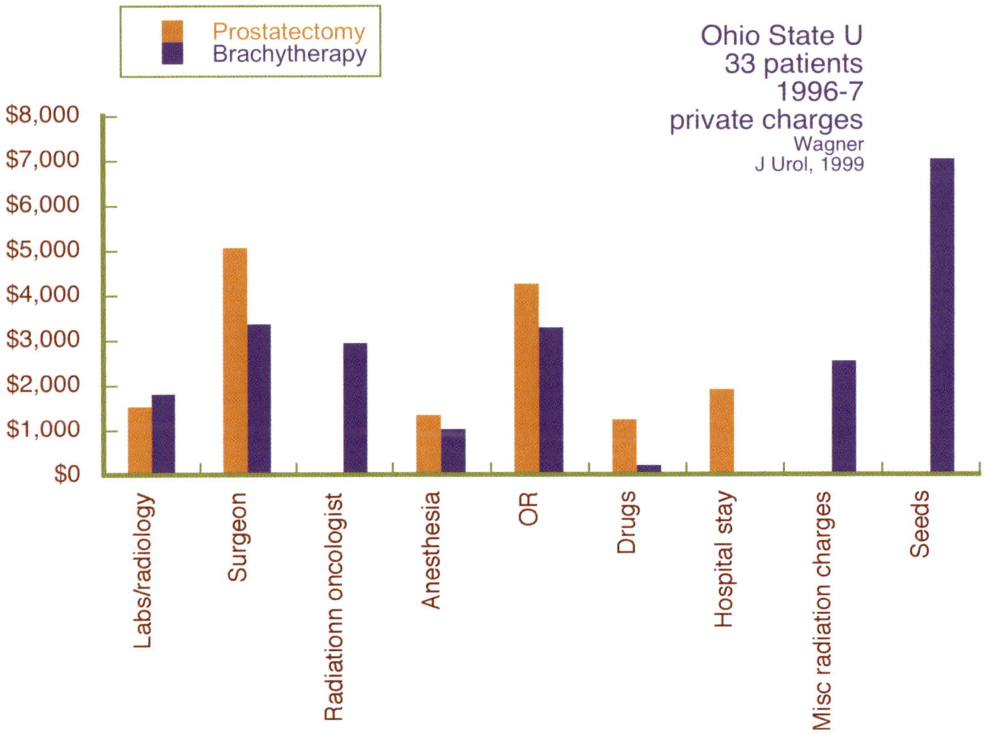

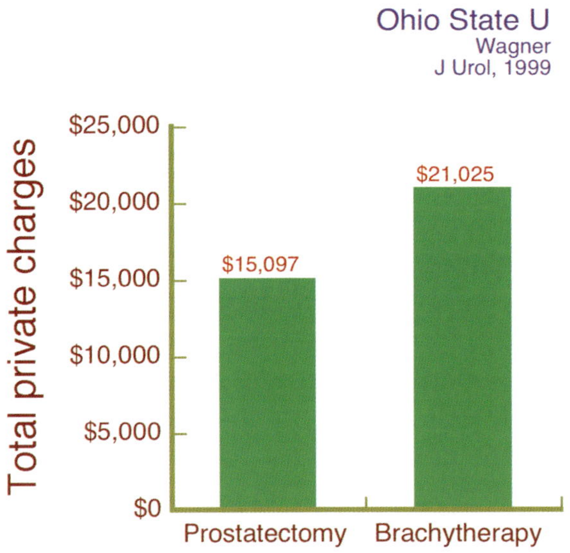

Figure 27-6. Breakdown comparison of private charges for prostatectomy versus brachytherapy at Ohio State University (above). Total charges for brachytherapy (left) were almost $6,000 higher, but included supplemental external beam radiation in some patients.

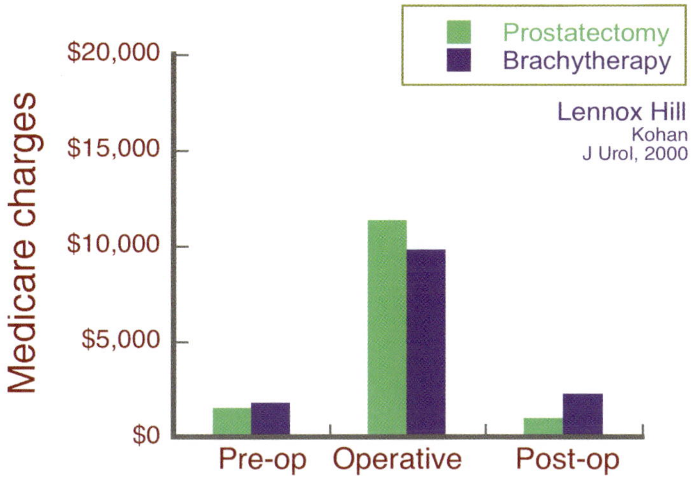

Figure 27-7. Breakdown comparison of Medicare charges for prostatectomy versus brachytherapy at Lenox Hill Hospital (above). Total charges between modalities were almost identical (lower).

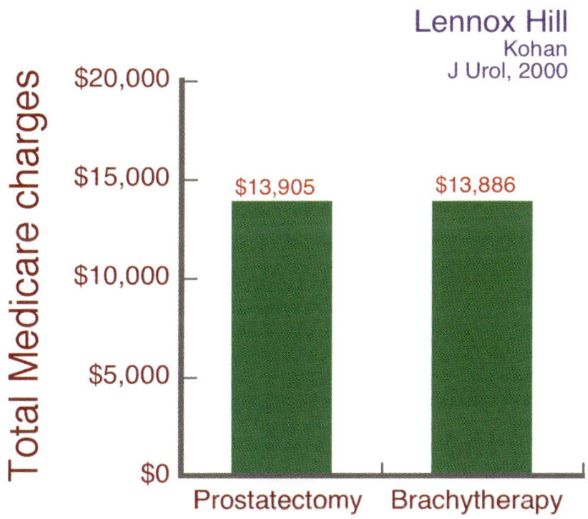

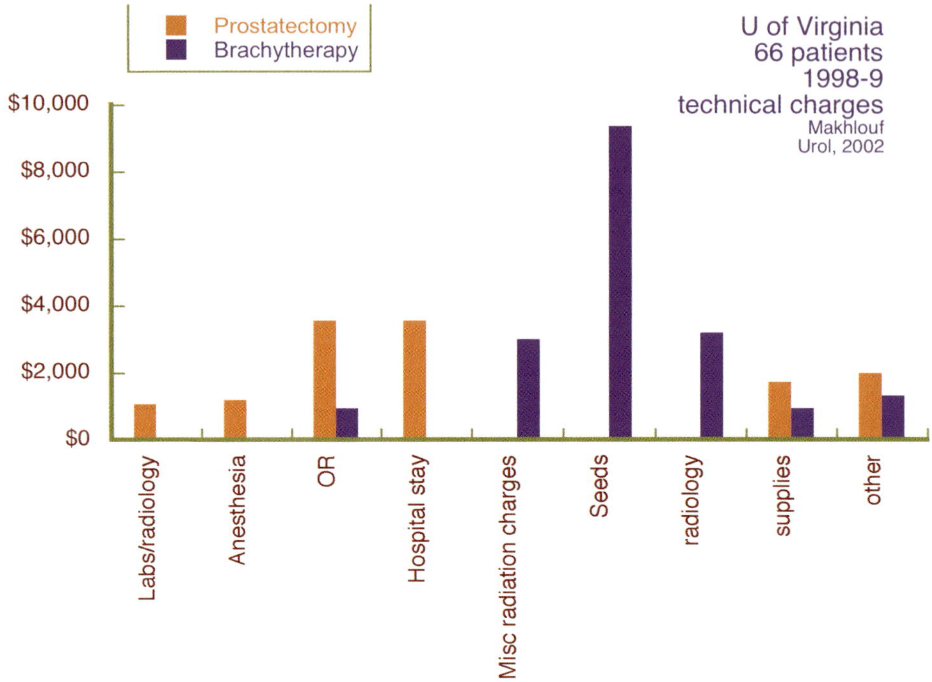

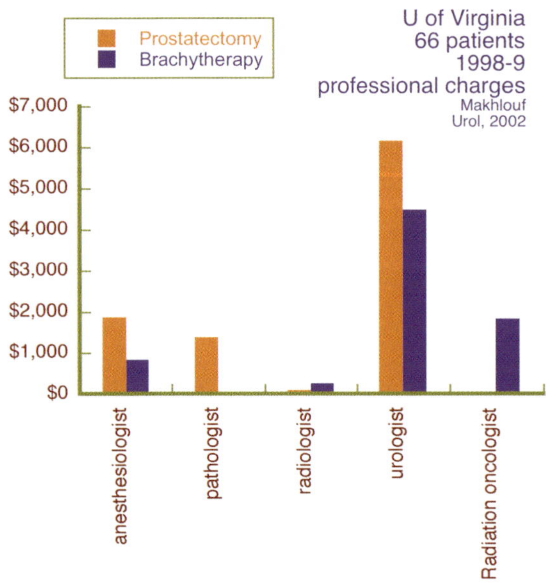

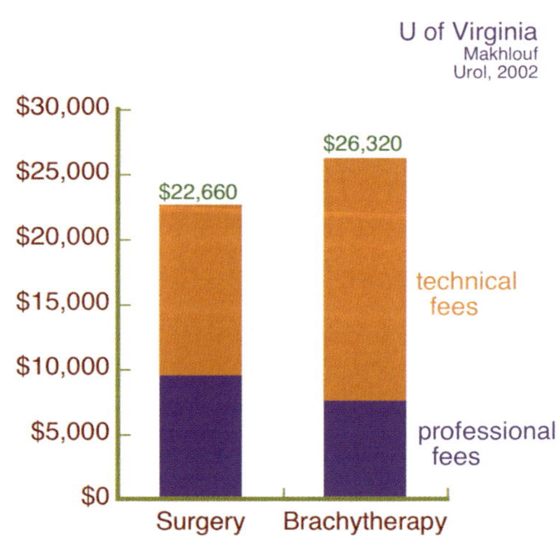

Figure 27-8. Detailed breakdown of private technical and professional charges.

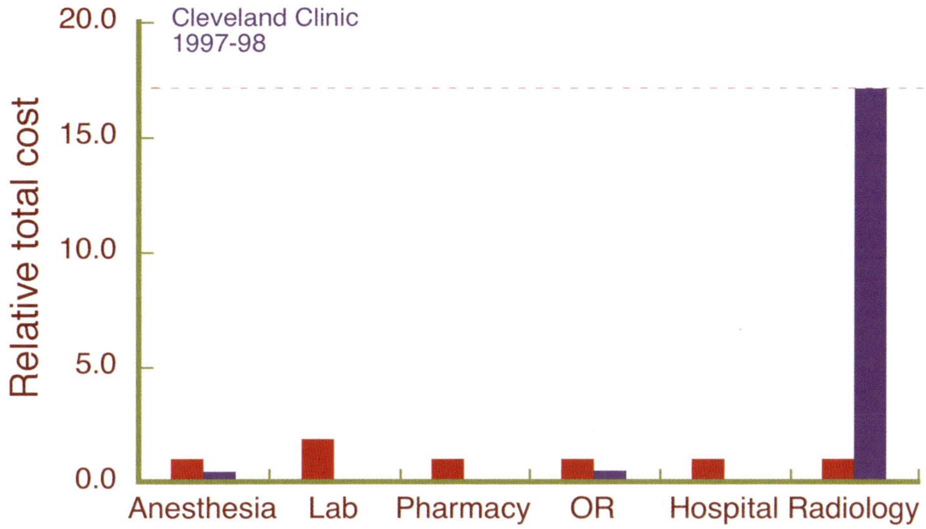

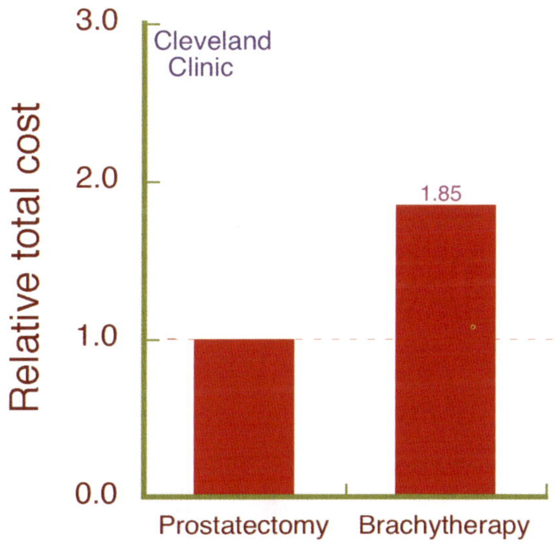

Figure 27-9. Alleged costs to perform prostatectomy compared to brachytherapy. This study is the first to use costs rather than charges. However, due to propriety concerns of the Cleveland Clinic Foundation, the brachytherapy figures were reported as relative to those of prostatectomy, rather than in actual dollars, making comparison to other hospitals difficult. Unfortunately, actual costs of a given procedure are difficult to separate from myriad other costs of a large, complex medical institution. These figures should be viewed skeptically.(CIEZKI)

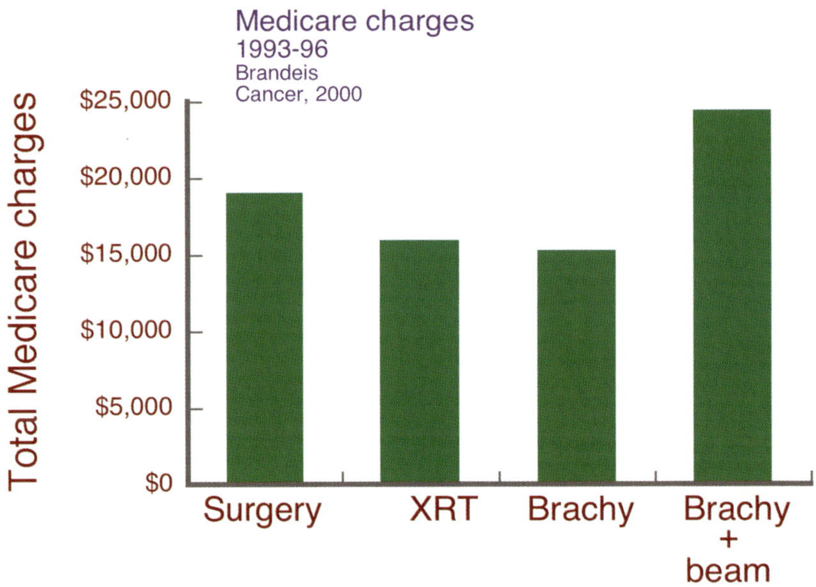

Figure 27-10. Total Medicare charges for prostatectomy, external beam radiation (XRT), transperineal implant, and implant+XRT. This data was from the 1990s.

Primary direct costs include those of the treatment itself: physician fees, operating room time, hospitalization, medication, laboratory fees, etc. These are the costs typically quoted by providers and typically used to calculate published comparisons between modalities.

Secondary direct costs are the insidious subsequent costs occasioned by treatment-related complications, accessory treatments, and treatment for recurrent disease. Secondary direct costs can be referred to as *hidden* costs, because they are not easily anticipated and are often ignored in providers' price quotes. Identifying secondary direct costs is crucial to determining the realistic, total consumer or societal cost of prostate cancer.

Indirect costs

Traditionally, indirect medical costs are the personal costs that a patient incurs by receiving treatment, including such things as travel costs and child care. *Lost wages* is the most easily quantified indirect cost and is the only one considered here.

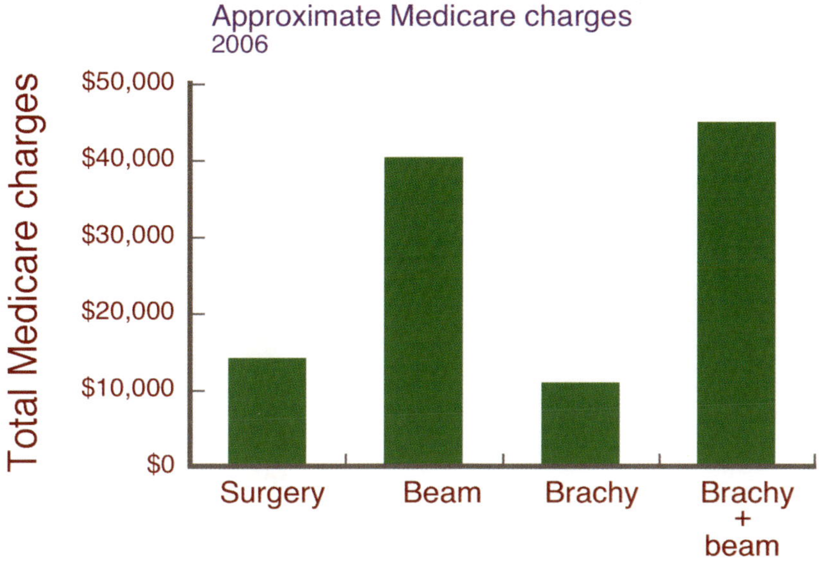

Figure 27-11. Approximate total 2006 Medicare charges for prostatectomy, external beam radiation (IMRT), implant, and implant+beam.

Table 27-3. Direct and indirect consumer medical costs.

Category	Example
Primary direct	hospitalization physician fees lab tests
Secondary direct	complications accessory treatments salvage therapy
Indirect (societal, personal)	lost wages

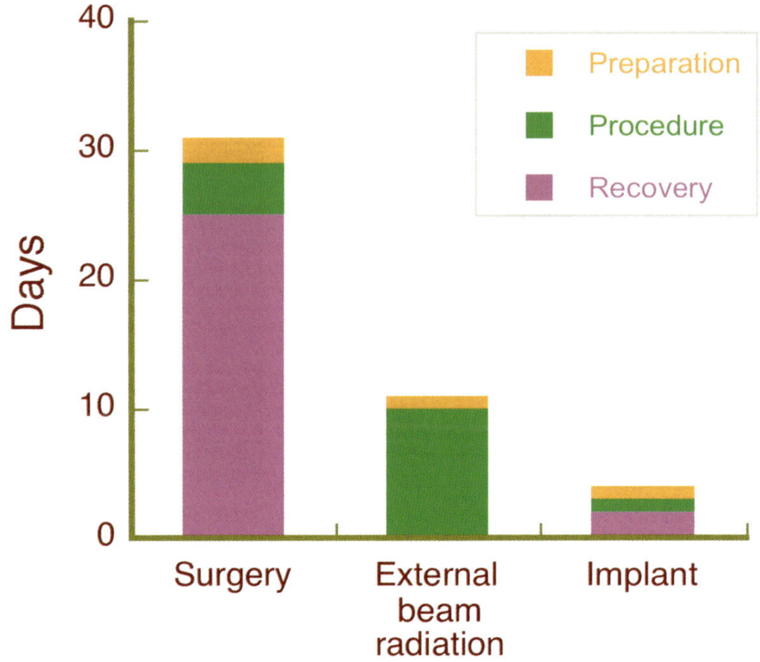

Figure 27-12. Work days missed with each modality. Numbers are estimations and could vary substantially, based on patient circumstances and physician policy regarding postoperative care.

Intangibles

As with most serious diseases and their treatments, there are substantial intangible costs to prostate cancer therapies, including physical discomfort, mental stress, and social disruptions. While clearly important, intangible medical costs are not easy to quantify and are not included in the cost considerations here. To date, indications are that relatively few major problems are associated with brachytherapy, and that it compares favorably to prostatectomy and external beam radiation.(BRANDEIS, HAN)

LOST WAGES

Perhaps the largest cost of treatment is related to lifestyle effects. Cancer-related lifestyle cost studies are still in their infancy.(YARBROFF) However, a relatively easily estimated factor is lost work time. Work time missed with an implant includes an office visit for treatment planning volume study and pre-anesthesia testing. The treatment itself, performed on an outpatient basis, requires one day off work. The at-home recovery time typically would be 1 to 3 days.

Work time missed with a prostatectomy includes time spent donating autologous blood, estimated at one day. The hospital stay is typically 3 to 5 days, in the absence of serious complications. The recovery time at home is generally 3 to 6 weeks, although some of that time could be spent working at home, depending on the nature of the patient's occupation.

Work days missed with beam radiation include those for simulation and for daily treatments. If one assumes a half day missed for simulation and plan verification and two hours missed for each of 40 treatments, a total of approximately eleven days would be missed.

Granted, these missed work estimates are sketchy. But few would argue that brachytherapy-related lost days compare favorably with external beam radiation or prostatectomy (**Figure 27-12**).

COST—THE ULTIMATE MEDICAL MYSTERY

Medical costs, incomes, and profits, especially from complex procedures, are difficult to quantify accurately. They vary by region and are constantly changing. And there is limited cost transparency. Patients seldom ask about charges, because of third party payers standing between the patient and provider.

The numbers given here are broad estimates. They are food for thought but suffer from substantial uncertainties. Brachytherapy, without supplemental hormonal therapy or beam radiation, is probably the most cost-effective therapy. But it is not necessarily the most lucrative for physicians or hospitals.

REFERENCES

1. Brandeis J, Pashos CL, Henning JM, Litwin MS. A nationwide charge comparison of the principal treatments for earlly stage prostat carcinoma. Cancer 2000; 89:1792-1799.

2. Carlsson P, Hjertberg H, Jonsson B, Varenhorst E. The cost of prostatic cancer in a defined population. Scand J Urol Nephrol Suppl 1989; 23:93-96.
3. Ciezki JP, Klein EA, Angermeier KW, Ulchaker J, Zippe CD, Wilkinson DA. Cost comparison of radical prostatectomy and transperineal brachytherapy for localized prostate cancer. Urol 2000; 55:68-72.
4. Cotter GW. Surgery or radiation therapy: A comparative cost analysis for early carcinoma of the prostate and breast. App Radiol 1990; January:25-28.
5. Han BH, Demel KC, Wallner KE, Young L. Patient reported short-term complications after prostate brachytherapy. J Urol 2001; (in press).
6. Hanks GE, Dunlap K. A comparison of the cost of various treatment methods for early cancer of the prostate. Int J Radiat Oncol Biol Phys 1986; 12:1879-1881.
7. Horwitz EM, Hanlon AL, Pinover WH, Hanks GE. The cost effectiveness of 3D conformal radiation therapy compared with conventional techniques for patients with clinically localized prostate cancer. Int J Rad Oncol Biol Phys 1999; 45:1219-1225.
8. Kohan AD, Armenakas NA, Fracchia JA. The perioperative charge equilvalence of interstitial brachytherapy and radical prostatectomy with 1-year followup. J Urol 2000; 163:511-514.
9. Lotan Y, Cadeddu J, Gettman M. The new economics of radical prostatectomy: Cost comparison of open, laparoscopic and robot assisted techniques. J Urology 2004; 172:1431-1435.
10. Makhlouf A, Boyd J, Chapman T, Theodorescu D. Perioperative costs and charges of prostate brachytherapy and prostatectomy. Urology 2002; 60:656-660.
11. Oncology. Prostate surgeries: Average charges throughout the United States, 1997. Oncology 2000; 14:371-378.
12. Palmer JS, Worwag EM, Conrad WG, al e. Same day surgery for radical retropubic prostatectomy: Is it an attainable goal? Urol 1996; 47:23-28.
13. Wagner TT, Young D, Bahnson RR. Charge and length of hospital stay analysis of radical retropubic prostatectomy and transperineal prostate brachytherapy. J Urol 1999; 161:1216-1218.
14. Wilson L, Tesoro R, Elkin E, et al. Cumulative cost pattern comparison of prostate cancer treatments. Cancer 2007.
15. Wodinsky HB, Jenkin RDT. The cost of radiation treatment at an Ontario regional cancer centre. Canadian Medical Association Journal 1987; 137:906-909.

16. Yabroff K, Davis W, Lamont E, et al. Patient time costs associated with cancer care. JNCI 2007; 99:14-23.

28

The Future

We are seeing today what seemed more fantasy than reality in the early 1990s: wide adoption of prostate brachytherapy as a prime treatment of choice for early-stage prostate cancer. Its resurgence initially met with substantial resistance from skeptical members of oncologic communities. With mounting evidence confirming its comparable efficacy and acceptable morbidity, even the most cautious oncologists are jumping on board. Early reports, generated by a few brachytherapy enthusiasts, have lead to a widespread interest by mainstream oncologists.

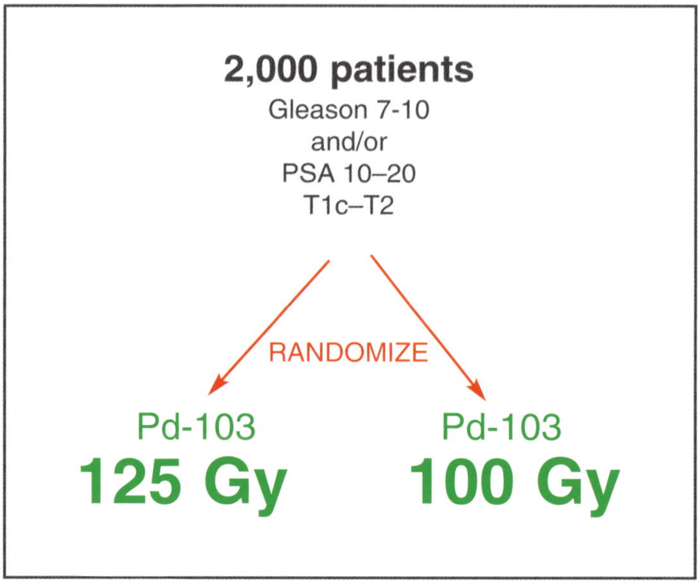

Figure 28-1. Design of a randomized trial comparing I-125 and Pd-103 for early stage, intermediate-risk cancers. The study was opened in 2006 and will have accrued all 2,000 patients by 2011.

QUALITY ASSURANCE

As is often the case with new techniques, early transperineal brachytherapy results have been published primarily by enthusiasts in the field, who have dedicated much of their time to perfecting the procedure. Results reported by early enthusiasts may not be representative of what is achieved as the technology and skills are adopted by less-specialized practitioners. Better-quality assurance will help brachytherapy to meet its full potential as a widely available, effective, and relatively cost effective treatment. Numerous investigators are helping to define and implement better quality brachytherapy.(HERSTEIN 07, STOCK 06, POTTERS, PAPAGIKOS, MERRICK, ORIO)

DOSE OPTIMIZATION

Current doses produce high cure rates with relatively favorable long-term complication rates. Although retrospective studies have helped define optimal doses, more rigorous studies could better optimize prescription doses. The first prospective dose reduction study should be concluded by 2009 (**Figure 28-1**). Fine-tuning studiesof this kind will be facilitated by the development intra-operative dosimetry.(GONG, ORIO 07)

ISOTOPE SELECTION

The search for the optimal isotope will continue. To date, most studies have been limited to retrospective studies, which are inherently subject to

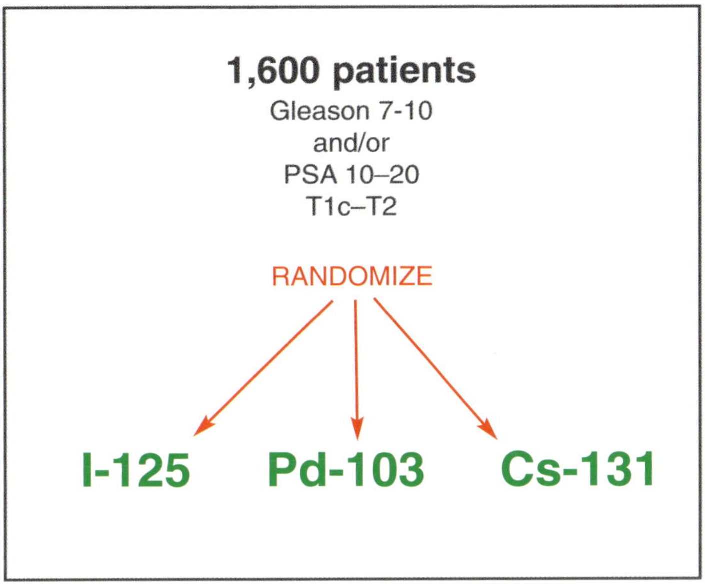

Figure 28-2. Design of a multi-institutional three-way randomized trial comparing I-125 and Pd-103 and Cs-131 for early stage, intermediate-risk cancers. The study was opened in 2007 and should have accrued all 1,600 patients by 2010.

patient selection bias, variable dose delivery and other, undefined factors. One large prospective randomized study has been completed, and at least one more is ongoing (**Figure 28-2**).(WALLNER 03)

SUPPLEMENTAL BEAM

The debate over the value of supplemental beam will likely continue through 2010. As in the case of isotope selection, most investigations have been retrospective, subject to patient selection bias, variable dose delivery and other undefined factors. Ongoing randomized studies should better answer this question.(MERRICK 03) The necessity for supplemental beam will be partly dictated by implant quality, so that its use will probably diminish as more brachytherapists improve their procedures.(ORIO 06)

HORMONAL THERAPY

We see the debate over adjuvant hormonal therapy continuing. There is little argument that hormonal therapy is inappropriate for low risk patients. Its role in intermediate and high risk patients, however, is a subject of continued controversy. As is the case for beam radiation, there is no question that adjuvant hormonal therapy delays biochemical recurrence.(STOCK 04, MERRICK 06) But it's effect on cancer-specific survival needs to be clarified.

ROOM TO IMPROVE

Serious rectal and urethral complications are very uncommon with current prescription doses. Even so, it's possible that current doses could go *lower*, without lowering the likelihood of cure. More trials like that in Figure 28-1 should help guide safe dose reduction.

Maintenance of sexual function has been the only major disappointment in the maturation of modern prostate brachytherapy. The initial assumptions that it would be markedly less likely to disturb sexual function were far too optimistic. Better maintenance of sexual function should be high on our list of priorities as the modality is studied. Minor changes in seed placements seem to have helped somewhat, but substantial improvements will require new thinking.(MERRICK 03)

RANDOMIZED TRIALS

Most would agree with the basic premise that brachytherapy is good at clearing cancer, with acceptable morbidity. The field is maturing. Clinical investigators are rapidly moving to prospective randomized trials, which will serve to "fine tune" brachytherapy (see Chapter 24).

WE REMAIN BULLISH

We're elated at the burgeoning number of reports confirming high biochemical tumor control rates, acceptable morbidity, and competitive societal cost of prostate brachytherapy. However, only when we have a quality assurance system in place, and have determined the optimal prescription doses, will we really know its full potential. Judging from what has been achieved with the present imperfect system, the results should be phenomenal.

Kent Wallner
Gregory Merrick
John Blasko
Michael Dattoli

REFERENCES

1. Gong L, Cho P, Han B, et al. Registration of prostate brachytherapy seeds with prostate anatomy for postimplant dosimetry. Int J Rad Oncol Biol Phys 2002; 54:1322-1330.

2. Herstein A, Wallner K, Merrick G, et al. There is a wide range of predictive dosimetric factors for I-125 and Pd-103 Prostate Brachytherapy. Am J Clin Onc 2007; in press.

3. Merrick G, Butler W, Wallner K, Galbreath R, Allen Z, Adamovich E. Androgen-deprivation therapy dies not impact cause-specific or overall survival after permanent prostate brachytherapy. Int J Rad Oncol Biol Phys 2006; 65:669-677.

4. Merrick G, Wallner K, Butler W. Minimizing prostate brachytherapy-related morbidity. Urol 2003; 62:786-792.

5. Merrick G, Wallner K, Butler W. Sexual dysfunction after prostate brachytherapy. Oncol 2003; 17:52-62.

6. Merrick G, Wallner K, Butler W, Blasko J. Permanent prostate brachytherapy: Is supplemental external-beam radiation therapy necessary? Oncol 2006; 20:514-525.

7. Orio P, Tutar I, Narayanan S, et al. Intra-operative ultrasound-fluoroscopy fusion can enhance prostate brachytherapy quality. (submitted) 2007.

8. Orio P, Wallner K, Merrick G, et al. Dosimetric parameters as predictive factors for biochemical control in patients with higher risk prostate cancer treated with Pd-103 and supplemental beam radiation. Int J Rad Oncol Biol Phys 2007; 67:342-346.

9. Papagikos M, deGuzman AF, Rossi P, CMcCullough D, Clark P, Lee WR. Dosimetric quantifiers for low-dose-rate prostate brachytherapy: Is V100 superior to D90? Brachytherapy 2005; 4:252-258.

10. Potters L, Cao Y, Calugaru E, Torre T, Fearn P, Wang X. A comprehensive review of CT-based dosimetry parameters and biochemical control in patients treated with permanent prostate brachytherapy. Int J Rad Oncol Biol Phys 2001; 50:605-614.

11. Stock RG, Cahlon O, Cesaretti J, Kollmeier M, Stone NN. Combined modality treatment in the management of high-risk prostate cancer. Int J Rad Oncol Biol Phys 2004; 59:1352-1359.

12. Stock RG, Stone NN, Cesaaretti J, Rosenstein B. Biologically effective dose values for prostate brachytherrapy: Effects on PSA failure and posttreatment biopsy results. Int J Rad Oncol Biol Phys 2006; 64:527-533.

13. Wallner K, Merrick G, True L, Sutlief S, Cavanagh W, Butler W. I-125 versus Pd-103 for low risk prostate cancer: Preliminary biochemical outcomes from a prospective randomized mulitcenter trial. Int J Rad Oncol Biol Phys 2003; 57:1297-1303.

index

S

T

U

V

W

Y

Z